Obstetrics

Daniel Haile
659 7456
Johns Hopkins
med School

Obstetrics

ESSENTIALS OF CLINICAL PRACTICE

SECOND EDITION

KENNETH R. NISWANDER, M.D.
Professor and Chairman,
Department of Obstetrics and Gynecology,
University of California, Davis, School of Medicine, Davis;
Director of Obstetrics and Gynecology,
University of California at Davis, Medical Center,
Sacramento

LITTLE, BROWN AND COMPANY   BOSTON

To Ruth, Sally, Dave, Phil, and Paul

Preface

It is a pleasure to be asked to revise a textbook. Such a request implies a degree of acceptance of the book by readers. The goal of this revised edition remains unchanged, to provide a short but comprehensive textbook for the junior medical student who is having his first clinical experience with the obstetric patient. The first edition apparently appealed to nursing students and other health professionals as well, and it is hoped that this edition will continue to do so.

The outline of the second edition remains unchanged, with an orientation that continues to emphasize the physiology and pathophysiology of the gravid patient and her fetus at the expense of a detailed description of the mechanics of the delivery process. Such technical details can be better learned in the delivery room.

A major updating has been necessary in several chapters to keep current with progress in obstetrics. Much of Chapter 12, which deals with abnormalities and diseases of the fetus, has been totally rewritten. Significant progress has been made in the recognition and treatment of the growth-retarded fetus. The sections on management of premature labor and premature rupture of the membranes have been rewritten. New information on contraception necessitated major changes in the chapter on fertility control. A few new illustrations have been added and several have been replaced to improve quality.

As with any task of this magnitude, many people have extended help to the author. The excellent portions of the book written by Drs. Levkoff, Purohit, and Jorgenson again are gratefully acknowledged. Some of the new illustrations were kindly supplied by Dr. Richard Oi and Dr. Harry Phillips. Ms. Helane Manditch-Prottas of Little, Brown and Company maintained the excellent copyediting supervision evident in the first edition. Finally, my secretary, Ms. Karen Sullivan, typed the entire manuscript with her usual unruffled excellence.

K. R. N.

Contents

Contributing Authors

Kenneth R. Niswander, M.D.
Professor and Chairman, Department of Obstetrics
and Gynecology, University of California, Davis,
School of Medicine, Davis; Director of Obstetrics
and Gynecology, University of California at Davis,
Medical Center, Sacramento

Ronald J. Jorgenson, D.D.S.
Professor of Clinical Genetics, Department of
Periodontics, The University of Texas Health
Science Center at San Antonio, Dental School

Abner H. Levkoff, M.D.
Professor of Pediatrics, Medical University of
South Carolina College of Medicine; Director of
Newborn Services, Medical University Hospital,
Charleston

Dilip M. Purohit, M.D.
Associate Professor of Pediatrics, Medical
University of South Carolina College of Medicine;
Associate Director of Newborn Services, Medical
University Hospital, Charleston

Obstetrics

The Placenta and the Fetus

The clinical practice of obstetrics begins at fertilization of the ovum, and it is at this point that we open our discussion. For a detailed consideration of the anatomy and physiology of the unfertilized germ cells, the endocrine and metabolic milieu in which they mature, and the disease states that result from malfunction in this prefertilization period, the reader is referred to a textbook of gynecology or of gynecologic endocrinology.

The Ovum

FERTILIZATION

The ovum completes its final meiotic division and extrusion of the second polar body after fertilization. The ampullary portion of the fallopian tube is the usual site of fertilization. The ovum is transported from the ruptured follicle to the fallopian tube by cilial action; it is transported down the tube primarily as a result of peristalsis. Sperm deposited in the vagina undergo a process called capacitation in the uterus and oviduct. This process is poorly understood but essential in mammals and probably in man to allow the sperm to penetrate the zona pellucida and the plasma membrane of the ovum. It seems well established that sperm deposited longer than 24 to 48 hours before ovulation are incapable of fertilizing the ovum. Sperm can be found regularly in the fallopian tube within a few hours of intercourse, transported there partly by their own motility but primarily by contractions of the female genital tract.

Fertilization probably should occur within 24 hours of ovulation if it is to be normal, and the formation of two pronuclei, one from the ovum and one from the sperm, can be noted. Each pronucleus contains a haploid chromosome content (23), resulting in a diploid chromosomal content (46) for the fertilized ovum. When the chromosomes of both nuclei come together (syngamy), fertilization is complete.

Surprisingly, the first cleavage of the fertilized ovum is not complete until about 30 hours after fertilization, but cleavage proceeds rapidly thereafter, with formation of a blastocyst on about the third day, soon after arrival in the uterine cavity. During its passage through the uterine tube, the fertilized ovum is propelled by the muscular action of the tube, a function that in turn is probably regulated by the levels of estrogen and progesterone. The developing blastocyst is probably nourished by energy sources both within itself and from tubal and uterine secretions. Implantation of the fertilized ovum apparently occurs about 6 or 7 days following fertilization, or about 20 to 21 days following the onset of the last menstrual period.

Most of the information regarding human fertilization and early fertilized ovum development has come from a crucial series of fertilized ova recovered by Hertig et al. [1–3] from surgical specimens. These investigators instructed about 200 normally ovulating women scheduled for elective hysterectomy to record carefully menstrual data and timing of intercourse prior to the surgical procedure. At the time of hysterectomy, meticulous search of the surgical specimen was rewarded with the recovery of many fertilized ova, which were then carefully studied. Some of this material is shown in Figures 1-1 to 1-3. Recently, in vitro fertilization of the human egg has been reported [4]. In at least one well-publicized patient, the ovum fertilized in vitro was implanted into the uterus and culminated in an apparently normal newborn. A number of clinics worldwide are attempting similar experiments.

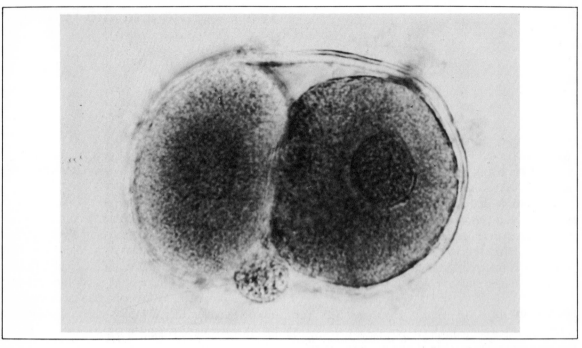

Fig. 1-1. Two-cell ovum, photographed by phase microscopy, found flushed from left fallopian tube (36–60 hours old). (From A. Hertig, J. Rock, E. Adams, and W. Mulligan. On the preimplantation stages of the normal ovum: A description of four normal and four abnormal specimens ranging from the second to the fifth day of development. Contrib Embryol 35:199, 1954. Courtesy of the Carnegie Institution of Washington, Department of Embryology, Davis Division.)

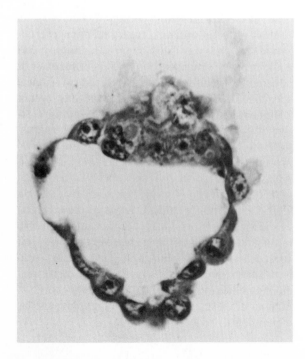

Fig. 1-2. Human 107-cell blastocyst recovered from uterine cavity (about fifth day). (From A. Hertig, J. Rock, E. Adams, and W. Mulligan. On the preimplantation stages of the normal ovum: A description of four normal and four abnormal specimens ranging from the second to the fifth day of development. Contrib Embryol 35:199, 1954. Courtesy of the Carnegie Institution of Washington, Department of Embryology, Davis Division.)

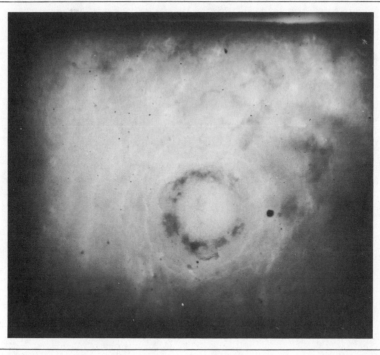

Fig. 1-3. Twelve-day ovulation age: Mouths of the uterine glands are prominent. (From A. Hertig and J. Rock. Two human ova of the pre-villous stage, having an ovulation age of about 11 and 12 days respectively. Contrib Embryol *29:127, 1941. Courtesy of the Carnegie Institution of Washington, Department of Embryology, Davis Division.)*

ENDOMETRIAL PREPARATION

To describe the preparation of the endometrium for implantation, a brief review of menstrual endometrial physiology is necessary.

The endometrium is highly responsive to ovarian secretion of estrogen and progesterone. Ovarian secretion of these substances is, of course, in turn dependent on the gonadotropic stimulation of the anterior pituitary hormones and on the release of these substances mediated through the hypothalamus. The developing follicle of the ovary secretes estrogen and smaller amounts of progesterone until ovulation. Thereafter, the corpus luteum increases the amount of progesterone secretion, continuing to secrete estrogen. In the absence of pregnancy, the regressing corpus luteum ceases to secrete its hormones. The endometrium sloughs as its hormonal support is withdrawn, and menstruation results.

Under the influence of the ovarian follicle, the endometrium undergoes the *proliferative (follicular) phase* of the cycle (Fig. 1-4). The endometrium thickens, and the endometrial glands increase in number. The endometrial cells change from a cuboidal type to a columnar variety, and mitotic activity is evident. The stroma is compact but begins to loosen somewhat as the time of ovulation is approached. With ovulation, the *secretory (luteal) phase* of the menstrual cycle is initiated. The glands become increasingly tortuous, until they assume a "sawtooth" appearance (Fig. 1-5). The cells lining the glands display subnuclear vacuolization at first, followed by the appearance of glycogen in the gland lumen as the nuclei resume their basilar location. The endometrial stroma gradually becomes edematous, and, as menstruation is approached, the stromal cells may show an early decidual reaction, a process that is greatly accelerated if pregnancy supervenes. *Menstruation* is probably initiated by vascular spasm under the influence of

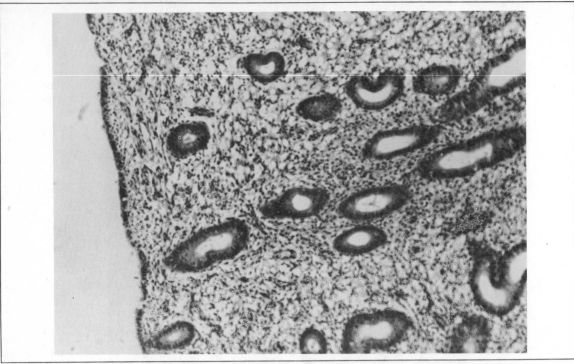

A

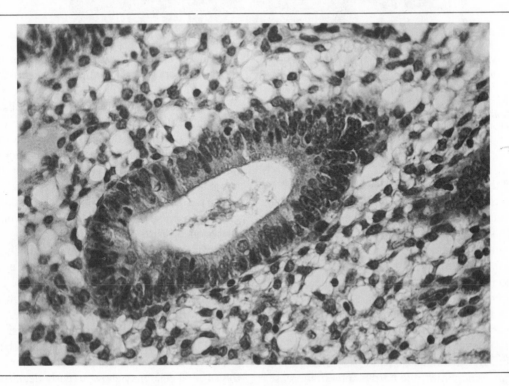

B

Fig. 1-4. Late proliferative endometrium. The glandular epithelium has become columnar, and there is begin-ning pseudostratification. The stroma is moderately dense.

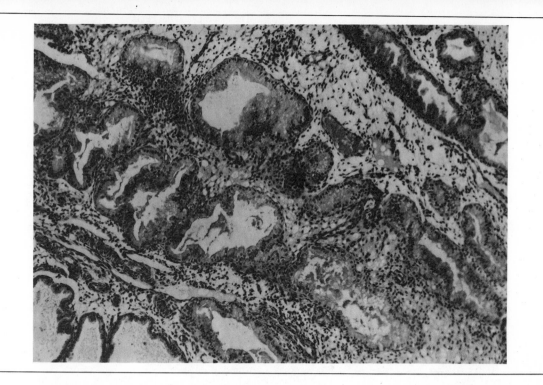

A

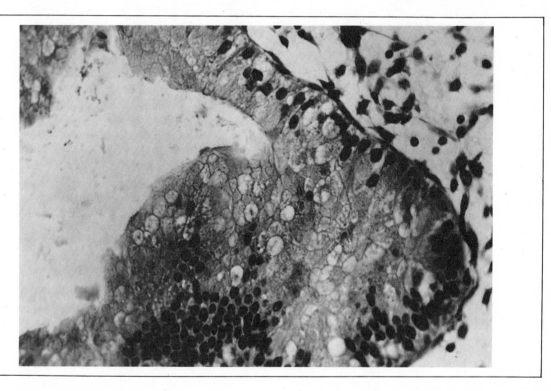

B

Fig. 1-5. Secretory endometrium about day 21 or 22. The glands are filled with secretion and have become more tortuous in shape. The stroma is less compact, due to edema fluid.

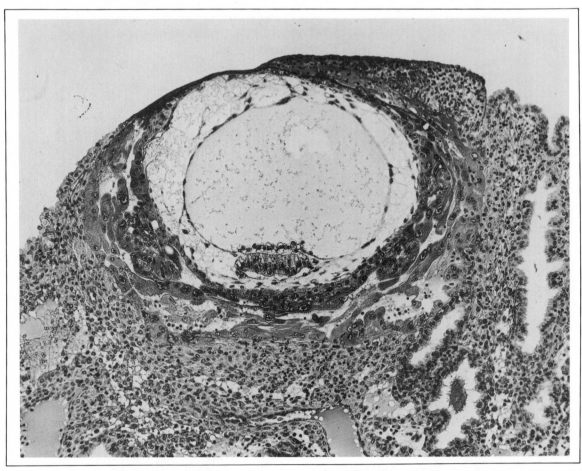

Fig. 1-6. Nine-day specimen. Dorsum of germ disk oriented toward top of picture. Some regeneration of epithelium is seen over the ovum. (From A. Hertig and J. Rock. Two human ova of the pre-villous stage, having an ovulation age of about 7 and 9 days respectively. Contrib Embryol 31:65, 1945. Courtesy of the Carnegie Institution of Washington, Department of Embryology, Davis Division.)

decreasing levels of ovarian hormones, and the functional layer of the endometrium is shed as the basal layer begins to repair the damage caused by the ischemic loss of superficial endometrium.

If pregnancy occurs, the corpus luteum does not regress, and ovarian steroid production is not interrupted. The decidual reaction becomes more intense as the stromal cells greatly enlarge with the increase in the amount of their cytoplasm. There is a deposition of glycogen in the decidual cells, and these cells and the endometrial glands form a rich source of energy for the ovum as it implants. Under certain circumstances, the endometrium may be inadequate for implantation; this is thought to be the result of inadequate corpus luteum secretion of progesterone [5]. The clinical aspects of this possi-

bility are discussed under causes of abortion in Chapter 5.

IMPLANTATION

Implantation in the human occurs most often on the midportion of the posterior or anterior uterine walls. The reason for this desirable choice of location is unknown, as are the reasons for the occasional lower implantation site as observed with

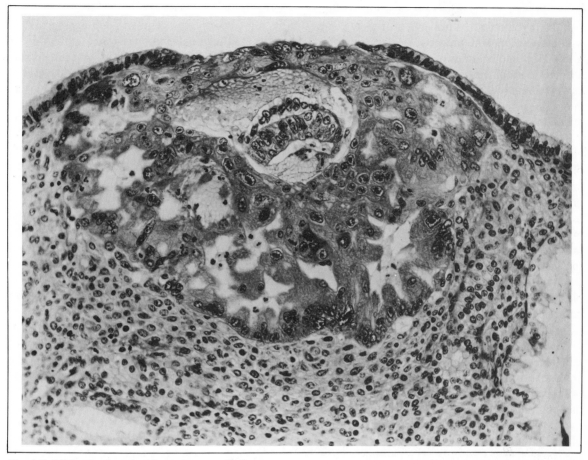

Fig. 1-7. Midsagittal section through ovum (12 days). Decidual reaction around ovum moderately prominent. (From A. Hertig and J. Rock. Two human ova of the pre-villous stage, having an ovulation of about 11 and 12 days respectively. Contrib Embryol *29:127, 1941. Courtesy of the Carnegie Institution of Washington, Department of Embryology, Davis Division.)*

placenta previa. Implantation occurs at a site between openings of the endometrial glands, and within about 48 hours the blastocyst has burrowed into the endometrium, with evidence of early healing of the broken endometrial surface by the proliferation of endometrial cells over it (Fig. 1-6). The implantation is a very superficial one, and the blastocyst bulges above the endometrial surface. By this time, the blastocyst can be seen to be composed of two elements: (1) the invading embryonic *trophoblast*, which has oriented itself to lie deeper in the endometrium than (2) the *inner cell mass*, which comes to lie nearer the endometrial surface (Fig. 1-7). While the embryonic trophoblast appears hyperplastic and active as it pursues its invasion, the inner cell mass looks atrophic.

By the twelfth day, the trophoblast consists primarily of large masses of actively invading syncytiotrophoblast, although a single inner layer of cytotrophoblast can be seen beneath the embryo. Some small spaces have begun to appear in the syncytiotrophoblast; these are primitive intervillous spaces. On succeeding days of development, the trophoblast invades the maternal capillaries, and the entry of maternal blood into the lacunae of the syncytiotrophoblast establishes a primitive circulation. At this point, for an unknown reason, invasion stops, and the decidua maintains itself as a barrier between the trophoblast and the myometrium. In the rare instance when invasion continues into the myometrium, a placenta accreta develops. Villous development proceeds as the trophoblast forms itself into columns of trophoblast tissue with an inner core of mesenchyme from the blastocyst cavity. Some of the villi thus formed lie free in the intervillous spaces, while others (anchoring villi) attach to the decidua.

The invasion of the trophoblast into the maternal circulation serves a twofold purpose at this stage of embryonic development. Maternal nutritive and excretory aid to the developing embryo is provided, and chorionic gonadotropin from the trophoblast can enter the maternal circulation to prolong the life of the corpus luteum and thus provide necessary continuing hormone support for the pregnancy. The proliferation of syncytiotrophoblast occurs over the entire surface of the blastocyst, but, soon thereafter, the proliferation ceases everywhere except immediately beneath the embryo, where the permanent placenta is formed.

At about the eighteenth day, a primitive circulation develops between the villi and the embryo, and angiogenesis occurs in the villi as well as in the primitive yolk sac, with fusion of these circulations on about the twenty-fourth day. Hematopoietic activity begins in the yolk sac, and the development of a primitive heart in the embryo soon allows establishment of a circulation. The chorion is formed as mesodermal fibroblasts come to line the inner surface of the trophoblast, and a chorionic cavity develops. The amniotic cavity forms as a space between the ectoderm and the chorionic membrane, and the cavity gradually surrounds the embryo completely. An umbilical cord develops from the allantois, which is derived from the body stalk formed from the primitive yolk sac.

The Placenta

Compared with the weight of the fetus, the placenta is proportionately larger early in pregnancy than at term, due to two factors. First, the placenta attains much of its size during very early pregnancy, at a time when the fetal growth rate is low. Second, although the placenta continues to grow throughout the remainder of pregnancy, the rate of growth of the fetus is much more rapid. At term, the ratio of

placental to fetal weight approximates 1:6 on the average. Poor placental growth during pregnancy is associated with delayed intrauterine growth of the fetus, which apparently results in inadequate support of fetal functions. While intrauterine growth retardation is a well-recognized condition in the newborn (small-for-dates baby), diagnosis of the phenomenon continues to be difficult to make in the fetus in utero (see Chap. 12).

APPEARANCE

The placenta at term is a discoid organ weighing between 500 and 600 gm. on the average and measuring about 15 cm. in diameter and about 2 cm. in thickness. The maternal surface of the placenta has a dark reddish color and is separated by decidual septa into an irregular number of subdivisions called cotyledons. The fetal surface is shiny and is traversed by many vessels of varying caliber and of both the arterial and the venous type (Fig. 1-8). The red color of the placenta is due primarily to the presence of the fetal blood, since most of the maternal intervillous blood is drained in the process of separation from the uterine wall following delivery.

The early villi contain a large amount of connective tissue and show two distinct types of surface epithelium, the inner cytotrophoblast (Langhans' layer) and the outer syncytiotrophoblast (Fig. 1-9). The cytotrophoblast consists of cells of definite borders, while the syncytiotrophoblast contains many nuclei without definite limiting cell membranes. As pregnancy advances, the villi become thinner, both as a result of additional branching and because of the decrease in the amount of connective tissue. The cells of Langhans' layer become less numerous and are usually present only in scattered locations in the term placenta.

Other changes in the placenta as it ages include a decrease in the thickness of the syncytium (Fig. 1-10), an increase in the number of capillaries, and a closer approximation of the blood vessels to the syncytium. These changes seem directed toward improving transfer across the placenta and probably serve as fetal safeguards. Deposition of fibrin on the surfaces of villi is common in late pregnancy and results in deprivation of maternal circu-

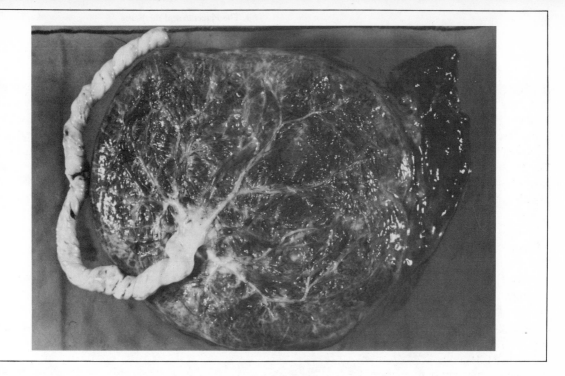

A

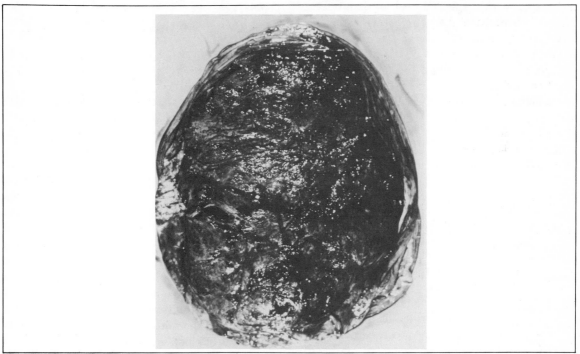

B

Fig. 1-8. Normal placenta. A. Fetal surface. B. Maternal surface.

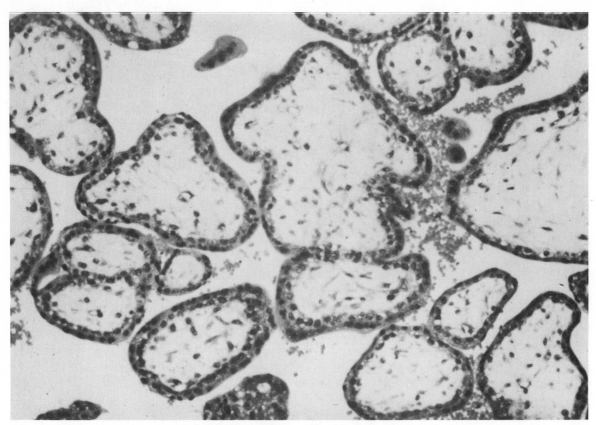

Fig. 1-9. Early placenta. Both syncytiotrophoblast and cytotrophoblast can be seen.

lation to the villus, but the large placental reserve usually prevents this event from being of clinical significance.

The location of placental endocrine function has been controversial. Recent evidence suggests a syncytial rather than a cytotrophoblast site [6]. It now appears that estrogen, progesterone, human chorionic gonadotropin (HCG), and human placental lactogen (HPL) are all secreted by the syncytium. This fact is not surprising when the histogenesis of the cells lining the villus is considered. The syncytium is presumably derived from the cytotrophoblast and functions as the mature form of these cells. As pregnancy progresses and the placenta ages, few cytotrophoblastic cells are seen, and the syncytium provides the major site of placental endocrine function.

CIRCULATION

The initial intervillous circulation is established very early in pregnancy when the invading syn-

cytiotrophoblast forms lacunae that are filled with myometrial venous blood from veins eroded by the trophoblast. Development of a fetal circulation through the growing villi follows soon thereafter. In the second month of pregnancy, the decidual spiral arteries are invaded, and a true intervillous circulation results. While little is known of placental circulation except in the term placenta, it is presumed that the circulation from two months' gestation to term is similar in terms of blood flow if not in terms of amounts of blood involved.

The fetal circulation through the placenta is simple. The two umbilical arteries arise from the fetal internal hypogastric arteries and pass through the umbilical cord to the surface of the placenta, where they fuse in most cases before dividing into many branching smaller vessels. The small vessels run

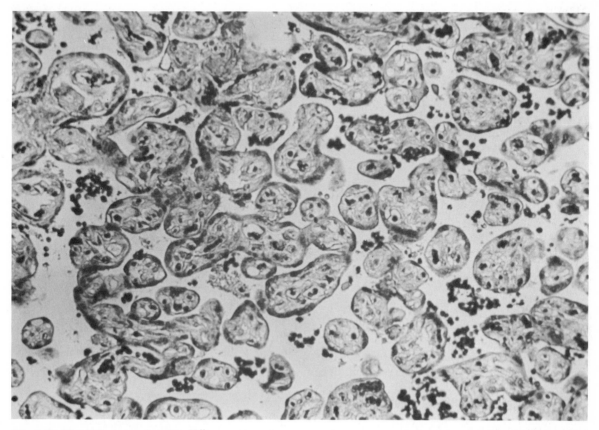

Fig. 1-10. Third-trimester placenta. Villi are numerous. Surfaces of the villi are composed almost entirely of syncytiotrophoblast of a very thin character.

over the fetal surface of the placenta and then enter the fetal villus after further branching into smaller arterioles. After passage through the villous capillaries, the blood is collected into venules and then into larger veins to be returned to the fetal heart through the umbilical vein.

The intervillous circulation is more complex and was incompletely understood until Ramsey and Harris [7] demonstrated its details using cineradiographic techniques with contrast dyes or anatomic corrosion preparations (Fig. 1-11). At term, as many as 20 spiral arterioles spurt blood into the intervillous space with a pressure probably not much lower than the systemic blood pressure. Not all spiral arterioles necessarily empty simultaneously into the intervillous space, and there is evidence that

not all areas of the placenta are necessarily receiving a maximal blood flow at all times. The head of pressure achieved by the blood entering the intervillous space allows a fountainlike flow of blood that bathes the villi before collecting in the basal plate and draining to decidual veins back to the maternal circulation. The mixing of intervillous blood is favored by the placement of the spiral arterioles at a right angle to the uterine wall, thus maximizing the inflow; the veins are generally parallel to the uterine wall, thus minimizing outflow. During a uterine contraction of moderate to high intensity, Ramsey and Harris's studies have clearly shown that the venous outflow of the intervillous space is zero. The potential deleterious effect of uterine tetany on fetal condition can be readily appreciated when one recognizes this fact.

Intervillous blood flow may be influenced by a number of factors. One such factor is uterine tone, as previously described, but only during hard pro-

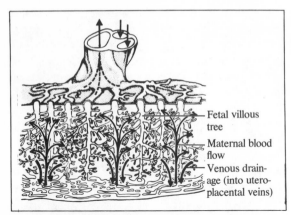

Fig. 1-11. Maternal intervillous circulation. (From E.
Ramsey, after Ranice W. Crosby. Courtesy of Carnegie
Institution of Washington, Department of Embryology,
Davis Division.)

longed contractions does this factor operate. The
placement of villi undoubtedly aids intervillous circulation and placental exchange, since the arterial
blood entering the intervillous space strikes many
villi, thereby causing blood disbursement. The
maternal blood pressure clearly affects the intervillous flow, and conditions causing maternal
shock, such as third-trimester bleeding, high spinal
anesthesia, and maternal hypotensive syndrome
from uterine pressure on the vena cava, must be
expected to cause an adverse effect on placental
exchange. Preeclampsia-eclampsia may be associated with spasm of the spiral arterioles and may
exert its well-known deleterious effect on the fetus
in this fashion. Poorly controlled oxytocin administration can also adversely affect intervillous circulation if uterine tetany occurs. The increasing
reluctance of obstetricians to administer oxytocin
without appropriate monitoring of fetal heart rate
and uterine contractions can be easily understood.

PLACENTAL EXCHANGE
The maternal and fetal circulations are known to be
totally separate, with no mixing of the two circulations possible under normal circumstances. Yet
nearly all substances are known to be transferred
from one circulation to the other, although in very
small amounts in many cases. The mechanisms by
which these transfers occur has been the subject of

intense study, resulting in an enormous biblio-
graphic accumulation over many years. The transfer of substances across the alveolar membrane of
the lung seems simple by comparison, since the
placenta performs so many functions other than gas
and water exchange. While much remains to be
learned, it is now clear that transfer across the
placenta can occur by a number of mechanisms:
simple diffusion, facilitated diffusion, active transport through a carrier system, and pinocytosis.

Classification of Physiologic Substances Passing the Placental Barrier

In 1957, Page [8] simplified the complexities of placental transfer with a classification based primarily
on the significance of a particular substance to the
fetus. Not surprisingly, he found that the most vital
substances passed the placental barrier at the highest rate, while substances less important for immediate fetal survival passed at much slower rates.
The classification is still a good one and is given
here in some detail. The four groups of substances
listed by Page are discussed in the sections that
follow.

GROUP I: SUBSTANCES CONCERNED WITH THE
MAINTENANCE OF BIOCHEMICAL HOMEOSTASIS OR
PROTECTION AGAINST SUDDEN DEATH. The rate of
transfer for these substances is measured in milligrams per second, and the predominant mechanism
of transport is rapid diffusion. Page [8] recognized
that with certain molecules (water, electrolytes),
equilibrium is reached between certain mols in the
two circulations. While the amount of water transferred in one direction across the placenta from
mother to fetus is enormous (500 mg. per second),
the net transfer is a very small fraction of the total
exchange. Sodium transfer peaks at about 36
weeks' gestation, reaching a level of 1 mg. per second from mother to fetus, a figure 70 times higher
than the rate per unit weight of the placenta at 10
weeks' gestation. This increase in sodium transfer
can be correlated with the anatomic changes in the
villus that improve placental exchange as pregnancy progresses.

Some substances in this group attain unequal
distribution between the two circulations, due to

differences in rates of removal, or different dissociation curves of the complex as formed, or both. Oxygen, for example, is in lower concentration in the fetal circulation because of the fetus's oxygen utilization. (Fetal hemoglobin is more nearly saturated with oxygen than is maternal hemoglobin.) Carbon dioxide provides another example but in the opposite direction. In certain other instances, there is unequal distribution between the two circulations because of placental destruction of the substance, such as potentially harmful amines. Epinephrine, for example, is rendered harmless through deamination by monoamine oxidase, which is present in the placenta.

GROUP II: SUBSTANCES CONCERNED PRIMARILY WITH FETAL NUTRITION. The rates of transfer of these substances is measured in milligrams per minute, and transfer is primarily through carrier systems in addition to diffusion. The carrier systems may operate equally in both directions (e.g., glucose), or they may operate against the concentration gradient (e.g., essential amino acids are more concentrated in fetal than in maternal plasma). In a third group, unequal distribution occurs because of molecular alteration during active transport (e.g., riboflavin). A precursor of free riboflavin enters the maternal surface of the placenta but cannot leave the fetal membrane. An enzyme splitting yields free riboflavin, which enters the fetal plasma and results in a level of free riboflavin that is 300 percent higher in the fetal plasma than in the maternal circulation. Similar systems operate on iron, magnesium, cobalt, and calcium.

GROUP III: SUBSTANCES CONCERNED PRIMARILY WITH MODIFICATIONS OF FETAL GROWTH AND MAINTENANCE OF PREGNANCY. The rate of transfer of these substances is measured in milligrams per hour and the predominant mechanism of transfer is very slow diffusion of relatively large molecules. Examples include steroid and protein hormones produced by the placenta or the maternal endocrine glands.

GROUP IV: SUBSTANCES OF IMMUNOLOGIC IMPORTANCE ONLY. The rate of transfer of these substances is measured in milligrams per day, and the mechanism of transport is by leakage through large pores or by droplet transfer by pinocytosis. In some cases, there is transfer of a whole cell (passage of fetal red blood cells causing the rare case of fetal anemia as well as isoimmunization against the Rh factor). In other cases, pinocytosis probably occurs (e.g., plasma proteins).

Passage of Drugs Across the Placental Barrier
The passage of drugs across the placental membrane is of clinical significance because of the well-known teratogenic effects associated with maternal ingestion of certain drugs (e.g., phocomelia from thalidomide, fetal goiter from propylthyrouracil; see Tables 3-3, 3-4, 3-5). Most pharmacologic agents do cross the placenta with ease, usually by passive diffusion. Few have been shown to harm the fetus, but many others are under suspicion in this regard. The frequently recommended proscription against the use of drugs in pregnancy, especially during the first trimester, would seem to be wise unless the mother's life or health is in danger. Drugs administered to the mother during labor may attain fetal levels that cause no harm as long as the maternal organism can detoxify them but may be harmful if a high level results in the neonate.

PLACENTAL HORMONES
The placenta is a rich source of hormones that are known or presumed to be necessary to maintain the pregnancy. The entire synthesis of certain of these hormones takes place in the placenta; with others, the fetal adrenal gland and the fetal liver (as well as the maternal adrenal gland) interact with the placenta in their synthesis. Such synthesis has been described as occurring in the "fetoplacental unit" [9]. More will be said of this concept when the production of estrogens is discussed.

Human Chorionic Gonadotropin
Human chorionic gonadotropin (HCG) was the first hormone shown to be produced by the syncytiotrophoblast of the placenta. It is a glycoprotein consisting of two dissociable subunits, an alpha subunit and a beta subunit. The alpha subunit is virtually

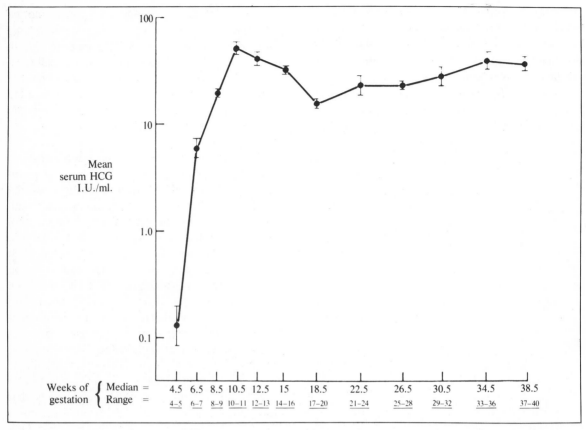

Fig. 1-12. Serum human chorionic gonadotropin concentrations during pregnancy as determined by radioimmunoassay. (From D. Goldstein et al. Radioimmunoassay of serum chorionic gonadotropin activity in normal pregnancy. Am J Obstet Gynecol *102:110, 1968.)*

identical to that found in luteinizing hormone (LH), but the beta subunit confers unique biologic properties as well as specificity in radioimmunoassays. In addition to its biologic effect, HCG is clinically useful, since the measurement of serum and urine levels of HCG provides the basis for currently used pregnancy tests (Fig. 1-12). The circulating level of HCG also is useful in determining the management of trophoblastic tumors as described in Chapter 12.

BIOLOGIC EFFECTS. The major known biologic effect of HCG is in maintenance of the corpus luteum of pregnancy. It can be shown to be present in the maternal serum as early as the eighth day following ovulation, just one or two days following implantation. The appearance of HCG at this time is essential for the continuation of the pregnancy; otherwise, the corpus luteum would regress and fail to

support the pregnancy with essential steroids. The luteotropic effect of HCG not only prolongs the life of the corpus luteum but also causes it to hypertrophy significantly.

Other biologic effects of HCG have been postulated but not proved. Stimulation of steroidogenesis in the fetal testis is one example. The serum level of HCG increases rapidly during early pregnancy, reaching a peak between the sixtieth and seventieth days of pregnancy, long after the need for the corpus luteum to maintain the pregnancy has passed. This suggests that it must have effects other than its luteotropic action. The level of

HCG drops precipitously at this time, following which a more gradual decrease in serum levels can be measured up to two weeks following delivery. Serum and urinary levels run in parallel fashion and at approximately equal levels.

MEASUREMENT. The methods for measuring HCG are either biologic or immunologic. The original Aschheim-Zondek (A-Z) pregnancy test used the presence of corpora lutea in the ovaries of immature mice as the end point of the assay for HCG. Other biologic tests are more rapid than the A-Z test but less accurate. Their end points include the presence of ovarian hyperemia in the rat and an increase in the weight of the immature rat uterus following stimulation with urine containing HCG. Less quantitative biologic tests use an ovulatory response in the South African toad or an ejaculatory response in the male American frog (*Bufo americanus*). Immunologic methods of measuring HCG are in common usage and include hemagglutination-inhibition and complement fixation tests as well as radioimmunoassay. Since these modern methods provide better quantification than the biologic tests, they are usually used when the quantity of the HCG rather than its mere presence is of importance, such as in trophoblastic disease. When the detection of exceedingly small levels of HCG is important (e.g., trophoblastic disease recurrence), measurement of the beta subunit is necessary since cross-agglutination with LH is not present.

USE IN DIAGNOSIS OF TROPHOBLASTIC DISEASE. Care must be exercised in using the serum or urinary levels of HCG to diagnose trophoblastic disease. Extremely high levels have been measured in normal pregnancies, and multiple gestation is particularly likely to cause high levels. An elevated HCG titer has also been reported to occur with severe Rh isoimmunization. Persistence of a high level beyond the sixtieth or seventieth day of pregnancy is suggestive of trophoblastic disease.

Human Placental Lactogen

Another glycoprotein hormone synthesized by the placenta was discovered in 1962 [10]. It was called human placental lactogen (HPL) because of its

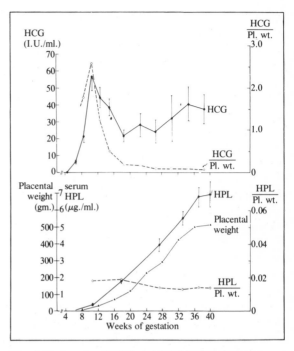

Fig. 1-13. Levels of HCG and HCS (HPL) during normal pregnancy. (From H. Selenkow et al. Measurements and Pathologic Significance of Human Placental Lactogen. In A. Pecile and C. Fenzi (Eds.), The Foeto-Placental Unit. Amsterdam: Excerpta Medica, 1969.)

lactogenic action but it is now known to have breast stimulating properties. It is nearly identical immunologically to the growth hormone produced by the pituitary gland with which it shares some similar metabolic effects.

Synthesis of HPL takes place in the syncytiotrophoblast and can be detected in the maternal serum as early as the sixth week of gestation. The level steadily rises throughout pregnancy and can be correlated with the weight of the placenta (Fig. 1-13). It is of great interest that the levels of the hormone are about 300 times greater in maternal blood than in umbilical vein blood, since this suggests that the major metabolic effects occur in the maternal organism rather than in the fetus. Measurements of serum or urinary levels use a radioimmunoassay procedure. Since the half-life of the hormone is very short, and since very high levels of the hormone occur in maternal serum, it is postulated that from 1 to 4 gm. of the material is synthesized daily by the placenta.

The biologic effects of HPL are of great interest, but the physiologic role the hormone plays during normal pregnancy is not entirely clear. While HPL has been shown to have prolactinlike activity in certain animals, its role in human breast development is obscure, especially since the serum level of the substance is zero after delivery, well before lactation is initiated. It has been suggested, but not proved, that HPL may act synergistically with HCG in providing the luteotropic activity that prolongs the corpus luteum during pregnancy [11]. It has growth-promoting activity, as well as certain diabetogenic effects similar to those of human growth hormone; HPL partially accounts for the diabetogenic effects of pregnancy, i.e., resistance to insulin, increased levels of serum insulin, impairment of glucose tolerance, and a rise in the level of circulating free fatty acids. It has been suggested that HPL may potentiate the effects of human growth hormone in these respects [12].

The clinical usefulness of HPL maternal blood measurements is suggested by several studies, although some authorities doubt their dependability [13]. Spellacy has defined a "danger" zone below 4 μcg per ml. after the thirtieth week of pregnancy [14]. Such levels predict a significant risk of fetal demise in hypertensive patients. Others have reported a higher risk of fetal distress or neonatal asphyxia with low levels of HPL [15]. The test is also useful in predicting the postterm dysmaturity syndrome with postterm pregnancy. It is less useful in managing the diabetic pregnancy.

Human Chorionic Thyrotropin
The placenta also secretes a third protein, human chorionic thyrotropin (HCT), with hormonal activity similar to that of the thyroid-stimulating hormone of the pituitary gland. The substance has been shown to be biologically capable of increasing the secretion of thyroid hormone. The levels of the hormone are high during early pregnancy, with a subsequent decrease to minimal levels near term. The physiologic role of this hormone during pregnancy is unknown.

Steroid Hormones
The placenta is a rich source of steroid hormones but, unlike the ovary, cannot synthesize the hormones de novo. Rather, both maternal and fetal organs provide the necessary precursors for the placental synthesis of the steroid hormones. This fact has led to the concept of the fetoplacental or the fetoplacental-maternal unit to account for the marked increase of steroid production during pregnancy. This concept is certainly valid for the production of estrogens and probably also for progesterone.

ESTROGENS. The syncytiotrophoblast is the site of secretion of placental estrogens. While many different estrogens are secreted by the placenta (at least 27 have been verified), the major estrogens are estrone, 17-β-estradiol, and estriol. Quantitatively, estriol is the most important. In the ovary, estriol is derived primarily from estrone and estradiol; in the placenta, all these hormones are derived directly from androgen precursors.

Both maternal and fetal precursors (dehydroepiandrosterone) are used by the placenta for the production of estrogens. While the maternal precursors predominate in early pregnancy, there is evidence that the fetal precursors are more important in later pregnancy. The maternal precursors are formed in the maternal adrenal gland, and the fetal precursors require an intact fetal adrenal gland and an intact fetal liver for their production. The estrogens secreted by the placenta gain access to the maternal circulation and can be measured both in maternal serum and maternal urine.

The high levels of estriol noted with normal pregnancy provide the basis for a useful clinical test of fetoplacental function. A fall in estriol excretion in the urine has come to suggest a defective placenta or a compromised or dead fetus. The levels of estriol excreted in the urine vary from hour to hour and even from day to day. To overcome this marked variation, it has become usual practice to measure the amount of estriol contained in a 24-hour sample of urine. More recently, a single sample of urine has been measured for estriol and creatinine simultaneously and an estriol-creatinine ratio determined. Creatinine is presumed to be excreted from the maternal kidney at a regular rate. All methods of correcting for variation in the urinary excretion of estriol are imperfect because of variation in kidney function. Changes in glomerular filtration rate and renal plasma flow induced by postural changes can cause a marked change in estrogen output. Indeed, the well-documented beneficial effect of bed rest on estrogen excretion may very well be due to the increase in urinary flow that follows bed rest. The use of serum levels of estriol offers little advantage over urinary measurements [16]. menahun

All these objections notwithstanding, measurement of urinary estriol excretion is a widely used measurement of fetal or placental function. Certain limitations must be imposed in the interpretation of estriol data, however, if clinical errors are to be avoided:

1. A single "normal" level of estriol, especially in a high-risk patient, should not lead the obstetrician into the mistake of failing to repeat the test.
2. A single "abnormal" reading must be confirmed before a clinical decision can be based even partially on the estriol levels.
3. Anencephaly with fetal adrenal hypoplasia results in a very low level of estriol excretion.
4. If the mother is receiving exogenous corticoids, estriol excretion is decreased, probably because of suppression of fetal ACTH.
5. A "normal" range of values should be developed by the particular laboratory performing the test, since the rate of recovery of estriol varies so widely with the method used.
6. The test should be used in conjunction with other placental function tests, especially the nonstress test and the oxytocin challenge test (see Chap. 12).

PROGESTERONE. Progesterone is essential for the maintenance of human pregnancy. The site of production during early gestation is the corpus luteum of pregnancy. Secretion of progesterone is assumed by the syncytium of the placenta as the corpus luteum regresses. The functional life span of the corpus luteum has been estimated at about 70 days. Gradually increasing levels of progesterone are detected in the serum during pregnancy until the last few weeks, when the rise gives way to a stable serum level (Fig. 1-14). While the corpus luteum can manufacture progesterone from acetate, the placenta requires maternal conversion of acetate to cholesterol or pregnenolone before it can synthesize progesterone.

Although progesterone is considered essential to the maintenance of pregnancy, the exact site of its action is not certain. It can be shown to decrease the amplitude and frequency of uterine muscle contractility, and it is presumed that it is this effect that keeps the uterus from contracting and expelling its contents during pregnancy. Why the uterus is allowed to contract at term (or prematurely in some cases) without a simultaneous decrease in serum progesterone is unknown. The hormone may reduce the excitability of uterine muscle, possibly by affecting the membrane potential of the myometrial fibers.

Progesterone has certain other important physiologic effects. It is responsible for the rise in basal body temperature that occurs with ovulation and during an ensuing pregnancy. This effect is thought to be mediated through the central nervous system. Progesterone is believed to have an effect on the development of breast lobules for lactation, but its precise role is uncertain. Progesterone may govern the depot fat storage known to occur during pregnancy. It may also cause the overbreathing of pregnancy, which leads to reduced alveolar and arterial P_{CO_2}. Progesterone causes sodium diuresis, apparently by antagonizing the effect of aldosterone at the renal tubule level. This action may explain the compensatory increase of circulating aldosterone described during pregnancy.

PLACENTAL IMMUNOLOGY
Since the fetus contains paternal genes foreign to the maternal host, an immunologic rejection reaction by the mother to the pregnancy might logically be expected. The mechanism that prevents such rejection remains one of the mysteries of biology. Many theories have been proposed to explain this

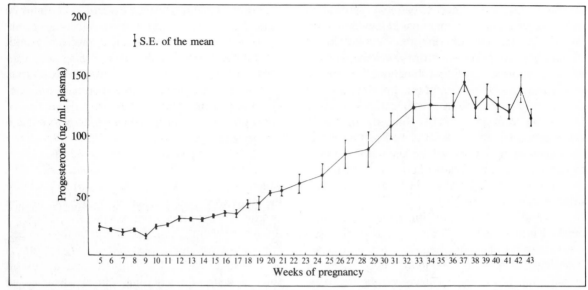

Fig. 1-14. Plasma progesterone concentrations during pregnancy. (From E. Johansson. Plasma levels of progesterone in pregnancy measured by a rapid competitive protein binding technique. Acta Endocrinol 61:607, 1969.)

lack of immunologic response, but a satisfactory explanation of the observation eludes the workers in this field.

One theory suggests that the fetus is immunologically immature, yet it is known that he can effectively synthesize IgM and IgG. The suggestion that the uterus might be an immunologically privileged site leaves unexplained the fact that extrauterine pregnancy, notably abdominal pregnancy, is not subject to rejection any more than is a uterine pregnancy. A third theory proposes that the anatomic separation of mother and fetus might explain the lack of immunologic rejection, and a more recent corollary suggests that fibrin deposited in the placenta provides an anatomic barrier. Since anatomic separation is not complete, and since fibrin is not deposited until the tenth week of pregnancy, these related theories fail to provide an explanation. Diminished immunologic reactivity of the mother is another theory that fails to provide a satisfactory explanation of the problem, since skin transplants of fetal tissue do, indeed, evoke the expected maternal rejection. A recent theory holds that sialomucins, which are known to coat trophoblastic cells, provide a chemical barrier to immunologic competency. Selective enzymatic destruction of the sialomucins does, indeed, result in

the ability of the previously immunologically inactive trophoblastic cells to express histocompatible antigens when transplanted. Most recently, protection of the fetus from maternal lymphocytic attack may be conferred by an immunosuppressive agent in the fetal serum (alpha fetoprotein?) or maternal serum [17]. New theories continue to be suggested, and the final word is yet to be written.

The Umbilical Cord

The umbilical cord forms in the body stalk from the allantois, a structure that develops in the primitive yolk sac. The vessels formed in the allantois of the body stalk fuse with the vessels that appear de novo in the primitive chorionic villi to establish the fetal circulation. Since the yolk sac also forms the gut of the fetus, it is not surprising that a herniation of the gut into the umbilical cord, an omphalocele, is occasionally noted in a newborn infant.

The cord runs from the anterior wall of the fetal abdomen to the placenta, where it inserts either centrally or somewhat eccentrically. If the cord inserts at the edge of the placenta, a *battledore* placenta results, but this insertion is thought to be of no clinical significance. Occasionally, the cord inserts into the fetal membranes, with the unprotected vessels traversing a variable distance through the thin membranes to the placenta. This is known as a *velamentous* insertion of the cord and is clinically significant, especially when the vessels in the membranes lie over the cervix (*vasa praevia*). Rupture of the membranes in this case may result in fetal hemorrhage that is often fatal (see Fig. 15-9).

STRUCTURE

The cord consists of three vessels, two arteries and one vein, supported by a gelatinous substance called Wharton's jelly and surrounded by a layer of amniotic membrane. The histologic appearance of the cord depends on the method of fixation, since the vessels appear small and insignificant if they are emptied before fixation but large and impressive if filled with blood before fixation. The cord may contain embryonic remnants of the allantois. False knots may appear in the cord as a result of folding of the tortuous vein with varicosity formation. True knots are noted, especially when the cord is long enough to allow movement of the fetus through a loop of cord. Sometimes, two or three or more knots are noted, but their clinical significance is uncertain. Since the cord is normally extremely erectile from the blood it contains, it seems unlikely that a knot can often tighten unless fetal death and lack of umbilical circulation has already occurred. Entwinement of the cord around the fetal neck or one or more of the fetal extremities seems equally unlikely to do harm to the normal fetus.

Cords vary markedly in length; a cord can be as short as 20 to 30 cm. or as long as 100 to 150 cm. The usual length is in the range of 50 to 70 cm. The diameter of the cord varies with the amount of Wharton's jelly it contains, but it is usually between 1 and 3 cm. Unusually long cords allow entanglements between fetus and cord, while an unusually short cord may prevent fetal descent during labor or cause a decrease in fetal circulation during fetal descent. Short cords are a rare cause of fetal distress.

The presence of only one artery and one vein in the umbilical cord is a disturbing finding, since an associated congenital anomaly is present in 15 to 20 percent of such cases. The presence of only two vessels in the cord occurs in about 1 percent of singleton pregnancies and should alert the pediatrician to search for a congenital abnormality in the infant.

BLOOD FLOW THROUGH THE CORD

The umbilical arteries arise from the common iliac arteries and are the main branches of the hypogastric arteries. They enter the umbilical cord at a blood pressure of about 60/30 mm. Hg and carry the fetal blood to the villi, where oxygenation of the blood occurs across the villous membrane (Fig. 1-15). The villous blood collects in one umbilical vein and is returned through the fetal liver to the fetal heart by one of two channels. Some blood passes through the hepatic veins, while a major portion is diverted to the ductus venosus. The ductus venosus has a sphincter mechanism that allows it to divert more blood through the hepatic veins should the situation demand it. Little is known about the nerve innervation of the umbilical cord or whether or not the cord is under a nervous influence.

The Fetal Membranes

The chorion and the amnion surround the fetus and adhere loosely to the inner uterine wall except in the area of the placenta, where the chorion comprises the major portion of the fetal part of this organ. Apart from the villous placenta, the membranes lie adjacent to the decidua capsularis or the decidua parietalis. The chorion probably is nourished by the underlying decidua, while the amnion receives most of its nourishment from the amniotic fluid. The chorion develops from the invading trophoblast, and the amnion differentiates either from the fetal ectoderm or possibly from the cytotrophoblast. The two membranes are adherent, but the attachment is a very loose one and can be

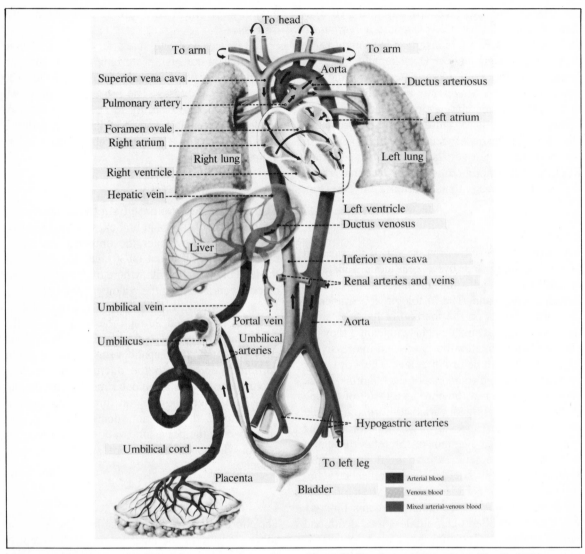

To head

To arm

To arm

Aorta

Superior vena cava

Ductus arteriosus

Pulmonary artery

Left atrium

Foramen ovale

Right atrium

Right lung

Left lung

Right ventricle

Hepatic vein

Left ventricle

Ductus venosus

Liver

Inferior vena cava

Renal arteries and veins

Umbilical vein

Portal vein

Aorta

Umbilicus

Umbilical arteries

Hypogastric arteries

Umbilical cord

To left leg

Placenta

Bladder

Arterial blood

Venous blood

Mixed arterial-venous blood

Fig. 1-15. Fetal circulation. (From Cervical Effacement and Dilatation, *Clinical Education Aid No. 1. Columbus, Ohio: Ross Laboratories, 1963.)*

easily broken. Layers of the two membranes are illustrated in Figure 1-16.

The amnion is less than 0.5 mm. in thickness, with a one-layered epithelium of cuboidal cells. The cells lining the amniotic sac may not secrete fluid but rather transfer it, although recent evidence suggests the possibility of a secretory property [18]. It is thought that the amniotic fluid, during early pregnancy at least, is primarily a product of the maternal plasma. In all likelihood, the amnion is primarily responsible for the formation of the amniotic fluid from the maternal plasma.

AMNIOTIC FLUID
The fluid-filled amniotic sac provides several important protective mechanisms for the fetus. It effectively protects the fetus against mechanical injury, regulates the temperature of the fetus, and provides a milieu in which the fetal extremities can grow and move without physical obstruction.

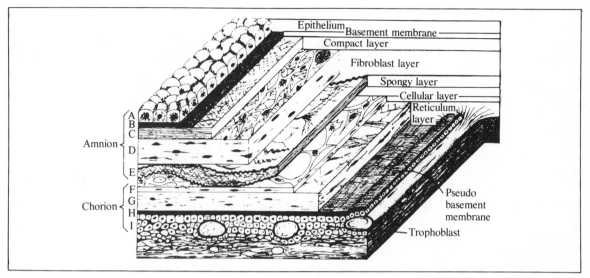

Fig. 1-16. Layers of the chorionic membrane. Composite drawing showing relations of various layers of amnion and chorion. (From G. Bourne. The microscopic anatomy of the human amnion and chorion. Am J Obstet Gynecol *79:1070, 1960.*)

During the first four months, the fluid is nearly identical in chemical content to maternal plasma, except for a lower protein level. The formation of the fluid is thought to result from diffusion of maternal plasma through the amniotic membrane, with smaller amounts supplied by the fetal skin or perhaps by the fetal trachea. At about four months, fetal swallowing and fetal urination apparently account for certain changes, including a higher level of kidney excretion products such as urea, creatinine, and uric acid and a decrease in osmolality, due probably to the lower osmolality of fetal urine. It is said that the fetus swallows about 500 ml. of fluid per day, and apparently about the same volume of urine from fetal urination passes into the fluid daily. When fetal deglutition is defective, as with esophageal atresia, hydramnios is noted. Not all hydramnios is associated with such defects, however. In similar fashion, oligohydramnios is often associated with congenital defects in the fetal kidney, presumably with decreased fetal urination.

There is a steady increase in the amount of amniotic fluid during pregnancy—from about 150 ml. at the sixteenth week to a maximum of 1000 to 1500 ml. at seven months. Thereafter, the amount of amniotic fluid decreases somewhat to about 700 to 800 ml. at term. Much lower volumes may be noted with the postmature infant syndrome. Of some clinical importance is the decrease in the bilirubin content of the amniotic fluid from its highest level at about 16 to 20 weeks' gestation to a zero or near zero level at 36 weeks. Absence of bilirubin in the amniotic fluid has been used as a test for fetal maturity.

A number of clinical uses of amniotic fluid analysis have been introduced in recent years. One major use is in the diagnosis of the severity of erythroblastosis fetalis and in determining the need for intrauterine transfusion (Chap. 12). Certain genetic abnormalities or metabolic defects of the fetus have also been diagnosed through an appropriate analysis of amniotic fluid (see Chap. 12), but the major use of amniotic fluid studies in clinical practice today is in the determination of fetal maturity (see Placental Dysfunction in Chap. 12).

The Fetus

FETAL DIFFERENTIATION

At about three weeks following ovulation, chorionic villi surround the ovum. At this point, the products of conception are referred to as the embryo and the early placenta. For the next five to six weeks, development of the embryo consists primarily of differentiation into the various organs and organ systems. It is during this crucial period that teratogenic factors can influence organ development. At about eight weeks after ovulation, differentiation is complete, and the embryo can now be called a fetus. Subsequent development consists of maturation of the fetal organs and growth.

During the embryonic period, any teratogenic influence must exert its effect at the precise moment of organ differentiation if an abnormality of that organ is to result. This fact explains the variation in stigmata induced by known teratogenic factors from one fetus to another. Rubella, for example, may induce a cardiac defect only if the infecting organism reaches the embryo at a crucial time. While precise time relationships have been noted in animal experiments, less exact information is available for the human. It is also important to note that full-blown maternal disease need not be present for a teratogen to exert its effect. Clinically insignificant or even unrecognized rubella, for example, can cause disastrous fetal effects if the infection occurs in a critical period.

FETAL GROWTH

Data on fetal growth and maturation are crucial to obstetrical care. The widespread use of fetal weight or length to appraise fetal development is apparent when one reads the older literature. These criteria were used not only because their end points were clear-cut and easy to measure, but also because a crucial disparity between fetal weight or length and physiologic maturity in many patients was not appreciated. The emphasis during the 1960s shifted from fetal weight to length of gestation as the criterion for assessing fetal maturity since a fetal weight that falls within the normal range can, in a particular case, actually be abnormally low. Appreciation of the interrelationship between these two parameters of fetal development in assessing fetal maturity has become increasingly evident [19]. The syndrome of the small-for-dates baby is now well recognized by neonatologists and to an increasing degree by obstetricians as well. Recent developments in fetal research have stressed the maturity of certain organ systems or functions as

the best criterion by which to judge fetal maturity, and these research data have been rapidly assimilated into clinical medicine. A discussion of fetal growth and maturity therefore must include not only fetal weight and length but also gestational interval and fetal organ maturity.

Fetal Weight and Length

The best data on fetal weight during the first 24 weeks of pregnancy remain those collected by Streeter [20] in the early part of this century. Streeter's data on increases in fetal weight during the latter half of pregnancy have been confirmed by a number of investigators in recent years. A consistency in the results, at least for clinical purposes, is evident. The greatest percentage increase in fetal weight occurs during the first few weeks of pregnancy, when 3-fold to 15-fold increases over four-week periods can be noted. Although the rate of increase in fetal weight gradually decreases as pregnancy progresses, the absolute increase in fetal weight rises as term is approached, and the fetal weight increases about 200 to 250 gm. weekly during the eight weeks preceding delivery at 40 weeks. The mean birth weight at term is 3300 gm. for infants in the United States, somewhat lower for black infants, and somewhat higher for male infants of either race.

The crown-to-rump length of the fetus also increases at a much more rapid rate during early pregnancy. A useful clinical estimate of gestational interval can be made from the crown-to-rump length, since this measurement is more consistent with gestational interval than is fetal weight. During the first five lunar months, the length may be divided by five to approximate the gestation in months.

As term approaches, the linear increase in fetal weight evident during the last trimester stops, and from 37 to 38 weeks until term, the increase in fetal weight proceeds at a much slower rate. This decrease in rate of growth begins earlier among patients from lower socioeconomic groups (environmental?) (Fig. 1-17), as well as with multiple births. It begins later with Swedish babies than with American babies. Whether or not this slowed growth is related to relative placental insufficiency

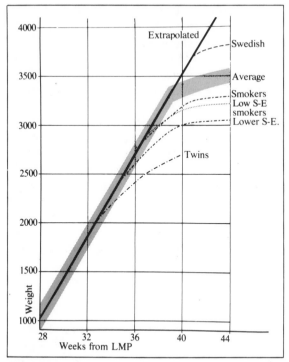

Fig. 1-17. Fetal growth curve from several population groups. (From P. Gruenwald. Growth of the human fetus. I. Normal growth and its variations. Am J Obstet Gynecol *94:1112, 1966.)*

is not known. Beyond 40 weeks, the growth rate slows even further, a fact that has been used to support the idea that the fetus eventually outgrows its placental support.

Factors Affecting Fetal Growth

Fetal growth is known to be affected by maternal nutrition, with many investigators reporting smaller infants with lower prepregnant weight of the mother or with lower maternal weight gain [21]. These studies were controlled for gestational interval, so that a shortened pregnancy does not explain the differences noted. Delayed intrauterine growth also occurs with uteroplacental insufficiency caused by such factors as maternal hypertensive disorders of pregnancy and severe maternal congenital heart disease. Many factors in the etiology of intrauterine growth retardation remain obscure (as discussed in Chap. 12).

Fetal Maturity

Recent observations have suggested that precise information on the degree of maturity of certain fetal organ systems can be obtained in a clinical setting while the fetus is still in utero. This information has already proved invaluable in the practice of obstetrics, and the clinical usefulness of these data is described in Chapter 12.

Perhaps the most valuable information has been accumulated on the degree of fetal lung maturity as measured by phospholipid concentration in the amniotic fluid. Gluck et al. [22] described a sharp increase in lecithin concentration in amniotic fluid with little or no rise in the concentration of sphingomyelin as fetal lung maturity is reached. Good correlation between the lecithin-sphingomyelin ratio and fetal lung maturity has been confirmed by numerous investigators, among them Lemons and Jaffe [23]. Recently it has been shown that the presence of phosphatidyl glycerol (PG) in the amniotic fluid of a fetus with a mature L/S ratio virtually eliminates the risk of hyaline membrane disease in the newborn [24]. Evaluation of lung maturity is especially important, since it is respiratory function more than any other organ function that determines survival of the infant born following a shortened gestation.

PHYSIOLOGY OF THE FETUS

Fetal Blood

Hematopoiesis occurs in the yolk sac of the very young embryo. This site of hematopoiesis is replaced by the liver, which reaches its peak function at four to five lunar months. The liver as the site of hematopoiesis is replaced by the bone marrow, which has assumed the exclusive hematopoietic function at term. While the very early fetal red blood cells are all nucleated, the percentage of nucleated cells in fetal blood has decreased to near zero at birth. The fetal hemoglobin levels have reached normal adult levels by mid-pregnancy and are higher at birth than adult levels (15 to 20 gm. per 100 ml.). Virtually all the hemoglobin of the very young fetus is hemoglobin F, identified by its resistance to alkaline denaturation. At term, the percentage of hemoglobin F has decreased to an average of about 65 percent, with the remainder in the adult form, hemoglobin A. Fetal hemoglobin has a greater affinity for oxygen than adult hemoglobin at any partial pressure of oxygen, and thus the fetus is protected against the relatively low partial pressures of oxygen that are normal to fetal blood.

Several of the accelerator factors of blood coagulation have been reported to be low in the fetus at term. Prophylactic vitamin K given to the mother during labor or to the infant immediately after birth prevents a further decrease in these factors and in the risk of hemorrhagic disease of the newborn. Fibrinolytic activity is said to be lower during fetal life, with a gradual rise to normal activity at term. According to one theory, this low level of blood fibrinolytic activity accounts for the predilection of the infant of shortened gestation to hyaline membrane disease, since the fibrin membrane laid down in the alveoli is not lysed as it is in the term infant [25].

Respiratory blood-gas analysis in the fetus is discussed in Chapter 12. Changes in the fetal circulation at birth are discussed in Chapter 13.

Respiratory System

The state of maturity of the pulmonary tract is the major determinant in the survival of the infant born before term. Recent investigations have suggested the possibility that intrauterine stress (increase in secreted adrenal cortical hormones?) or corticosteroid administration to the mother may accelerate the maturation of the fetal lungs to some degree. However, there remains a definite physiologic time limit on the ability of the lung to support extrauterine existence [26].

During the first half of pregnancy, the lung is composed of bronchi lined by a low columnar or cuboidal epithelium without alveolar structure and with poorly vascularized connective tissue support. Gradually, bronchioles form and are surrounded by connective tissue that becomes vascularized with numerous capillaries. As term approaches, alveoli appear, and the alveolar epithelium becomes more and more sparse, until little more than the capillary endothelium separates the capillary from the air sac. When sufficient alveoli are formed, extra-

uterine existence is possible. While this event usually occurs at about 28 weeks' gestation, it is highly variable. The newer tests of lung function, which depend on the measurement of various amniotic fluid substances, accurately identify the time at which the lung is sufficiently mature to sustain life.

There is good experimental evidence of fetal respiratory movement. As long ago as 1946, Davis and Potter [27] demonstrated thorium oxide (Thorotrast) in the fetal lungs following intraamniotic injection of the substance. The reason for the respiratory movement remains obscure, however. Some have suggested that the intrauterine respiratory activity prepares the lungs for the first extrauterine breath. Others have credited the bronchial tree with an excretory function in utero, a theory that is yet to be proved.

Urinary Tract

The fetal kidney is known to excrete as early as the fourth or fifth month, and in the latter half of pregnancy, urine is apparently excreted in sufficiently large amounts to alter the amount and composition of amniotic fluid appreciably. In similar fashion, the hypotonicity (low sodium, potassium, chloride) and high concentration of urea and creatinine seen in fetal urine is mirrored in changes in the composition of amniotic fluid. In early pregnancy, the amniotic fluid closely approximates the composition of the fetal plasma; in later pregnancy, the electrolyte composition falls as the concentration of urea and creatinine increases.

While there is evidence that the fetal kidney is immature even at term (limited pH control, low osmolality), the function is always adequate for fetal survival unless there is a severe abnormality of the urinary tract. When urethral obstruction is present in utero, urine back pressure can cause hydronephrosis with destruction of the renal parenchyma.

Gastrointestinal System

Swallowing and peristalsis begin at least as early as the end of the first trimester. The injection of radiopaque dye into the amniotic sac preceding in-

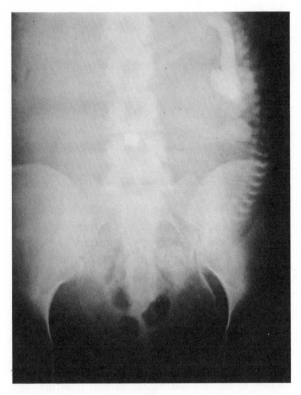

Fig. 1-18. Iodine dye concentrated in the fetal descending colon a number of days following injection of dye into the amniotic sac.

trauterine fetal transfusion for severe Rh hemolytic disease has allowed numerous observations of gastrointestinal tract function from as early as the twenty-fifth week of pregnancy. The dye can regularly be seen in the normal fetus at this gestation as early as two hours after injection. It has been noted that a live fetus in poor condition from the hemolytic disease often fails to ingest the dye. The dye can be seen in the large bowel a few days after initial swallowing (Fig. 1-18).

The term fetus swallows about 450 ml. of amniotic fluid per 24 hours. This fluid is absorbed from the fetal gut into the fetal circulation and excreted through the fetal kidney. It is likely that fetal swallowing is useful in removing insoluble debris from the amniotic fluid, such as desquamated fetal cells, vernix caseosa, and lanugo hair. Mixed with bile pigments added in the duodenum, this debris col-

lects in the bowel as meconium. Intrauterine expulsion occurs apparently only with anal sphincter relaxation, usually caused by a fetal hypoxic episode. With breech presentation, pressure on the fetal abdomen during delivery frequently causes the expulsion of meconium. As noted in the section on hydramnios in Chapter 12, obstruction of fetal swallowing, as with duodenal atresia or other congenital anomaly of the upper gastrointestinal tract, is a frequent accompaniment of hydramnios.

The fetal liver, even at term gestation, lacks certain functional capabilities present in the adult. Of special importance is the minimal ability of the fetal liver to conjugate free bilirubin to allow its excretion in the bile; this function may be necessary after birth to clear the neonatal circulation of bilirubin. The deficiency is of vital importance in the normal premature infant, in whom liver immaturity may be severe, and in the infant of any gestational age with hemolytic disease, when excessive bilirubin is formed. While there is evidence that barbiturates may increase fetal or neonatal conversion of bilirubin to a soluble state by increased glucoronyl transferase activity in the liver, the practical impact of this observation is uncertain at this time.

Bilirubin is formed in large amounts in the fetus from hemoprotein such as cytochrome P_{450} and, to some extent, from red cell hemoglobin. The exact pathway by which bilirubin enters the amniotic fluid is uncertain, but it is known that less and less bilirubin is found in the amniotic fluid of a normal fetus as gestation increases and term is approached. The fetal liver is somewhat less capable than the adult liver of conjugating the circulating free bilirubin; the conjugated bilirubin is excreted into the small bowel, accounting for the brownish color of meconium. Unconjugated bilirubin readily crosses the placenta to the mother, where the maternal liver conjugates it for excretion. At birth, this maternal liver function is lost to the neonate, and free bilirubin circulating in the newborn in excessive amounts may cause deposition of bilirubin in certain areas of the brain, which is clinically recognized as brain damage (kernicterus). The importance of fetal liver maturation can easily be appreciated.

Nervous System

Electroencephalograms (EEG) obtained on the fetus in utero show brain activity well before term [28]. Changes in the fetal EEG produced by noise or other stimulation can also be demonstrated. Intrauterine hypoxia in the experimental animal quickly causes changes in the fetal EEG that disappear following relief from the hypoxic state. The return to a normal EEG, however, occurs much more slowly than is the case with hypoxia-induced fetal heart rate changes. Whether or not this sequence of events has applicability to the problem of brain damage that may result from intrauterine hypoxia is unclear at this time. Recent evidence suggests that intrauterine hypoxia is rarely the cause of clinical brain damage in a surviving human infant [29].

The Endocrine System

There is evidence suggesting activity of a number of fetal endocrine glands before birth, although the importance of these functions in maintaining fetal health is uncertain in many instances.

PITUITARY. The fetal pituitary gland apparently is functional from early in pregnancy. Adrenocorticotropic hormone (ACTH) is produced and is necessary for the growth of the fetal adrenal gland. Experimental decapitation of an animal fetus causes atrophy of the fetal adrenals, and anencephaly in the human fetus is similarly associated with atrophic fetal adrenals. The normal fetal adrenal gland is remarkably large; at birth, it is nearly as large as the kidney. This hypertrophy is primarily in the "fetal zone" of the cortex, an area that rapidly atrophies after birth without evidence of adrenal insufficiency. Of clinical importance is the major role played by the fetal adrenal gland in the production of estriol, since the measurement of this substance in maternal urine has been used clinically as a test of fetoplacental function (see Chap. 12).

The fetal pituitary also secretes growth hormone, but the function of this substance in the fetus is unknown. Maternal growth hormone is also seen in high levels in cord blood. Decapitation of an animal

fetus does *not* interfere with normal growth of that fetus.

THYROID. Thyroid-stimulating hormone (TSH) is secreted by the fetus beginning in early pregnancy. The fetal thyroid gland concentrates maternally administered iodine, and the gland is functional from early in pregnancy. Active thyroid substances cross the placental barrier poorly, and the fetus apparently depends on its own thyroid gland for essential support.

PANCREAS. The fetal pancreas secretes insulin from early pregnancy and responds to hyperglycemia by an increase in the secretion of insulin. It is likely that the fetal pancreatic hypertrophy that occurs with maternal diabetes mellitus results from maternal (and therefore fetal) hyperglycemia. Due to this pancreatic hypertrophy, the infant of a diabetic mother is a likely candidate for hypoglycemia at birth.

TESTIS AND OVARY. While the testis has been shown to secrete androgens during fetal life, the ability of the fetal ovary to synthesize steroids has not been demonstrated.

Fetal Immunology

The immunologic competence of the human fetus has been demonstrated conclusively [30]. The ability to produce antibodies develops gradually through fetal and early extrauterine life. While the fetus is able to produce immunoglobulin M (IgM), the immunoglobulin G (IgG) found in fetal blood is largely, if not exclusively, of maternal origin. Full adult reactivity to antigens is not reached in the child until a number of years after birth.

The thymus gland is the first site for immunologic reactivity in the fetus, and microscopic changes in this gland suggest activity as early as 12 to 14 weeks. Subsequent sites of intrauterine immunologic function include the lymph nodes, spleen, and bone marrow. The precise role of each site is unknown.

IgG is transferred with ease across the placental

barrier, and maternal IgG in the fetal circulation provides the major protection against infectious diseases in early extrauterine life. Not all maternal IgG is advantageous to the fetus, however. The IgG antibodies against the Rh factor provide a prime example of fetal damage from maternal antibodies.

IgM may also be found in the fetal circulation, and since maternal IgM does not cross the placenta, the globulin must be of fetal origin. While low levels of IgM in the fetal circulation are the rule, high levels may follow intrauterine infection, a fact which is of clinical use. Intrauterine syphilis, rubella, cytomegalovirus infection, and other infections will give rise to a high level of IgM in the fetus. Some newborn nurseries now include a determination of IgM levels on newborn sera as a routine screening procedure.

References

PLACENTA AND FETUS

1. Hertig, A., and Rock, J.   Two human ova of the pre-villous stage, having an ovulation age of about 11 and 12 days respectively. *Contrib Embryol* 29:127, 1941.
2. Hertig, A., and Rock, J.   Two human ova of the pre-villous stage having developmental age of about 7 and 9 days respectively. *Contrib Embryol* 31:65, 1945.
3. Hertig, A., Rock, J., Adams, E., and Mulligan, W.   On the preimplantation stages of the normal ovum: A description of four normal and four abnormal specimens ranging from the second to the fifth day of development. *Contrib Embryol* 35:199, 1954.
4. Edwards, R. G.   Studies in human conception. *Am J Obstet Gynecol* 117:587, 1973.
5. Hughes, E., Lloyd, C., Van Ness, A., and Ellis, W.   The Role of the Endometrium in Implantation and Fetal Growth. In E. Engle (Ed.), *Pregnancy Wastage*. Springfield, Ill.: Thomas, 1953.
6. Thiede, H., and Choate, J.   Chorionic gonadotropin localization in the human placenta by immunofluorescent staining. *Obstet Gynecol* 22:433, 1963.
7. Ramsey, E., and Harris, J.   Comparison of uteroplacental vasculature and circulation in the rhesus monkey and man. *Contrib Embryol* 38:59, 1966.
8. Page, E. W.   Transfer of materials across the human placenta. *Am J Obstet Gynecol* 74:705, 1957.
9. Acevedo. H., Strickler, H.. Gilmore, J., Vela, B., Campbell, E., and Arras, B.   Urinary-steroid profile

as an index of fetal well being. *Am J Obstet Gynecol* 102:867, 1968.
10. Josimovich, J., and MacLaren, J.   Presence in the human placenta and term serum of a highly lactogenic substance immunologically related to pituitary growth hormone. *Endocrinology* 71:209, 1962.
11. Josimovich, J.   Maintenance of pseudopregnancy in the rat by synergism between human placental lactogen and chorionic gonadotropin. *Endocrinology* 83:530, 1968.
12. Josimovich, J., and Atwood, B.   Human placental lactogen (HPL), a trophoblastic hormone synergizing with chorionic gonadotropin and potentiating the ancholic effects of pituitary growth hormone. *Am J Obstet Gynecol* 88:867, 1964.
13. Josimovich, J., Kosor, B., Boccella, L., Mintz, D., and Hutchinson, D.   Placental lactogen in maternal serum as an index of fetal health. *Obstet Gynecol* 36:244, 1970.
14. Spellacy, W., Cruz, A., and Kalra, P.   Oxytocin challenge test results compared with simultaneously studied serum human placental lactogen and free estriol levels in high risk pregnant women. *Am J Obstet Gynecol* 135:917, 1979.
15. Letchworth, A., and Chard, T.   Placental lactogen levels as a screening test for fetal distress and neonatal asphyxia. *Lancet* 1:704, 1972.
16. Speroff, L., Glass, R. H., and Kase, N. G.   *Clinical Gynecologic Endocrinology and Infertility* (2nd ed.). Baltimore: Williams & Wilkins, 1978.
17. Billingham, R.   From transplantation biology to reproductive immunobiology. In R. Wynn (Ed.), *Obstetrics and Gynecology Annual*. New York: Appleton-Century-Crofts, 1978. Vol. 7, p. 6.
18. Danforth, D., and Hull, R.   The microscopic anatomy of the fetal membranes with particular reference to the detailed structure of the amnion. *Am J Obstet Gynecol* 75:536, 1958.
19. Westphal, M., and Joshi, G.   The interrelationship of birthweight, length of gestation, and neonatal mortality. *Clin Obstet Gynecol* 7:670, 1964.
20. Streeter, G.   Weight, sitting height, head size, foot length, and menstrual age of the human embryo. *Contrib Embryol* 11:143, 1920.
21. Niswander, K., Singer, J., Westphal, M., and Weiss, W.   Weight gain during pregnancy and prepregnancy weight: Association with birth weight of term gestation. *Obstet Gynecol* 33:482, 1969.
22. Gluck, L., Kulovich, M., Borer, R., Brenner, P., Anderson, G., and Spellacy, W.   Diagnosis of the respiratory distress syndrome by amniocentesis. *Am J Obstet Gynecol* 109:440, 1971.
23. Lemons, J., and Jaffe, R.   Amniotic fluid lecithin/sphingomyelin ratio in the diagnosis of hyaline

membrane disease. *Am J Obstet Gynecol* 115:233, 1973.

24. Gluck, L. Evaluation of fetal lung maturation by analysis of phospholipid indicators in amniotic fluid. In *Lung Maturation and the Prevention of Hyaline Membrane Disease, Proceedings of the Seventieth Ross Conference on Pediatric Research,* Ross Laboratories, Columbus, Ohio, 1976. Pp. 47–49.

25. Ambrus, C., Weintraub, D., Niswander, K., and Ambrus, J. Studies on hyaline membrane disease. II. The autogeny of the fibrinolysin system. *Pediatrics* 35:91, 1965.

26. Freeman, R., Bateman, B., Goebelsmann, U., Arce, J., and James, J. Clinical experience with the amniotic fluid lecithin/sphingomyelin ratio. II. The L/S ratio in "stressed pregnancies." *Am J Obstet Gynecol* 119:239, 1974.

27. Davis, M., and Potter, E. Intrauterine respiration of the human fetus. *JAMA* 131:1194, 1946.

28. Rosen, M., and Scibetter, J. The Human Fetal Electroencephalogram. In *Perinatal Factors Affecting Human Development.* Washington, D.C.: Pan American Health Organization, 1969. P. 137.

29. Niswander, K., Gordon, M., and Drage, J. The effect of intrauterine hypoxia on the child surviving to 4 years. *Am J Obstet Gynecol* 121:892, 1975.

30. Smith, R. Development of Fetal and Neonatal Immunologic Function. In N. Assali (Ed.), *Biology of Gestation,* Vol. 2, *The Fetus and Neonate.* New York: Academic, 1968. P. 321.

Additional Readings

Abdul-Karim, R. Fetal physiology. *Obstet Gynecol Surv* 23:713, 1968.

Assali, N. (Ed.). *Biology of Gestation,* Vol. 2. New York: Academic, 1968.

Boyd, J., and Hamilton, W. *The Human Placenta.* Cambridge, Eng.: Heffer, 1970.

Brown, W., and Bradbury, J. A study of the physiologic action of human chorionic hormone: The production of pseudopregnancy in women by chorionic hormone. *Am J Obstet Gynecol* 53:749, 1947.

Evans, M., Mukherjee, A., and Schulman, J. Human in vitro fertilization. *Obstet Gynecol Surv* 35:71, 1980.

Langman, J. *Medical Embryology* (3rd ed.). Baltimore: Williams & Wilkins, 1975.

Moore, K. L. *The Developing Human: Clinically Oriented Embryology.* Philadelphia: Saunders, 1973.

Noyes, R., Hertig, A., and Rock, J. Dating the endometrial biopsy. *Fertil Steril* 1:3, 1950.

Ostergard, D. The physiology and clinical importance of amniotic fluid: A review. *Obstet Gynecol Surv* 25:297, 1970.

Simmer, H. Placental Hormones. In N. Assali (Ed.), *Biology of Gestation.* New York: Academic, 1968. Vol. 1, p. 290.

Wynn, R. Morphology of the Placenta. In N. Assali (Ed.), *Biology of Gestation,* Vol. 1, *The Maternal Organism.* New York: Academic, 1968. P. 93.

2

Metabolic Changes

WEIGHT GAIN

Much has been written about weight gain during pregnancy, and it can fairly be said that the attempt to minimize weight gain during pregnancy has obsessed a generation or two of American obstetricians. The idea that excessive weight gain predisposes to the development of preeclampsia-eclampsia seems to have had its genesis in the misinterpretation of World War I data from Germany during the food blockade. An observed decrease in the incidence of eclampsia in Germany during that period of time was thought to have resulted from the decrease in the food available to pregnant women as well as to the population in general [1]. Actually, the decrease in the incidence of eclampsia *preceded* the decrease in food availability, and the incidence of eclampsia rose to prewar levels *before* the food situation had improved. The more plausible explanation for the eclampsia observation is the decrease in the number of primigravid births in Germany at that time. Since preeclampsia-eclampsia is almost exclusively a disease of the primigravida, a shift toward multigravidity in an obstetrical population might be expected to decrease the incidence of the disease.

The average weight gain during pregnancy in a group of patients who eat to satiety is nearly impossible to determine, since dieting during pregnancy is virtually universal. A reliable estimate of this figure is 25 to 28 pounds (11.3 to 12.7 kg), but the *mean* weight gain (Fig. 2-1) should not be taken as the normal weight gain, since about half the patients will have gained more than the average. The average maternal weight gain in patients with preeclampsia-eclampsia is better documented. Chesley [2] has pointed out the lack of correlation between weight gain and preeclampsia-eclampsia. He suggests that 72 percent of women who have a total pregnancy weight gain of 30 pounds (13.6 kg.) or more will show no evidence of a hypertensive disorder; conversely, 88 percent of patients in whom preeclampsia develops will have gained less than 30 pounds. The rate of weight gain in normal patients varies widely. A weight gain of only 2 pounds (0.9 kg.) during the first trimester is usual, while much larger gains occur in the second and third trimesters. It is not possible to set an upper limit on "normal" weight gain per week, but gains in excess of 2 pounds should be viewed with concern since the excessive weight gain *may* be a sign of preeclampsia-eclampsia. A careful search for other evidence of the syndrome should be undertaken. In most cases, the excessive weekly weight gain will not have been a sign of impending preeclampsia-eclampsia.

Most of the increase in maternal weight during pregnancy can be accounted for. The fetus at term weighs between 7 and 8 pounds (3400 gm.) on the average; the placenta weighs about 1½ pounds (650 gm.); the amniotic fluid weighs nearly 2 pounds (800 gm.); and the increase in uterine size accounts for almost 2½ pounds (1135 gm.). The increase in breast size may add about a pound and the increased blood volume, 3 pounds (1350 gm.). Perhaps 3½ pounds of maternal weight gain can be accounted for by an increase in extracellular fluid. The remaining 7 pounds (3345 gm.) probably results from maternal storage of fat, a normal occurrence in the first half of pregnancy (Fig. 2-2). There is little evidence that a normal weight gain is maintained after pregnancy. There is no evidence to support the common contention that childbearing per se causes an increase in body weight. There is good evidence, however, that body weight in-

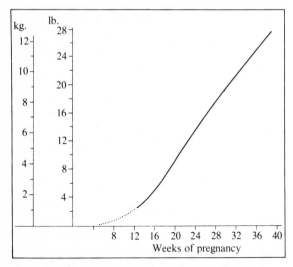

Fig. 2-1. Mean weight gain in pregnancy of 2868 normotensive primigravidas. (From A. Thomson and W. Billewicz. Clinical significance of weight trends during pregnancy. Br Med J *1:243, 1957. By permission of Hugh Clegg, Editor,* British Medical Journal.)

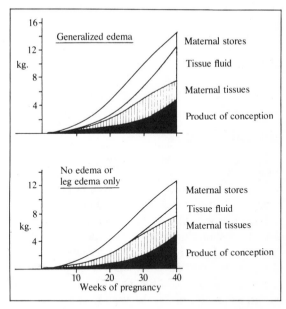

Fig. 2-2. The components of weight gain in normal pregnancy. (From F. Hytten and I. Leitch. The Physiology of Human Pregnancy *[2nd ed.]. Oxford, Eng.: Blackwell, 1971. P. 363.)*

creases with aging, whether or not childbearing occurs.

FAT STORAGE

Fat storage is a recognized phenomenon in pregnancy. The storage occurs primarily during the first half of pregnancy and amounts to about 7½ pounds (3.4 kg.) on the average. The fat storage portion of total weight gain dominates the first half of pregnancy, and the increase in fetal size accounts for most of the weight gain in the latter half of pregnancy. The precise location of the storage of the fat is unknown, but certain deductions are possible from the measurement of skin-fold thicknesses over certain sites of the body (Fig. 2-3).

It is not difficult to postulate a reason for the accumulation of body fat during early pregnancy. It is probably a protective mechanism to provide a measure of safety for mother and fetus should food become scarce later in pregnancy. While such a happening is rare in modern Western societies, this has not always been so and is not universally so even today. The accumulation of fat might be considered a disadvantage in contemporary Western culture.

Fat storage may be encouraged by progesterone as observed to occur in the rat, but this relationship has not been proved in the human.

NITROGEN BALANCE

Pregnancy has traditionally been considered a period of positive nitrogen balance, with some authorities suggesting a total accumulation of protein in the amount of 515 gm. of nitrogen [3]. This effect may be mediated by the anabolic steroidlike effect of progesterone. While some of the increase can be accounted for in the form of additional hemoglobin and plasma protein, increase in uterine size, and fetal growth, the site of the remainder remains a mystery. Recent evidence suggests a much more modest accumulation of protein by the maternal organism, namely, about 6 gm. of protein daily over the last 10 weeks of pregnancy [4].

WATER METABOLISM

Total body water increases continuously during pregnancy. While much of this increased water can

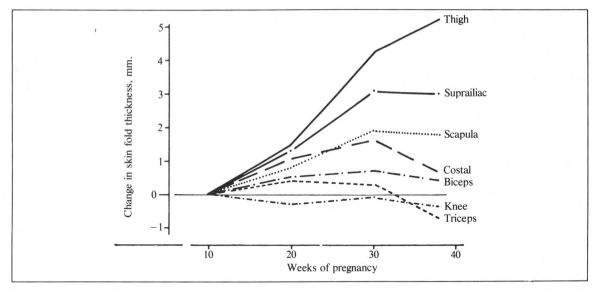

Fig. 2-3. Increase in skin-fold thickness at seven sites in pregnancy. (From F. Hytten and I. Leitch. The Physiology of Human Pregnancy [2nd ed.]. Oxford, Eng.: Blackwell, 1971. Fig. 11-3. From data of N. Taggart et al. Br J Nutr 21:439, 1967.)

be accounted for by the increase of plasma volume, the increase in the size of the uterus and breasts, and the fetal components, there remains about 2½ liters that cannot be accounted for by any of these factors. The 2½ liters is largely extracellular accumulation, which probably occurs in the form of edema.

The nature of edema in pregnancy remains an enigma, especially since acute toxemia of pregnancy is so frequently accompanied by clinical edema. Hytten and Leitch [5], however, suggest that edema in pregnancy should be considered a normal phenomenon that is perhaps mediated by an estrogen effect on the ground substance of the connective tissue. A retrospective study of 24,079 single pregnancies without hypertension revealed some evidence of edema in nearly 40 percent [6]. Robertson [7] suggests that edema is universal in pregnancy. Of great interest is a study of Thomsen et al. [6], in which women who exhibited edema without hypertension not only delivered larger babies but experienced a lower perinatal mortal-

ity than did patients without edema. Therefore, edema, even in the hands and face, is not necessarily a pathologic finding in pregnancy. Edema with the additional findings of hypertension and albuminuria is, of course, another matter.

MINERAL METABOLISM
The maternal organism and fetus store sodium, potassium, and calcium during pregnancy. The sites of storage are shown in Table 2-1. The mother and fetus also require large amounts of iron during pregnancy. It is interesting to note that iron is the one substance known to be absorbed in increased amounts from the small intestine during pregnancy. Authorities disagree on the exact amounts involved, but there is no doubt that (1) the development of the fetus and placenta demands a large amount of iron (300 to 450 mg.), (2) the expansion of the red cell mass requires iron (290 to 500 mg.), and (3) a blood loss of at least 500 ml. with normal delivery should be added to the need for iron (150 to 450 mg.). When the normal loss of ingested iron from the gastrointestinal tract and the frequent depletion of maternal iron stores preceding pregnancy are taken into account, one can easily understand Pritchard and Scott's [8] suggestion that pregnant patients should be given an iron supplement.

Table 2-1. Storage of Minerals During Pregnancy

Site	Na (mEq.)	K (mEq.)	Ca (gm.)
Fetus	290	154	28.0
Placenta	57	42	0.65
Amniotic fluid	100	3	Negligible
Uterus	80	50	0.22
Breasts	35	35	0.06
Plasma	140	4	0.12
Red cells	5	24	0.38
"Edema fluid"	240	8	0.25
Total	947	320	29.66

Source: Modified from F. Hytten and I. Leitch. *The Physiology of Human Pregnancy* (2nd ed.). Oxford, Eng.: Blackwell, 1971, P. 368.

CARBOHYDRATE METABOLISM

Glucose homeostasis during pregnancy is complex and incompletely understood, yet the frequent association of diabetes mellitus and pregnancy makes glucose metabolism an important area for the obstetrician to study. The central factor governing the maternal changes in glucose metabolism during pregnancy is probably that the fetus uses only glucose for its energy needs and that a constant supply of glucose by the maternal organism is essential for fetal survival and well-being.

The fasting level of blood glucose in pregnancy is slightly lower than in the nonpregnant person (68 mg. per 100 ml. versus 76 mg. per 100 ml.). The circulating levels of insulin are slightly increased during pregnancy, and the insulin response to glucose administration is even greater during pregnancy than in the nonpregnant person. Both the oral glucose tolerance test (GTT) and the intravenous glucose tolerance test (IVGTT) have been used in pregnant patients to identify abnormalities of glucose metabolism. Each test has certain limitations. The GTT is less reliable during pregnancy because of delayed glucose absorption from the gastrointestinal tract. The IVGTT fails in part to evoke an important stimulus of insulin release, the production of glucagon from the intestinal mucosa.

Thus, the delay in return to normal blood levels of glucose following the GTT is not experienced with the IVGTT.

The exaggerated insulinogenic response to glucose loading during pregnancy provides a possible explanation for the well-known phenomenon of "gestational" diabetes. It is easy to imagine a maternal pancreas with a borderline capability of secreting sufficient insulin that simply is inadequate for the physiologic response needed in pregnancy. A postulated "antiinsulin substance," particularly in late pregnancy, may add to the explanation; the mechanism of this well-recognized antagonism is unknown. Possibilities include protein binding of insulin, secretion of a placental antiinsulin substance (human placental lactogen), or raised levels of corticosteroids. It is not surprising that pregnancy first reveals the diabetic trait in certain women in whom frank diabetes is destined to develop subsequently. Whether or not pregnancy causes diabetes remains an unsettled question.

The cause of the unusually large babies observed with frank diabetes as well as with gestational diabetes is another point of conjecture. The simplified explanation that the exposure of the fetus to high levels of glucose during pregnancy leads to the large-baby syndrome is no longer tenable. A more plausible explanation centers around the well-known antagonism to insulin in normal pregnancy that is exaggerated in diabetes. The antagonist (a polypeptide?) interferes with muscle glycogen deposition induced by insulin but does not interfere with lipogenesis. The fetal pancreatic overdevelopment reported by various groups of investigators might result as an overcompensation to the insulin antagonism as the fetal pancreas secretes increasing amounts of insulin to overcome the high levels of glucose resulting from maternal hyperglycemia. The insulin effect on glycogen storage is blocked, but lipogenesis proceeds without interruption, and a large baby results.

Changes in glucose homeostasis in pregnancy similar to those described above have been noted in patients on combination birth control pills containing an estrogen and a progestin. This observation, coupled with evidence that progesterone increases the plasma insulin response to glucose administration in the monkey, has led to the speculation that the changes are due to the increased levels of sex steroids known to be associated with pregnancy.

Cardiovascular Physiology

Physicians have long been aware of significant alterations in cardiovascular physiology induced by pregnancy. Recent studies, however, have suggested that many of these recognized changes occur earlier in pregnancy than previously thought and may result from hormonal rather than mechanical factors [9].

HEART

Whether or not heart size increases during pregnancy remains uncertain, but an increase of about 10 percent seems possible. This change may be accounted for by dilatation or by actual hypertrophy. One investigator favored the hypertrophy theory, since he found the heart still enlarged two months into the puerperium [10]. Some investigators have suggested that the risk of delivering a small baby is increased if the heart volume fails to increase during pregnancy [11]. This idea, however, has been refuted by recent evidence [12]. The position of the heart is altered by the growing uterus, and x-ray studies demonstrate that the heart is pushed upward and rotated forward. Other x-ray findings that might suggest heart disease in a nonpregnant patient but are simply the physiologic changes of pregnancy include indentation of the anterior wall of the esophagus, straightening of the upper left cardiac border, and increased prominence of the pulmonary conus. Most ECG studies reveal a definite deviation in the electrical axis of the heart to the left.

A rapid rise in cardiac output occurs during the first trimester, with little change thereafter. Contrary to the findings of earlier studies, cardiac output during the last trimester apparently remains stable and does not decrease. In recent studies, the cardiac output has been measured with the patient in the lateral recumbent rather than in the supine position, a technique that explains the difference in experimental results [13]. This technique eliminates the decreased venous return to the heart caused by uterine pressure on the vena cava. The increase in cardiac output is apparently brought about both by an increase in the stroke volume, which is related to increased blood volume, and by an increase in the pulse rate, which approximates 15 per minute in late pregnancy. There is a further increase in cardiac output with each contraction during labor, a finding far more noticeable in the supine than in the lateral recumbent position. Immediately after delivery, there is a large increase in cardiac output secondary to expulsion of uterine blood into the systemic circulation. The augmented burden on the heart during this period is associated with an increased risk of cardiac decompensation.

A slight fall in both the systolic and diastolic pressures occurs during early and mid-pregnancy, but a return to nonpregnant levels is reported to occur in late pregnancy. In measuring blood pressure with a sphygmomanometer, allowance should be made for the hypotension brought about by uterine blockage of the vena cava when the patient is in the supine position. Any rise of 30 mm. Hg or more systolic or 15 mm. Hg or more diastolic during pregnancy should be accepted as evidence of disease, usually preeclampsia, until proved otherwise.

It has been well documented that pressure in the femoral and other veins of the lower extremities increases markedly during pregnancy. Pressure in the veins of the arms, however, is not altered. The explanation for this discrepancy can be found in the pressure exerted on the vena cava by the enlarging uterus; after delivery, the high venous pressure drops precipitously to normal levels. While the high venous pressure in the lower extremities and perineal area undoubtedly predisposes to the development of varicosities of the legs, vulva, and anus, the distensibility of the veins also is a factor in whether varicosities will develop or not. McCausland et al. [14] measured the distensibility of the veins of the hands in groups of pregnant patients and reported that in women with varicose veins the distensibility was much greater than in those without varicosities.

BLOOD CHANGES

The blood volume increases markedly during pregnancy, reaching a maximum level on the average that is almost 50 percent higher than in the nonpregnant state. However, there is a wide variation in this increase from patient to patient, with some patients showing little change and others nearly double the blood volume. The increase begins in the first trimester and rises sharply into late pregnancy, when it reaches a plateau that shows little change until delivery. The increase in blood volume undoubtedly serves to fill the increased vascular bed provided by the enlarging uterus and placenta.

Plasma Volume and Erythrocytes

The increase in blood volume results both from an increase in plasma volume and an increase in red cell mass. The plasma volume increase occurs earlier than the increase in red cell mass and is greater overall. This results in a physiologic dilution of the red cell mass beginning early in pregnancy. During the last few weeks of pregnancy, however, the red cell mass increase continues while the plasma volume remains stable, and the dilution becomes less pronounced. The red cell mass at term is between 250 and 450 ml. greater than in the nonpregnant state. The result of the hemodilution is a drop in hemoglobin concentration from an average of about 13.3 gm. per 100 ml. in normal nonpregnant women to 12.1 gm. at term. The drop in hemoglobin concentration is most marked when the plasma volume reaches its highest point (at about 34 weeks), after which the hemoglobin concentration increases slightly until term. As Pritchard and Scott [8] noted, however, supplemental iron medication is still necessary during pregnancy if lower hemoglobin concentration values are to be avoided, since the fetus, as well as the mother, requires large amounts of iron.

The increase in total red cell mass is accounted for by the increased production of red blood cells, not by a delay in their destruction during pregnancy. It is interesting to note that the degree of increase in plasma volume is directly related to the birth weight of the child. In a study by Hytten and Paintin [12], many women with a history of fetal death or abortion or who gave birth to an underweight child displayed much smaller increases in pregnancy plasma volume than expected.

Leukocytes

The leukocyte count is also increased during pregnancy, but the reason for this change is not evident. The change may be estrogen-induced. An average nonpregnant value of 7100 white blood cells per cubic millimeter rises to a mean value of 10,500 in late pregnancy. Values up to 25,000 cells per cubic millimeter are common during labor. Most of the increase is accounted for by an increase in the number of polymorphonuclear cells, with only a slight increase in lymphocytes. No change in the number of monocytes or eosinophils has been reported. It is important to remember this physiologic leukocytosis when attempting to use the leukocyte count in evaluating the presence of infection in the pregnant patient. A shift of the differential white blood cell count toward more immature polymorphonuclear cells might suggest infection, since pregnancy per se does not cause such a change.

Blood Clotting and Lysis

While certain changes in the blood clotting and lysing systems occur during pregnancy, the precise clinical significance of these changes remains obscure. Serum fibrinogen increases from a mean nonpregnant level of about 300 mg. per 100 ml. to about 400 to 450 mg. per 100 ml. at term. Wide normal variations occur in both these figures. Other factors (VII, VIII, IX, and X) also are increased. The platelet count shows little change. The changes reported can be partially, but not entirely, induced by the administration of estrogen and progesterone to the nonpregnant patient. While this change to a "hypercoagulable" state might suggest the possibility of an increased risk of thrombophlebitis during pregnancy, in actuality, the risk during pregnancy is low, and during the puerperium, when these values are returning to normal, it is increased.

No satisfactory explanation for this apparent paradox is available. Fibrinolytic activity has been reported to diminish during pregnancy.

Blood Gases, pH, and Electrolytes

The hyperventilation that occurs in pregnancy is progesterone-induced and results both from a slight increase in the respiratory rate and an increase in the tidal volume (see Respiratory Function). Hyperventilation results in a lower blood CO_2 tension. A reduction in the plasma bicarbonate level compensates for the respiratory alkalosis. In this fashion, the acid-base balance is maintained, and little change in blood pH results. There are few other electrolyte changes in the blood during pregnancy, with only a slight decrease in the plasma potassium and no apparent change in calcium, magnesium, or chloride.

Proteins

The proteins show substantial changes in pregnancy. The total serum proteins fall from a nonpregnant level of about 7 gm. to about 6 gm. per 100 ml. The decrease is almost totally in the albumin fraction, which drops about 1 gm. The alpha-1, alpha-2, and beta globulin fractions all show increases during pregnancy, but it is not clear whether these changes are due to an absolute increase or to a proportionate increase of the total proteins as the albumin fraction decreases. The levels of gamma globulin apparently remain unchanged or decrease very slightly. The reason for these changes in the protein fractions of the blood is unknown.

Lipids

The total lipid content of the blood is raised from about 650 to 700 mg. per 100 ml. of serum to 1000 mg. per 100 ml. at the end of pregnancy. The serum cholesterol fraction of the lipids rises from about 180 mg. per 100 ml. early in pregnancy to about 260 mg. per 100 ml. late in pregnancy. The phospholipid fraction rises in much the same way as cholesterol. Lipid is carried in the blood attached to protein, and the lipoproteins can be differentiated into α-lipoproteins and β-lipoproteins, depending on whether they migrate electrophoretically with the alpha or beta globulins. The relative proportion of β-lipoprotein increases during pregnancy, so that the β-α lipoprotein ratio increases. Neither the cause nor the physiologic effect of these lipid changes is understood.

Respiratory Function

During pregnancy, there is an increase in tidal volume (the volume of gas inspired or expired with each normal breath) with either no change or a slight increase in the respiratory rate (Fig. 2-4). The result is in an increase in the minute volume (the amount of air inspired and expired in 1 minute). The increase in tidal volume is accomplished at the expense of decreased expiratory reserve with little or no change in the inspiratory reserve [15]. The vital capacity is probably unchanged, while the residual volume (the gas remaining in the lungs and airways at the end of a maximal expiration) is decreased. These changes are apparently induced to ensure good respiratory exchange for the sake of the fetus.

The increase in total ventilation (tidal volume times respiratory rate) is accompanied by an increased alveolar ventilation; this in turn leads to a lowering of alveolar CO_2 concentration and alveolar and arterial CO_2 tension. This physiologic change may be due to the stimulatory effect of progesterone on the respiratory center; it begins even before the first skipped menstrual period. The change may represent an adaptation to the needs of the fetus and probably assists in fetal placental CO_2 exchange. Another respiratory system finding in pregnancy is the marginally reduced airway resistance and related increased airway conductance that occurs in the last trimester of pregnancy. This is probably related to hormonal or chemical changes rather than being secondary to primary mechanical alterations.

The anatomic changes in the rib cage and diaphragm induced by pregnancy have been observed to occur long before any mechanical pressure from the enlarging uterus could account for their development. The ribs flare and increase the subcostal angle from about 68 to 103 degrees in late preg-

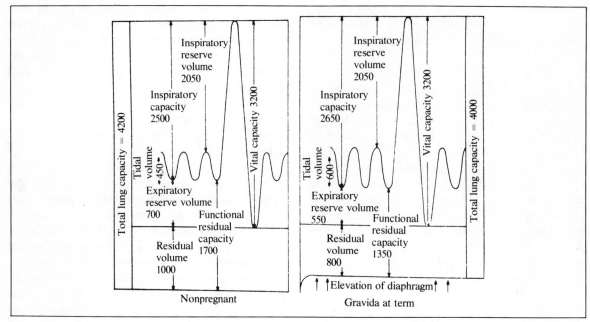

Fig. 2-4. Pulmonary volumes and capacities during pregnancy, labor, and the postpartum period. (From E. A. Leontic. Med Clin North Am 61:1, January, 1977.)

nancy. The transverse diameter of the chest increases by about 2 cm., and the diaphragm is elevated, sometimes as much as 4 cm., above the nonpregnant level. The excursion of the diaphragm does not decrease during pregnancy but simply occurs from a higher level. The increased lung markings noted on chest roentgenograms during pregnancy are due to the hypervolemia of pregnancy, which causes an increased pulmonary blood volume.

The overall effect of these respiratory system changes is that respiratory function is as efficient in pregnant as in nonpregnant women. The compensated respiratory alkalosis is accompanied by minor alterations in electrolyte concentrations, notably decreased plasma bicarbonate and sodium concentrations.

The mucous membranes of the mouth and nose also exhibit pregnancy changes that are extremely marked in some patients. The hyperemia of these mucous membranes, which is probably estrogen-induced, results in swelling of the mucous membrane to such a degree that nasal breathing may be difficult, much as with an allergic rhinitis. Nosebleeds are common during pregnancy, probably

as a result of the hyperemia. A great increase in postnasal drip disturbs some patients, even to the point of gagging. The patient can be reassured that these symptoms will disappear at the end of pregnancy.

Gastrointestinal Function

MOUTH

Some, but not all, investigators have shown an increase in the production of saliva during pregnancy [16]. Others have suggested that the ptyalism noted by many pregnant patients may be due simply to the inability of a nauseated pregnant woman to swallow a normal amount of saliva [17]. One investigator, whose findings have not been confirmed by other observers, noted a decrease in the pH of the saliva, possibly explaining the increase in dental caries experienced by many patients [18]. It is generally agreed that changes in calcium metab-

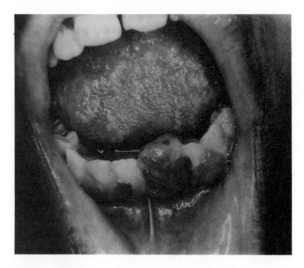

Fig. 2-5. Pyogenic granuloma of the gum. These "tumors" are much more common during pregnancy.

olism related to pregnancy do not account for caries in adult teeth.

Edema and hypertrophy of gingival tissue occur during pregnancy and may be so marked that a "tumor" of the gums, an epulis, may develop and require surgical removal (Fig. 2-5). Gingivitis is common, and an increase in peridontal disease is reported to occur, with loss of gingival attachment and an increase in tooth mobility. The mechanism for this change is uncertain, but the edema may be due to increased levels of estrogen during pregnancy.

ESOPHAGUS AND STOMACH
There is an apparent decrease in contractile activity of the entire gastrointestinal tract, possibly related to the hormonal changes of pregnancy. There is a decrease in the secretion of acid and pepsin by the stomach, which may account for improvement in the symptoms of peptic ulcer patients during pregnancy. It has also been suggested that an increase in mucin secretion may underlie the frequently observed favorable effect of pregnancy on the symptoms of peptic ulcer. Both estrogens and progesterones produce a decrease in pressure in the lower esophageal sphincter, and this probably accounts for the increased frequency of reflux of gastric contents during pregnancy, which results in heartburn. Heartburn is often associated with an actual esophagitis in the lower third of the esophagus, but in many patients, only thinning of the epithelium is present.

INTESTINES
Absorptive and secretory functions of the small intestine during pregnancy have not been studied in any detail, and little or no information is available on the effects, if any, of pregnancy. It is surprising that only one nutritive substance, iron, has been shown to be absorbed in increased amounts during pregnancy. There is increased absorption of water from the large bowel, which may acount in part for the constipation noted by many patients. Sodium also is absorbed in increased amounts from the large bowel.

LIVER AND GALLBLADDER
The results of most laboratory tests utilized in the evaluation of hepatobiliary integrity are normal during pregnancy. Estrogens can produce cholestasis, with a decrease in bile flow and sodium sulfobromopthalein (Bromsulphalein) (BSP) excretion. While BSP excretion by the liver is decreased during pregnancy, the ability of the liver to extract and store BSP and some other substances is increased, and the BSP test results are therefore "normal." The level of alkaline phosphatase is increased markedly during pregnancy; the increase is due most often to production by the placenta, not to a change in hepatobiliary function. The levels of serum glutamic oxaloacetic transaminase (SGOT) and serum glutamic pyruvic transaminase (SGPT) decrease slightly during pregnancy and more sharply in the postpartum period [19]. Liver biopsies have failed to show a difference between the liver during pregnancy and in the nonpregnant state. It should be noted, however, that estrogens can impair liver function in the absence of liver disease and can worsen liver function in the presence of active progressive liver disease. It is therefore possible that pregnancy may have an adverse effect

on some forms of liver disease, especially on chronic active hepatitis.

Although the relationship between pregnancy and cholelithiasis is controversial, there is evidence that the incidence of gallstones is higher in women than in men and possibly even greater in multiparous women. It is probable that pregnancy reduces the mean age at which gallstones occur but has little effect on the overall frequency in women. Cholesterol stone formation is intimately related to the ratio of cholesterol to total bile acid in bile and perhaps to stasis within the gallbladder. The results of studies of bile composition in pregnant women have been variable, and animal studies to date have not shown a definite lithogenic effect of pregnancy on bile composition. However, the gallbladder empties poorly during pregnancy, and oral cholecystograms may not visualize it well.

Urinary Tract Function

During pregnancy, there is an increase in glomerular filtration rate (GFR) of about 50 percent and a slightly smaller increase in renal plasma flow. The mechanism for these changes is not understood, and both physiologic functions return to normal after delivery. One result of this change in kidney function is that solutes are excreted through the glomerulus in greatly increased amounts. If tubular reabsorption is not increased, the level of these solutes in the urine is increased substantially, with a concomitant decrease in serum levels. This occurs, for example, with plasma urea nitrogen and serum creatinine, which are substantially lower in the serum during pregnancy. The mean plasma urea nitrogen during pregnancy is 8.7 mg. per 100 ml. compared to 13.1 mg. in nonpregnant subjects. Another example of clinical importance is glucose. Since tubular reabsorption of the increased amounts of glucose filtered by the glomerulus is relatively fixed, glycosuria during pregnancy is not uncommon. However, the clinician cannot assume that glycosuria in a pregnant patient is due to a normal increase in glomerular filtration, since diabetes mellitus also causes glycosuria and must be excluded before attributing the finding to a physiologic change.

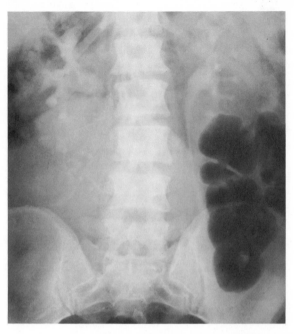

Fig. 2-6. Hydronephrosis of pregnancy. Normal kidney calyces on the right. Note sharp details. Kidney on the left (patient's right kidney) shows blunted calyces typical of hydronephrosis. Hydronephrosis is more commonly noted in right kidney, as in this case.

The cause for the mild hydroureter and hydronephrosis (Fig. 2-6) noted in most pregnant patients continues to be controversial. Two theories have been proposed: (1) that the dilatation is hormonally induced, probably by progesterone, and (2) that the dilatation is mechanically caused by pressure on the ureters. Favoring the endocrine theory is the appearance of dilatation as early as the fourth month, before significant uterine pressure could be applied. Further, in the monkey, the dilatation continues with a functioning placenta even after removal of the fetus. Convincing evidence that obstruction, either by an enlarging uterus or by dilatation of the ovarian vein plexus or the iliac artery, may be the primary cause of the upper urinary tract dilatation has also been presented. The ureteric tone above the pelvic brim, where obstruction would presumably occur, is higher than normal during pregnancy but decreases when the woman lies on her side. The ureteral dilatation is usually more severe on the right, probably because pressure on the left ureter is cushioned by the sigmoid colon. After a careful review of the available literature, Hytten and Leitch [20] concluded that "the concept of toneless sagging ureters, their smooth muscle paralyzed by progesterone, is no longer tenable."

Whatever the cause of the ureteral dilatation, it has important clinical consequences. The asymptomatic bacteriuria noted so commonly during pregnancy frequently progresses to frank infection, due partially, no doubt, to urinary stasis. Another consequence of the increase in "dead space" in the upper urinary tract is the confusion that is caused in the interpretation of kidney function tests. Indeed, the changes in the urinary system are so marked and so confusing during pregnancy that evaluation of kidney function is best reserved for the period between pregnancies if a delay is clinically feasible.

Endocrine Function

PITUITARY GLAND

The pituitary gland enlarges during pregnancy, and the increase in size apparently begins early in pregnancy. Both acidophilic and basophilic cells have been reported to increase in number. Follicle-stimulating hormone continues to be excreted during pregnancy but at low levels. Human growth hormone (HGH) is apparently at normal nonpregnant levels during pregnancy, although not all authorities agree on this finding [21]. The concentration of HGH in the fetal blood has been reported to be three times the maternal level, yet both the mother and the fetus can apparently function well throughout pregnancy without HGH. Assays of HGH are complicated by the presence in the maternal serum of human placental lactogen (HPL), which is produced by the trophoblast in increasing amounts during pregnancy and has metabolic effects similar to those of HGH, as well as immunologic similarities. The precise role of these hormones in the reproductive process remains uncertain.

THYROID GLAND

The elevated basal metabolic rate (BMR) long known to be associated with pregnancy was mistakenly thought to indicate a hyperthyroid state during gestation. It is now known that the increased oxygen uptake revealed by the BMR can be accounted for by the needs of the fetus for oxygen, and thus this test is unreliable in gauging thyroid function during pregnancy.

The greatly increased levels of estrogen during pregnancy increase the thyroxine-binding globulin (TBG) of the serum. Increased amounts of thyroxine are bound to the TBG to become metabolically inactive. A compensatory increase occurs in the secretion of thyroid-stimulating hormone from the anterior pituitary gland, and the thyroid gland is stimulated to produce more thyroxine, which results in hyperplasia of the gland. An enlargement of the gland to two to three times normal size during pregnancy can be appreciated by palpation of the gland.

Because of these changes, thyroid function tests during pregnancy must be interpreted with care. As previously pointed out, the increase in BMR almost universally seen during pregnancy is an effect of oxygen consumption by the fetus and not a hyperthyroid state of the mother. As one might expect from the thyroid gland hyperplasia, protein-bound iodine (PBI), butanol extractable iodine (BEI), and total thyroxine (T_4) are all increased above nonpregnant levels in maternal serum. The increased levels do not indicate hyperthyroidism, however, since the substances are protein-bound and are not metabolically active.

Another test that is useful in the evaluation of thyroid function, especially during pregnancy, is triiodothyronine (T_3) resin uptake. Radioactive T_3 is equilibrated in vitro with a sample of serum from the patient, and a resin is added to the resulting mixture. The results of the test indicate the degree of saturation of TBG by circulating thyroxine. With hyperthyroidism, the T_3 uptake is elevated, indicating TBG saturation and an increased availability of metabolically active thyroxine. In pregnancy, the increased levels of thyroxine do not fully saturate the increased TBG, and the T_3 uptake is lower

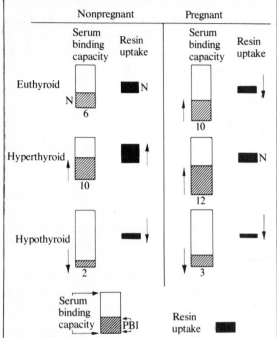

Fig. 2-7. *Protein-bound iodine, resin uptake, and protein-binding capacity of serum for thyroxine in pregnant and nonpregnant euthyroid, hyperthyroid, and hypothyroid states. (N = normal; ↑ = increased; ↓ = decreased.) A theoretical PBI value in µg./100 ml. is included with each rectangular representation of the binding capacity. Note the increased thyroxine-binding capacity in normal pregnancy and in nonpregnant hypothyroidism. (From E. Furth and A. Pagliara. Thyroid Hormones. In F. Fuchs and A. Klopper [Eds.]. Endocrinology of Pregnancy. New York: Harper & Row, 1971. P. 216.)*

than normal. These tests are summarized in Figure 2-7. An elevated PBI or T_4, together with a lowered T_3 uptake, suggests a euthyroid state during pregnancy.

ADRENAL GLAND
There is no evidence that the secretion of adrenocorticotropic hormone (ACTH) is increased during pregnancy, although there is no doubt that secretion of corticosteroids rises during pregnancy. Attempts to implicate a placental source of ACTH

to account for the increased adrenal corticosteroids have not been successful.

Plasma levels of cortisol increase twofold to fourfold during pregnancy, and this is accompanied by an increase in transcortin, the protein that binds cortisol in plasma. All the increased cortisol secretion, however, is not bound, and increased levels of free cortisol also are observed during pregnancy. These physiologic changes are partially reproduced by the administration of estrogen to a nonpregnant subject.

Secretion of aldosterone is also increased during pregnancy. The increased production of aldosterone is reflected in an increased urinary excretion, probably mediated through the activity of the renin-angiotensin system, whose activity is greatly increased during pregnancy. Although the effects of the increased aldosterone are uncertain, the high levels may protect the organism against the sodium-losing effects of progesterone, which occur at the level of the distal convoluted tubule of the kidney. If sodium intake is restricted, further increases in the levels of aldosterone result.

SEX-STEROID-BINDING GLOBULIN
In pregnancy, there is also an increase in the sex-steroid-binding globulin (SBG), the protein that binds circulating estradiol and testosterone. This contributes to increased levels of both testosterone and estradiol measured in pregnancy.

Reproductive Tract
VULVA AND VAGINA
Most of the changes in the vulva during pregnancy are due to a marked hyperemia. This may produce a mild vulvar edema or varicosities of the vulva that, on occasion, may be severe. The vagina becomes hyperemic and changes color from pink to blue to violet (Chadwick's sign). It is this vascularity beneath the mucous membrane, as well as the change in the submucosal connective tissue, that allows the vagina to distend sufficiently to permit easy passage of the fetal head during labor.

Vulvar varicosities are surprisingly infrequent compared with varicosities in other locations (anus, lower extremities) that are also exposed to the increased venous pressure resulting from uterine pressure on the vena cava. Vulvar varicosities are almost unknown in the primigravid patient and are rare in the multigravida. Phlebitis in the varicosities is extremely rare, and the only symptoms attributable to their presence are pressure and the feeling that the patient is "sitting on something." The symptoms are relieved by the recumbent position. Even large varicosities disappear completely after delivery.

The squamous epithelium of the vagina is thickened during pregnancy, and large numbers of cells are desquamated. These cells are recognized primarily as being intermediate and parabasal in type under the influence of progesterone. Some investigators have tried to correlate a "good" vaginal smear (one with many parabasal cells) with the likelihood that the pregnancy is a "good" one (unlikely to terminate with abortion), presumably a measurement of progesterone effect. A vaginal smear read in this manner has not proved to be a useful clinical tool.

UTERUS

The uterine fundus and the uterine cervix function as if they were individual organs. Thus, it is necessary to consider the pregnancy changes in these two portions of the uterus separately.

Uterine Fundus

Uterine growth occurs throughout pregnancy, but the type of growth varies so markedly from one trimester to another that generalizations cannot be made. The overall growth can be described in terms of weight (from 50 to 100 gm. to about 1100 gm.). During the first three months, this growth is due to hypertrophy of the individual muscle cells and probably also to the formation of new muscle cells (hyperplasia). Many mitotic figures can be seen during this time period. Subsequent to the third month and proceeding to term, the uterine musculature grows by hypertrophy. Early growth of the uterus occurs at a more rapid rate than demanded by the growth of the fetus and placenta, and this is apparently a hormonal effect; the growth in the second and third trimesters occurs in re-

sponse to the markedly increased rate of growth of the conceptus. During the first trimester, the uterus is greatly softened, thus providing a useful sign in the diagnosis of early pregnancy. Subsequently, the uterus is much firmer as it becomes more and more distended by the conceptus.

The symmetry and shape of the uterus also change as growth proceeds. A nonpregnant flattened shape is replaced by a more globular shape. During the last trimester especially, the upper portion of the fundus distends more rapidly than does the portion lying inferior to the attachment of the tubes and round ligaments. The result is an increase in the convexity of the upper fundus and an insertion of the tubes and round ligaments at an appreciably lower level than previously noted. Dextrorotation of the uterus, due apparently to the presence of the sigmoid colon on the left, is also a constant finding. It becomes clinically important at the time of cesarean section, since the dextrorotation may be so extreme that the left broad ligament lies directly beneath a lower midline abdominal incision.

The individual uterine muscle cells increase enormously in length and in width, resulting in an increase in total uterine musculature of about 100-fold. The uterine fundus decreases in thickness from about 1 cm. at four months' gestation to about 0.5 cm. at term. This decrease in uterine-wall thickness is due to stretching caused by the growing intrauterine contents. As term is approached and as labor begins, the fundal musculature again increases in thickness. With each uterine contraction, the muscle cell in the active fundus shortens; following the contraction, an incomplete return to the precontraction length is apparent (brachystasis). The result is a thickening of the contracting fundal portion of the uterus as the fetus is pushed downward into the noncontracting lower uterine segment. This process is described in more detail in Chapter 9.

Recognition of the changes described in the fundus can be applied to the clinical care of patients. The diagnosis of early pregnancy is based primarily on the physical findings of uterine enlargement and softness in a patient with an appropriate history. The uterine enlargement may be difficult to appreciate if the uterus is extremely softened by hyperemia, as it frequently is. It should be remembered that multiparity per se causes slight uterine enlargement, and thus the finding of uterine enlargement may be less useful in the multiparous patient. The fundus fills the pelvis at three months' gestation and can be felt as an abdominal organ in most patients by this time. It reaches the level of the umbilicus by mid-pregnancy and the level of the xiphoid process of the sternum at 36 to 38 weeks. Thereafter, the height of the fundus may decrease as the presenting part enters the pelvis.

Little is known about the amount of uterine blood flow during pregnancy. The best estimate is that its value increases from about 50 ml. per minute at 10 weeks to between 200 and 600 ml. per minute at term. The spiral arterioles gradually become straightened as pregnancy progresses, and these arterioles deliver arterial blood to the intervillous space. Venous blood from the intervillous space and from the remainder of the uterus returns to the vena cava through the ovarian veins and the broad ligament to the hypogastric veins. The veins of the uterus and broad ligament are enormously dilated during pregnancy and bleed briskly when cut at the time of cesarean section. Rarely, one of the large veins ruptures spontaneously, and a catastrophic event, intraperitoneal hemorrhage, results.

Uterine Cervix

The cervix becomes markedly hyperemic early in pregnancy, thus demonstrating certain physical changes that are most useful to the clinician for the diagnosis of early pregnancy. The cervix changes color from pink to blue to purple, a finding that becomes increasingly marked as pregnancy progresses. Especially useful as a clinical sign is softening of the lower uterine segment, due apparently to hyperemia (Hegar's sign). This softening can become so extreme in certain cases that the fundus and cervix feel to the examiner like separate and distinct organs.

The endocervical glands hypertrophy during pregnancy and there is a marked increase in the amount of cervical secretions. The cervical secretions plug the cervical canal, providing a barrier to ascending infection from the vagina as pregnancy progresses. As labor begins, the cervical mucus, together with cells from some of the cervical glands, is extruded from the cervix as a "mucus plug," a useful sign of impending labor.

The vagina and the ectocervix are covered by stratified squamous epithelium. The endocervical epithelium, on the other hand, is of a tall, columnar, mucinous variety. The two types of epithelium meet at the squamocolumnar junction, a junction of varying anatomic location. The usual location is at the external os of the cervix or a short distance onto the ectocervix. Diethylstilbestrol exposure during intrauterine life has the effect of extending this junction much farther down onto the cervix or even onto the vagina as vaginal adenosis.

During reproductive life, there is continual replacement of columnar epithelium by squamous metaplastic epithelium. This process results in the squamocolumnar junction eventually being well within the cervical canal. The exact location varies from woman to woman. The area where these metaplastic changes occur is known as the transformation zone.

Under the influence of pregnancy the cervix hypertrophies and everts, thus exposing more columnar epithelium that has not undergone metaplastic change. The pink, glistening appearance of the stratified squamous epithelium is replaced by the reddish, velvety appearance of the columnar epithelium. A similar eversion occurs in patients on combination estrogen/progesterone birth control pills, suggesting that the change may be hormonally mediated.

A second cellular event in the cervix during pregnancy of even greater importance is the basal cell hyperplasia that occurs with increased frequency in a population of pregnant women. A disturbing change in the Pap smear results. The reason for the hyperplasia is uncertain, and the frequency with which it persists following the completion of the pregnancy remains in dispute. What is certain is that the pathologic change is more frequent during pregnancy than in nonpregnant patients and that care must be exercised in differentiating the lesion from an atypical hyperplasia or even a carcinoma in situ. Most pathologists are of the opinion that the basal cell hyperplasia is likely to regress following pregnancy and that the lesion is rarely a cause for worry. However, the final word has not been written on the problem.

OVARIES AND FALLOPIAN TUBES

The corpus luteum of pregnancy is of crucial importance to the maintenance of pregnancy in many animals. It probably is equally crucial in human beings, but for a short time only. During pregnancy, the corpus luteum, on about the eighth day of its existence, begins to undergo the regressive changes expected when pregnancy does not occur. The regression lasts only briefly, however, since the developing trophoblast makes HCG available to the corpus luteum through the mother's bloodstream to replace the anterior pituitary hormone support.

The corpus luteum develops rapidly, and during the first few weeks of pregnancy, it typically enlarges to a diameter of 2 to 2½ cm. Removal of the corpus luteum of pregnancy very early in human pregnancy probably results in abortion. However, a corpus luteum has been removed as early as the forty-first day of gestation without abortion. The corpus luteum reaches its anatomic peak at about 6 or 7 weeks after the last menstrual period, and gradual atrophy begins at this point. After the completion of the pregnancy, the corpus luteum is replaced by a corpus albicans, as are other corpora lutea. Functionally, the trophoblast and the developing placenta take over the hormonal functions of estrogen and progesterone secretion from the corpus luteum at a very early stage, with maximal function of the corpus luteum ending probably about six weeks after the last menstrual period (LMP).

A decidual reaction is frequently noted on the surface of the ovaries as well as in areas of the pelvis covered by peritoneum. While the decidual reaction may in some cases represent a hormonal reaction to pregnancy in areas of prior endometriosis, in other instances, the reaction undoubtedly arises by metaplasia of the germinal epithelium or of the peritoneum. On the ovary, the tiny red areas may bleed easily and appear to be the site of fine adhesions that have been disrupted.

Few pregnancy changes have been noted in the fallopian tubes except for the hyperemia present in all pelvic organs. The tubal mucosa may be flattened, and there may be small patches of decidual reaction both in the endosalpinx and on the peritoneal surface of the tubes.

BREASTS

The breasts undergo hypertrophy during pregnancy, and breast enlargement, together with tingling and increased sensitivity, is a useful symptom of early pregnancy. A yellowish substance, colostrum, may be manually expelled from the breasts in some patients. Also, in early pregnancy, the nipples become more erectile, and the areola around the nipple becomes increasingly pigmented—markedly so in patients with a dark complexion. Hypertrophy of the sebaceous glands is characterized by the development of Montgomery's follicles, which are multiple small, raised papules in the breast areola, a finding that constitutes another useful sign of early pregnancy but is of greater use in the primigravid patient than in the multigravida. Lactation is discussed in Chapter 14.

DURATION OF PREGNANCY

The mean length of pregnancy in the human female is about 280 days, or 40 weeks, counting from the first day of the LMP. While only about 1 woman in 20 will deliver precisely on the expected date of confinement (EDC), about two-thirds will deliver within 10 days of the EDC, that is, between 10 days before and 10 days after the EDC.

Premature labor is usually defined as labor occurring before 38 completed weeks of gestation. The hazards of premature labor to the fetus and newborn are well recognized and increasingly great with decreasing gestation. Postmature labor is usually defined as labor occurring beyond 42 weeks. About 10 to 12 percent of white gravidas will begin labor beyond 42 weeks. Postmature labor is associated with an increased perinatal mortality rate, due

berkurang/susut

perhaps to waning placental support of the fetus [22].

The mean gestational interval among women with regular 28-day cycles is 280 days. With longer intermenstrual intervals, the mean gestational interval is proportionately longer. Since the interval between ovulation and the *following* menstrual period is relatively constant at about 14 days, a woman with a 35-day cycle, for example, might be expected to have a gestational interval of about 287 days. The mean gestational interval also varies with race. Black women, for example, have a mean gestational interval of only about 272 days. It is not known whether this difference is due to genetic factors or to socioeconomic or other factors.

To calculate the EDC in a regularly menstruating woman with 28-day cycles, Naegele's rule is utilized: Add seven days to the date of the LMP and subtract three months. For example, if the LMP began on May 7, the EDC is February 14.

LMP ~ Date +7 ~ Tarinya lahir
Month -3 ~ Bulnya "

References

1. Eclampsia rare on war diet in Germany (editorial). *JAMA* 68:732, 1917.
2. Chesley, L. Weight changes and water balance in normal and toxic pregnancy. *Am J Obstet Gynecol* 48:565, 1944.
3. Macy, I., and Hunscher, H. An evaluation of maternal nitrogen and mineral needs during embryonic and infant development. *Am J Obstet Gynecol* 27:878, 1934.
4. Hytten, F., and Leitch, I. *The Physiology of Human Pregnancy* (2nd ed.). Oxford, Eng.: Blackwell, 1971. P. 387.
5. Ibid., p. 348.
6. Thomsen, A., Hytten, F., and Billewicz, W. The epidemiology of oedema during pregnancy. *J Obstet Gynaecol Br Commonw* 74:1, 1967.
7. Robertson, E. The natural history of oedema during pregnancy. *J Obstet Gynaecol Br Commonw* 78:520, 1971.
8. Pritchard, J., and Scott, D. Iron Demands During Pregnancy. In L. Hallberg, H. Harworth, and A. Vannotti (Eds.), *Iron Deficiency: Pathogenesis, Clinical Aspects, Therapy.* New York: Academic, 1970. P. 173.
9. Kerr, M. Cardiovascular dynamics in pregnancy and labor. *Br Med Bull* 24:20, 1968.
10. Ihrman, K. A clinical and physiological study of pregnancy in a material from Northern Sweden. VII The heart volume during and after pregnancy. *Acta Soc Med Ups* 65:326, 1960.
11. Racha, C., Johannson, C., Lind, J., and Vara, P. Heart volume during pregnancy with special consideration of its reduction. *Ann Paediat Fenn* 3:65, 1957.
12. Hytten, F., and Paintin, D. Increase in plasma volume during normal pregnancy. *J Obstet Gynaecol Br Commonw* 70:402, 1963.
13. Ueland, K., Novy, M. J., Peterson, E. N., and Metcalfe, J. Maternal cardiovascular dynamics: IV. The influence of gestational age on the maternal cardiovascular response to posture and exercise. *Am J Obstet Gynecol* 104:856, 1969.
14. McCausland, A., Hyman, C., Winsor, T., and Trotter, A. Venous distensibility during pregnancy. *Am J Obstet Gynecol* 81:472, 1961.
15. Leontic, E. Respiratory disease in pregnancy. *Med Clin North Am* 61:111, 1977.
16. Kullander, S., and Smesson, B. Studies in saliva in menstruating, pregnant and post-menopausal women. *Acta Endocrinol* (Kbh) 48:329, 1965.
17. Hytten, F., and Leitch, I., op. cit., p. 168.
18. Buhs, A. *Zahnkaries, Speichel, und Schwangerschaft: klinisch-experimenteller Beitrag zum Kariesproblem.* Leipzig: Barth, 1959. Pp. 1, 42, 96. (Sammlung-Meusser; Abhandlungen aus dem Gebiete der klinischen Zahnheilkunde, Heft 42.)
19. Goodlin, R. *Care of the Fetus.* New York: Masson, 1979.
20. Hytten, F., and Leitch, I., op. cit., p. 141.
21. Yen, S., Samaan, N., and Pearson, O. Growth hormone levels in pregnancy. *J Clin Endocrinol Metab* 27:1341, 1967.
22. Browne, J. Postmaturity. *Am J Obstet Gynecol* 85:573, 1963.

Additional Readings

Gaensler, E. Lung Displacement, Abdominal Enlargement, Pleural Space Disorders, Deformities of the Thoracic Cage. In W. Fenn and H. Rahn (Eds.), *Handbook of Physiology.* Section 3. *Respiration,* Vol. 2. Washington, D.C., American Physiological Society, 1965.
Hytten, F., and Leitch, I. *The Physiology of Human Pregnancy* (2nd ed.). Oxford, Eng.: Blackwell, 1971.

3

Diagnosis and Management of Pregnancy

Diagnosis

The diagnosis of pregnancy is usually inferred from certain subjective observations made by the patient herself. The physician is able to confirm the presumption of pregnancy by noting objective signs. The presence of certain of these signs allows a definitive diagnosis of pregnancy, while others permit only a presumptive diagnosis. In special circumstances, laboratory aid will be sought in confirming the diagnosis.

SUBJECTIVE OBSERVATIONS

Cessation of Menses

Cessation of menses is the first subjective evidence of pregnancy in most patients. The symptom is reliable only if the patient has previously experienced regular menstrual flows. The longer the period of amenorrhea in such a patient, the more reliable is the symptom. It should be remembered, however, that there are many reasons other than pregnancy for amenorrhea and that some patients experience menstruallike bleeding even during pregnancy. The symptom is therefore only presumptive evidence of pregnancy.

The most common cause for a lack of menses in the absence of pregnancy is psychogenic amenorrhea, a symptom seen frequently in the patient who either wants very badly to become pregnant or who is afraid of becoming pregnant. Changes in the patient's environment may also provoke a period of amenorrhea. Going away from home for the first time, for example, to college, frequently brings on amenorrhea. Anatomic and endocrinologic causes for amenorrhea must also be ruled out.

Bleeding during pregnancy in an amount sufficient to alarm the patient occurs in about 25 percent of patients; in many cases it occurs in the first trimester. Few of these patients ultimately abort; most continue the pregnancy uneventfully. The cause of bleeding in many cases is unknown. While bleeding during pregnancy is frequently benign, the symptom should always be thoroughly investigated to rule out a significant cause. The bleeding may be due to a pathologic pregnancy, abortion, or ectopic pregnancy; or it may be due to a local cause, such as a benign lesion of the cervix or even a carcinoma.

Breast Changes

Fullness and tingling of the breasts or sensitivity of the nipples are frequent complaints of early pregnancy but are of doubtful value in the diagnosis.

Nausea

Nausea with or without vomiting is almost universal during early pregnancy. While the complaints may conform in timing to the traditional "morning sickness," in severe cases the nausea may be constant. The symptoms usually disappear late in the first trimester.

Bladder Irritability

Bladder irritability may be a symptom of early pregnancy, caused by pressure of the enlarging uterus on the bladder. The complaint disappears when the uterus rises out of the pelvis, only to reappear near term when the fetal head descends into the pelvis. The complaint is usually a minor one and extreme frequency of urination should suggest a pathologic condition of the urinary tract.

Distention of the Lower Abdomen

Distention of the lower abdomen is a very early complaint of some pregnant women. Enlargement of the uterus would seem to explain this symptom,

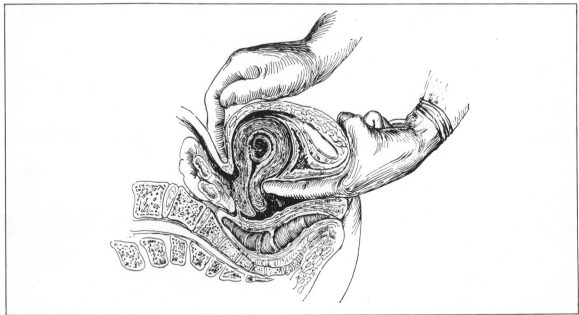

Fig. 3-1. Hegar's sign. The softness and compressibility of the lower uterine segment can be so extreme that the fundus and cervix may even feel like separate organs. (From J. R. Willson, C. T. Beecham, and E. R. Carrington. Obstetrics and Gynecology [5th ed.]. St. Louis: Mosby, 1975.)

but the "bloating" frequently precedes any significant uterine enlargement and may be due to bowel distention.

Quickening

Quickening, the sensation of fetal movement, is usually noted by the patient about the sixteenth to eighteenth week of pregnancy, although some patients have reported this sensation much earlier. Of greater reliability is the observation of fetal movement by a person other than the patient herself.

Fatigue

Fatigue is a symptom of early pregnancy that is especially useful for diagnosis because it is so universally experienced and because it is not ordinarily part of the folklore of pregnancy. The patient "knows" she is supposed to experience the preceding symptoms, but fatigue is a symptom to which she pays little attention.

OBJECTIVE SIGNS

Changes in the Uterus, Cervix, and Vagina

Changes in the uterus, cervix, and vagina provide the most useful evidences of early pregnancy, al-though the evidence is only presumptive, not positive.

HEGAR'S SIGN. The earliest indication is Hegar's sign (Fig. 3-1), which is softening of the lower uterine segment, due apparently to engorgement with blood. The softening allows compression of the area between the cervix and the fundus, sometimes to a degree that gives the impression that the cervix and fundus are totally separate organs. The sign is evident as early as one to two weeks after the skipped period. It may be seen with conditions other than pregnancy, notably when a period is delayed due to prolonged corpus luteum activity, but usually to a minimal degree.

ENLARGEMENT AND SOFTENING OF THE FUNDUS. Enlargement, or softening of the fundus, *or both* provides additional evidence of pregnancy. The softening may be so extreme that it is difficult to feel the fundus at all. The sign may be difficult to elicit if the uterus is retroverted. Enlargement of the uterus is an especially useful sign of pregnancy between 8 and 12 weeks, since the enlargement is progressive, a fact easily noted with repeated examinations.

SOFTENING OF THE CERVIX. Softening of the cervix is a common finding with early pregnancy but is less reliable than Hegar's sign in making a diagnosis. The softening occurs two or three weeks later than Hegar's sign and occasionally is not noted at all.

CHADWICK'S SIGN. Engorgement of the pelvic organs also may cause a bluish discoloration of the cervix or of the vagina (Chadwick's sign) sometimes to an extreme degree. These signs also occur later than Hegar's sign.

Breast Changes

While not diagnostic, certain objective breast changes induced by pregnancy may be useful, especially in the primigravida. The areola may become darkened, and the follicles of Montgomery around the nipple may become prominent. The breasts may appear engorged, with many tiny bluish venules. It may be possible to expel colostrum, a thick yellowish fluid, from the breasts by massage but only later in pregnancy. Colostrum may be present for months or even years following a previous pregnancy.

Braxton Hicks Contractions

Irregular contractions of the uterus known as Braxton Hicks contractions occur sporadically from very early pregnancy. Their usefulness as an aid to pregnancy diagnosis is doubtful.

Fetal Movement

Fetal movement can be experienced by the examiner as early as the sixteenth week by gentle palpation of the fundus. This objective evidence of fetal activity constitutes a positive sign of pregnancy when it is felt.

Ballottement of the Fetus

Pushing the internal examining fingers sharply against the lower uterine pole may cause the fetus, which is floating in a large amount of amniotic fluid, to bump against the distal uterine wall and return again to the examining fingers. Ballottement of the fetus may be experienced as early as the fifth month and is definite evidence of pregnancy.

Fetal Heart Sounds

The fetal heart sounds (FHS) can sometimes be heard through a fetoscope as early as the sixteenth or seventeenth week of pregnancy; they can be heard consistently by the nineteenth or twentieth week. Obesity or an unusual fetal position may delay the recognition of this positive sign of pregnancy. To be diagnostic, the FHS must be counted at the same time the maternal pulse is palpated and found to be at a different rate. Although the fetal heart rate is usually 120 to 140 beats per minute and is thus easily distinguished from the maternal pulse, tachycardia in the mother or bradycardia in the fetus may confuse the findings.

The FHS may be heard with ultrasonic equipment as early as the twelfth week of pregnancy. The instrumentation is based on the Doppler principle of sound conduction, in which the frequency of a sound returning from a moving object either increases or decreases, depending on the direction toward which the object is moving. The change in pitch is registered by a receiving crystal. The movement of the fetal cardiac muscle or pulsations of maternal arteries can be recognized with relative ease. Several commercial devices for this purpose are on the market.

Other sounds heard during auscultation of the pregnant fundus include the funic souffle, the uterine souffle, and fetal movements, but none is of diagnostic importance. The funic souffle is synchronous with the FHS and is probably due to the rush of blood through the umbilical arteries. The uterine souffle is synchronous with the maternal pulse and is due to blood flow in the uterine ar-

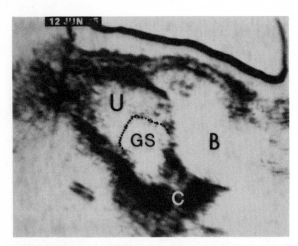

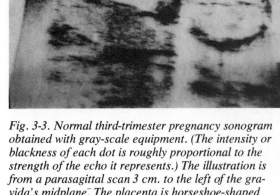

Fig. 3-2. Gray-scale sonogram taken sagitally through midplane of gravida. The slightly enlarged uterus superior and posterior to the maternal bladder contains a sonolucent (i.e., fluid-filled) structure, the gestational sac. The size of the sac is consistent with an 8- to 10-week pregnancy. Scattered echos within the sac (better seen in an adjacent scan through the sac) are produced by the fetus. A fetal skull is not yet identified. (B = bladder; U = uterus; GS = gestational sac; C = cervix.)

Fig. 3-3. Normal third-trimester pregnancy sonogram obtained with gray-scale equipment. (The intensity or blackness of each dot is roughly proportional to the strength of the echo it represents.) The illustration is from a parasagittal scan 3 cm. to the left of the gravida's midplane. The placenta is horseshoe-shaped and extends both anteriorly and posteriorly in the uterine corpus. The fetal skull, with its midline echo, is seen adjacent to the superior wall of the maternal urinary bladder.

teries. Fetal movements are heard with some regularity late in pregnancy and are easily recognized.

LABORATORY AIDS

Ultrasonography
A sonogram (Figs. 3-2, 3-3) will allow recognition of a gestational sac much earlier than a roentgenogram displays the fetal skeleton. The factors of early recognition and greater safety to the fetus will undoubtedly encourage increasing use of the sonogram as the necessary expensive equipment for its use becomes available in all hospital centers.

Roentgenographic Diagnosis
The diagnosis of pregnancy is usually certain by the eighth to the tenth week, but this is not universally so. If the FHS cannot be heard, or if a possible complication obscures the usual evidences of pregnancy, the clinician may ask for the help of the radiologist. As early as the fourteenth to sixteenth

week, and with regularity by the eighteenth to twentieth week, the fetal skeleton may be seen on a carefully taken abdominal film, preferably an oblique film to minimize overlapping of the fetal skeleton and maternal pelvic bones. This technique is especially applicable to cases of suspected fetal demise because the roentgenogram reveals certain signs of fetal death, notably, overlapping of the fetal skull bones.

Pregnancy Tests
Laboratory recognition of the high levels of human chorionic gonadotropin (HCG) produced by the placenta is the basis of several reliable tests for pregnancy. Laboratory confirmation of the clinical diagnosis of pregnancy will rarely be necessary in the usual patient, but certain problem situations are best handled with the aid of a laboratory test. Total reliance on the test is unwise, since the laboratory can be just as wrong or just as uncertain as

Table 3-1. Biologic Tests for Pregnancy

Test	End Poin	Duration of Test
Aschheim-Zondek (mouse)	Corpus luteum formation	5 days
Friedman (rabbit)	Corpus luteum formation	48 hours
Ovarian hyperemia (rat)	Hyperemia of immature ovary	12–18 hours
Frog test	Extrusion of eggs from cloaca	24 hours
Male toad test	Microscopic extrusion of sperm	2–5 hours

the clinical examination. While pregnancy tests approach 100 percent reliability, skepticism toward an unexpected result is warranted.

The available laboratory tests employ either a bioassay or an immunoassay identification of HCG. The newer immunoassay methods are currently more popular, but the bioassay techniques still have applicability in certain situations. The HCG may be identified in the serum or in other body fluids as well as in the urine, the commonly used method.

BIOASSAY METHODS. The pregnancy tests depend on HCG-induced changes in the gonads of the test animal. The details of some of the more commonly used methods are listed in Table 3-1. Since none of these tests is in current common use, the technical details have been omitted. The interested reader can find these details in older texts.

IMMUNOASSAYS. The immunologic identification of HCG is complicated by the cross-reactivity between HCG and luteinizing hormone (LH) secreted by the pituitary. A test sensitive enough to measure low concentrations of HCG may be positive, due not to HCG but to LH (false-positive test for pregnancy). A less sensitive test will not measure LH but will also fail to identify low concentrations of HCG (false-negative pregnancy test).

For many reasons, however, the immunologic tests have largely replaced the bioassay methods in spite of these disadvantages. They are equally accurate; they are usually quicker; they require no animal housing facilities; they avoid the occasional uncertainties of biologic systems; and they are frequently cheaper. So little equipment is required for some that they can be performed even in the small office.

Hemagglutination-Inhibition Test. Antiserum collected from a rabbit immunized against HCG will cause agglutination of HCG-coated red blood cells. If, however, urine containing HCG is added to the antiserum before mixing it with the red blood cells, the HCG will bind the antiserum and prevent agglutination of the red blood cells (positive test). If the urine contains no HCG, agglutination of the red blood cells occurs (negative test).

Latex Agglutination Test. The latex agglutination test (Fig. 3-4) is a modification of the hemagglutination-inhibition test; HCG-coated latex particles replace the HCG-coated red cells. The test is performed on a slide and is easily done in the office. Failure of an HCG antiserum mixed with an unknown urine to cause agglutination of the latex particles indicates the presence of HCG in the urine (positive test). The test can be completed in 3 minutes and has a high degree of accuracy.

Radioimmunoassay. The radioimmunoassay is a highly sensitive test used primarily for research needs or for quantitative measurements of HCG as required in the follow-up of patients with trophoblastic disease; HCG in urine competes with radioactively labeled HCG for binding sites on the antibody. The test can detect levels as low as 10 ImU per milliliter of HCG. Since the beta subunit of HCG is used, cross reactivity with LH is not a problem.

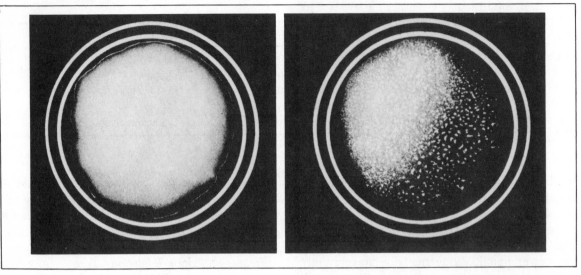

Fig. 3-4. Latex agglutination pregnancy test. Positive test (no agglutination) is at the left. Negative test (agglutination) is shown on the right.

Management of Pregnancy

GOAL

The primary goal of prenatal care is to assure that the mother remains healthy and that the fetus is maintained in the best possible intrauterine environment to permit optimal extrauterine development.

The idea that the pregnant woman should receive special medical attention during gestation is a relatively new one historically, dating back only to the turn of the present century. The first goal of prenatal care became maintenance of maternal health, and, as this goal was approached, an increasing interest developed in fetal care during pregnancy. Over the last few years, interest has centered around monitoring of the fetal condition during pregnancy, as well as around the development of techniques that might favorably alter the intrauterine environment. Without doubt, increasingly sophisticated techniques of fetal monitoring and therapy of fetal disease will continue to evolve.

Another important development in prenatal care is the recognition that only a small percentage of the total pregnant population accounts for a large percentage of pregnancy complications. While it is not always possible to identify the woman who will deliver a damaged fetus or a sick newborn, it is now common practice to select the gravida in any obstetrical population who are most likely to deliver a fetus at risk. Indeed, this triage function of prenatal care has developed sufficiently in some centers to permit the separation of women at high risk during pregnancy into a separate clinic for intensive care. Through this mechanism, the high-risk patient can get special attention, while the patient at low risk receives more routine care. Emphasis in the latter group is on the identification of a pregnancy complication that necessitates the patient's transfer to the high-risk group. More will be said later about the identification of high-risk patients.

INITIAL OFFICE VISIT

Diagnosis of Pregnancy

Confirmation of a presumption of pregnancy is a major reason for a visit to the physician's office. The patient will usually have made the diagnosis herself because of a period of amenorrhea and other symptoms suggesting pregnancy. Objective signs of pregnancy that may suggest the diagnosis include changes in the size and consistency of the uterus during early pregnancy and detection of fetal movement or fetal heart sounds in mid-pregnancy. Laboratory confirmation of the diagnosis can usually be obtained within two weeks of the skipped period. Methods for making the diagnosis are discussed earlier in this chapter.

Medical History

PRESENT PREGNANCY. Since the patient has presented herself to the physician primarily to discuss her present pregnancy, she should be encouraged to describe not only the symptoms that have suggested the diagnosis, but also how she feels about being pregnant.

Menstrual History. When did the last menstrual period (LMP) start? The previous period? When did the menarche occur? How long does her usual menstrual period last, and at what interval do menstrual periods appear? A history of regular periods at 28-day intervals suggests that pregnancy occurred on about the fourteenth day of the cycle. On the other hand, if the menstrual periods occur at grossly irregular intervals, it may be impossible to determine an expected date of confinement (EDC) on the basis of menstrual history.

Expected Date of Confinement. The EDC can usually be determined by referring to Naegele's rule: Count back three months from the first day of the LMP and add seven days. For example, if the LMP began on September 15, the EDC can be calculated to be June 22, which is 40 weeks from the LMP. Term gestation, however, includes a period between 37 and 42 weeks from the LMP, and thus few women will deliver precisely on the EDC.

Factors other than information on the LMP will be needed if an appropriate EDC is to be arrived at in the patient with irregular periods. A history of isolated coitus will occasionally be elicited and is most useful. Ovulation occurs about 14 days before the next menstrual period. A history of prolonged but regular intermenstrual intervals will allow the addition of an appropriate number of days, using Naegele's rule.

Without one of these historical aids, the EDC

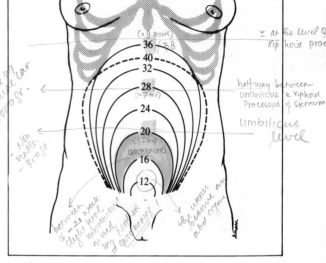

Fig. 3-5. Fundal height as felt by abdominal examination at various weeks of gestation.

will of necessity be determined by physical examination. How large is the uterine fundus by pelvic examination? There is a rough correlation between uterine size and length of gestation (Figure 3-5). The FHS are usually heard first at about eighteen to nineteen weeks gestation. A fetal heart rate (FHR) Doppler instrument will detect the FHR as early as ten to twelve weeks. Fetal movement is usually experienced by the gravida first at about sixteen to eighteen weeks. Ultrasonographic measurement of the biparietal diameter of the fetal skull will also help date the pregnancy.

PREVIOUS PREGNANCIES. Since a poor pregnancy outcome is much more likely to occur in a patient who has already had such an outcome, a careful history of previous pregnancies is important.

Length of Gestation. Inquire about the length of gestation when the prior pregnancy was terminated. A woman who has delivered prematurely in a previous pregnancy is more likely to do so again than are other gravidas. Try to determine a cause for abortion or premature labor from the history.

Birth Weight. Did the birth weight of prior children correspond to the length of gestation? Recall that birth weights of successive pregnancies of the same parentage tend to increase. A small fetus may indicate a "small-for-dates" baby or may be due to an incorrect EDC. Can the reason for a small-for-dates baby be elicited? If the birth weight of a prior child was excessive (over 9 pounds), a search for overt or gestational diabetes mellitus is essential.

Fetal Outcome. Was the child born alive? Were there evidences of abnormalities during the nursery course? Was the baby anemic or jaundiced after delivery? Has he developed normally?

Labor. Was labor spontaneous or induced? Why was labor induced? Was labor unusually short or unusually long?

Presentation and Type of Delivery. Was delivery accomplished spontaneously, with forceps, or by cesarean section? Why was an operative procedure necessary? What drugs or procedures were used for analgesia and anesthesia? Were there any complications from them?

Complications. The patient should be asked about any complications that occurred with the birth of previous children.

During Pregnancy. During a prior pregnancy, did the patient have high blood pressure, albumin in the urine, swelling of the hands and face, excessive weight gain, or any other signs or symptoms of acute toxemia? Were there any bleeding episodes during pregnancy? Did she have any complicating concurrent disease during pregnancy?

During Labor. Did the patient suffer high blood pressure, albumin in the urine, or convulsions during labor? Was bleeding excessive at any time? Did she make normal labor progress, or was it necessary to stimulate her labor? What methods were used to stimulate labor?

During the Postpartum Period. Was there excessive bleeding? Were there any evidences of acute toxemia? Any elevation in temperature? How long was she hospitalized?

Nursing. If the patient previously failed to nurse, was this by choice or by necessity?

HISTORY OF PRIOR ILLNESS. *Medical*. Concurrent disease of the cardiorespiratory, gastrointestinal, or endocrinologic organ systems is frequently of great import during pregnancy. In addition to a history of prior illness of these and other organ systems, a careful inquiry about body functions to detect an undiagnosed disease is essential. Organic disease may have a deleterious effect on pregnancy, causing an increased risk of maternal death or of perinatal loss; and in similar fashion, the pregnancy may cause a deterioration in the disease process. Although few disease states demand pregnancy interruption in contemporary practice, exceptions to this rule do occur.

In most instances, any underlying organic disease will have been recognized before the onset of pregnancy, but the obstetrician is sometimes the first physician able to make the diagnosis. The patient may have ignored obvious symptoms, and, in some instances, pregnancy itself may have unmasked previously unrecognized disease. Two examples will illustrate the latter possibility. Gestational diabetes mellitus is now a well-recognized disease and a frequent one in certain populations. The gestational diabetic patient will manifest hyperglycemia and have a positive oral glucose tolerance test result only during pregnancy. A second example is the patient with chronic hypertensive vascular disease with normal blood pressure between pregnancies and elevated blood pressure during pregnancy. These two examples are fundamentally different, however, since most patients in whom gestational diabetes mellitus develops fail to have frank diabetes in later years. Hypertension during pregnancy, however, is a frequent forerunner of chronic hypertension.

A history of sensitivity to drugs may provide useful information for prenatal care. A history of a prior mismatched blood transfusion may explain the development of hemolytic disease in the fetus, either from the Rh antigen or an unusual antigen.

Surgical. A history of a previous appendectomy will greatly simplify the differential diagnosis should symptoms of acute abdominal disease develop during pregnancy. Prior surgery on the spine may make spinal or epidural anesthesia unwise.

Of special importance is a history of prior gynecologic surgery. Illegal or even legal abortion may predispose to an incompetent cervical os. Prior cesarean section, myomectomy, or hysterotomy may necessitate delivery by cesarean section. Surgery involving the cervix may predispose to mid-trimester abortion. History of surgery on the pelvic floor may necessitate cesarean section if the surgical repair is not to be damaged.

FAMILY HISTORY. If the physician can elicit a history of hereditary disease in the family, it may be possible to determine whether or not the fetus in utero also has the disease. The methods used for analysis of amniotic fluid in such cases is described in Chapter 12.

A family history of diabetes mellitus is a frequent precedent to the development of diabetes in the pregnant patient. Such a history, especially if elicited in conjunction with a history of previously exceptionally large babies, a child with a congenital anomaly, or a history of prior perinatal death, demands a 2-hour postprandial blood sugar determination and sometimes an oral glucose tolerance test as well.

Physical Examination

A general physical examination is important because the patient will frequently not have undergone a recent previous examination, and unexpected findings, often of a serious nature, may be revealed at this time.

GENERAL APPEARANCE. Does the patient have typical female contours and wide hips that suggest an ample pelvis, or are her hips narrow? Is she seriously underweight, and does she show other evidences of nutritional lack?

SKIN. Is there evidence of skin disease? Is there skin pallor, and does it suggest anemia? Does the skin or conjunctival surfaces reveal jaundice?

HEAD AND NECK. Mild diffuse enlargement of the thyroid gland during pregnancy may be normal. A nodule in the thyroid gland, however, demands investigation. Careful palpation of cervical nodes may uncover the rare case of lymphatic disease. Inspection of the nasal and oral mucous membranes will reveal the normal hyperemia and engorgement of pregnancy.

HEART AND CHEST. Although heart murmurs due to changes in blood volume are frequently noted during pregnancy, careful evaluation of the murmur, together with a carefully taken cardiorespiratory history, will usually allow the recognition of nonphysiologic murmurs. Physical examination of the chest is usually unremarkable, except for flaring of the ribs and elevation of the diaphragm in later pregnancy.

BREASTS. Palpation for masses is as essential in the pregnant as in the nonpregnant patient. The adequacy of the nipples for nursing should be noted.

ABDOMEN. Abdominal-wall tone may be poor, especially in multiparas. Diastasis recti is a common finding in multiparas. Is there any evidence of herniation? Any abdominal mass that should be investigated? Are any abdominal scars consistent with the medical history? Can the fundus of the uterus be felt, and is the size compatible with the length of gestation by menstrual history?

EXTREMITIES. Examination for varicosities of the lower extremities should be made with the patient standing. Varicose veins may be asymptomatic or produce only mild discomfort; or they may be the site of thrombophlebitis during the ensuing pregnancy or in the postpartum period. Deep tendon reflexes may be hyperactive in the preeclamptic patient.

PELVIC EXAMINATION. *Soft Tissue.* Physical examination of the female genitalia must be performed in a systematized fashion to avoid overlooking an important abnormal finding. A mental "checklist" of a step-by-step procedure will assure completeness.

After inspecting and palpating the external genitalia, a speculum of appropriate size (usually a medium-sized Graves' speculum) is inserted deep into the vagina. Warm water can be applied to the speculum to ease insertion, but use of a lubricant should be avoided, since it interferes with the reading of a Papanicolaou (Pap) smear. When deep penetration into the vagina has been achieved, the speculum is opened, and the cervix usually comes easily into view. The vagina and cervix are inspected for abnormalities. A smear should be taken by the technique preferred by the laboratory the physician uses. Some pathologists request a "pooled" specimen from the posterior fornix of the vagina, while others prefer scrapings from the squamocolumnar junction of the cervix. A smear and culture for *Neisseria gonorrhoeae* can be taken from the external os of the cervix.

Bimanual Examination. Bimanual examination is performed by inserting the index and middle fingers of one hand into the vagina while the other hand provides abdominal counterpressure on the pelvic organs in a manner that allows palpation of the pelvic organs with the internal fingers (Fig. 3-6). Pressure of the vaginal fingers posteriorly on the perineum causes no discomfort to the patient, but pressure anteriorly on the urethra or on the periosteum of the symphysis pubis may elicit pain. The fingers palpate the cervix and enter the anterior fornix of the vagina. The gentle upward pressure of these fingers is opposed by downward counterpressure on the pelvic organs by the abdominal hand. In this manner, the uterine fundus should be felt and its size, shape, and position determined. If the uterus is retroverted, palpation of the fundus may be better appreciated with the internal fingers in the posterior fornix of the vagina. Next, the fingers palpate immediately adjacent to the fundus to seek the ovary on each side. Normal ovaries cannot always be felt, but any enlargement or fixation should be recognized.

Pelvic examination is completed by inserting the middle finger in the rectum and the index finger in the vagina and repeating the preceding maneuvers (rectopelvic examination). This additional technique allows recognition of any rectal abnormalities and permits better palpation of any abnormalities that may lie behind the uterus.

CHECKLIST. The checklist should include the following:

External Genitalia. Is the hair distribution normal? Are the external genitalia normal in appearance? Is the clitoris of normal size? Are the labia minora normally soft and pliable? Are there tumors or ulcerations? Is there any redness suggesting infection? Is the introitus adequate? Is there significant discharge exuding from the vagina?

Vagina. Is the vagina normally soft and pliable? Any evidence of a septum? Any redness or discharge to suggest infection? Are there tumors?

Cervix. Does the cervix appear normal? Are any lacerations well healed? Any polyps? Is the cervix swollen or edematous, suggesting infection? Is the mucous membrane a normally pink color? Is there an abnormality of the transition zone? Any tumorous growth? Any blood exuding from the os?

Bimanual Examination. Does the vagina feel normal, without evidence of septum or tumor? What is the consistency of the cervix? Of the lower uterine segment? Of the fundus? Is the uterus enlarged? Is the uterus of normal shape? Is the uterus anteverted or retroverted? Is the uterus freely moveable? Can the adnexa be felt? What is the size of the ovary? Is the ovary moveable or fixed? Any swelling of the uterosacral area or parametrial area? Is pain elicited on motion of the cervix?

BONY PELVIS. Evaluation of the adequacy of the bony pelvis for vaginal delivery is an important facet of prenatal care and is performed at the initial office examination as well as during an office visit near term. The method for evaluating the bony pelvis is described in Chapter 9.

Laboratory Tests

A serologic test for syphilis should be performed at the initial office visit and again during the seventh or eighth month of pregnancy. At least one test is required by all states. If maternal syphilis is dis-

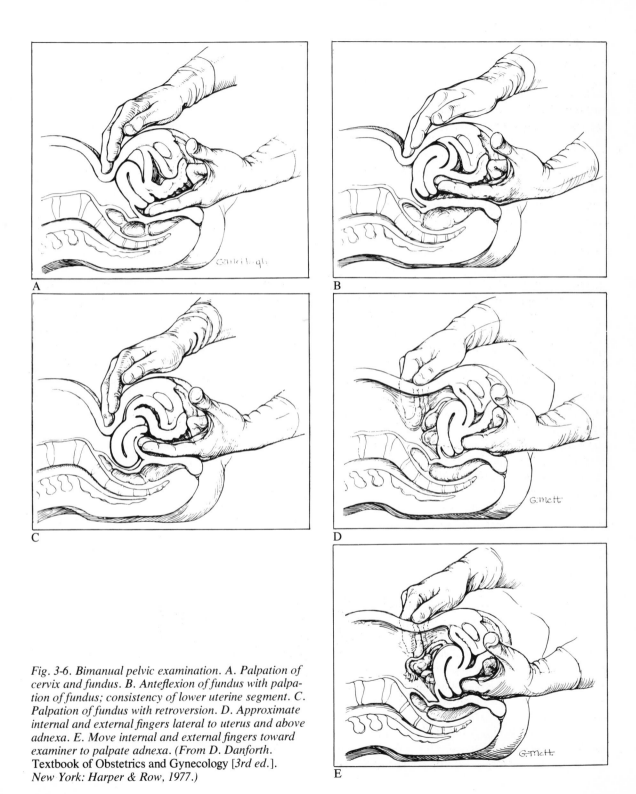

Fig. 3-6. Bimanual pelvic examination. A. Palpation of cervix and fundus. B. Anteflexion of fundus with palpation of fundus; consistency of lower uterine segment. C. Palpation of fundus with retroversion. D. Approximate internal and external fingers lateral to uterus and above adnexa. E. Move internal and external fingers toward examiner to palpate adnexa. (From D. Danforth. Textbook of Obstetrics and Gynecology *[3rd ed.]. New York: Harper & Row, 1977.)*

covered before mid-pregnancy, treatment will prevent congenital syphilis in the fetus. Cervical and rectal cultures for gonococci are performed routinely by some clinics. Although the yield from this routine procedure may be low, prevention of gonococcal ophthalmia neonatorum is an important result.

A hemoglobin or hematocrit determination should be ordered at the time of the first office visit. A low value demands repetition; and if the low value persists, a hematologic investigation is indicated.

An ABO blood type and Rh determination is performed on all pregnant patients unless the type and Rh factor are known from a previous pregnancy. A routine search for atypical antibodies is recommended for all patients. The serum of the Rh-negative patient is screened for Rh antibodies.

Urinalysis will detect proteinuria, indicating the possibility of acute toxemia of pregnancy or of kidney disease. Glycosuria during pregnancy is common and frequently physiologic but demands investigation to rule out maternal diabetes mellitus.

A Pap test is performed annually on all patients over the age of 20 whether or not they are pregnant. For best results, the technique for obtaining the smear should be discussed with the pathologist.

A chest roentgenogram to rule out tuberculosis is no longer recommended routinely. It should be reserved for the patient with a positive TB skin test.

Emotional Support
Pregnancy is a major life event for most patients. It is essential that the physician provide an opportunity for the patient to discuss her joys, her misgivings, and her plans. She may want to discuss the effect of the pregnancy on other children, on her relationship with her husband, and on her general social adjustment. She will want to discuss analgesia and anesthesia, and she may express a preference for one method over another. She may ask the physician's advice on breast feeding or request a medical regimen to prepare for successful nursing. While pregnancy and delivery are usually physiologic rather than pathologic events, they engender strong emotional reactions and cannot be

taken casually. Pregnancy is normal for everyone but the patient herself.

SUBSEQUENT VISITS
The prenatal patient is seen monthly during the first six months, every two weeks during the seventh and eighth months, and weekly during the ninth month of pregnancy. More frequent visits may be indicated if complications develop. The initial visit may be lengthy, but subsequent visits are usually brief.

History
The patient should be asked about unusual symptoms, especially evidences of impending abortion, acute toxemia, or third-trimester bleeding.

Physical Examination
The weight of the patient is recorded in the same state of dress at each examination. The blood pressure is recorded with the patient in the same position on each visit. Ankle, pretibial, facial, or hand edema is identified.

Abdominal examination is carried out with the patient in the supine position. The examination allows identification of the lie of the fetus, the fetal heart tones, and abnormalities in the size and shape of the uterus.

Physical examination of other parts of the body is performed as necessary.

CARE OF THE FETUS
The physician must constantly remember that he is caring for the fetus as well as for the mother. Fetal condition can be assessed by history, by physical examination, and by the utilization of certain laboratory tests.

A history of decreased fetal activity may precede fetal death. The gravida should be asked at each prenatal visit about fetal movements, and she should be encouraged to report any decrease noted between visits. Such a history is an indication for fetoplacental function tests as described in Chapter 12.

Since some infections are potentially deleterious to the fetus, the mother should be instructed to

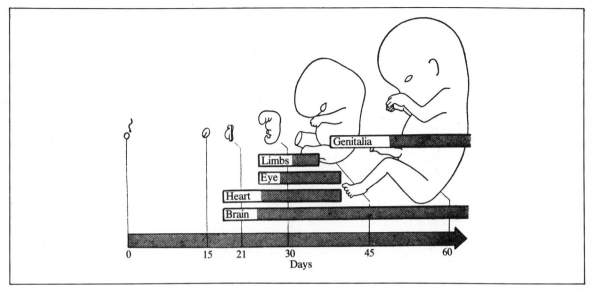

Fig. 3-7. *Organogenesis and critical phases of drug interference with embryonic development. (From H. Tuchmann-Duplessis. Reactions of the Foetus to Drugs Taken by the Mother. In* Foetal Autonomy [*A Ciba Foundation Symposium*]. *London: Churchill, 1969.)*

avoid infection if at all possible. A number of viral diseases are known or suspected to be teratogenic and are especially hazardous. A few drugs are known to be teratogenic and a number are *suspected* of this hazard (Fig. 3-7; see Table 3-3). It seems best, therefore, to avoid all drugs taken for trivial reasons during pregnancy. Indicated drugs may be used with due regard for their teratogenic potential.

When abdominal palpation suggests an excessively large fetus, suspicion of an incorrect EDC or of a multiple pregnancy should be raised. Also to be ruled out are certain congenital fetal anomalies, notably hydrocephalus, polyhydramnios, and other causes of an enlarged uterus. An unusually small fetal size for gestational age presents an even more complex problem. One plausible explanation for a small fetus is an incorrect EDC. Methods for identifying a small-for-dates baby are discussed in Chapter 12.

On rare occasions, other fetal defects can be recognized. An unusually slow fetal heart rate suggests congenital heart block, for example.

Laboratory procedures may allow evaluation of fetal condition. A roentgenogram of the abdomen will identify some congenital anomalies, and it will also make possible estimation of gestational age by noting the presence of certain bony epiphyses. Laboratory tests of amniotic fluid will allow accurate estimation of gestational age or maturation of certain organ systems, notably the lungs (see Chap. 12). Severity of Rh disease can also be estimated by identifying the level of bilirubinoid substances in the amniotic fluid (Chap. 12).

PREPARATION FOR LABOR

The multipara should be admitted to the hospital as soon as her contractions are occurring at regular intervals. Admission of the primigravid patient may be delayed until the contractions are regular and occurring at 4- to 5-minute intervals. Telephone consultation with the physician is frequently essential if unnecessary or premature hospitalization is to be avoided. The patient should seek advice from the physician if any of the following danger signals appear during the prenatal course:

Table 3-2. Recommended Daily Dietary Allowances for Girls and Women at Various Ages, with Added Allowances for Pregnancy

Item	Recommended Daily Allowances for Nonpregnant Women by Age					Recommended Daily Allowances Added for Pregnancy
	12–14 Yr.	14–16 Yr.	16–18 Yr.	18–22 Yr.	22–35 Yr.	
Calories (kcal.)	2300	2400	2300	2000	2000	200
Protein (gm.)	50	55	55	55	55	10
Vitamin A (I.U.)	5000	5000	5000	5000	5000	1000
Vitamin D (I.U.)	400	400	400	400	. . .	0
Vitamin E (I.U.)	20	25	25	25	25	5
Ascorbic acid (mg.)	45	50	50	55	55	10
Folacin (mg.)	0.4	0.4	0.4	0.4	0.4	0.4
Niacin (mEq.)	15	16	15	13	13	2
Riboflavin (mg.)	1.4	1.4	1.5	1.5	1.5	0.3
Thiamine (mg.)	1.2	1.2	1.2	1.0	1.0	0.1
Vitamin B_6 (mg.)	1.6	1.8	2.0	2.0	2.0	0.5
Vitamin B_{12} (μg.)	5	5	5	5	5	3
Calcium (gm.)	1.3	1.3	1.3	0.8	0.8	0.4
Phosphorus (gm.)	1.3	1.3	1.3	0.8	0.8	0.4
Iodine (μg.)	115	120	115	100	100	25
Iron (mg.)	18	18	18	18	18	30–60
Magnesium (mg.)	350	350	350	350	300	150

Source: Modified from Maternal Nutrition and the Course of Pregnancy (Summary Report). Washington, D.C.: National Academy of Science, 1970.

1. Leakage of amniotic fluid.
2. Any vaginal bleeding.
3. Evidence of acute toxemia of pregnancy: edema of the hands or face, blurring of vision, headache, epigastric distress, or convulsions.
4. Chills, or fever, or both.
5. Abdominal pain.

NUTRITION DURING PREGNANCY

Any approximation of the dietary needs of the pregnant patient can be seen in Table 3-2, which lists daily dietary allowances recommended by the Food and Nutrition Board of the National Research Council. Underweight patients or young gravidas with incomplete growth may require much larger allowances. Ideally, the physician or his assistant should take a full diet history, then approve or correct it as needed. A good rule of thumb is to encourage a pregnant patient to eat at least the following each day:

Milk: 1 pint
Citrus fruit or tomato: 1 serving
Lean meat, fish, poultry, eggs, beans, cheese: 2 servings
Leafy green vegetables: 1 serving
Yellow vegetables: 1 serving

If what should be eaten rather than what should be avoided is emphasized, better nutrition will result.

Specific Requirements

PROTEIN. Protein intake should be increased by 10 gm. per day, with most of the protein in the form of animal protein (meat, milk, cheese, poultry, eggs, fish). Although it has been suggested that a high-protein pregnancy diet may decrease the likelihood of many complications of pregnancy, this theory remains unproved.

MINERALS AND VITAMINS. Certain minerals may need to be added to the diet to satisfy nutritional requirements. One quart of cow's milk (skim milk may be preferred) contains 1.0 gm. of calcium, which is close to the 1.2-gm. daily requirement recommended for most patients. Some blacks, Orientals, and Chicanos are unable to digest milk because of a lactase deficiency resulting in intolerance to the lactose in milk. If the patient cannot or will not drink milk, she should be encouraged to eat green, leafy vegetables, whole grain foods, whole fish (sardines), and fermented cheeses if tolerated. Supplementation in the form of calcium lactate may also be prescribed.

Supplemental iron is recommended to prevent depletion of maternal iron storage, frequently already inadequate, during the last half of pregnancy. A daily increment of 30 mg. of iron in the form of oral ferrous gluconate or ferrous fumerate will fulfill this requirement. To prevent the development of megaloblastic anemia of pregnancy due to inadequate folate intake, 1 mg. of oral folic acid should also be added to the diet. It has been observed that the amount of iodine in the typical American diet is much greater at the present time than it was several decades ago. The usual recommendation that iodized salt should be used in areas with iodine deficiency is presently under study.

Other minerals and vitamins are usually found in adequate amounts in a good diet and do not need to be taken separately. Little harm will result from the multivitamins and mineral pills so often taken during pregnancy. However, the cost of these preparations cannot be justified for most patients, and some patients assume that they do not need to eat a balanced diet if they take their vitamins.

Weight Gain
Obstetricians for the past 50 years have encouraged pregnant patients to limit their pregnancy weight gain, sometimes severely. Recent evidence has

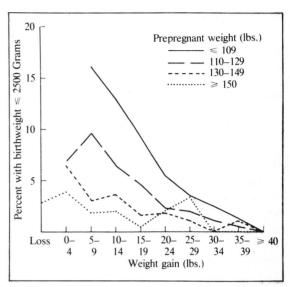

Fig. 3-8. Percent of cases with birth weight ≤ 2500 gm. by weight gain and gravida's prepregnant weight (white patients). (From K. Niswander, J. Singer, M. Westphal, and W. Weiss. Weight gain during pregnancy and pre-pregnancy weight. Obstet Gynecol *33:482, 1969.)*

shown this practice to be both unnecessary and unwise, and severe weight restriction is no longer recommended by most physicians [1]. The practice was based on the long-held belief that excessive weight gain predisposes the gravid patient to acute toxemia of pregnancy, a belief now known to be untrue. Current advice to pregnant patients stresses *what should be eaten,* not *what should be avoided.* A weight-reducing diet is distinctly contraindicated in most pregnant patients.

In recent years, there has been a rediscovery of the finding that increased maternal weight gain results in an increased mean birth weight of the offspring. The risk of delivering a low-birth-weight child (less than 2501 gm.) is greatly increased if the gravida experiences a small weight gain during pregnancy, especially if she is of small prepregnant weight. The same relationship is noted among women of greater prepregnant weight, but the differences are less striking than with low prepregnant weight (Fig. 3-8). Chase [2] has said that the difference between the lower neonatal mortality of certain Western European countries and the higher rate experienced in the United States may be based primarily on the higher rate of low-birth-weight infants in the United States. She suggests that an arithmetic increase of 1 percent in infants weighing less than 2501 gm. causes a relative increase of 10 percent in mortality in the first week. With these findings in mind, the implications of restricted maternal weight gain on perinatal outcome seem obvious.

Recent studies have also suggested another hazard of poor maternal nutrition. There is evidence that the human fetal brain develops by an increase in both the number of brain cells and the size of the cells. These events are dependent on good maternal nutrition. Inadequate nutrition during pregnancy may actually decrease the number of brain cells that develop in the fetus in utero; and the decrease is thought to be permanent. If the expected increase in the number of brain cells fails to occur, a permanent decrease in the number of cells results. While this result can only be inferred in the human, it has been observed in animals [3]. The implications of this observation, if true in the human, are enormous.

Of equal importance to fetal development is the nutritional status of the woman before she becomes pregnant. Prepregnant weight is a strong determinant of mean newborn weight. The physician may not be able to influence this important factor in pregnancy outcome but should be aware of it. Eastman and Jackson [4] have suggested that the pregnant patient with a low prepregnant weight and a low weight gain by midpregnancy should be considered a high-risk patient and treated accordingly.

While severe weight restriction is no longer tenable, the search for an "ideal" weight gain continues, but it is doubtful that such a figure exists. Chesley [5] has written that the average weight gain in nontoxemic patients, excluding gain due to fat, is 28.7 pounds (13 kg.)—conception products, 11.2 pounds (5085 gm.); uterine growth, 2.5 pounds (1135 gm.); breast growth, 3 pounds (1360 gm.); protein retention, 4.0 pounds (1800 gm.); blood volume, 3.5 pounds (1600 gm.); and interstitial water increase, 4.5 pounds (2100 gm.). If 28.7 pounds is the mean weight gain, it naturally follows that half of nontoxemic patients will gain more than that amount. Any attempt to limit *all* pregnant patients to a weight gain of 28.7 pounds will obviously lower this mean weight gain of normal pregnancy. While obesity is not advisable, an attempt at weight loss should *follow* pregnancy, when no ill effect on the fetus will result.

Salt Restriction and Diuretics
Routine sodium restriction during pregnancy has been recommended and practiced widely in the past in an attempt to reduce the likelihood that acute toxemia will develop. The presumed relationship between excessive sodium intake and the *initiation* of acute toxemia is now seriously questioned. Indeed, the Committee on Maternal Nutrition of the National Research Council [6] suggests that sodium restriction in late pregnancy may put undue stress on the adrenal cortex, since this organ attempts to compensate for sodium lack. This hazard has been shown in animals, but it has not been demonstrated with certainty in human subjects.

Diuretic drugs similarly are no longer recommended during pregnancy either to prevent or to treat acute toxemia. Their effectiveness in this regard has not been shown. Thiazide diuretics have been associated with maternal death in a few cases, due apparently to electrolyte depletion and pancreatitis.

COMMON COMPLAINTS
Nausea and Vomiting
ETIOLOGY. Nausea, vomiting, or both are the most common complaints experienced by the pregnant patient. The etiology of the symptom is unknown. Although there is an emotional component in many patients, the case for a physiologic cause is excellent. The author has seen patients with nausea and vomiting who had no reason whatsoever to suspect pregnancy.

HYPEREMESIS GRAVIDARUM. While the nausea is typically experienced on arising in the morning and

[handwritten:] Weight gain in Pregnancy is usually in the range of 10-12 Kg or 24-28 lbs.

improves as the day proceeds, the symptom may persist all day long in some patients. Dehydration is rare, but, when it is present, a diagnosis of *hyperemesis gravidarum* is justified. This disease was common in previous generations but is rare today. Hospitalization may be necessary because of severe dehydration, and nonspecific therapy in the form of parenteral fluids and sedation is frequently sufficient to provide improvement in the symptom.

TREATMENT. Innumerable remedies have been prescribed for the nausea and vomiting of pregnancy. The large number of therapies tried suggests the inadequacy of all treatments. A sympathetic physician, however, can usually do much to relieve the symptom. Concern that vomiting may harm the pregnancy is a major worry of many patients, and reassurance that this is not so is sometimes sufficient to relieve the symptom. On occasion, the patient will become nauseated following ingestion of certain foods peculiar to her particular pregnancy, and avoidance of these foods may relieve the symptom. This is true of coffee for many patients, or fatty foods for others. Sometimes, the ingestion of dry soda crackers or unbuttered bread immediately on arising will relieve the symptom. The mere avoidance of food until 10 or 11 A.M. will sometimes prevent the development of the symptom. While many drugs reputed to relieve the symptom are on the market, most patients will not demand drug therapy because of the current concern about the teratogenic effects of drugs taken during the first trimester of pregnancy. Certain of these drugs, however, are thought to be safe and may be prescribed (e.g., Bendectin).

Heartburn

Heartburn, a common symptom of pregnancy, is apparently due to relaxation of the cardiac sphincter which allows gastric contents to regurgitate back into the esophagus. Some investigators think that an actual esophagitis is necessary before the symptom is manifested. The frequency of the symptom is probably related to the general relaxa-tion of the gastrointestinal musculature so evident during pregnancy. The symptom occurs most commonly when the patient is lying flat in bed or assumes some other position that encourages gastric reflux.

Treatment with various antacids (such as Maalox, Amphogel, and Gelusil) is highly effective but short-acting. Sodium bicarbonate is an effective therapy and is widely utilized by patients. However, it should be avoided because of the large sodium intake associated with its use.

Constipation

Constipation is caused primarily by relaxation of the bowel musculature during pregnancy. Treatment is unnecessary unless the patient complains of abdominal cramping or bowel pressure. The best treatment is a change in dietary habits, with a substantial increase in roughage foods (cereals, fruits, and vegetables). Laxative foods, such as prunes, dates, and figs, may be effective, and the patient should be encouraged to drink large amounts of fluid. Stool softeners or bulk laxatives, especially when taken on a regular basis, may relieve the symptom. Harsh laxatives should be avoided, especially near term, since these drugs are thought to encourage the onset of labor. Mineral oil is contraindicated, since it prevents the absorption of fat-soluble vitamins from the gastrointestinal tract.

Ptyalism and Pica

Some pregnant women complain of ptyalism (excessive salivation), and neither the cause nor an effective treatment for this complaint is known. Pica can be defined as the ingestion of materials that are not usually considered food and have no caloric value. Pica is common among certain groups of people. Starch, clay, baked earth, and other substances may be ingested. It is likely that the symptom is not physiologic but rather results from the patient's having heard old wives' tales about the value of the substance in pregnancy. While pica is usually not harmful in itself, the substitution of nonnutritious materials for foods may cause undernourishment. The practice should be

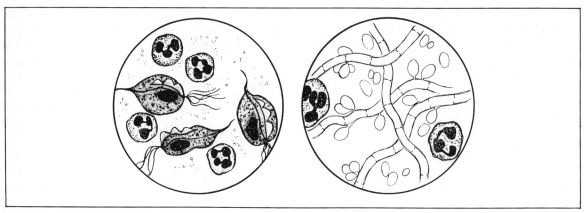

Fig. 3-9. Causes of vaginitis. Microscopic confirmation of Trichomonas vaginalis (left) and Candida albicans (right). (From K. Niswander. Obstetric and Gynecologic Disorders: A Practitioner's Guide. Flushing, N.Y.: Medical Examination Publishing Co., 1975.)

discouraged by explaining the hazards to the patient.

Urinary Frequency

Urinary frequency occurs most notably with early pregnancy, as the enlarging uterus presses on the bladder, and near term, when the descending presenting part causes bladder pressure. If the frequency is accompanied by urgency, dysuria, hematuria, or other urinary symptoms, urinary tract diseases should be suspected. Investigation of the complaint will usually lead to the diagnosis of urinary tract infection, which should be treated appropriately. In the absence of disease, the symptom usually requires no therapy.

Leukorrhea

When the vaginal discharge that most women normally experience is sufficiently disturbing to necessitate medical advice, the symptom can be called leukorrhea. Vaginal discharge normally increases during pregnancy because the amount of material secreted by a normally hyperactive cervix increases. If the patient complains about the discharge, or if other symptoms such as pruritus also develop, a diagnostic work-up and treatment are necessary.

TRICHOMONAS VAGINALIS INFECTION. If the vaginal discharge is bubbly and a yellowish-green color, or if the cervix or upper vagina displays the typical

"strawberry" spots, a diagnosis of Trichomonas vaginalis infection should be entertained. The diagnosis is established by identifying the organism on a glass slide under the high power of the microscope. A small amount of vaginal material is placed on the slide and diluted with a small amount of warm normal saline solution. The organism is pear-shaped, flagellated, and highly motile to the eye (Fig. 3-9). While 20 to 30 percent of pregnant patients harbor the organism in the vagina, an infection actually develops in only a few.

Treatment of Trichomonas infection can be local or systemic metronidazole (Flagyl), or sulfanilamide vaginal cream. Flagyl is known to cross the placenta and it is not recommended systemically during pregnancy, especially during the first trimester. Sulfanilamide cream will provide some relief of symptoms.

CANDIDAL INFECTION. As with Trichomonas vaginalis, Candida albicans, the causative agent of candidal infection (Fig. 3-9), can be identified from the vagina in many pregnant patients, but an infection develops in relatively few. The symptoms are likely to be acute and severe, with vaginal and vulvar burning and itching and a profuse white chunky discharge that resembles cottage cheese. Examination usually reveals a markedly reddened vagina, and vulvitus is a commonly associated finding. The symptoms are aggravated by intercourse, and the male may experience mild itching and redness of the penis following exposure. Local mycostatin or gentian violet in various forms uniformly gives symptomatic relief. No systemic therapy is indicated. While the symptoms are usually easily relieved, flare-ups throughout pregnancy are to be expected, and treatment during pregnancy should be considered symptomatic rather than curative. After the completion of the pregnancy, the disease can usually be eradicated.

NONSPECIFIC INFECTION. If neither *Trichomonas* nor *Candida* can be identified as the cause of the symptoms, a nonspecific infection should be suspected. It is likely that the seemingly nonspecific infection may be caused by a bacterium, *Hemophilus vaginalis*. Treatment with a local sulfonamide cream is usually effective in eradicating this infection.

Sometimes no causative organism can be identified, and therapeutic agents must be nonspecific of necessity. The application of petroleum jelly to the vulva to provide protection to the vulvar skin may help relieve the symptoms if vulvar irritation is prominent. If douching is to be prescribed (2 tablespoons of white vinegar in a douche bag full of water), the patient should be warned to insert the douche tip no more than an inch through the introitus and to avoid closing the labia during douching. Air emboli have been reported with douching during pregnancy.

Varicosities of the Extremities

Varicosities of the lower extremities may make their first appearance during pregnancy, primarily because the enlarging uterus obstructs the venous return from the lower extremities in various degrees. While the major etiologic factor with varicose veins is probably familial, pregnancy is certainly an aggravating factor. Relief from the symptoms of varicosities can be provided by frequent elevation of the legs or by application of an elastic stocking. There is no evidence that such therapy actually improves the varicosities, but symptomatic relief can be dramatic. It is likely that the collapse of the distended and tortuous varicosities provided by the elastic stocking helps in the prevention of thrombophlebitis. Neither surgery nor the injection of thrombosing substances is recommended during pregnancy.

Occasionally, the varicosities involve the vulva and perineum. Treatment is unsatisfactory, but various perineal pressure devices have provided some relief.

Varicosities of the Hemorrhoidal Veins

Hemorrhoids are a variant of varicosities of the lower extremities, with a similar familial etiology. Hemorrhoids occur with great frequency during pregnancy, undoubtedly because of venous obstruction by the enlarging uterus. They frequently disappear following the termination of the pregnancy.

The diagnosis is an easy one to make, since the dilated tortuous veins are easy to see at the anal opening. The patient sometimes complains of rectal bleeding but more frequently complains of itching or burning around the anus. Therapy during pregnancy is largely limited to conservative measures. Gentle manual replacement of hemorrhoids is occasionally helpful; hot sitz baths or local compresses may give symptomatic relief, and topical anesthetics are helpful in some cases. Surgical therapy is prescribed only when thrombosis occurs in the hemorrhoids, a complication that produces very severe pain. After spraying of the hemorrhoids with a topical anesthetic, the thrombosed vein is opened with a small scalpel, and the clot is evacuated. Almost instantaneous relief is usual.

Headache

Headache is as common during pregnancy as it is in the nonpregnant state. It rarely indicates serious disease, but a persistent headache may require the same diagnostic work-up necessary in a nonpregnant patient. Headache is a symptom of severe acute toxemia of pregnancy.

Sinus congestion is a common cause of headache during pregnancy because of the hormonally induced increased vascularity of the nasal mucosa. The edematous mucosa mimics the changes seen with allergy. Blockage of the tiny sinus openings may lead to sinusitis if infection supervenes. Treatment with various antihistamines is effective in shrinking the mucosa and relieving the symptoms. Some investigators, however, have suggested that antihistamines are potentially teratogenic and should not be used during early pregnancy.

Edema

Edema of the lower extremities is extremely common in pregnancy, especially during late pregnancy, and edema of the hands and face is not rare. Most edema in pregnancy is benign and is due apparently to the sodium and water retention that is related to the secretion of ovarian and placental steroid hormones. Obstruction of venous and lymphatic return from the leg by the enlarging uterus is also a major etiologic factor.

Edema may be associated with acute toxemia of pregnancy; in this case, the edema is not benign. Elevation of the blood pressure and albuminuria are nearly always associated with toxemic edema.

Benign edema should be treated only if the patient demands it. Elevation of the legs will relieve edema by reducing the venous blockage caused by the uterus. Restriction of sodium intake will produce diuresis with temporary decrease of edema and may be helpful. Diuretic substances, notably the thiazides, have been used in the past in the treatment of edema, but they are no longer recommended. Potassium depletion and acute pancreatitis in the gravida and thrombocytopenic purpura in the newborn are reported complications of thiazide therapy.

Backache and Pelvic Pressure

The symphysis pubis and sacroiliac articulations are synarthrotic joints and permit almost no motion in the nonpregnant adult. The pelvis functions essentially as a single entity, although it is composed of three separate bones. During pregnancy, however, the joints loosen, probably under the influence of relaxin, a pregnancy hormone secreted by the corpus luteum. The physiologic advantage of this change is that additional room is allowed the fetus during its passage through the birth canal. The disadvantage is a functionally unstable pelvis in the pregnant patient. This results in the well-known symptoms of low backache, pelvic pressure, and sciatica.

During normal pregnancy, the protuberant abdomen forces the gravida to throw her shoulders back to maintain her balance. The neck is flexed slightly to compensate and to maintain the head in erect position. The effect of these changes is to increase the normal curvature, both of the lumbar and the cervicothoracic spine. A snug maternity girdle will reduce the abdominal protuberance and minimize the compensating spinal changes. A similar therapeutic effect can be obtained by suggesting that the woman wear shoes with wide 2-inch heels. The heels cause her to throw her shoulders into a more anterior position, thus reducing the lumbar lordosis.

Other therapeutic suggestions for these pelvic complaints include local heat to the back, which decreases discomfort by relaxing muscle spasm. Less walking will help some patients, but if the symptom is severe, strict bed rest or hospitalization may become necessary.

Leg Cramps

Many pregnant patients complain of severe cramps in the gastrocnemius muscles during pregnancy. The cause of this complaint is unknown, but one theory suggests that it is due to a relatively reduced level of diffusable serum calcium, or to a relatively increased level of serum phosphorus, or to both. If this theory is correct, a treatment that decreases phosphate intake (milk and dicalcium phosphate tablets are high in phosphate) and increases the intake of calcium in a nonphosphate form (calcium lactate) might be therapeutic. Immediate relief of the symptoms may be obtained by massaging the calf muscles gently and attempting to flex the foot passively.

Abdominal Pain

Abdominal pain may be due to a significant pathologic condition in the abdomen and must always be considered a serious complaint. This is especially true during pregnancy, when the diagnosis of abdominal disease is unusually difficult. Abdominal pain, however, is not always of serious import. Common causes of benign pain include painful contractions of the uterus, especially during the third trimester (Braxton Hicks contractions), and round-ligament tension.

Tingling of Extremities

Some pregnant patients complain of a "pins-and-needles" sensation of the hands or feet, "as if the circulation is shut off." This complaint frequently persists and is resistant to treatment. The etiology is unknown, but the symptom is apparently not a serious one. Reassurance is usually adequate to satisfy the patient.

HABITS

Drugs

A large number of drugs are suspected of exerting a teratogenic effect during pregnancy. Although few of these relationships have been established with certainty, it is clear that a physician should prescribe a drug during early pregnancy only if there is a compelling reason for its use. Equal care with the prescription of drugs should be exercised during the last half of the menstrual cycle, when a woman might be pregnant. Tables 3-3, 3-4, and 3-5 list drugs known or suspected of teratogenicity with recommendation for use or nonuse. Special care should be taken with these medications.

Travel

Travel during pregnancy used to be interdicted by physicians, but this no longer seems reasonable, since no adverse effect of automobile, train, or plane travel on pregnancy has been established. There are reasons for restricting travel under certain circumstances. A patient with vaginal bleeding or cramping during early pregnancy should not travel simply because she might abort away from home. Travel late in pregnancy is uncomfortable,

Table 3-3. Risk Outweighs Benefits
in the First Trimester

Drug	Effects Reported
Thalidomide	Limb, auricle, eye, and visceral malformations
Serotonin	Increase of anomalies
Phenmetrazine	Skeletal and visceral malformations
Tolbutamide	Increase of anomalies
Chlorpropamide	Increase of anomalies
Streptomycin	Eighth nerve damage, micromelia, multiple skeletal anomalies
Tetracycline	Inhibition of bone growth, micromelia, syndactyly, discoloration of teeth
Iodide	Congenital goiter, hypothyroidism, mental retardation
Chloroquine	Retinal damage, eighth nerve damage
Methotrexate (for psoriasis)	Multiple anomalies
Meclizine	Multiple anomalies
LSD	Chromosomal abnormalities, increase of anomalies
Amphetamines	Transposition of great vessels, cleft palate
Trimethadione	Multiple anomalies
Paramethadione	Multiple anomalies
Diphenylhydantoin	Multiple anomalies
Sex steroids	VACTERL syndrome
Diethylstilbestrol	Clear cell adenocarcinoma of vagina and cervix, genital tract anomalies
Ethanol	Fetal alcohol syndrome
Bishydroxycoumarin	Skeletal and facial anomalies, mental retardation
Sodium warfarin	Skeletal and facial anomalies, mental retardation
Podophyllin (in laxatives)	Multiple anomalies
Acetazolamide	Limb defects

Source: F. Howard, and J. Hill. Drugs in pregnancy. *Obstet Gynecol Surv* 34:643, 1979.

Table 3-4. Risk Versus Benefits
Uncertain in the First Trimester

Drug	Effects Reported
Gentamicin	Eighth nerve damage
Kanamycin	Eighth nerve damage
Lithium	Goiter, eye anomalies
Benzodiazepines	Cardiac defects
Thiouracil	Goiter, hypothyroidism, mental retardation
Propylthiouracil	Goiter, hypothyroidism, mental retardation
Barbiturates	Increase of anomalies
Cannabis	Increase of anomalies
Quinine	Increase of anomalies
Septra or Bactrim	Cleft palate
Diazoxide	Increase of anomalies
Cytotoxic drugs	Increase of anomalies
Pyrimethamine	Increase of anomalies
Metronidazole	None
EDTA	Increase of anomalies
Atromid S	None

Source: F. Howard and J. Hill. Drugs in pregnancy. *Obstet Gynecol Surv* 34:643, 1979.

Table 3-5. Benefit Outweighs Risk
in the First Trimester

Drug	Effects Reported
Clomiphene	Increase of anomalies, neural tube effects, Down's syndrome
Glucocorticoids	Cleft palate, cardiac defects
General anesthesia	Increase of anomalies
Tricyclic antidepressants	CNS and limb malformations
Haloperidol	Limb malformations
Sulfonamides	Cleft palate, facial and skeletal defects
Rifampin	Spina bifida, cleft palate
Idoxuridine	Increase of anomalies
Antacids	Increase of anomalies
Hydralazine	Increase of anomalies
Monoamine oxidase inhibitors	None
Salicylates	CNS, visceral and skeletal malformations
Acetaminophen	None
Heparin	None
Isoproterenol	None
Terbutaline	None
Theophylline	None
Phenothiazines	None
Bendectin	None
Antihistamines	None
Insulin	Skeletal malformations
Penicillins	None
Chloramphenicol	None
Isoniazid	Increase of anomalies
Imipramine	CNS and limb anomalies
D-Penicillamine	Connective tissue defect

Source: F. Howard and J. Hill. Drugs in Pregnancy. *Obstet Gynecol Surv* 34:643, 1979.

and long trips should be discouraged for this reason alone.

Employment

Pregnant patients should be encouraged to continue their employment under most circumstances. Some jobs demand excessive physical activity, and the pregnant patient may simply not feel up to it. Excessive fatigue may adversely affect the uteroplacental circulation. In the final analysis, the decision of the woman regarding work during pregnancy should be supported.

Clothing

Loose-fitting, conventional clothing will be sufficient for most pregnant women during early gestation. Later, it will be necessary in many instances to purchase special maternity garments for comfort. A maternity girdle is useful in many patients, since it provides support for the unstable pregnant pelvis. Panty girdles or garters to hold up the stockings should be avoided, since edema will be exaggerated.

Smoking

An increase in the incidence of low-birth-weight infants and an increase in the perinatal mortality rate has been reported by many investigators [7]. The effects are dose-related. Certain maternal complications also occur with greater frequency in smokers (abruptio placentae, placenta previa). Certainly pregnant women should be encouraged not to smoke. If smoking is continued, the number of cigarettes per day should be sharply curtailed.

Alcohol Ingestion

Alcohol readily crosses the placenta and in some patients alcohol ingestion is now known to result in certain features in the neonate that have come to be known as the "fetal alcohol syndrome" [8]. The major features of the syndrome are prenatal and postnatal growth retardation, mental deficiency, small head size, and minor anomalies of the face, eyes, heart, joints, and external genitalia. The fetus is apparently susceptible to the syndrome throughout the major part of gestation. A large alcoholic intake also exerts a deleterious effect through poor maternal nutrition. An infant born of a chronic alcoholic mother may experience withdrawal symptoms during the perinatal period.

Sexual Activity

Interdiction of intercourse during the last month of pregnancy has long been prescribed by physicians. The danger envisaged by the physicians was an increased risk of infection and of premature labor. Recent studies have shown the infrequency with which these effects occur, and it is no longer common for physicians to interdict coitus. Orgasm may be hazardous late in pregnancy in patients who have previously experienced premature labor according to one group of investigators, who feel that they have been able to induce labor in an occasional patient at term by self-induced orgasm [9]. There is evidence that orgasm causes the uterus to contract. Interdiction of coitus should probably be limited to the occasional patient who has previously given birth to a premature infant and to the patient with ruptured membranes.

Bathing

The major hazard of bathing during pregnancy is that the patient may be injured by slipping and falling in the bathtub or shower. It has been shown that bathwater does not enter the vagina, so that the concern about bathing causing infection no longer seems justified.

Douching

Fatal air embolism from douching has been reported during pregnancy. To minimize this risk, the patient should introduce the douche tip no more than an inch into the vagina and allow the liquid to run freely from the vagina without holding the labia closed.

Care of the Teeth

Essential dental work may be performed during pregnancy without restriction. Only local anesthesia should be used unless an expert anesthesiologist administers an indicated general anesthetic, thus assuring adequate oxygenation. The effects of intrauterine hypoxia, which may result from general anesthesia, may be damaging to the fetus.

IMMUNIZATION

Immunization with live virus should be avoided in pregnant women unless there is a disease epidemic or other compelling reason for the inoculation. Immunization with the dead poliomyelitis virus, however, is recommended, since poliomyelitis is more severe in the pregnant than in the nonpregnant patient. Rubella vaccine should be avoided during pregnancy, since the effects on the fetus are unknown.

High-Risk Pregnancy

With the recognition that a high percentage of bad pregnancy outcomes occur in a small percentage of gravida, the concept of a high-risk pregnancy was introduced into clinical medicine. Identification of the gravida at high risk permits intensive monitoring of her pregnancy, both during the prenatal course and during labor. The patient at low risk can receive more routine care, unless an event of pregnancy or labor changes her status to high risk. The problem thus becomes one of recognition of the high-risk patient. Several ways of detecting such patients have been proposed.

Table 3-6. Identification of High-Risk Gravida: Prenatal Factors

Risk Factor	Score[a]	Risk Factor	Score[a]
I. *Cardiovascular and renal*		8. Infant > 10 pounds	5
1. Moderate to severe toxemia	10	9. Multiparity > 5	5
2. Chronic hypertension	10	10. Epilepsy	5
3. Moderate to severe renal disease	10	11. Fetal anomalies	1
4. Severe heart disease, Class II–IV	10	IV. *Anatomic abnormalities*	
5. History of eclampsia	5	1. Uterine malformation	10
6. History of pyelitis	5	2. Incompetent cervix	10
7. Class I heart disease	5	3. Abnormal fetal position	10
8. Mild toxemia	5	4. Polyhydramnios	10
9. Acute pyelonephritis	5	5. Small pelvis	5
10. History of cystitis	1		
11. Acute cystitis	1	V. *Miscellaneous*	
12. History of toxemia	1	1. Abnormal cervical cytology	10
		2. Multiple pregnancy	10
II. *Metabolic*		3. Sickle cell disease	10
1. Diabetes ≥ Class A-II	10	4. Age ≥ 35 or ≤ 15	5
2. Previous endocrine ablation	10	5. Viral disease	5
3. Thyroid disease	5	6. Rh sensitization only	5
4. Prediabetes (A-I)	5	7. Positive serology	5
5. Family history of diabetes	1	8. Severe anemia (< 9 gm. Hgb)	5
		9. Excessive use of drugs	5
III. *Previous histories*		10. History of TB or PPD ≥ 10 mm.	5
1. Previous fetal exchange transfusion for Rh	10	11. Weight < 100 or > 200 pounds	5
2. Previous stillbirth	10	12. Pulmonary disease	5
3. Post-term > 42 weeks	10	13. Flu syndrome (severe)	5
4. Previous premature infant	10	14. Vaginal spotting	5
5. Previous neonatal death	10	15. Mild anemia (9–10.9 gm. Hgb)	1
6. Previous cesarean section	5	16. Smoking ≥ 1 pack per day	1
7. Habitual abortion	5	17. Alcohol (moderate)	1
		18. Emotional problem	1

[a]Score greater than 20 identifies a patient in a high-risk category. Scores are additive.
Source: Modified from C. Hobel, M. Hyvarinen, D. Okada, and W. Oh. Prenatal and intrapartum high risk screening. I. Prediction of the high risk neonate. *Am J Obstet Gynecol* 117:1, 1973.

RISK FACTORS

Certain factors seem of extreme importance in assessing the risks of a poor pregnancy outcome. A maternal age below 15 or over 35, for example, is known to be associated frequently with perinatal death. Other important factors that can be recognized during prenatal care include a poor reproductive history (previous abortion, premature labor, fetal death, neonatal death, congenital anomaly), concurrent disease (e.g., diabetes mellitus, chronic hypertensive vascular disease, heart disease), generative tract disorders (uterine malformation, small pelvis), and miscellaneous factors. During labor, the presence of premature rupture of the membranes, placenta previa, premature separation, or the development of toxemia, uterine dysfunction, abnormal presentation, prolapse of the umbilical cord, or a number of other events warrants management of a gravida as a high-risk patient. Hobel et al. [10] published a system of iden-

Table 3-7. Identification of High-Risk Gravida: Intrapartum Factors

Risk Factor	Score[a]	Risk Factor	Score[a]
I. *Maternal factors*		3. Post-term > 42 weeks	10
1. Moderate–severe toxemia	10	4. Meconium stained amniotic fluid (dark)	10
2. Hydramnios or oligohydramnios	10	5. Meconium stained amniotic fluid (light)	5
3. Amnionitis	10	6. Marginal separation	1
4. Uterine rupture	10		
5. Mild toxemia	5		
6. Premature rupture of membrane > 12 hr.	5	III. *Fetal factors*	
7. Primary dysfunctional labor	5	1. Abnormal presentation	10
8. Secondary arrest of dilation	5	2. Multiple pregnancy	10
9. Demerol > 300 mg.	5	3. Fetal bradycardia > 30 minutes	10
10. MgSO$_4$ > 25 gm.	5	4. Breech delivery total extraction	10
11. Labor > 20 hours	5	5. Prolapsed cord	10
12. Second stage > 2½ hours	5	6. Fetal weight < 2500 gm.	10
13. Clinical small pelvis	5	7. Fetal acidosis pH ≤ 7.25 (Stage I)	10
14. Medical induction	5	8. Fetal tachycardia > 30 minutes	10
15. Precipitous labor < 3 hours	5	9. Operative forceps or vacuum extraction	5
16. Primary cesarean section	5	10. Breech delivery, spontaneous or assisted	5
17. Repeat cesarean section	5	11. General anesthesia	5
18. Elective induction	1	12. Outlet forceps	1
19. Prolonged latent phase	1	13. Shoulder dystocia	1
20. Uterine tetany	1		
21. Pitocin augmentation	1		
II. *Placental factors*			
1. Placenta previa	10		
2. Abruptio placentae	10		

[a]Score greater than 20 identifies a patient in a high-risk category. Scores are additive.
Source: Modified from C. Hobel, M. Hyvarinen, D. Okada, and W. Oh. Prenatal and intrapartum high risk screening. I. Prediction of the high risk neonate. *Am J Obstet Gynecol* 117:1, 1973.

tifying such patients and the screening factors suggested by Hobel are listed in Tables 3-6 and 3-7. In 1974, at the time of initial publication of this system, a score of 10 or greater effectively identified a high-risk population shown to be at risk of perinatal morbidity and mortality. The highest perinatal mortality occurred in patients identified as high risk at both prenatal and antepartum assessments (145 per 1000 compared with 3 per 7000 in the low-risk category). A recent reassessment of this tool for identifying high-risk gravida has shown that changes in obstetrical practice have necessitated a revision in the cut-off score [11]. Severe preeclampsia, for example, was a good predictor in 1977.

Improved medical management of the disease, improved neonatal care, and the more frequent utilization of cesarean section probably account for this difference. Similar examples could be cited. Hobel [11] currently recommends that the list of factors should remain unchanged, but that the score identifying a high-risk gravida should now be established at 20 or greater.

MONITORING
The tools for monitoring the pregnancy of the high-risk gravida are described in detail in Chapters 9 and 12. Prenatal monitoring includes an initial history and physical examination, an assessment of

high risk factors as described on page 68, subsequent historical information and reevaluation of high risk factors, and appropriate examination of the gravida. A decrease in fetal movement or a suspicion of intrauterine growth retardation or other abnormality at any antenatal visit demands further assessment of the fetus (e.g., estriol determination, nonstress test, oxytocin challenge test, serum level of human placental lactogen). Assessment of fetal age or maturity (e.g., ultrasonography for fetal size, amniocentesis for lecithin/sphingomyelin ratio) and identification of a fetal abnormality or abnormal presentation (ultrasound is usually the best laboratory tool) may be needed. Intrapartum evaluation will include continuous fetal heart rate monitoring, fetal scalp blood sampling, and other tools. The obstetrician may seek consultation with physicians with appropriate expertise to improve the care of the patient. A neonatologist in particular should be consulted regularly during prenatal care and labor to insure continuous care of the fetus and neonate.

References

1. Niswander, K. Should pregnant patients gain more weight? *Postgrad Med* 48:133, 1970.
2. Chase, H. *International Comparison of Prenatal and Infant Mortality: United States and Six Western European Countries.* U.S. Public Health Service Publication No. 1000, Series 3, No. 6. Washington, D.C.: U.S. Government Printing Office, 1967. P. 63.
3. Winick, M. Cellular changes during placental and fetal growth. *Am J Obstet Gynecol* 109:166, 1971.
4. Eastman, N., and Jackson, E. Weight relationships in pregnancy. I. The bearing of maternal weight gain and prepregnancy weight on birth weight in full term pregnancies. *Obstet Gynecol Surv* 23:1003, 1968.
5. Chesley, L. Weight changes and water balance in normal and toxic pregnancy. *Am J Obstet Gynecol* 48:565, 1944.
6. Maternal Nutrition and the Course of Pregnancy. Washington, D.C.: National Academy of Science, 1970.
7. ACOG Technical Bulletin #53, September, 1979.
8. Mulvihill, J., and Yeager, A. Fetal alcohol syndrome. *Teratology* 13:345, 1976.
9. Goodlin, R., Schmidt, W., and Creevy, D. Uterine tension and fetal heart rate during maternal orgasm. *Obstet Gynecol* 39:125, 1972.
10. Hobel, C., Hyvarinen, M., Okada, D., and Oh, W. Prenatal and intrapartum high risk screening. I. Prediction of the high risk neonate. *Am J Obstet Gynecol* 117:1, 1974.
11. Hobel, C. Personal communication, 1980.

Additional Readings

Guilbeau, J., and Turner, J. The effect of travel on interruption of pregnancy: An analysis of 1917 cases with minimum journeys of 300 miles. *Am J Obstet Gynecol* 66:1224, 1953.

Osofsky, H. Relationships between nutrition during pregnancy and subsequent infant and child development. *Obstet Gynecol Surv* 30:227, 1975.

Pugh, W., and Fernandez, F. Coitus in late pregnancy. *Obstet Gynecol* 2:636, 1953.

Whalley, P., Scott, D., and Pritchard, J. Maternal folate deficiency and pregnancy wastage. I. Placental abruption. *Am J Obstet Gynecol* 105:670, 1969.

Howard, F., and Hill, J. Drugs in pregnancy. *Obstet Gynecol Surv* 34:643, 1979.

4

Medical and Surgical Complications of Pregnancy

Virtually any disease can occur during pregnancy, although disease states with higher incidence in the very young or the old are, of course, less likely to occur during the reproductive years. The physiologic changes in pregnancy frequently alter the signs and symptoms of a disease, thus complicating the diagnostic and therapeutic problems encountered. Understanding these changes is of equal importance to the obstetrician caring for the pregnant patient and to the consultant who must monitor the disease during pregnancy. The presence of a fetus must also be considered in the choice of therapy during pregnancy, and the effects of drugs or other therapeutic regimens on the fetus as well as on the mother must be kept in mind. For these reasons, this chapter will emphasize the relationship between pregnancy and intercurrent disease. How do pregnancy changes affect the diagnostic plan for a disease? What is the effect of the disease on the mother and on the fetus? Do the anatomic and physiologic changes inherent in pregnancy adversely affect the disease? Are the drugs or other treatments usually prescribed for the disease appropriate during pregnancy?

Another problem may arise when pregnancy occurs in a patient already known to have a particular disease. If pregnancy is expected to affect the patient's disease adversely, should the pregnancy be terminated? Or, even more basically, should the patient with a particular disease be advised against becoming pregnant at all? Will the disease of the mother or potential mother be transmitted genetically to the baby? If so, can the disease in the fetus be recognized early enough to permit the choice of abortion if this solution is desired?

When information is available, we will attempt to answer these questions for the diseases commonly encountered during pregnancy.

Diseases of the Cardiovascular System

HEART DISEASE

Heart disease during pregnancy continues to be a major cause of maternal mortality. It occurs in about 1 percent of pregnant patients and in most instances is of rheumatic origin [1]. An increasingly greater percentage of pregnant cardiac patients have congenital heart disease, since the life of such patients can now be successfully prolonged into the childbearing years with surgical therapy. The remaining few cases include hypertensive cardiovascular disease, coronary artery disease, the heart disease of thyrotoxicosis, syphilitic heart disease, primary myocardial disease, and a number of other rare conditions. If the disease is recognized early in pregnancy, and if the patient is well managed, the risk of maternal mortality should be increasingly remote.

Diagnosis

The diagnosis of heart disease is complicated by certain physiologic changes of normal pregnancy. An apical or a pulmonic systolic murmur is heard in many, if not most, pregnant patients. While these functional murmurs, due to such factors as the increased blood volume of pregnancy, must not lead the physician to overdiagnosis, an intensity greater than grade 2/4 demands that organic disease must be seriously considered. It is sometimes difficult to determine whether the movement of the cardiac apex to the left on physical examination signals cardiac enlargement or merely a physiologic change of pregnancy due to elevation of the heart. The differentiation is important, since true cardiac enlargement must be considered a definite sign of heart disease. The changes in respiratory function described in Chapter 2 frequently cause respiratory symptoms (including dyspnea) suggestive of cardiopulmonary disease when in fact no decrease in pulmonary function can be measured. Similarly, edema of the lower extremities, another sign of cardiac failure, is nearly universal among pregnant patients.

Pregnancy may cause the patient to seek medical advice for the first time in many years, and the obstetrician may be able to recognize a disease of the heart not previously suspected by the patient. However, care to avoid overdiagnosis in a patient suspected of having heart disease is of great psychological importance. When the diagnosis is seriously in doubt, the woman should be treated as a cardiac patient during pregnancy, reserving definitive evaluation for the postpartum period. However, a noninvasive approach by electrocardiography now allows diagnosis during pregnancy, especially in patients with cardiac valvular abnormalities. As with most medical diseases encountered during pregnancy, appropriate consultation should be sought.

The diagnosis of valvular heart disease rests on the recognition of a diastolic murmur and some degree of cardiac enlargement. Systolic murmurs usually are to be considered normal during pregnancy, although a loud murmur is likely to be due to a pathologic condition of the heart. Congenital heart disease is suggested by a loud ventricular systolic murmur with an associated thrill along the left sternal border (ventricular septal defect) or by a continuous murmur at the base of the heart (patent ductus arteriosus). Less common congenital lesions may produce other murmurs and may or may not be associated with cyanosis. Burwell and Metcalfe [2] have suggested certain criteria, any one of which will confirm the diagnosis of heart disease: (1) a diastolic or continuous heart murmur, (2) definite cardiac enlargement, (3) a loud systolic murmur associated with a thrill, or (4) a severe arrhythmia. In the absence of any of these criteria, the diagnosis is best delayed until the postpartum period. An abnormal ECG is also helpful in confirming the diagnosis.

Classification of Patients for Prognosis and Management

The classification proposed by the New York Heart Association for estimating the functional capacity of a patient with cardiac disease is in wide use. While certain important factors—the presence of serious cardiac arrhythmias, a recent history of acute rheumatic fever, and the effects of concurrent medical disease—are not included in the classification, it provides the best means available of dividing patients into functional categories for management recommendations.

FUNCTIONAL CLASSIFICATION.

Class I: Cardiac patients with no limitation of physical activity. No symptoms of cardiac insufficiency or angina are experienced at any time.

Class II: Cardiac patients with slight limitation of activity. More than ordinary physical activity causes fatigue, palpitation, dyspnea, or anginal pain not experienced when at rest.

Class III: Cardiac patients with marked limitation of activity. While asymptomatic at rest, ordinary physical activity provokes the symptoms of fatigue, palpitation, dyspnea, or anginal pain.

Class IV: Cardiac patients unable to perform any physical activity without discomfort. Symptoms of cardiac unsufficiency may even occur at rest.

THERAPEUTIC CLASSIFICATION.

A. The patient needs no restriction.

B. The patient is restricted to ordinary activity only.

C. The patient is restricted to milder ordinary activity.

D. The patient is restricted to complete rest.

Cardiac Decompensation

The appearance of cardiac decompensation during pregnancy greatly worsens the prognosis for both mother and baby. Measurements of cardiac output and plasma volume during pregnancy made earlier suggested that a peak risk of cardiac failure might be expected at about seven months' gestation, but these physiologic measurements are now known to have been wrong. The cardiac output increases during early pregnancy and then maintains this elevation at a more or less stable level through the remainder of pregnancy. The plasma volume increases to a maximum at about 34 weeks, although it may increase more slowly until term. The risk of cardiac failure thus persists. Certainly, there is no decrease in plasma volume during late pregnancy as reported by earlier investigators. Cardiac decompensation must be guarded against *throughout pregnancy,* especially in the postpartum period, when the contracted uterus expels its blood into the general circulation. Cardiac failure during labor is surprisingly infrequent.

Treatment

Treatment of heart disease in pregnancy is based primarily on the following guidelines: (1) prevention of cardiac decompensation if at all possible, (2) vigorous treatment of decompensation should it occur, and (3) never allowing a successfully treated decompensated patient to go home from the hospital before delivery.

Patients in Functional Classes I and II may be treated on an ambulatory basis throughout most of pregnancy. Their condition should be carefully monitored with visits every two weeks or weekly both to the obstetrician and to the cardiologist, since incipient heart failure must be recognized early. Although few of these patients will decompensate, the seriousness of the exception to this rule justifies a vigilant attitude toward all patients. Prevention of decompensation is accomplished in a number of ways: (1) First and foremost, the patient should be given specific directions about permitted activity. She may do light housework unless she tires, but climbing stairs or engaging in other vigorous activities (e.g., shopping) should be avoided. She should have at least 8 to 9 hours of sleep nightly, and she should rest in bed for an hour after each meal. (2) She should carefully avoid exposure to anyone with an infection, since even an upper respiratory infection may induce respiratory embarrassment and produce stress on the cardiovas-

cular system. (3) Weight gain and excessive fluid retention should be controlled with careful diet, including a low salt intake. Excess weight may tip the scales toward cardiac decompensation. (4) The iron stores should be maintained with exogenous iron medication. Frequent blood counts should be done to rule out anemia, which might cause a compensatory increase in cardiac output; this in turn might precipitate cardiac failure.

Minor signs or symptoms of early decompensation include basilar chest rales that do not disappear with coughing, exertional dyspnea, orthopnea, hemoptysis, persistent cough, or progressive edema. While cardiac failure may occur suddenly and without apparent warning, the presence of one or more of these signs or symptoms allows early recognition of incipient failure in some patients. The vital capacity of the lungs normally increases during pregnancy, and measurement of the vital capacity at each office visit may predict incipient heart failure.

Patients with Class III heart disease or those with a history of previous decompensation should be warned of the hazard of pregnancy, so that pregnancy can be avoided if the patient chooses this course of action. Should she inadvertently become pregnant, therapeutic abortion should be considered. If she chooses to take the risk of pregnancy, she must be put on bed rest immediately and expect to spend many days in the hospital during the remainder of pregnancy. An increase in overt heart failure occurs in about one-third of these patients; this is a complication that demands immediate hospitalization. Stress is placed on early recognition of increased heart failure if it cannot be avoided altogether. Some physicians insist on continuous hospitalization of Class III patients throughout pregnancy, regardless of the degree of heart failure. This course of action is undoubtedly wise, but convincing the patient of this fact is often difficult. Acute toxemia of pregnancy is a particularly hazardous complication in a cardiac patient.

Initial hospital treatment of acute cardiac failure with pulmonary congestion or edema includes strict bed rest, oxygen, morphine sulfate, parenteral diuretics, and frequently digitalis. Continuing management includes continuing hospitalization, sodium restriction, diuretic therapy, and digitalis. Although recovery to a cardiac compensated state may take a few days and may require maintenance diuretic and digitalis therapy, most patients will respond well to treatment. The temptation to allow the patient to return home following her recovery should be vigorously resisted, since decompensation will usually recur on home treatment.

Regardless of her heart status, a cardiac patient should be admitted to the hospital at least a week before labor is expected. Spontaneous onset of labor should be awaited; labor should not be induced. Cardiac status should be reevaluated at this time to detect any deterioration that may have accompanied the changes of late pregnancy. Vaginal delivery should be anticipated, although the second stage of labor should be abbreviated to reduce the vigorous work of bearing-down efforts. Cesarean section is associated with a higher morbidity and mortality and should be utilized for obstetric indications only. Sedation during labor should be used in moderate doses to ally the patient's apprehension. While continuous epidural analgesia gives excellent and desirable pain relief, the hazards of a hypotensive episode following its use should be recalled. Hypotension in the gravid patient may decrease or even terminate uterine blood flow, and in patients with cardiac shunts due to congenital lesions, hypotension may allow a right-to-left shunt of blood, with a fatal outcome.

Should cardiac failure occur during labor, treatment is directed toward the heart disease (e.g., digitalis, oxygen) rather than toward a traumatic operative delivery. A hasty or unwise obstetrical maneuver will aggravate the heart failure and should be avoided unless there is a strong obstetrical indication for it. If the cervix is fully dilated, a rapid vaginal delivery is usually wise to avoid the exertion of maternal pushing in the second stage of labor. Incomplete cervical dilatation, however, should contraindicate a vaginal delivery in the heart disease patient just as in patients without medical complications. Cesarean section is performed for obstetri-

cal indication, not because the heart disease is severe.

The puerperium is also a time of hazard for the cardiac patient because the blood from the contracted uterus is returned to the general systemic circulation at this time, and the mobilized interstitial fluid from body tissues also enters the systemic circulation. The same meticulous observation of the patient's vital signs (blood pressure, pulse, respirations, skin color) exercised during labor should be continued for at least the first two postpartum days. In patients with cardiac lesions predisposing to infective endocarditis, antibiotic medication is mandatory during the puerperium, as it is during labor. If the patient's condition warrants it, there is no reason why she should not nurse if she so desires.

The treatment of Class IV patients is almost identical to that given patients with cardiac failure in any class, i.e., continuous hospitalization with a cardiotonic regimen. Whether or not therapeutic abortion should be offered to such a patient is uncertain, since the abortion itself may prove as much of a strain as continuation of the pregnancy, especially if the pregnancy is too far advanced to warrant the suction abortion technique.

Therapeutic Abortion in Cardiac Patients

The decision regarding therapeutic abortion in a cardiac patient should be primarily the patient's, and the obstetrician and the cardiologist should supply to the patient and her family all the pertinent information on which the decision should be based. Factors to be considered include not only the immediate risk of pregnancy to the patient but also the ultimate energy cost to her generated by the care of the child following delivery. She should be informed of the emotional and financial cost engendered by the long hospitalization that may be required during pregnancy, as well as the increased risk of early death that her condition entails. The likelihood that life expectancy is not adversely affected by a successful abortion is another factor she may wish to consider. In the final analysis, she will probably base her decision on the effect the pregnancy will have on her husband and on her other children, if any, as well as on the strength of her desire to have the baby. While the physician can evaluate the medical risks involved, the social and emotional factors are so private and so unique in a particular patient that he should not seek to impose his opinion too vigorously.

If termination of pregnancy is selected, the simplest procedure available should be chosen. For a gestation of less than twelve weeks, suction curettage is usually best, followed by an abdominal tubal ligation if the patient desires it and if her condition warrants it. Abortion by hypertonic saline solution may be hazardous because of sodium overloading of the circulation. Abortion by intra-amniotic prostaglandin is safer. Abdominal hysterotomy carries with it a substantially greater risk than suction abortion and is rarely necessary. Prophylactic antibiotics to minimize the risk of infective endocarditis are essential at the time of surgery.

Fetal and Neonatal Outcome

With most cardiac disease in pregnancy, even when successfully treated cardiac failure supervenes, the perinatal mortality rate is only slightly increased, with the increase due primarily to the effects of prematurity. There is also evidence that the child is unlikely to suffer any brain damage from the potential intrauterine hypoxia to which he may have been subjected [3]. An exception to this rule occurs with severe cyanotic congenital heart disease. The fetal outcome can be predicted by observing the level of the compensatory polycythemia that develops in the mother as a result of hypoxia. If the cardiac disease is of sufficient severity to increase the patient's hematocrit to above 60 vol%, there is an increased risk of abortion, intrauterine growth retardation, premature labor, and perinatal death. With a hematocrit below 60 vol%, the fetal risk is apparently not increased.

Surgical Repair

Whether to perform cardiac surgery during pregnancy, to interrupt the pregnancy and perform the needed surgery after termination, or to treat severe cardiac disease with intensive medical treatment and allow continuation of the pregnancy remains a therapeutic dilemma. In the final analysis, the decision will probably depend on the experience of the particular medical team caring for the patient. While good results have been reported following mitral valvulotomy during pregnancy, postoperative death remains a possibility, and some have suggested that intensive medical management will accomplish the same results. Of major concern if heart surgery is to be performed during pregnancy is the effect of potential hypoxia on the fetus. Hypoxia at a critical time in fetal development (usually during the first trimester) may increase the risk of a congenital malformation. Another therapeutic problem complicating cardiac surgery is the need for anticoagulant therapy in patients receiving prosthetic valve replacement and the effect of this therapy on the fetus. Dicumarol crosses the placental barrier with ease and may cause a severe hemorrhagic diathesis in the fetus. Since heparin does not cross the placenta with ease, it should be used in preference to dicumarol in pregnant patients. The drug should be discontinued for delivery, and bleeding complications in the mother can be treated with protamine sulfate. Either heparin or dicumarol can be used in the postpartum patient, with due care to avoid bleeding.

Treatment in Congenital Heart Disease

Congenital heart disease is seen with increasing frequency during pregnancy as earlier surgical repair has allowed the patient to reach childbearing age. *Patent ductus arteriosus* poses few problems if it has been surgically closed previously; if still patent, it may be closed during pregnancy to prevent a possible right-to-left shunt from a hypotensive episode from whatever cause, especially conduction anesthesia. *Coarctation of the aorta*, while rare, poses a serious problem during pregnancy. Heart failure, infective endocarditis, and even rupture of the aorta above the point of obstruction are all possibilities. The fetal outcome in various *cyanotic congenital heart diseases* will depend primarily on the level of the compensatory hematocrit reading, as mentioned, while the major maternal danger is the development of a right-to-left shunt in a patient with a previous left-to-right shunt. Therapeutic abortion may well be considered in these patients.

Antibiotic Medication

Prophylactic treatment with an appropriate antibiotic (usually penicillin or ampicillin) should be prescribed at the time of labor and delivery for any patient with a valvular or congenital cardiac lesion, no matter how mild. Infective endocarditis is a common problem at this time and should be prevented. The treatment of endocarditis during pregnancy is the same as in the nonpregnant patient, i.e., a careful blood culture, followed by treatment with an appropriate antibiotic in large doses. Treatment is usually entirely successful.

Treatment in Postpartal Cardiomyopathy

Postpartal cardiomyopathy is a term that describes a syndrome occurring between the second and twentieth week postpartum. The signs and symptoms are those of congestive heart failure. The etiology remains obscure, but a virus or antimyocardial antibodies of fetal origin have been suggested as possibilities. Treatment must be initiated early and includes complete bed rest. Subsequent pregnancies may cause an exacerbation of the disease. Even with intensive care, the mortality is 15 to 50 percent [4].

ARTERIAL DISEASE

Raynaud's disease, characterized by attacks of peripheral cyanosis, especially of the fingers, is not aggravated by pregnancy and, in fact, may be improved by it. The patient should not receive ergot medication to induce uterine contractility after delivery because of the well-known arterial spasm induced by large doses of ergot, especially in the hypersensitive patient. Dissecting aneurysm of the aorta or splenic artery, while rare, seems to have a predilection for the pregnant patient. Death usually follows the typical cardiovascular collapse, which is most likely to occur in the third trimester, presumably because of the great increase in blood volume or changes in the aortic media. Some cases of dissecting aortic aneurysm have been reported with coarctation of the aorta. Intracranial vascular accidents, mostly due to aneurysm, are common and are discussed under Disorders of the Nervous System.

DISEASES OF THE VEINS

Varicose veins are frequently seen during pregnancy (see discussison in Chap. 3). Thrombophlebitis and pulmonary embolus are not usually seen during pregnancy and are discussed in Chapter 14, on the puerperium. If thrombophlebitis is recognized during pregnancy, heparin, not dicumarol, is the anticoagulant that should be prescribed, as previously noted. The occasional use of vena caval ligation to prevent recurrent emboli has been reported not to interfere with subsequent development of the pregnancy in spite of the massive placental separation experimentally produced by Mengert and coworkers [5] with vena caval obstruction at the time of repeat cesarean section.

Diseases of the Blood

ANEMIA

The frequency with which anemia will be diagnosed during pregnancy depends on the level of hemoglobin required for the diagnosis and the type of population treated. A reasonable cutoff point to justify the diagnosis of anemia is 10 gm. of hemoglobin per 100 ml. of blood, or a hematocrit of 34 vol%. These levels would be low if applied to a population of men or nonpregnant women, since the hemodilution of pregnancy causes a lower "normal" level. While the red cell mass expands in pregnancy, the plasma volume increases at a greater rate, thus producing a dilution of the red blood cell mass, especially in the middle trimester.

The incidence of anemia noted in a particular clinic will also depend on the racial background and socioeconomic level of the population served. Poor nutrition before pregnancy, noted especially in the lower socioeconomic groups of patients, may have decreased the iron stores to the point where the amount of iron available cannot keep up with the increased erythropoiesis of pregnancy. A high percentage of black patients in the clinic will result in a higher incidence of anemia, since sickle cell anemia is largely limited to the black race. Other socioeconomic or racial factors may similarly affect the frequency with which the diagnosis of anemia is made.

No attempt will be made to discuss all the types of anemia that may occur in the general population and thus in pregnant patients. The major anemias, for our purposes, may be classified according to whether they occur as a result of pregnancy or whether they simply occur in a pregnant woman. Among the anemias related causally to pregnancy are iron deficiency anemia and the megaloblastic anemia of pregnancy. The anemias that may occur during pregnancy include hereditary anemias (sickle cell anemia and related disorders), thalassemia, and acquired anemia (aplastic anemia).

Iron Deficiency Anemia

The amount of iron needed by the pregnant patient is about 800 mg.; 300 mg. goes to the fetus, and 500 mg. is necessary for the additional hemoglobin synthesis required for the normal and expected expansion of the maternal red cell mass. Since many patients enter pregnancy with inadequate body iron stores, iron deficiency anemia is a common predictable consequence if exogenous iron medication is not prescribed. For this reason, most authorities recommend iron medication throughout pregnancy [6]. The iron can be taken in the form of oral ferrous sulfate (300 mg. three times a day to supply 200 mg. of iron), or another oral preparation, or intramuscularly (iron-dextran). Since the oral preparations are as effective as the parenteral medication in restoring iron stores and correcting anemia, the parenteral iron should be used only if severe anemia is detected near term with insufficient time to correct the anemia before labor, or if the patient cannot tolerate oral iron or refuses to take it regularly. Periodic laboratory determinations should be made to assure that the anemia has improved, thus, in effect, confirming the correctness of the diagnosis of an iron deficiency cause. In addition to a rise in hemoglobin, the peripheral blood will contain new red blood cells that may be polychromatophilic or basophilic. A rise in the reticulocyte count can also be expected.

The diagnosis of iron deficiency anemia is frequently a matter of excluding other forms of anemia. In addition to lowered hemoglobin and hematocrit levels, the serum iron concentration in iron deficiency is usually low; and if the anemia is severe, erythrocytic hypochromia and microcytosis may be noted. Although usually not necessary for the diagnosis, a bone marrow smear will show hemosiderin in the absence of iron deficiency anemia. A peripheral blood smear may help to rule out aplastic anemia or megaloblastic anemia of pregnancy, and a sickle cell preparation should be made on all black patients. The presence of bilirubin in the serum, evidenced by a yellow color in the fluid above the packed cells in the hematocrit tube, will suggest a hemolytic process.

Treatment of iron deficiency anemia consists almost exclusively of iron medication. The therapy should be continued for six months beyond delivery to restore normal iron stores. The iron medication is primarily for maternal well-being, since the iron stores of the infant of even a severely anemic gravida will usually be normal. Blood transfusion to correct iron deficiency should be reserved for the patient whose anemia results from acute blood loss, not poor iron stores. In patients with severe long-standing anemia, hypervolemia and cardiac insufficiency may be induced by the anemia.

Megaloblastic Anemia of Pregnancy

Megaloblastic anemia is a rare complication of pregnancy in areas of the world with adequate nutrition. The disease is due to a deficiency of folic acid, which is almost always the result of a deficient intake of uncooked green, leafy vegetables and animal protein; occasionally it is due to deficient absorption or utilization of folic acid. The daily adult requirement for folic acid increases from a level of 50 to 100 μg. per day before pregnancy to 300 to 400 μg. per day in late pregnancy. The fetus effectively extracts folic acid from maternal blood (as it extracts iron), so that it is rarely anemic, even with severe folic acid deficiency and megaloblastic anemia in the mother.

The disease is usually detected in the third trimester of pregnancy, when maternal folic acid requirements are at their maximum. The anemia may be very severe, with a hemoglobin level of 3 to 5 gm. per 100 ml. not an uncommon finding. The patient will experience symptoms of anemia (e.g., easy fatigability), but these may be surprisingly mild. The diagnosis can be suspected when the peripheral blood contains hypersegmented polymorphonuclear white blood cells and macrocytic red blood cells. Peripheral megaloblasts may be seen. The diagnosis is confirmed by bone marrow biopsy, which will reveal the typical megaloblastic erythropoiesis. Thrombocytopenia and leukopenia are commonly noted with severe disease.

Prophylactic treatment of megaloblastic anemia of pregnancy should be part of prenatal care, since adequate nutrition can be expected to prevent the disease. Most authorities recommend routine supplementation of the pregnancy diet with 1 mg. of folic acid daily. While folic acid can mask an undiagnosed pernicious anemia due to a lack of vitamin B_{12}, the extreme rarity of this disease during pregnancy justifies prophylactic treatment of the much more likely folic acid–deficient state.

Treatment of megaloblastic anemia of pregnancy consists primarily of the administration of 1 mg. of folic acid daily and corrections in the patient's diet to eliminate the deficiency. Within a few days, a marked hematologic response can be expected, with a sharp increase in the reticulocyte count. Since iron deficiency is commonly associated with folic acid deficiency, supplemental iron should also be furnished to the patient. Between pregnancies, the patient should have careful dietary instructions to avoid a repetition of the disease in her next pregnancy.

Sickle Cell Disease

The normal person inherits a normal hemoglobin gene (A) from each of his parents and is characterized electrophoretically as having type A-A hemoglobin. A black child may inherit type A hemoglobin from one parent and type S (sickle cell) hemoglobin from the other; as a result, he will have sickle cell trait (S-A). This pattern is observed in

about 8 percent of American blacks and is not usually associated with anemia. If the child inherits S hemoglobin from both parents, he has sickle cell disease (S-S), a serious abnormality characterized by anemia and recurrent bouts of excruciating abdominal and joint pain (sickle cell crises). Sickle cell disease complicating pregnancy is a rare but very serious threat both to the mother and to the fetus. Also serious in the pregnant woman is S-C disease, which results from a combination of an S hemoglobin gene and a C hemoglobin gene; the homozygous C-C state (hemoglobin C disease) is usually much less severe and results only in a mild anemia. Hemoglobin C–thalassemia disease is usually equally mild; sickle cell–thalassemia disease, however, parallels sickle cell disease in severity.

The diagnosis of sickle cell trait is made by adding a drop of sodium metabisulfite to a drop of peripheral blood; if the trait is present, sickling will be demonstrated. A diagnosis of sickle cell disease requires hemoglobin electrophoresis. The fetal loss from abortion, fetal death, or neonatal death is said to approach 50 percent with S-S disease. Expert management has reduced maternal mortality to near zero, but the risk must be kept in mind constantly. The pregnancy is characterized by anemia, attacks of abdominal and bone pain when a hemolytic crisis occurs (probably related to obstruction of the microcirculation), and infections. The crises are said to be more likely to occur late in pregnancy, during labor, and during the puerperium. The treatment of the crisis continues to be a matter of some dispute. Some authorities prefer to transfuse such patients only when the hemoglobin drops below 7 gm. per 100 ml. Others feel that repeated small transfusions are of value. All agree that supplemental folic acid and probably iron should be prescribed throughout pregnancy, since the intense hematopoiesis requires them.

Delivery should be accomplished in the least traumatic fashion possible, and hypoxia should be avoided at all costs, since a sickling crisis may accompany the hypoxia. Cross-matched blood must be available before delivery to combat the effects of any excessive blood loss effectively and quickly. Postpartum sterilization should be encouraged in these patients because of the expected decrease in life span as well as the hazard of subsequent pregnancies. Oral contraception is probably contraindicated because of the increased risk of vascular occlusion.

Sickle cell–hemoglobin C disease and sickle cell–thalassemia disease are equally serious to the pregnant woman. The clinical picture in these diseases is similar to that of sickle cell disease, and similar therapies are prescribed. While these diseases are less common than sickle cell disease, their hazards must not be underestimated.

Thalassemia

The heterozygous form of thalassemia, thalassemia minor, is characterized by a hypochromic microcytic anemia. Differentiation from an iron deficiency anemia can be made by the presence of a normal serum iron and excessive amounts of bilirubin in the serum, suggesting a hemolytic process. The disease is congenital and occurs primarily in Mediterranean peoples, although it has been recognized in non-Mediterranean whites and blacks on occasion. The disease results from abnormalities in hemoglobins, and fetal hemoglobin and A-2 hemoglobin are found in increased amounts. The homozygous form of the disease (thalassemia major) results in a very severe anemia that is usually fatal during childhood. For this reason, only thalassemia minor is seen in patients of reproductive age.

The pregnancy outcome in patients with thalassemia minor is usually good. Iron and folic acid are prescribed during pregnancy. Transfusion is reserved for blood loss, since repeated blood transfusion may result in hemochromatosis. No medical therapy for the disease is available.

Aplastic Anemia = Acquired Anemia

While rare at any time and certainly during pregnancy, aplastic anemia has been reported to complicate pregnancy. In some cases, the anemia has antedated the pregnancy, while in others it has been reported to appear initially during pregnancy. Bleeding from the associated thrombocytopenia and infection constitute the major hazards of the disease. There is no known effective treatment,

although corticosteroids may provide some help, and transfused blood will prolong the life of the patient. A careful history and physical examination should be performed in an attempt to find an extrinsic cause (a drug?) or an intrinsic cause (hidden infection?) for the disease. Therapeutic abortion should be offered to the patient in the hope of improving the disease, although the effectiveness of this procedure is uncertain.

OTHER DISEASES OF THE BLOOD

Thrombocytopenic Purpura

Thrombocytopenic purpura may be idiopathic or secondary to a known cause (e.g., infection, allergy, radiation, drugs). Removal of the cause is essential as part of the treatment of the disease. The idiopathic variety is less frequent and is a rare complication of pregnancy. Modern treatment has lowered the perinatal mortality to about 20 percent and there is virtually no maternal mortality [7]. The cause of the idiopathic variety remains an intriguing problem. An isoagglutinin in the bloodstream of many patients has been identified by some investigators, while others find the antibody in only a small percentage of cases [8]. Transfer of the isoagglutinin to the fetus has been recognized in up to three-fourths of the newborns and has resulted in congenital thrombocytopenia. While the significance of the isoagglutinin is uncertain, the major cause of neonatal mortality is intracranial hemorrhage from purpura [9]. Bleeding from a circumcision can be avoided by delaying the procedure until the platelet count returns to normal.

Prednisone may be an effective agent in helping restore the platelet count toward normal, although not all investigators have recognized this effect. Careful delivery of the baby to avoid lacerations usually results in minimal bleeding during delivery. The fundus must be carefully massaged during the postpartum period to avoid postpartum bleeding. Transfusion of fresh platelets may be of use if bleeding ensues or if major surgery (cesarean section) is necessary. However, major surgery should be avoided if at all possible.

Leukemia

Chronic leukemia, especially myelogenous leukemia, is more likely to complicate pregnancy than is acute leukemia, but both forms of the disease in pregnancy are rare; it seems unlikely that pregnancy exerts an adverse effect on leukemia. The perinatal mortality in these cases, however, is high, due primarily to premature labor, which probably results from the debility of the mother. The chronic form of the disease carries a better fetal prognosis than does the acute form.

The diagnosis is usually an easy one to make. The choice of therapy is made largely without considering the pregnancy. Radiotherapy may be prescribed for the chronic form of the disease and is not contraindicated during pregnancy. The fetus should be shielded from the radiation by lead.

Antimetabolites (vincristine, mercaptopurine, methotrexate) have been given in the second and third trimesters without evident deleterious effect on the fetus, but their use should be avoided if possible during the first trimester. Prednisone may be of some value as a therapeutic agent. Careful avoidance of infection is mandatory in these patients. Labor should be awaited and vaginal delivery performed except when there are obstetrical indications for cesarean section.

Congenital leukemia in an infant born of a leukemic mother has not been reported. Congenital leukemia in the infants of nonleukemic mothers has, however, been reported. The meaning of these observations is uncertain.

Hodgkin's Disease

Hodgkin's disease is said to have no deleterious effect on a pregnancy. The presence of abdominal disease that must be treated during pregnancy, however, could make therapeutic abortion advisable in some patients. The mother's wishes regarding pregnancy interruption should be considered in any form of the disease. She may be concerned with factors other than the effect of the disease on the pregnancy. Treatment during pregnancy will usually be in the form of x-radiation, and this can be used safely if the fetus is shielded with lead. Blood transfusion may also be required. The ob-

servation that 10 percent of fetuses are afflicted with Hodgkin's disease transplacentally raises the question of a viral etiology of the disease. Labor and delivery are managed as in patients without the disease.

Diseases of the Respiratory System

Pregnancy changes in the respiratory system during normal pregnancy should be remembered when considering pulmonary disease. The rib cage flares, and both the transverse diameter of the chest and the substernal angle increase. Increased total and alveolar ventilation results in a lowering of blood carbon dioxide tension. Oxygen consumption is increased, especially in late pregnancy, but not as greatly as the increase in total ventilation. A slight reduction in airway resistance is seen during the third trimester of pregnancy. The overall effect is a well-sustained respiratory efficiency during pregnancy.

Acute Pulmonary Disease

BACTERIAL PNEUMONIA. The modern treatment of bacterial pneumonia has greatly minimized the seriousness of this disease both in nonpregnant and pregnant patients. The lessons of the past should not be forgotten, however, and the extremely high maternal and fetal risk should pneumonia be untreated must be kept in mind. Prompt diagnosis of the disease and immediate hospitalization of the pregnant patient for appropriate treatment are as important today as they ever were. The fetus withstands hypoxia poorly, the oxygen should be used without delay if respiratory embarrassment is detected in the mother. An increase in the risk of abortion, premature labor, and perinatal death can be expected if the mother is inadequately treated, or if the disease fails to respond to antibiotics.

VIRAL DISEASE. Viral disease of the lungs can also be devastating, as in the influenza epidemic of 1918, when maternal mortality was extremely high, largely as a result of complicating bacterial pneumonia. Although antibiotic agents are of no value in viral infection per se, they markedly reduce the risk of secondary bacterial invaders, and their use should be encouraged when the patient has severe chest involvement following a viral respiratory infection. Furthermore, during the 1957 epidemic of Asian influenza, pregnant women were at greater risk of dying than were nonpregnant women of similar age. Most of the deaths were the result of a complicating bacterial pneumonia, frequently by coagulase-positive staphylococci. Except when this complication occurs, the perinatal outcome in viral pulmonary disease should be good.

Chronic Pulmonary Disease

ASTHMA. Asthma is not uncommon during pregnancy, and the prevailing point of view is that pregnancy exerts no particularly deleterious effect on the disease. Our own experience suggests a less optimistic outlook, since 4 of our 277 patients with asthma complicating pregnancy died either during pregnancy or during the first postpartum year [10]. The effect of the disease on the fetal outcome was also evident, with a twofold increase in the perinatal mortality. Nor was the increased frequency with which the children of asthmatic mothers experienced a severe respiratory illness during the first year of life reassuring. However, the children did not show any increased incidence of neurologic abnormalities at 1 year of age.

Most drugs used to treat asthma in nonpregnant patients can also be prescribed during pregnancy. One exception to this rule is medication containing iodine, since iodine readily crosses the placenta and may induce a congenital goiter in the fetus if given in large doses. Many preparations for the treatment of asthma contain iodine, and this fact must be kept in mind. Cortisone is frequently prescribed for asthmatic patients, and its use appears to be safe during pregnancy.

Labor and delivery should be managed as with normal patients. Status asthmaticus at any time during pregnancy, however, should be treated vigorously, since it may exert an adverse effect both on mother and fetus. Cesarean section should be reserved for obstetrical indications. The question of therapeutic abortion is rarely raised but may be justified in a severely asthmatic patient. If abortion is to be performed using a prostaglandin, especially prostaglandin $F_{2\alpha}$, the drug should be administered with extreme caution, since these compounds can cause severe bronchospasm in asthmatic persons.

PULMONARY TUBERCULOSIS. Pulmonary tuberculosis during pregnancy is less prevalent in the United States than it once was, although the disease has by no means been eradicated. The more favorable prognosis enjoyed currently by the pregnant patient with pulmonary tuberculosis is based primarily on the effectiveness of drug therapy in arresting the disease. The chemotherapeutic agents used so successfully in nonpregnant patients can also be used during pregnancy.

Many clinics perform a routine tuberculin skin test on all pregnant patients. A chest roentgenogram should be ordered on positive reactors. Routine chest x-ray studies in all patients no longer seems wise, since the yield of positive tests is so low. Shielding of the fetus during x-ray exposure is important.

The changes in lung markings induced by the pulmonary changes of pregnancy may confuse the radiographic picture. Sputum examination may reveal the tuberculosis bacillus on direct smear, but a time-consuming culture may be necessary to identify the organism. When the diagnosis has been made, treatment with isoniazid, ethambutol, and streptomycin is indicated. The known hazard of a streptomycin-induced fetal abnormality of vestibular or auditory function must be considered if this drug is used. Isoniazid is teratogenic in animals.

Tuberculosis rarely exerts an unfavorable effect on a pregnancy, and congenital tuberculosis in the fetus is very rare. Pregnancy is usually tolerated well by the tuberculous patient, and therapeutic abortion is not indicated unless there is severe interference with cardiopulmonary function. Tuberculosis in extrapulmonary locations usually poses no special problems, since a favorable response to chemotherapy can also be expected in these patients. Tuberculosis of the female internal genitalia is rarely associated with an intrauterine pregnancy, since sterility is the rule. When pregnancy does occur, it usually terminates by abortion or by tubal implantation.

During pregnancy the tuberculous patient is treated at home unless she is infectious. Labor and delivery are managed with the usual analgesic and anesthetic techniques, although it is best to avoid lung irritants (e.g., ether). The newborn infant should be isolated immediately, and breast feeding should be avoided. Tuberculosis in the infant almost always results from exposure to the mother after birth, not from an intrauterine infection.

BRONCHIECTASIS. Bronchiectasis exerts no unfavorable effect on pregnancy, and the disease is rarely aggravated by the pregnancy. Since the disease is chronic but with frequent acute pneumonic exacerbations, active medical management is essential. Postural drainage and antibiotics for acute infection remain the major therapeutic tools. When the disease is limited to one lobe, lobectomy may be curative, although the desirability of performing this operation during pregnancy is uncertain. Conduction anesthetics are preferred to inhalation anesthetics for delivery.

Pulmonary Resection
Provided the residual functional capacity of the lungs is adequate, pregnancy will pose no special problem for a patient who has had a pulmonary lobe or an entire lung resected because of cancer. The patient's respiratory behavior furnishes a good index of pulmonary function, although a more precise determination should be made. A patient with *pulmonary fibrosis* has the same prognosis as the patient who becomes pregnant following pulmonary resection if the residual pulmonary capacity is similar.

Diseases of the Urinary Tract

INFECTIONS
An infection in the urinary tract may be limited to the bladder (cystitis); less commonly, the upper urinary tract is also involved in the infection (acute pyelonephritis). In some cases, the infection be-comes chronic (chronic pyelonephritis) although a history of a preceding acute process is not always elicited. Asymptomatic bacteriuria is present in many pregnant patients and is a frequent cause of acute pyelonephritis in pregnancy. Since ultimate kidney function may be at stake, all urinary tract infections should be thoroughly investigated and vigorously treated. These diseases are the most common serious complications of pregnancy and the postpartum period.

Cystitis
Cystitis is an inflammation of the bladder caused by bacteria. While bacteria are not found in normal human bladder urine, a number of factors predisposing to the development of urinary tract infection are present during pregnancy or the puerperium. A single catheterization always introduces bacteria into the bladder, and cystitis results in a number of such cases. In pregnancy, the hyperemic bladder is traumatized during delivery and becomes atonic in the postpartum period, thus presenting an ideal circumstance for the initiation of infection. Further, in about 5 percent of patients, an asymptomatic bacteriuria is present during pregnancy, even without the introduction of infection by catheter, and a clinical urinary tract infection develops fully in 40 percent of these patients.

Cystitis is characterized by symptoms of dysuria, urgency, and frequency. A clean catch urinalysis usually shows a variable number of white blood cells, and red blood cells may also be seen. Bacteria are evident in the urinary sediment of those patients with high colony counts. Although cystitis occurs in the absence of infection of the upper tract, an ascending infection may, of course, follow. Treatment of acute cystitis is similar to the treatment of acute pyelonephritis.

Acute Pyelonephritis
Acute pyelonephritis usually results from an ascending infection, although a blood or lymph-borne infection can occur. The disease causes an inflammation of the interstitial connective tissue of the kidney, usually without involvement of the nephron. In most adequately treated cases, the kidney

lesion heals completely, but recurrent or persistent disease may lead to chronic pyelonephritis. The acute disease occurs in 2 to 3 percent of pregnant or postpartum patients, with a peak incidence in the last trimester of pregnancy and the early postpartum period. Symptoms may first appear during labor.

The diagnosis is usually an easy one to make, although acute appendicitis or postpartum intrauterine infection may need to be differentiated. The onset is frequently abrupt, with the symptoms of acute cystitis, a backache in one or both lumbar areas, fever, and chills. Secondary gastrointestinal symptoms may also occur. The temperature is frequently elevated to 103° F. (39.4° C.) or even higher, and tenderness is elicited when the costovertebral angle is jarred. While history and physical examination are usually typical, urinalysis will show many white blood cells with numerous bacteria. Culture of the urine is indicated, and in most cases, *Escherichia coli* will be recovered. Occasionally, another coliform bacterium will be the offending organism, as will the staphylococcus or streptococcus. Since the patient's clinical picture will not permit therapeutic delay to await the culture report, the chosen antibiotic may need to be changed when the culture report is received.

Asymptomatic Bacteriuria

Asymptomatic bacteriuria is recorded in about 5 percent of pregnant patients examined routinely in the first trimester. The diagnosis is made only when a clean-voided specimen is found to contain more than 100,000 organisms per milliliter of urine. Most authorities think that all pregnant patients should have a urine culture early in pregnancy. Of patients with bacteriuria, 40 percent will experience one or more attacks of acute pyelonephritis during pregnancy or in the postpartum period. Antibacterial therapy in this group of patients will reduce the risk of the development of acute pyelonephritis to 1 to 2 percent. While early investigations suggested that asymptomatic bacteriuria also accounted for a sharp increase in the number of women entering labor prematurely [11], this risk is apparently not as great as previously feared [12]. Unpublished data of

the author suggest a persisting relationship between frank acute pyelonephritis and premature labor, however.

In some cases of asymptomatic infections, bacteriuria is present only in the bladder urine, while in other cases the upper tract urine is involved as well. In the 60 percent of patients with bacteriuria who do not experience an attack of acute pyelonephritis during pregnancy, the bacteriuria is probably limited to the bladder urine. Since it is difficult to tell with available clinical tools which patients with bacteria have kidney involvement, most authorities recommend antibiotic treatment of all patients with asymptomatic bacteriuria. The choice of drugs is discussed below.

Catheterization also predisposes to urinary tract infection. One study has shown a 9 percent incidence of urinary tract infection in patients catheterized before delivery [13]. Most obstetricians no longer practice this routine. If catheterization is necessary either before delivery or in the postpartum period, an antibiotic should be prescribed for three or four days to reduce the risk of subsequent infection.

Treatment of Urinary Tract Infections

The treatment of urinary tract infection can be accomplished on an ambulatory basis with asymptomatic bacteriuria or when the infection is limited to the bladder. Patients with acute pyelonephritis are sick enough to require hospitalization, and for many reasons they should be managed in the hospital. Acute pyelonephritis is one of the major causes of septic shock, and careful monitoring of blood pressure, pulse, and urinary output is essential during the acute phase of the disease. Clinical improvement is usually evident within 24 to 48 hours after the onset of therapy. A poor clinical response to therapy suggests (1) a causative organism that is not sensitive to the prescribed antibiotic or (2) an obstructive or congenital lesion of the urinary tract that interferes with pregnancy. Obstructive pyelonephritis is a urologic emergency, since irreparable renal damage occurs within hours. Immediate drainage of the blocked infected kidney is necessary. Except for this rare but serious complication, a complete investigation of the urinary tract should be delayed until after delivery.

The choice of antibiotic must be made initially on the assumption that the causative agent is *E. coli,* a diagnosis that is correct at least 75 percent of the time. The antibiotic can be changed if necessary to a more appropriate choice when the culture and sensitivity reports are available. An *E. coli* infection responds most readily to a sulfonamide, nitrofurantoin, or ampicillin. Any choice the physician makes will have certain disadvantages. He must carefully weigh the various possibilities before the decision is made. Ampicillin exerts no known ill effect on the fetus, but gastrointestinal side effects occur. Nitrofurantoin is safe for most patients but may lead to hemolytic anemia in patients whose erythrocytes are deficient in glucose 6-phosphate dehydrogenase, which occurs most commonly among black patients. Sulfonamides compete with bilirubin for albumin-binding sites and may cause kernicterus in the neonate born to a mother taking the drug. The drug should never be used near term or in the patient whose labor might be expected to begin prematurely.

Tetracycline is an effective drug in many cases of acute pyelonephritis, but two hazards are recognized with this drug: it may yellow the deciduous teeth of the child or, more seriously, cause maternal liver damage if kidney excretion is impaired. A few deaths in pregnant women have been reported from this cause.

The seriousness of urinary tract infection or of asymptomatic bacteriuria is sufficiently great to warrant taking a risk with the prescribed drug. The risk can be minimized if individual patient factors are considered. The chosen drug should be administered for a minimum of ten days, although the symptoms of the disease will usually disappear within a day or two of initial administration. A repeat urine culture should be performed after therapy is discontinued and retreatment instituted if the culture is positive. Recurrence of acute pyelonephritis is common enough to warrant this precaution. An intravenous pyelogram is indicated following delivery in all patients with upper tract disease during pregnancy. A more complete urologic evaluation may be necessary in a few. The physician must be certain that a chronic pyelonephritis is not present before he can reassure the patient of her normalcy.

Chronic Pyelonephritis
Chronic pyelonephritis is preceded by an acute infection in the urinary tract in less than half of the patients. The pathological changes in the kidney may be relatively mild, or they may be severe, with scar tissue in the renal cortex and fibrosis of Bowman's capsule. In severe cases, kidney function may be markedly impaired; the functional reserve determines the effect of a pregnancy on the kidney disease. The symptoms of the chronic pyelonephritis may be those of kidney insufficiency, or there may be no symptoms at all. Acute pyelonephritis is a common complication that may further injure the kidney. In some cases, therapeutic abortion may be the best course, since severe kidney impairment or bouts of superimposed acute infection may prove hazardous. Treatment is directed toward eliminating the offending microorganism if the pathologic condition in the kidney is not severe. If severe kidney damage is present, the treatment is less satisfactory and is directed toward preservation of as much kidney function as possible.

GLOMERULONEPHRITIS
Acute Glomerulonephritis
Acute glomerulonephritis usually follows a streptococcal infection that has occurred two to three weeks before the onset of the disease. The disease is characterized by the acute appearance of edema, hematuria, cylinduria, albuminuria, and hypertension. Progression of the disease may lead to evidences of kidney failure or the complication of hypertension. Treatment of the disease is nonspecific, except for the use of an antibiotic effective against streptococci. Terminal renal failure develops in a few patients, but most patients recover without kidney damage; chronic glomerulonephritis develops in a small percentage. A history of complete recovery from the disease usually indicates an uneventful pregnancy. The appearance of the disease during pregnancy is rare, and insufficient data are available to predict maternal and

fetal outcome. The importance of the disease rests in the diagnostic confusion it may cause if it appears during the third trimester. However, differentiation from acute toxemia of pregnancy is usually possible by the persistence of hematuria and the presence of red cell casts.

Chronic Glomerulonephritis

Chronic glomerulonephritis may appear following an attack of acute glomerulonephritis, or it may manifest itself without any such history. The disease may be asymptomatic except for persistent proteinuria; at the other end of the scale, renal failure may be the first manifestation of the disease. Hypertension is a frequent complication of chronic glomerulonephritis, and the disease complex is not always easy to differentiate from acute toxemia. The pregnancy outcome depends primarily on the severity of the kidney damage and the presence or absence of superimposed acute toxemia, a frequent complication.

Treatment of chronic glomerulonephritis varies from symptomatic therapy to dialysis in some patients. Irreversible severe chronic glomerulonephritis necessitating dialysis may also require that therapeutic abortion be performed early in pregnancy. Delayed intrauterine growth, due apparently to inadequate placental development, can be monitored with urinary estriol levels, although severe kidney disease may interfere with the excretion of estriol in the urine and thus invalidate the test. In this case, serum estriol levels may be useful. Better evaluation of fetoplacental function is provided by the nonstress test (NST) and the oxytocin challenge test (OCT) described in Chapter 12.

OTHER DISEASES OF THE KIDNEY

Renal Tuberculosis

Renal tuberculosis associated with pregnancy is no longer considered to carry a bad prognosis as once thought. The factor primarily determining the effect of the pregnancy on the disease is the degree of renal function. Good renal function usually implies a good outcome.

Renal tuberculosis, long quiescent, may be reactivated during pregnancy. The diagnosis should be suspected in a patient with pyelonephritis that either fails to respond to antibiotic therapy or is associated with pyuria in an acid urine but with a negative urine culture. Demonstration of the tubercle bacillus in the urine may be possible, although a parenchymal "cold abscess" may be isolated from the urinary tract, resulting in a negative urinary sediment test. Treatment consists primarily of appropriate chemotherapy. Therapeutic abortion is indicated if kidney function is seriously impaired. Pregnancy should not be recommended following nephrectomy for renal tuberculosis in a nonpregnant patient for at least two years following the operation. In the interim, normal kidney function should be established in the remaining kidney.

Pregnancy with a Solitary Kidney

Renal tuberculosis, pyonephrosis, urinary calculi, kidney tumors, and other diseases may necessitate unilateral nephrectomy. Whether or not pregnancy is wise following nephrectomy is a question posed occasionally. The answer to the question primarily concerns the function of the remaining kidney. A thorough functional evaluation is therefore indicated before advice is given. In any event, if the remaining kidney is pelvic in location, pregnancy is contraindicated. If the solitary kidney has normal function, pregnancy can be recommended. The increase in glomerular filtration rate and renal plasma flow associated with normal pregnancy provides more than enough kidney reserve for the pregnancy. The kidney should be periodically evaluated during pregnancy. If the solitary kidney is functioning below normal, pregnancy is contraindicated. If accidental pregnancy should occur, a therapeutic abortion may be necessary. If hypertension should develop late in pregnancy, early induction of labor is mandatory.

Urinary Calculus

Urinary calculi associated with pregnancy are unusual in spite of the urinary stasis that accompanies dilatation of the ureters and kidney pelvices in pregnancy. One possible explanation for this observation is that inhibitors of urinary calculus formation are increased in the urine of pregnant women. The symptoms the calculus elicits in the pregnant patient depend on the stage of gestation in which it occurs. During early pregnancy, before dilatation of the upper urinary tract has become extreme, the symptoms may be those that occur in the nonpregnant patient, that is, ureteral colic, hematuria, and sometimes fever. Later in pregnancy, ureteral colic is likely to be absent while evidence of pyelonephritis is much more prevalent. Indeed, the likelihood of associated infection is a major hazard of the disease, since repeated infection may lead to permanent kidney damage. The possible association of urinary calculi with pyelonephritis is one of the major reasons why a postpartum urologic evaluation in patients with infection is recommended.

The diagnosis may be suggested by the symptomatology, or the disease may be silent, with discovery of the stone made by an abdominal x-ray film taken for an unrelated reason. The treatment will depend on kidney function, the presence or absence of infection, and gestational age at which the diagnosis is made. If the stone is passed spontaneously, minimal subsequent treatment is required. If the stone is discovered during the first five months of pregnancy and does not pass spontaneously, surgical removal is recommended to prevent the hazards of infection and reduction in kidney function. If the diagnosis is made later in pregnancy, removal of the stone can be delayed if infection can be prevented or controlled and if kidney function is near normal. The enlarged uterus obstructs the surgical approach to a lower ureteral stone, and open surgical removal may be impossible beyond seven months' gestation. If kidney function appears compromised, a nephrostomy may be necessary to prevent destruction of the kidney. Pregnancy following successful treatment of a prior kidney stone is usually uncomplicated and is not contraindicated.

Anomalies of the Urinary Tract
Anomalies of the urinary tract may be discovered before pregnancy, when an associated abnormality of the genital tract is investigated, or during pregnancy, when the cause for pyelonephritis is sought. The anomalies may be relatively innocuous, consisting of duplication of the ureter or kidney pelvis or segmented ureter; or they may have potentially more serious consequences, i.e., horseshoe kidney, pelvic kidney, or polycystic disease of the kidney. With the less serious disorders, pregnancy can usually be expected to progress normally unless kidney function has decreased or unless repeated bouts of pyelonephritis occur. With displacement of the kidney, especially if a second normal kidney is not present, repeated bouts of pyelonephritis with potential serious damage to the kidney should be anticipated. With luck, kidney function will have been evaluated before pregnancy. Consideration should be given to therapeutic abortion in these cases if kidney function is impaired or if repeated infection occurs. When obstruction of delivery by a pelvic kidney occurs, which it rarely does, delivery by cesarean section may be necessary.

The seriousness of polycystic renal disease during pregnancy is directly related to the amount of kidney function already destroyed by the disease process. The disease may be discovered for the first time during pregnancy, necessitating a complete urologic evaluation before a treatment plan can be chosen. A serious decrease in kidney reserve, especially if hypertension is an associated finding, may require interruption of the pregnancy.

Pregnancy Following Renal Transplantation
While pregnancy following renal transplantation has been reported in a number of cases, the danger both to the mother and to the fetus is evident [14]. Immunosuppressive therapy must be continued during the pregnancy, or the kidney will be lost. Hypertension or proteinuria has developed during the pregnancies of these patients with some frequency, although other patients seem to have withstood pregnancy with little difficulty. Intrauterine growth retardation, premature delivery, and other abnormalities have been noted in the infants [15].

Endocrine Disorders
DIABETES MELLITUS
Diabetes mellitus associated with pregnancy is largely a disease of the postinsulin era. Before insu-

lin became available, few diabetic patients achieved pregnancy, either because of the frequently associated amenorrhea or because their general nutritional state was so poor. Of the few who became pregnant, about a fourth died, and the perinatal loss is said to have been 50 percent. The availability of insulin improved this prognosis, so that the maternal mortality approaches zero today. While the perinatal mortality is much lower than it was in the preinsulin era, it remains distressingly high. Although the best clinics report rates as low as 3 to 6 percent, the overall mortality in recent years has been 10 to 15 percent. Because of the diabetogenic effect of pregnancy, there is a group of patients in whom abnormal glucose tolerance develops during pregnancy with no prior evidence of diabetes. The term we prefer to use for the disease in these patients is *gestational diabetes*. Others use the term chemical diabetes to illustrate that the disease becomes evident only when certain laboratory tests are performed, not from any symptoms that the patient experiences. In most cases, the abnormal metabolism reverts to normal after completion of the pregnancy. Not all these patients have "prediabetes," since only about 25 percent will ultimately develop frank diabetes in later life. They are treated as diabetic during pregnancy, however, since as a group they will experience an increase in perinatal mortality unless the disease is carefully monitored during antenatal care.

Diagnosis

Many pregnant patients with diabetes mellitus knew of their diabetic state before pregnancy and present no diagnostic challenge. In a few patients, detectable frank diabetes will first develop during pregnancy, with the classic clinical manifestations of excessive hunger and thirst and polyuria, confirmed by massive glycosuria and ketonuria. In mild cases, however, the diagnosis will be less obvious; indeed, even the criteria on which to make the diagnosis in the bulk of patients remain in dispute.

Certain bits of information from the history will help identify patients who should be investigated for the presence of diabetes. A patient with a family history of diabetes is a likely candidate for the dis-

ease. If she has had a poor reproductive history (unexplained fetal death or a congenitally defective child) or has delivered an unusually large baby, she is suspect. The presence of glycosuria always demands a diagnostic evaluation, but in many cases the glycosuria will have resulted from the spillage of lactose, especially in late pregnancy, or will occur as a normal variant due to pregnancy changes in the kidneys (see p. 38). Glucose filtration through the glomerulus is greatly increased in pregnant women, but the reabsorption of glucose through the distal tubule usually prevents spillage into the urine. In some instances, the reabsorption is insufficient, and glycosuria results. Lactose is not identified by most of the commercially available kits (Clinistix, TesTape) for measuring reducing substances in the urine, so that a positive test is evidence that there is glycosuria.

Frank diabetes is diagnosed when the fasting blood sugar level is above 130 mg. per 100 ml. on repeated samplings. Gestational diabetes, however, is associated with a normal or near-normal fasting level of blood glucose, and detection requires further testing. With gestational diabetes, the 2-hour postprandial level of blood glucose will be elevated. If the fasting level is above 90 mg. per 100 ml. and the 2-hour postprandial level greater than 145 mg. per 100 ml., after an oral glucose load (see below), a diagnosis of gestational diabetes is justified.

The glucose tolerance can be measured following oral ingestion of glucose (GTT) or after intravenous injection of glucose (IVGTT). During pregnancy, absorption of glucose from the gastrointestinal tract may be delayed, with a subsequent delay in blood absorption. The result is an overdiagnosis of diabetes and a disturbing number of false-positive results. The IVGTT, on the other hand, is much less sensitive and thus is less likely to give false-positive diagnoses. The price of this advantage, however, is a higher risk of false-negative tests. Many clinicians prefer to screen patients suspected of being diabetic with the GTT and confirm a positive test by the IVGTT during pregnancy.

The confusion in arriving at a diagnosis of diabetes in pregnancy is further complicated by the lack of agreement on criteria for interpreting the results of the glucose tolerance test. Felig [16] accepts the following criteria for diagnosis of diabetes by the GTT:

	Blood Glucose (mg./100 ml.)	
Time	Pregnant*	Nonpregnant
Fasting	90	100
1 hour	165	170
2 hours	145	120
3 hours	125	110

The figures apply to whole venous blood and subjects given a 100 gram oral dose of glucose. If plasma rather than whole blood is used for analysis, the values should be increased by 15 percent.

Classification

Assessment of the severity of diabetes is important for many reasons. Perinatal mortality is higher with severe disease. Severe diabetes may be adversely affected by pregnancy, while less severe disease does not carry this hazard. Classification of the severity of the disease in an individual patient will allow prediction of both the perinatal and maternal outcomes.

An increase in insulin requirement is usual in diabetic patients and may not measure the severity of the disease. Indeed, no change or a decrease in the insulin requirement in a particular patient may predict a bad outcome. The best classification of the severity of diabetes was proposed by White [17] many years ago and refined by her since that time. It is based primarily on the age of the onset of the disease, the duration of the disease, and the amount of vascular involvement caused by the disease:

Class A: Diagnosis on the basis of glucose tolerance test only (gestational diabetes).
Class B: Onset of clinical diabetes after the age of 20; duration less than 10 years; no evidence of vascular disease.

*The diagnosis of diabetes is established if two or more values exceed the limits shown.

Class C: Onset of clinical diabetes between the ages of 10 and 19; duration 10 to 19 years; no evidence of vascular disease.
Class D: Onset of clinical diabetes before the age of 10, or duration of 20 or more years, or x-ray evidence of vascular disease in the legs, or retinitis.
Class E: Same as group D, with x-ray evidence of arteriosclerosis of the pelvic vessels.
Class F: Diabetic nephropathy.
Class R: Active retinitis proliferans.

Only about 10 percent of diabetic patients will be in Class D or have more severe diabetes. The diabetes may seem to progress during pregnancy, with retinal vessel change or proteinuria appearing for the first time. Certain types of retinal changes disappear; a few (e.g., retinitis proliferans) do not revert to normal following termination of pregnancy.

Effect of Pregnancy on Diabetes

Why pregnancy should exert a diabetogenic effect is a question of great interest. The evidence for the phenomenon is convincing: an exaggerated insulinogenic response to glucose loading; an elevated serum insulin level; and an abnormal glucose tolerance test result in many women known to be normal previously. The mechanism for the effect may be related to the apparent need for an exaggerated insulinogenic response to glucose loading. A maternal pancreas with a borderline capability of secreting insulin may simply not have the reserve to keep up with insulin requirements, but without the stress of pregnancy, the pancreas may be adequate. The effect of insulin is opposed probably by two mechanisms during pregnancy: (1) the action of insulinase, an enzyme in the placenta that inactivates insulin and (2) the action of human placental lactogen (HPL), an insulin antagonist (an effect that may be its primary function).

Many pregnancy factors affect the management of diabetes. Most obvious is the increase in insulin requirement that occurs with most pregnancies; the increase is frequently as much as 50 to 200 percent. Although the insulin requirement may fluctuate, a drop in insulin requirement may in some cases predict fetal demise. Furthermore, the insulin requirement may be markedly affected by the nausea and vomiting of early pregnancy, infection during pregnancy, and labor. With nausea and vomiting, the patient may fail to ingest an adequate diet, thus running the risk of a hypoglycemic reaction. Infection in the diabetic gravida leads to insulin resistance and ketoacidosis in a remarkably short time. Labor may be equally disturbing to carbohydrate balance, since the lack of food intake and muscular activity so characteristic of this period may markedly change insulin needs. Careful monitoring of insulin requirements during pregnancy, especially in times of stress, will minimize, but not eliminate, the hazard of adverse metabolic effects on the fetus.

Effects of Diabetes on Pregnancy

Diabetes is associated with many maternal complications, and its intensification of certain effects increases both maternal and fetal risk. Among the potential maternal effects are toxemia of pregnancy, ketoacidosis, hydramnios, and retinal changes. The fetal effects of the disease include excessively large babies (occasionally a very small baby), increased neonatal risk of respiratory distress syndrome, increased risk of congenital anomaly, and likely inheritance of the diabetic gene. While maternal mortality, with good medical supervision, is relatively low, the perinatal mortality experienced by most clinics remains at 10 to 15 percent.

The incidence of what appears to be toxemia is increased fourfold or fivefold in the presence of diabetes, but whether the disease is acute toxemia of pregnancy or a hypertensive disease superimposed on the vascular disease so common in diabetic patients is uncertain. The effect is perhaps the same, since the disease certainly increases maternal and fetal hazard. Ketoacidosis occurs in many diabetic gravidas because of frequent changes in insulin requirements due to nausea and vomiting, infection, or other factors. The maternal hazard of ketoacidosis is well known. The fetal hazard is also great; maternal ketoacidosis probably accounts for many of the fetal deaths.

Hydramnios occurs more commonly than with normal pregnancy; some authors quote an incidence of 20 percent. Hydramnios is associated with an increased fetal hazard, partly because the hydramnios itself is evidence that the fetus is in poor condition and partly because hydramnios often terminates in premature labor.

Progressive retinal change is a particularly disturbing development, since this is probably the one maternal effect of diabetes in pregnancy that is not reversible after delivery. Furthermore, the retinal vascular changes are evidence, usually, of a generalized vascular pathologic state, and a strong association between retinal change and poor fetal prognosis is evident. The retina shows sclerosis of the vessels, "cotton-wool" exudates, and hemorrhages. Frequent observation of the fundi is essential to recognize the progressive changes. The retinal changes may lead to sudden blindness, and for this reason alone they may justify abortion. Indeed, a diabetic patient with retinal disease should not become pregnant at all.

Excessive size of the infant is a frequent accompaniment of diabetes and may cause fetopelvic disproportion. The excessive size is thought to result from the hyperglycemia of the mother and the consequent fetal hyperglycemia. Since insulin, either endogenous or exogenous, does not cross the placenta in significant amounts, the fetal pancreas must secrete additional insulin to metabolize the blood glucose. The resulting macrosomatia involves all fetal organs except the brain, and the fetal pancreas shows hypertrophy at autopsy. Although most babies delivered of diabetic women are large, with severe diabetes (Class D or worse), an infant who is small for gestational age may result. The mechanism for this delayed intrauterine growth is probably a vascular deficiency, with poor fetoplacental circulation.

The large size of the infant may be misleading, since delivery is frequently accomplished before 37 weeks' gestation. In spite of his large size, the infant functions as a premature, and the respiratory distress syndrome is commonly seen in these infants. The hypertrophy of the fetal pancreas with excess insulin secretion will produce a severe hypoglycemia in most infants. For these reasons, the risk of neonatal death is greatly increased. The recent literature also emphasizes the frequency with which a congenital anomaly is seen in the infant born of a diabetic mother; the increase is about threefold [18].

Since diabetes is an inherited disease, the infant is likely to inherit the trait or the actual disease. Although the evidence for the disease may not become apparent for many years, this hazard must be explained to the parents of the child. The risk of the development of diabetes appears to be highly dependent on whether or not the disease is present in other family members.

Management of Diabetes

Close supervision of the patient with diabetes is crucial. The careful monitoring of the disease should be shared by an internist and an obstetrician, both of whom should be especially interested in diabetes in pregnancy. The intricacies of diabetic management during pregnancy should be explained to the patient, so that she can watch for danger signs herself. The hazard of nausea and vomiting or of infection should be especially emphasized, since early medical attention may make the difference between ketoacidosis and fetal death or live birth. She should know that glycosuria is present in many normal patients during pregnancy and that more than the usual amount of glycosuria should be observed before altering insulin dosage. She should be told that hydramnios frequently precedes fetal death by only a short interval and that she should report any excessive abdominal growth.

OFFICE VISITS. Office visits at least as frequent as twice a month for the first two trimesters and weekly in the last trimester are mandatory. The obstetrical examination at each office visit should include observation for hydramnios and for hypertension, or proteinuria, or both, as well as for the usual determinations of fetal size, fetal heart rate, and fetal position. The urine should be examined for glucose and acetone as well as for protein, and levels of blood glucose, serum urea nitrogen, and

serum carbon dioxide should be determined periodically to evaluate metabolic function. The retinas should be examined at each visit.

DIET AND INSULIN. Close dietary supervision is important with diabetes in pregnancy, just as it is in the nonpregnant patient. Indeed, careful dietary control usually precludes the need for insulin in patients with gestational diabetes. Excessive weight gain should be avoided, but weight loss may be unwise. The help of a nutritionist should be sought for dietary instruction, and deviation from the prescribed diet should be reported immediately, since a change in insulin requirement will probably result. Long-acting insulins are usually prescribed and are satisfactory in most patients. In the gravida with unstable diabetes, or in the presence of nausea and vomiting or an infection in any gravida, it may be necessary to change the insulin to a short-acting type. The marked variation noted in insulin requirement in most diabetic gravidas is carefully observed, and changes in dosage are made accordingly. While an increase in insulin requirement is most usual and is often marked, this is not always the case, and frequent checks of blood glucose and urinary acetone are essential.

HOSPITALIZATION. Ideally, a diabetic patient should be hospitalized at periodic intervals to check the diabetic control more closely. In practice, this is difficult to achieve and perhaps unnecessary. At the very least, the appearance of an infection, or severe vomiting, or toxemia should be treated as an emergency with immediate hospitalization. The diabetic patient should also be hospitalized for a week before delivery; those with severe disease should be hospitalized earlier.

COMPLICATIONS. The presence of a severe complication requires special care. Kidney failure or severe hypertension and heart failure may develop in patients with vascular disease. Delayed intrauterine growth may be evident (see Chap. 12). Assessment of kidney and cardiac function may be required, and the results may necessitate a change in delivery date and method. It is in these patients in particular that urinary estriol determinations or oxytocin challenge tests (OCT) for fetoplacental condition and various methods of determining fetal maturity may find their greatest usefulness (see Chap. 12).

STEROID HORMONES. The use of increasingly large oral doses of estrogen and progesterone in pregnant diabetic women has been recommended to correct the hormone "imbalance" [17]. A much higher perinatal survival rate has been reported following the use of this therapy. The apparent cause-and-effect relationship between administration of the drugs and the improved perinatal result is probably spurious, however. The meticulous medical care given these patients may have been a more important factor in the improved result than was the steroid therapy. Attempts to repeat these therapeutic results in other clinics have failed to show the same effect [19]. Most obstetricians doubt the efficacy of the steroids and do not use them in pregnant diabetic patients.

DELIVERY. Selecting the proper time for delivery is of vital importance if perinatal mortality is to be avoided. Delivery too early will result in a premature infant who may die of the effects of a respiratory distress syndrome. Delivery too long delayed may be preceded by fetal death from the effects of an episode of ketoacidosis or from some other cause. Although certain generalizations can be made, individual circumstances will alter the decision. In the absence of complication, delivery of the Class A (gestational) diabetic patient should be performed at term. In this instance, urinary estriol determinations or OCTs may be helpful. With frank uncomplicated diabetes, delivery should be accomplished at 37 to 38 weeks' gestation. A poor obstetrical history or the development of a complication will necessitate another choice. If an unexplained fetal death has occurred in a previous pregnancy, a shorter gestational interval for delivery may be chosen (perhaps 35 weeks). If hypertension and albuminuria or hydramnios develop, or if repeated attacks of acidosis occur, immediate delivery is indicated if the gestation is beyond 32 weeks. While neonatal deaths will occur under these circumstances, the risk is less than the risk of fetal death if delivery is delayed.

The method of delivery is also controversial. Some clinics prefer induction of labor and vaginal delivery in most patients, reserving cesarean section only for special indications. Others deliver most diabetic women by cesarean section. Induction of labor should probably be tried if the patient has not been previously delivered by cesarean section, if the parity is less than five, if the pelvis is clinically adequate, and if the pelvic factors (presentation, condition of cervix) seem favorable. This set of circumstances will be present more often in Class A diabetic patients, who are usually delivered at term. If induction fails, or if the circumstances necessary for induction are not present, delivery should be by cesarean section. Most clinics deliver a large proportion of frank diabetic patients abdominally.

If induction is elected, careful monitoring of the fetal heart rate (FHR) and uterine contractions is indicated. Any serious deviation from a normal pattern necessitates cesarean section. Conduction anesthesia is preferred whether the delivery is vaginal or by section. An anesthesiologist and a pediatrician in the delivery room are essential.

There has been increasing interest in monitoring diabetic pregnancy with urinary estriol levels. Some authorities now suggest that a series of normal estriol levels, if done at least every other day, are indicative of adequate fetoplacental function and that delivery may be postponed in such patients in the absence of a complication. The same reassurance is provided by OCTs at about five-day intervals. The advantages of this delay are increased fetal maturity and avoidance of the hazards of early induction or cesarean section. Few authorities would suggest delay in delivery in severe diabetes. A major objection to the use of urinary estriol determinations in selecting delivery time is that they are unreliable before 32 to 34 weeks of pregnancy. If their use is restricted to the less severe case, however, this objection seems inappli-

Table 4-1. Trends of Course of Pregnancy by Class of Diabetes Mellitus

Class of Diabetes Mellitus	Spontaneous Abortion Rate	Degree of Hydramnios	Excessive Weight Gain	Pre-eclampsia	Large Placenta	Heavy Birth Weight	Fetal Loss			Congenital Anomalies	Diabetes Mellitus Intensification
							Intra-uterine	Intra-partum	Neo-natal		
A	N	+	+	+	++++	++++	+	++++	+	+	+
B	N	++++	++++	++++	++++	++++	++	++++	+	+	++++
C	N	+++	+++	+++	+++	+++	+	++	++	+	+++
D	+	++	++	++	++	++	+++	+	+++	+	+
E	++++	++	++	++	+	+	++++	+	++++	+	+
F	++++	±	0	?	0	0	++++	+	++++	+	±
R	++++	±	0	Super-imposed?	0	0	++++	+	++++	+	±

Source: P. White. Pregnancy and diabetes, medical aspects. *Med Clin North Am* 49:1015, 1965.

cable. A large clinical trial will be required before the role of urinary estriols in the selection of the best time for delivery in the diabetic patient is clarified.

The clinician is also faced with an uncertain gestational interval with many diabetic pregnancies. In addition to the prevalent uncertainty about menstrual dates, certain other factors may confuse the gestational interval in diabetes. The excessive size of the infant may suggest a longer gestation than the menstrual dates allow, while the small infant of a mother with severe diabetes may lead the clinician to suspect a shorter gestational interval than originally calculated. In these circumstances, the various tests for fetal maturity should be employed. Of special use is amniotomy and measurement of the amniotic fluid for bilirubin, creatinine, and the lecithin-sphingomyelin ratio. Details of this test are given in Chapter 12.

Maternal and Fetal Prognosis

Few maternal deaths occur in well-managed diabetic pregnancies, although the maternal mortality rate is much higher than in the nondiabetic population. Most maternal deaths result from the complications of the disease—vascular disease or hypertension. The high perinatal death rate is divided about equally between fetal and neonatal deaths. Many of the fetal deaths are unexplained, although some follow an episode of ketoacidosis. A few fetal deaths occur in the intrapartum period as a result of

difficult delivery, especially from impacted shoulders. The neonatal deaths in a well-supervised nursery are largely the result of the respiratory distress syndrome or congenital anomalies. Both fetal and neonatal deaths are more likely to occur with the more severe degrees of diabetes. The risks of various maternal and fetal events in each class of diabetic patient as proposed by White are shown in Table 4-1.

THYROID DISEASE

Disorders of the thyroid gland in pregnancy are rare. However, the marked changes in thyroid function during normal pregnancy complicate the task of arriving at a correct diagnosis when such a disorder does occur. The importance of thyroid disease in pregnancy lies primarily in its potential harm to the fetus either from the disease itself or from the maternal therapy prescribed.

Hyperthyroidism

Hyperthyroidism is seen in only about 0.1 percent of gravida pregnant women, since infertility is the rule among hyperthyroid patients, due to their high rate of menstrual disorders. Unrecognized or inadequately treated hyperthyroidism in pregnancy is associated with a high fetal loss. If the diagnosis is made prior to pregnancy, successful treatment has usually been instituted, and the hazard of the pregnancy under these circumstances is not great. If the disease is suspected during pregnancy because of persistent tachycardia and exophthalmos, thyroid function tests should be interpreted with full knowledge of the changes in these tests induced by normal pregnancy. Thus the protein-bound iodine should be above 12 μg. per 100 ml. in hyperthyroidism, which is markedly higher than the non-pregnant euthyroid level and higher than the level induced by normal pregnancy. Similarly, the T_3 resin uptake may not show the typical decrease noted with a euthyroid pregnancy; with hyperthyroidism in pregnancy, it may be recorded at normal or increased levels. Some of the symptoms that suggest a diagnosis of hyperthyroidism in the non-pregnant patient may be normally experienced by the pregnant patient and are less helpful as diagnostic aids during pregnancy. Breathlessness and heat intolerance are examples of such symptoms.

The treatment of hyperthyroidism during pregnancy is controversial. All authorities agree that a maternal euthyroid state should be attained to protect both mother and fetus but not on the best method for achieving this goal. Some authorities recommend the administration of propylthiouracil in doses adequate to induce euthyroidism. The addition of thyroxine to this regimen to provide the fetus with this hormone has been recommended by some. Recent evidence has cast doubt on the advisability of this combination of drugs, because propylthiouracil readily crosses the placenta, while thyroxine crosses only in very small amounts. Thus, the mother may be successfully treated for hyperthyroidism, but depression of the fetal thyroid with the antithyroid medication may induce a dangerous hypothyroid state or congenital goiter in the fetus. It has recently been recommended that the propylthiouracil be given in small doses to reduce the maternal hyperthyroidism but not over-correct it [20]. No thyroxine is added to this regimen.

A good case can be made for thyroid surgery during pregnancy to treat maternal hyperthyroidism. The arguments for such treatment include the relative safety of the surgery for the mother and the absence of ill effects on the fetus. The surgery should be preceded by a short course of propylthiouracil and Lugol's solution to induce a eu-thyroid state. Thyroxine may be given to the mother postoperatively as needed. Long-term iodine medication is contraindicated because of the possibility of inducing a goiter in the fetus.

Hypothyroidism

Hypothyroidism in pregnancy is even more rare than hyperthyroidism, and patients with full-blown myxedema probably never become pregnant. There is some evidence that pregnancy may induce hypothyroidism in a patient who had borderline thyroid function before pregnancy. The fear of the development of cretinism in the fetus of a hypothyroid mother is the chief medical concern. Cretinism, however, can occur without maternal hypothyroidism, apparently as a result of an aberration in the embryonic development of the fetal thyroid gland. There is evidence also that maternal hypothyroidism increases the risk of congenital malformation in the fetus. The diagnosis of hypothyroidism during pregnancy is suggested by failure of the total T_4 and protein-bound iodine to rise as expected during normal pregnancy. Thyroxine should be administered to the mother.

PARATHYROID DISEASES

Pregnancy appears to increase parathyroid activity, which may account for the greater incidence of hyperparathyroidism in females as opposed to males. Nevertheless, the association of pregnancy with parathyroid disease is very rare.

Hyperparathyroidism

Hyperparathyroidism in pregnancy results from hyperplasia or adenoma of the parathyroid gland. The diagnosis is made by the presence of hypercalcemia, hypercalciuria, and a low serum phosphorus resulting from a large urinary excretion of phosphorus. The hypercalciuria may cause nephrolithiasis, with subsequent kidney damage. Marked bone resorption occurs because of withdrawal of calcium from the bone, and x-ray examination frequently shows decalcification and cyst formation in the bone. Treatment is extirpation of the offending parathyroid hyperplasia or adenoma. Tetany in the newborn can be treated with calcium and vitamin D, although the tetany is self-correcting.

Hypoparathyroidism

Hypoparathyroidism in pregnancy usually follows a thyroidectomy in which parathyroid tissue was inadvertently removed. Low urinary phosphorus excretion and a high level of serum phosphorus accompany a fall in serum ionizable calcium. Muscular irritability or even full-blown tetany can occur in the mother. The fetus preferentially withdraws calcium from the maternal circulation, thus increasing the severity of the disease. Treatment with calcium and dihydrotachysterol to promote phosphorus excretion is adequate. The fetus usually sustains no damage.

ADRENAL DISEASE

Adrenal Hypofunction

Adrenal hypofunction (Addison's disease) was rarely associated with pregnancy before the advent of replacement therapy, but the association is no longer so uncommon as it once was. The maintenance dose of cortisone needed for treatment of the disease before pregnancy is continued during pregnancy, although the required dose may decrease slightly during the second and third trimesters. Careful monitoring of steroid needs is essential during pregnancy, especially if nausea and vomiting cause an electrolyte disturbance, and also during labor and delivery, when the stress associated with these events usually results in a need for additional hormone replacement. Infection and blood loss are poorly tolerated by patients with adrenal hypofunction, and early treatment of either complication is mandatory. The fetus usually does well if the maternal disease is adequately managed.

Adrenal Hyperfunction

Adrenal hyperfunction due to Cushing's syndrome is rarely associated with pregnancy because of infertility in patients with this disease. If the patient has been treated by adrenalectomy, her problems during pregnancy are essentially those of adrenal hypofunction. Adrenal hyperplasia due to the ad-

renogenital syndrome is successfully treated with suppressive cortisone medication. Subsequent to such treatment, a few patients have become pregnant, and an essentially uneventful pregnancy can be anticipated. Suppressive cortisone medication should be continued and can be used safely through pregnancy.

Pheochromocytoma

Pheochromocytoma is a dangerous tumor of the adrenal medulla that causes paroxysmal attacks of hypertension associated with such symptoms as severe headache, palpitation, and tachycardia. In the few cases of the tumor in pregnant women that have been reported, the maternal and fetal loss was very high. The disease should always be included in the differential diagnosis of any patient with fluctuating hypertensive episodes during pregnancy, or when the evidence of acute toxemia is not typical. The diagnosis is supported by a finding of markedly elevated urinary catecholamines. Treatment may include an infusion of phentolamine to lower the blood pressure, surgical extirpation with continuation of the pregnancy, or abortion with subsequent treatment of the tumor. A high mortality attends all forms of treatment, and individualization of treatment is mandatory.

PITUITARY DISEASE

Diabetes Insipidus

Diabetes insipidus results from a deficiency of antidiuretic hormone (vasopressin) from the posterior pituitary gland and is rarely associated with pregnancy. Pregnancy, labor, and delivery are usually uncomplicated in such cases, and a good pregnancy outcome can be anticipated. Vasopressin replacement can be continued during pregnancy, although urine volume is said to be more difficult to control in pregnant than in nonpregnant patients.

Diseases of the Gastrointestinal Tract and Liver

ACUTE SURGICAL ABDOMINAL DISEASE

Surgical disease of the abdominal organs occurs during pregnancy with about the same frequency experienced in the nonpregnant population. The physician caring for obstetrical patients must therefore expect to see an occasional patient with an acute abdominal disease demanding an immediate surgical procedure. The special circumstances surrounding such an event in pregnancy makes it difficult to arrive at a diagnosis. Displacement of other abdominal organs by the enlarging uterus may change the location of pain or obscure the expected physical findings. Abdominal pain may be incorrectly interpreted as being uterine in origin. Reluctance to perform an abdominal operation because of a presumed increased risk of premature labor or perinatal loss likewise contributes to the frequent delays in treatment occurring with acute abdominal disease in pregnancy.

With these facts in mind, it cannot be too strongly stated that the major hazard of acute abdominal disease during pregnancy is the *failure* to operate when indicated. Abdominal surgery rarely does the fetus any harm, but failure to treat an abdominal disease frequently leads not only to maternal danger but also to abortion, premature labor, and perinatal death. If a reasonable doubt exists about the presence of an acute surgical abdominal disease in a pregnant patient, the best therapeutic plan is to operate. If an error in diagnosis cannot be avoided, it is best to overdiagnose with this group of diseases. While any disease can occur, the most common are acute appendicitis and intestinal obstruction.

Acute Appendicitis
Acute appendicitis occurs about once in every 1000 pregnancies, either during pregnancy or in the immediate puerperium [21]. The chief hazard is failure to make the diagnosis early enough to avoid rupture of the appendix and peritonitis; this is most likely to occur late in pregnancy or during the puerperium, when the large uterus or the relaxed abdominal musculature obscures the physical findings. Furthermore, the presenting complaints of nausea and vomiting and abdominal distention are commonly encountered in normal pregnancy. While a complaint of periumbilical pain may be helpful in early pregnancy, later in pregnancy, the symptom may be attributed to uterine irritability. With

the displacement of the cecum upward and to the right by the uterus, the characteristic radiation of the pain to the right lower quadrant may not occur. Leukocytosis is present in normal pregnancy, but a shift of the polymorphonuclear cells to more immature forms may be a helpful laboratory finding. The change in the clinical picture of appendicitis during pregnancy may make its differentiation from renal colic, kidney infection, a twisted adnexal lesion, or degeneration of a uterine myoma more difficult than usual.

Since the hazards of appendiceal perforation far outweigh the hazards of laparotomy, surgery should be performed as soon as the diagnosis is made. While delay of a few hours to await a more definite clinical picture may be warranted, persistence of a suggestive clinical picture demands surgical intervention. Surgery does not appreciably increase the fetal risk if hypoxia from anesthesia or other factors is meticulously avoided. While some physicians have used parenteral progesterone in the postoperative period to decrease uterine irritability—and presumably the risk of premature labor—the evidence for the efficacy for this therapy is unconvincing. Cesarean section at the time of appendectomy should be avoided because of the risk of infection. Labor will do no harm to a well-closed abdominal incision, even in the immediate postoperative period.

Maternal mortality in reported series of acute appendicitis complicating pregnancy is alarmingly high, especially in late pregnancy and in the puerperium. A recent paper recorded an overall maternal mortality of 2 percent and a maternal mortality of 7.3 percent in the third trimester [22]. The disease is associated with a prematurity rate of 17 percent and the perinatal mortality rate is increased. Failure to make an early diagnosis accounts for the major part of this mortality. Surgical delay must be avoided if this maternal mortality is to be lowered. Fetal loss results from abortion and premature labor and is more likely to occur because of failure to operate before appendiceal rupture and peritonitis develop than from the surgical procedure itself. Again, early diagnosis and operation can be expected to decrease the fetal risk.

Intestinal Obstruction

Intestinal obstruction during pregnancy is usually due to stretching by the enlarging uterus of adhesions formed from previous surgery. Other causes include volvulus, either of the small intestine or of the sigmoid colon, or other antecedents of intestinal obstruction encountered in nonpregnant patients. While the disease is rare in pregnancy, a high maternal and fetal risk has been reported, due primarily to failure either to make the diagnosis or to operate early enough. As with appendicitis, delay in performing necessary surgery is far more hazardous than an operation performed on the basis of an incorrect diagnosis.

Intestinal obstruction should be suspected in any patient with persistent vomiting and abdominal pain. While excessive bowel activity can usually be recognized by peristaltic rushes elicited by auscultation, a large uterus may obscure this finding. The clinician should not hesitate to order an x-ray film of the abdomen, which will usually reveal the stepladder pattern of air and fluid typical of bowel obstruction. Differentiation from the paralytic ileus that may result from ureteral colic or other lesions can be aided by noting whether or not the diminished peristaltic activity characteristic of ileus is present. Treatment of bowel obstruction may be by continuous bowel suction if the obstruction is partial, or by operation if the obstruction is complete.

PEPTIC ULCER

The symptoms of a preexisting peptic ulcer frequently subside or improve during pregnancy, perhaps because of the concurrent decrease in acid secretion by the stomach. Under exceptional circumstances, however, the symptoms of the ulcer are aggravated during pregnancy, and perforation or bleeding can occur. The treatment either of symptomatic uncomplicated peptic ulcer or of a complication of the ulcer are the same during pregnancy as in the nonpregnant patient. Indicated surgery should be performed without delay.

PANCREATITIS

Pancreatitis during pregnancy is rare. The diagnostic tests (serum amylase, etc.) and therapy (monitoring of fluid and electrolyte balance, nasogastric suction) are similar to those necessary in the nonpregnant patient. Maternal and perinatal mortality are both high. Of importance, however, is the reported relationship between the development of pancreatitis and the use of either tetracycline medication or thiazides during pregnancy. While rare, this complication of drug therapy in pregnancy is important because of the seriousness of the disease.

ULCERATIVE COLITIS

It is important to consider the emotional makeup of the pregnant patient with ulcerative colitis if a prediction regarding the effect of pregnancy on the disease is to be attempted. Indeed, psychogenic factors rather than physiologic ones probably account for any change in the course of colitis in pregnancy. Pregnancy appears to have little effect on the course of active disease, and the frequency of relapse is the same in pregnant and nonpregnant young women. In some patients the disease definitely improves during pregnancy. In others a flare-up of symptoms may occur, most often about the third month of gestation or during the puerperium. While quiescent disease during pregnancy exerts no deleterious effect on the pregnancy, the devastating pathologic changes in maternal fluid balance and nutrition with severe disease take their toll both in maternal risk and in perinatal mortality.

In general, therapy should be directed toward the diseased bowel and not toward the uterus. Total colectomy and ileostomy may be necessary if medical management fails. Therapy during pregnancy is little different from that employed for the nonpregnant patient, but the potential effects of medication, especially steroids, on the fetus must be taken into account. If steroids are administered, the dosage probably should be increased for two to four weeks following delivery to prevent the puerperal increase in symptoms occasionally encountered. Spontaneous labor and vaginal delivery can be anticipated. Cesarean section is recommended only for obstetrical indications.

Advice to the patient with ulcerative colitis concerning the feasibility of becoming pregnant should be based primarily on the length of time during which the disease has been quiescent. Certainly, pregnancy can be more safely undertaken if the patient has been symptom-free for a full year or two than if she has just recovered from an acute attack. A completely informed approach to the pregnancy decision must await an expansion of our knowledge of the factors that influence the course of this disease and the development of more effective therapy.

REGIONAL ILEITIS

Crohn's disease is not likely to exert any adverse effect on the pregnancy unless significant nutritional disturbances are present, and the effect of the pregnancy on the disease is usually not remarkable. Only a few patients experience an increase in symptoms, and no increased risk of maternal mortality has been reported. In the absence of malnutrition, the disease has no effect on the incidence of abortion, low birth weight, and fetal death.

CARCINOMA OF THE BOWEL

While carcinoma of the bowel is a rare disease in pregnancy, the importance of the lesion lies in the need to differentiate the rectal bleeding it causes from common hemorrhoidal bleeding. Since a high percentage of bowel carcinomas can be palpated with the examining finger, rectal bleeding should not be assumed to have been due to hemorrhoids without at least rectal palpation and probably sigmoidoscopy. Other associated symptoms of rectal carcinoma, i.e., tenesmus and a change in bowel habits, are later manifestations. The treatment of bowel cancer in pregnancy is surgical, just as in the nonpregnant patient. During the third trimester, cesarean section will be necessary before definitive bowel surgery can be performed. Pregnancy probably exerts no deleterious effect on the disease.

LIVER DISEASE

Viral Hepatitis

Viral hepatitis is an increasingly common complication of pregnancy. It may be transmitted to the patient either by the ingestion or parenteral administration of the infecting organism. There are two hepatitis viruses, with varying incubation periods and clinical courses. Hepatitis B virus is the infecting agent in long-incubation hepatitis (formerly called serum hepatitis) and hepatitis A virus, in the short-incubation form of the disease (formerly called infectious hepatitis). The severity of viral hepatitis in the pregnant as well as in the nonpregnant patient varies from a fulminant, often fatal, form to a mild form that may produce minimal symptoms. It is clear that in most cases of viral hepatitis, the patient is anicteric, and the condition may go undiagnosed. Pregnancy apparently exerts no unfavorable effect on the course of the disease; maternal mortality is not increased in a well-nourished population. A report from India indicates maternal mortality from hepatitis twice as high in pregnant women as in nonpregnant, probably because of the nutritional impoverishment of the patient population [23]. There is also an increase in fetal death and prematurity rates. The fetus may acquire the disease from contamination with maternal blood or feces at delivery.

The symptoms of early or mild viral hepatitis are essentially those of early pregnancy, i.e., tiredness, anorexia, nausea, and vomiting. Hyperbilirubinemia is usually present and may be clinically evidenced by jaundice. With more severe disease, fever is usual, and the liver is enlarged or tender. Since most of the results of the laboratory tests used to evaluate the hepatobiliary system are not altered by normal pregnancy, such tests may be useful in helping to establish the diagnosis. The most marked changes will be seen in serum glutamic-pyruvic transaminase (SGPT) and serum glutamic-oxaloacetic transaminase (SGOT) levels. Rarely, the clinical picture will be of extremely acute illness, with a rapid downhill course leading to lethargy, delirium, coma, and death (fulminant hepatitis). Treatment is nonspecific and supportive. The effect of therapeutic abortion on the course of the disease remains controversial. Since the patient who is most likely to require the procedure is already in a precarious clinical condition, most authorities warn against abortion.

The pathologic picture in viral hepatitis varies from mild portal and lobular inflammation to massive necrosis. While most patients with massive necrosis die, recovery, with parenchymal regeneration, occurs in 10 to 15 percent. In other instances, death is avoided, but permanent fibrosis and disrupted hepatic architecture lead to cirrhosis.

Treatment includes complete bed rest and adequate nutrition—parenteral nutrition if the patient cannot tolerate food orally. If labor supervenes, drugs that are metabolized in the liver should be avoided or employed in reduced dosage. There is no evidence that corticosteroids exert a beneficial effect on viral hepatitis.

The outcome of viral hepatitis is unpredictable, and essentially nothing is known about the factors underlying mild versus severe or fatal episodes. Type A hepatitis can be transmitted orally or parenterally. It tends to have a more acute onset than does type B hepatitis and a very low mortality except in the uncommon fulminant form. It has an incubation period of two to six weeks and occurs at a younger average age than does type B hepatitis. The hepatitis-associated antigen (HAA) is not found in this type of hepatitis, and chronic or late sequelae do not appear to occur. Type B hepatitis is commonly transmitted parenterally, but infection can occur by the fecal-oral route as well. Its clinical onset is usually more gradual than that of type A hepatitis, with an incubation period of six weeks to six months. It carries a higher overall mortality, is HAA-positive in 50 to 60 percent of cases, and carries a risk of progression to chronic liver disease in the form of subacute hepatic necrosis (bridging necrosis), chronic active hepatitis, and macronodular cirrhosis.

Acute Steatosis of Pregnancy

Acute steatosis of pregnancy is a rare disorder, occurring primarily in the third trimester and characterized by a massive accumulation of fat within the liver, associated with minimal necrosis and little or no inflammation. Although the spontaneous form is of unknown cause, it bears a striking pathological and clinical resemblance to tetracycline toxicity. Maternal mortality is high.

Tetracycline Toxicity

Tetracycline toxicity is manifested by a fatty liver, often with liver failure, azotemia, and pancreatitis. Most, though not all, cases occur during pregnancy and appear to be the result either of excessive dosage of tetracycline or depressed renal function leading to high serum and tissue levels of tetracycline. Anorexia, nausea, vomiting, abdominal discomfort, and jaundice are present, and the clinical picture resembles that of viral hepatitis. Laboratory abnormalities include hyperbilirubinemia, hypoprothrombinemia, and varying, but often marked, elevation of SGOT. Fetal and maternal mortality is high, with coma and shock the terminal event. Treatment for acute steatosis of pregnancy, whether or not it is related to tetracycline administration, is supportive, including dialysis.

Recurrent Cholestasis of Pregnancy

Recurrent cholestasis of pregnancy occurs in the third trimester and is characterized by pruritus, anorexia, nausea, and often jaundice. Pathologically, there is an intrahepatic cholestasis, which will be reflected in the clinical laboratory primarily by an increase in bilirubin, alkaline phosphatase, and cholesterol; SGOT elevations are minimal. Estrogens are believed to be responsible, since they are markedly elevated at this time and are known to produce an impairment in hepatic excretory function. The syndrome tends to recur with each subsequent pregnancy or with the administration of estrogen-containing compounds in the nonpregnant state. The maternal course is benign and requires no treatment. If pruritus is severe, cholestyramine administration may be helpful. Recent evidence suggests an increased perinatal mortality risk [24].

GALLBLADDER DISEASE

Although cholelithiasis is much more frequent in women than in men, and cholelithiasis requiring surgery is more common in women who have borne children than in nulligravidas, neither cholelithiasis nor cholecystitis is common during pregnancy. There is no explanation of this apparent paradox.

When an attack of acute cholecystitis occurs during pregnancy, management should not be influenced by the pregnancy. If surgery is indicated, it should be performed without delay. Abortion rarely follows needed surgery. All the complications of gallstones found in nonpregnant women may also occur with pregnancy and should be managed without respect to the pregnancy.

Disorders of the Reproductive Tract

DISEASES OF THE VULVA, VAGINA, AND CERVIX

Varicosities

Vulvar varicosities of any severity are uncommon during pregnancy but are more common in multiparas than in primigravidas. Symptoms include a sense of heaviness or local irritation. Complications are rare but include bleeding, either spontaneous or from the trauma of delivery. While injection of a sclerosing solution into the varicosities has been reported to be of help, we prefer symptomatic treatment with bed rest and a perineal pressure device to be worn while the patient is ambulatory. Varicosities in this location usually disappear after delivery.

Bartholin's Gland Infection and Cyst Formation

Infection in Bartholin's glands may be due to gonococci or to a number of other pathogenic organisms. Abscess formation is frequently the first clinical evidence of the disease, and severe pain and tenderness are experienced by the patient. If an abscess forms during pregnancy, incision and drainage is indicated to attempt to prevent ascending infection from rupture of the abscess during labor. The incision is made at the mucocutaneous junction, and the wall of the abscess cavity should be sutured to the adjoining skin or mucous membrane to provide marsupialization. A rubber or gauze drain should be inserted and maintained in the cavity until granulation is complete.

A cyst of a Bartholin's gland duct is usually pre-

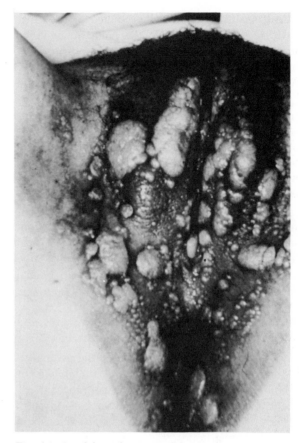

Fig. 4-1. Condyloma latum (syphilis).

ceded by a Bartholin abscess. The treatment in the nonpregnant patient is incision and marsupialization. It may be wise to postpone the surgery until after delivery, since the cyst is rarely large enough to obstruct labor and since elective surgery is better performed when the patient is not pregnant.

Condyloma Acuminatum

Condyloma acuminatum of the vulva and vagina, which is of uncertain etiology, must be differentiated from condyloma latum due to the *Treponema pallidum* of syphilis (Fig. 4-1). Condylomata lata are small *flat* papules that are highly contagious and show the causative organism when smeared on a slide and identified by a dark-field examination. Condylomata acuminata, on the other hand, are usually somewhat pointed papules that may become confluent to the point of involving large areas of skin or vaginal mucous membrane. Either lesion can also occur on the cervix. Condylomata acuminata seem to occur in patients with poor vaginal and vulvar hygiene, and the appearnace of the lesion on the genitalia of the male partner is common.

Treatment of condyloma latum is parenteral penicillin in adequate dosage. Treatment of condyloma acuminatum is local, either with podophyllin in 25% solution for small lesions or, in extensive lesions, with dessication by electrocautery or cryocautery. Extensive vaginal lesions occasionally disappear or improve markedly with a topical sulfonamide cream. If the lesions involve large areas of the vagina at the time of labor, abdominal delivery may be necessary to prevent hemorrhage from lacerations.

Other Vaginal Problems

VAGINITIS. Vaginitis is common during pregnancy and is usually due to a *Trichomonas, Candida,* or *Hemophilus* organism, as in the nonpregnant patient. Conventional treatment of vaginitis in pregnancy is notoriously unsuccessful. Mycostatin vaginal suppositories, for example, suppress the symptoms of candidal vaginitis very quickly, but the disease recurs after discontinuation of the treatment. The therapy of vaginitis during pregnancy must therefore be considered symptomatic until the pregnancy terminates.

VAGINAL CYSTS. Vaginal cysts, usually due to embryologic rests (Gartner's duct or the müllerian duct), seldom cause serious trouble during pregnancy, since they are usually small. Rarely, the cyst may be large enough to obstruct labor and require excision. Extremely rare tumors, such as a carcinoma or sarcoma of the vagina, may occur during pregnancy. The treatment is appropriate tumor therapy, with little regard for the pregnancy.

Carcinoma of the Cervix

Invasive carcinoma of the cervix is preceded by a noninvasive carcinoma (carcinoma in situ) in most cases. Carcinoma in situ is thought to remain noninvasive in most instances for many years, but it is not likely to regress to a normal histologic state. In similar fashion, carcinoma in situ is usually preceded by dysplasia of the cervix, but not all cervical dysplasia proceeds to carcinoma in situ. Indeed, many dysplastic lesions are thought to revert to a histologically normal state.

In discussing carcinoma of the cervix during pregnancy, it is necessary to consider not only invasive carcinoma but also the lesions thought to precede the invasion. Certain histologic changes that are pregnancy-induced must also be considered, notably basal cell hyperplasia, since this lesion presents a problem in differential diagnosis.

INVASIVE CERVICAL CARCINOMA. Invasive carcinoma of the cervix during pregnancy has increased in frequency in recent years, probably due to improved case-finding techniques. The incidence of the disease varies widely from clinic to clinic, depending primarily on the type of patient population served. However, an average incidence of 1 case per 1500 to 2000 deliveries is a reasonable estimate. Since the disease is usually preceded by a noninvasive carcinoma, the diagnosis of invasion during pregnancy implies that a cervical lesion has been present for some time and has been overlooked, either because the patient has failed to have routine pelvic examinations or because a Pap test has not been performed. The importance of routine cancer screening examinations cannot be overemphasized.

Diagnosis. The diagnosis of invasive carcinoma may be suspected when the patient presents the usual symptom of the disease, i.e., abnormal vaginal bleeding, especially on contact. Although most pregnant patients who report vaginal bleeding during pregnancy will be found to be experiencing an abortion or have benign cervical disease, this is not always so. Thus, any abnormal bleeding should be thoroughly investigated with a pelvic examination and Pap smear. In some cases of early invasive carcinoma of the cervix, no symptoms will be present, and the diagnosis will be made only by routine Pap smear and biopsy. This set of circumstances is discussed under the diagnosis of preinvasive carcinoma. The examination of the patient may reveal an obvious ulceration of the cervix, or, in some cases, the cervix may appear entirely normal. The diagnosis is established by punch biopsy of the obvious lesion or by biopsy of an area of the cervix found to be abnormal by colposcopic examination.

Treatment. Treatment of invasive carcinoma of the cervix will vary, depending on the extent of the disease and on the length of gestation at the time the diagnosis is made. If the diagnosis is established during the first trimester of pregnancy, external radiation to the cervix and to the pelvis is begun without regard to the pregnancy. Within two to four weeks, abortion usually occurs, following which radium in appropriate dosage is applied to the cervix. If abortion fails to occur, hysterotomy is essential, since the radiation will have adversely affected the fetus.

If the diagnosis is made during the middle trimester, abdominal hysterotomy is followed by external radiation and radium therapy. If the diagnosis is made after 28 weeks of gestation, a delay of a few weeks probably will not unfavorably affect the prognosis, and delivery by cesarean section at 34 to 36 weeks' gestation, followed by external radiation and radium, may be chosen by the patient. Some clinics perform a radical hysterectomy and a pelvic node dissection in place of radiation therapy for patients with stage 1B and stage 2A disease, and the results are equally good. The participation of an experienced cancer surgeon, however, is absolutely essential in this instance, just as an experienced radiologist is needed for radiotherapy. Stage 1A (early stromal invasion) may be treated by a total hysterectomy with excision of a wide cuff of vagina. With this one exception, there is no place for simple hysterectomy in the treatment of invasive carcinoma of the cervix.

Prognosis. The prognosis of invasive carcinoma of the cervix in pregnancy is unchanged, stage for stage, from the prognosis in nonpregnant patients of the same age. One exception to this rule is suggested by reports of lower five-year survival rates when the diagnosis is made very late in pregnancy or during the puerperium. The reason for this variation is uncertain, but failure to make the diagnosis early seems a likely explanation.

CARCINOMA IN SITU AND DYSPLASIA OF THE CERVIX. *Diagnosis*. The diagnosis of carcinoma in situ or dysplasia of the cervix must be made on the basis of routine Pap smears, since neither disease causes any symptoms. Routine Pap smear during pregnancy will yield about 3 to 5 patients per 1000 with carcinoma in situ and a larger number with cervical dysplasia of some degree. The incidence of carcinoma in situ is highest among multiparas who began childbearing at an early age. The diagnosis is based on certain histologic criteria, which include a specific alteration of the cells of the cervical squamous epithelium *throughout the entire thickness* of the epithelium with demonstration of an intact basal membrane (Fig. 4-2). Dysplasia is diagnosed when the cellular changes are similar but fail to extend through the entire thickness of the epithelium. The interested reader is referred to a more complete description of the histology of these lesions in a gynecologic text.

The diagnosis in a particular patient is suggested, first of all, by the reading of the Pap smear. A Class I report indicates that no malignant cells were seen; with Class II there are abnormal cells, but they are not malignant; a Class III smear contains suspicious cells, but they are not definitely malignant; with a Class IV smear, definite malignant cells were seen by the cytologist, and with Class V the malignant cells were seen in greater numbers and sometimes in more bizarre form. To generalize, patients with Class I and Class II smears are usually free of malignant disease; some patients with Class III smears will exhibit cervical dysplasia or occasionally carcinoma in situ; Class IV patients will usually have carcinoma in situ; and patients with Class V smears may have carcinoma in situ or invasive carcinoma. A report of a Class III, IV, or V smear demands a repeat smear; if the original report is confirmed, histologic investigation is essential.

To establish a histologic diagnosis (1) take multiple punch biopsies of all suspicious areas that fail to stain with Lugol's solution, (2) perform a cold-knife conization under anesthesia with excision of the

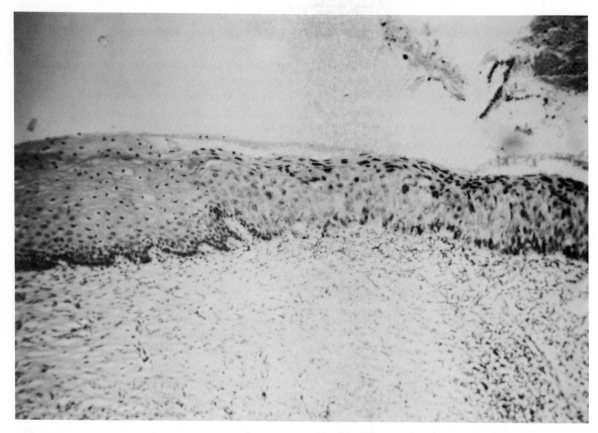

Fig. 4-2. Microscopic appearance of carcinoma in situ of the cervix. Normal cervical squamous epithelium is on the left; carcinoma in situ is on the right.

squamocolumnar junction as well as all nonstaining areas, (3) biopsy all areas that appear suspicious through a colposcope. Colposcopically directed biopsies offer the most precise diagnosis and the least trauma. If a colposcope is unavailable, another method may be used.

The histologic findings usually reflect the lesion predicted by the Pap smear report. If there is a discrepancy, further diagnostic steps are indicated. If cervical dysplasia, for example, is the pathologic diagnosis on a patient with a Class V smear, it is essential either to take more punch biopsies or to request the pathologist to cut more sections from the cone specimen. It should be remembered that the cervix may contain invasive carcinoma, carcinoma in situ, and simple dysplasia in different portions.

Treatment. When it is certain that the cervix contains no lesion more serious than carcinoma in situ, a treatment plan should be formulated. It is usually best to follow the status of the lesion by repeat Pap smears and pelvic examinations throughout the remainder of the pregnancy and to allow vaginal delivery. A change in the lesion, of course, may alter this plan of management. Further investigation of the lesion in the puerperium will dictate further treatment. If there is no progression of the disease, the treatment for carcinoma in situ may be by cryotherapy, by therapeutic conization, or by simple hysterectomy with excision of a 2-cm. vaginal cuff, depending on the seriousness of the diagnosis. Dysplasia may be treated, usually with cryotherapy. Inadequate destruction or a recurrence of the disease will be revealed by repeated Pap smears posttherapy.

During normal pregnancy, hyperplasia of the basal cells of the cervix may be so intense under the influence of estrogen that a confusing Pap-smear picture may result. Since basal cell hyperplasia is thought to be a reversible lesion, it is important that this pathologic change be differentiated from dysplasia or carcinoma in situ. Biopsy of the cervix should allow the pathologist to make the appropriate diagnosis.

DISPLACEMENT OF THE UTERUS

Anteflexion

Extreme anteflexion of the uterus in early pregnancy is common and is rarely of clinical significance. Later in pregnancy, a relaxed abdominal wall may permit protrusion of the uterus anteriorly, sometimes to an extreme degree in the multigravida. If the protrusion is severe, the longitudinal axis of the uterus may assume a right angle to the pelvic inlet. Abnormal positions of the fetus are common with anteflexion, and a transverse lie or lack of engagement with a longitudinal lie may be noted. The patient may experience backache and pelvic discomfort, as well as extreme fatigue. A well-fitted girdle or a tight abdominal binder may sometimes compensate for the poor abdominal muscle support and correct the pathologic condition, thus allowing better fetopelvic orientation.

Retrodisplacement

Uterine retroflexion, or retroversion, is commonly seen among nonpregnant patients. Since there is no evidence that the condition predisposes to infertility, as once thought, it is not surprising that a retrodisplacement of the uterus is a frequent finding in early pregnancy. The retrodisplacement rarely causes difficulty, although the diagnosis of very early pregnancy is less certain than with an anterior position of the uterus. In most instances, the retrodisplacement is corrected as the uterus enlarges and requires more room to grow than that provided by the pelvic cavity. In rare cases, incarceration of the retroverted uterus in the pelvis is seen, resulting in urinary symptoms as the major patient complaint. As the uterus enlarges, the cervix is pushed increasingly anteriorly toward the bladder and urethra, and incomplete emptying of the bladder results. If the incarceration is not corrected, complete urinary retention develops, necessitating catheterization. With the patient in the knee-chest position and with a tenaculum on the anterior lip of the cervix to provide countertraction, vaginal pressure on the posterior wall of the uterus will usually correct the displacement. Occasionally, anesthesia is required for the maneuver; every more rarely, simple measures will fail, and a laparotomy will be necessary.

Prolapse of the Uterus

Pregnancy in a patient with procidentia is extremely rare, partially, at least, because coitus is impossible unless the uterus is manually replaced. Pregnancy in patients with lesser degrees of prolapse is not uncommon, and the lesion rarely causes any difficulty. While the prolapse may be evident for the first 12 to 16 weeks of gestation, the enlarging uterus eventually rises out of the pelvis and draws the cervix up with it; but if the pregnancy has taken place with complete procidentia, this event will not occur, and if the uterus cannot be replaced manually, abortion is inevitable.

Treatment of partial prolapse of the uterus during pregnancy with a well-fitting pessary is usually possible. Sometimes, the degree of relaxation of the vaginal walls will not permit retention of the pessary. Hygienic care of the protruding cervix is important, since infection is an ever-present threat.

Torsion of the Pregnant Uterus

While rare, torsion of the pregnant uterus is important because of its clinical picture, which can be confused with abruptio placentae or some other abdominal catastrophe. Abdominal pain and shock are the major symptoms. The treatment is immediate laparotomy with detorsion in early pregnancy and cesarean section near term. Hysterectomy is frequently necessary. The condition is associated with some other pelvic abnormality in 80 percent of cases, i.e., bicornuate uterus, uterine fibromyomas, pelvic adhesions, or previous uterine suspension. The maternal mortality has been reported as high as 50 percent, with an even higher perinatal mortality.

UTERINE MYOMAS

Uterine myomas are very common tumors, especially in the black race. In the vast majority of instances, they do not interfere with conception, pregnancy, or labor. In a minority of cases, however, they complicate the reproductive process by interfering with conception, causing early abortion, predisposing to abnormal presentations, producing symptoms of abdominal disease during pregnancy, obstructing labor, or complicating the puerperium.

While most patients with uterine myomas experience no difficulty in achieving pregnancy, some patients are infertile, especially those with submucous myoma that interferes with endometrial physiologic processes. If pregnancy is achieved in these patients, the risk of abortion is increased, due to interference with nidation or with the blood supply to the conceptus. Myomas may also confuse the diagnosis of early pregnancy, since uterine enlargement is noted both with pregnancy and with a myoma, and because softness of the uterus may not be appreciated when tumors are present.

Uterine myomas usually enlarge during pregnancy, and degeneration of a myoma, perhaps as it outgrows its blood supply, may be a consequence. Red, or carneous, degeneration is particularly likely to occur during pregnancy, producing a clinical picture of abdominal pain, uterine tenderness, mild leukocytosis, and a slightly elevated temperature. Surgery is not necessary if the diagnosis can be established, although the differential diagnosis from more serious abdominal disease is not always easy. After sedation and rest for a day or two, the symptoms of the degeneration usually subside.

The presence of uterine myomas predisposes to an abnormal presentation, especially breech presentation. The tumors may also interfere with uterine contractility and cause uterine dysfunction during labor. In some instances, they obstruct the birth canal sufficiently to prevent vaginal delivery. Prediction during early pregnancy whether or not a particular myoma will cause pelvic obstruction is at best uncertain, and the diagnosis of obstructed labor should not be made until the patient is at term or in labor. While a myoma in the lower uterine segment may enlarge during pregnancy, it may also rise above the pelvic brim and cause no complication whatsoever. Cesarean section is necessary in an obstructed labor.

Management of the third stage of labor and the puerperium may be complicated by the presence of myomas. If the tumor is submucous, separation of the placenta may be incomplete, and manual removal may be necessary. During this procedure, the myoma may be torn loose from the uterus, with severe hemorrhage as a consequence. Transfusion and immediate hysterectomy are usually necessary to manage the patient. The puerperium may be complicated by postpartum bleeding from poor uterine contractility or by degeneration of a myoma, causing diagnostic confusion with other intra-abdominal disease.

The role of myomectomy before pregnancy, during pregnancy, or at the time of cesarean section remains an unsettled issue. Myomectomy to improve fertility or to prevent an early pregnancy loss due to abortion is probably best reserved for the patient with a submucous myoma. With careful patient selection, a judicious myomectomy apparently increases the chances of pregnancy and decreases the risks of abortion. Delivery by cesarean section is probably wise in these patients, just as in patients who have had a previous section. There are few advocates of myomectomy during pregnancy unless major degeneration has necessitated laparotomy. Myomectomy at the time of cesarean section performed either because of obstructed labor or for another indication is considered unwise by most clinicians because of the risk of hemorrhage or postoperative infection. Although the procedure seems a good one in certain instances, a hysterectomy is probably a better operation for most patients.

Infections

While pregnant women seem no more susceptible to most infections than others, an infectious disease in pregnancy is frequently more severe than in nonpregnant patients. Acute infection during pregnancy may adversely affect the pregnancy in a number of ways. The maternal mortality is increased with many diseases; the risk of abortion, premature labor, and fetal death is also increased. Some diseases (notably rubella, cytomegalovirus disease, and herpes simplex) are teratogenic. Transplacental spread of viral, bacterial, fungal, and parasitic disease has been shown to occur even with diseases presumed not to be teratogenic. Antibiotic medication has altered the course of bacterial disease and of viral disease complicated by superimposed bacterial disease, but most viral diseases continue to run a typical course.

VIRAL DISEASES
Rubella
Rubella (German measles) is a mild and innocuous disease in the nonpregnant individual but of enormous consequence when it occurs during pregnancy. Gregg [25], in 1942, first reported an association between rubella during early pregnancy and serious congenital malformation in the infant. Gregg's observations have subsequently been confirmed by many investigators, and only the degree of risk has been argued.

The earlier in the pregnancy the maternal infection occurs, the higher the risk of effects on the fetus. Maternal infection during the first month is followed by embryopathy in perhaps 35 percent of cases, with a decrease to about 10 to 15 percent in the third month. Hardy et al. [26] have shown a risk even after the twelfth week of pregnancy. Since viremia may persist for many weeks following rubella infection, the risk of embryopathy is great when the infection occurs just before pregnancy begins.

Unless rubella occurs during an epidemic, it may

be especially difficult to diagnose because of minimal physical findings. The unreliability of data from the history regarding previous rubella infection has been demonstrated in pregnant women. For this reason, many clinics now perform a rubella antibody titer to identify women at risk for rubella during pregnancy. A negative or low titer suggests susceptibility to the disease; a high titer suggests immunity; and a rising titer suggests a recent active infection. This information may be vitally important, especially during an epidemic, when therapeutic abortion is a consideration because of presumed infection during pregnancy.

Fetal infection may lead to a variety of malformations, including congenital heart disease, deafness, cataracts or other eye lesions, thrombocytopenia and anemia, hepatosplenomegaly, and bone changes. Intrauterine growth retardation is common, and microcephaly is particularly common with disease after the third month. A newborn so affected may shed the virus for many weeks or months and thus be a source of spread. The administration to the gravida of immune gamma globulin, presumably containing a high titer or rubella antibody, has not consistently reduced the risk of fetal infection. Indeed, there is some evidence that the gamma globulin may mask the signs and symptoms of maternal disease yet not prevent the embryopathy.

Immunization against rubella by the use of live attenuated virus is now feasible. The immunization should *not* be done during pregnancy, since the virus has been shown to lodge in the fetus, with unknown effects. If the vaccine is to be used in a woman of childbearing age, she *must* agree to avoid pregnancy with an effective contraceptive for two to three months following the injection. If pregnancy should occur, or if the patient proves to have been pregnant at the time of the injection, abortion should probably be recommended. The immediate portpartum period is an ideal time for immunization.

Cytomegalovirus
Cytomegalovirus infection usually produces no recognizable symptoms in the mother yet may have

a devastating effect on the fetus, including microcephaly, hydrocephaly, cerebral calcification, blindness, and seizures. Fortunately, although 3 percent of women excrete cytomegalovirus during pregnancy, only a few deliver an abnormal infant.

Herpesvirus Hominis

According to Sever [27], transplacental passage of the herpesvirus, though rare, may occur, with resultant microcephaly, cerebral calcification, and retinal dysplasia in the newborn. More commonly, infection in the newborn results from passage through a birth canal infected with herpes (Fig. 4-3). Generalized herpes in the newborn may result, with involvement of the spleen, liver, lungs, and adrenals and an almost universally fatal outcome. Cesarean section is usually recommended when genital herpes is recognized within four weeks of delivery, to minimize the risk of fetal infection. No safe and effective treatment for genital herpes is in general use.

Influenza

The availability of antibiotic medication has greatly improved the prognosis for pregnant women who have influenza. The main cause of death in the 1918 pandemic was a complicating pneumonia or other bacterial invasion. Although antibiotics are ineffective against the virus, bacterial complications may be prevented by their use, and if they occur, the disease will respond to such medication. The incidence of the disease during an epidemic has been shown to be higher in infants, debilitated people, and pregnant women. It was shown in the 1957 epidemic of Asian influenza that pregnant women are more likely to experience severe disease than are nonpregnant women. Of women of childbearing age dying of the disease, 50 percent were pregnant [28]; these deaths occurred despite the availability of antibiotics. The need for vigorous treatment of the disease when it occurs in pregnant women is evident. During an epidemic, immunization of pregnant women seems a wise precaution for maternal safety. No teratogenic potential of influenza has been recognized. The abortion risk is said to be increased by this disease.

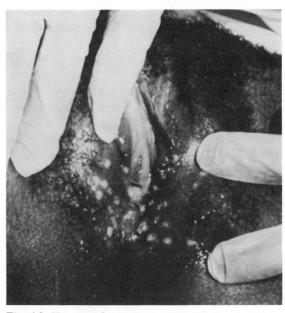

Fig. 4-3. Herpes vulvae.

Other Viral Diseases

Mumps occurs in only about 1 in 1000 pregnant women in a nonepidemic year. An increased risk of abortion or congenital defect if the infection occurs early in pregnancy is suspected but not proved. *Measles* is much less common during pregnancy than mumps, because most young girls either have had the disease during childhood or have been immunized before bearing children. An increased risk of abortion or of a congenital defect is suspected but not shown conclusively to result from measles during pregnancy. *Poliomyelitis* is both more frequent and more severe in pregnant than in nonpregnant women. Fortunately, the disease has become a rarity because of routine immunization. *Smallpox* is virtually nonexistent in the United States because of vaccination but is associated with an extremely high fetal mortality; intrauterine infection of the fetus occurs. During an epidemic, vaccination should be encouraged, since the hazards of maternal cow pox viremia are almost certainly less than those of maternal smallpox. *Chickenpox* rarely complicates pregnancy but may have a fulminant course that ends in death.

BACTERIAL DISEASE

Bacterial disease during pregnancy is likely to respond to an appropriate antibiotic, usually with minimal maternal or fetal harm. Severe, long-standing acute infection is associated with an increased risk of abortion or premature labor, perhaps because of the resultant hyperthermia.

Both *scarlet fever* and *erysipelas* are rare during pregnancy. The causative organism of both diseases, *Streptococcus pyogenes,* is sensitive to penicillin, and treatment is usually rapidly curative. Of extreme importance is the isolation of such a patient from other obstetrical patients, since an epidemic of puerperal sepsis may ensue from spread of the organism. Recently, a less virulent group B streptococcus (*S. agalactiae*), a normal constituent of the vaginal flora in as high as 25 percent of women, has become a common cause of perinatal infection. Infection during passage through the birth canal may result in serious neonatal infection, especially in the premature infant.

Typhoid fever rarely complicates pregnancy because the disease has been largely eradicated by public health measures and immunization procedures. When the disease has occurred in the past, an extremely high fetal mortality (75 percent) and a high maternal mortality (15 percent) has resulted. Chloramphenicol is an effective treatment, and a much reduced fetal and maternal risk should attend its use. Immunization of gravidas with killed typhoid bacteria is certainly warranted during an epidemic.

Listeria monocytogenes is thought to be a cause for abortion. Late in pregnancy, transplacental or ascending infection from the vaginal tract can lead to serious and often fatal infection in the newborn.

VENEREAL DISEASE

Syphilis

Syphilis is a serious complication of pregnancy. If it is not treated, fetal infection will lead to the ravages of congenital syphilis. If the disease is diagnosed before 16 weeks' gestation and treated

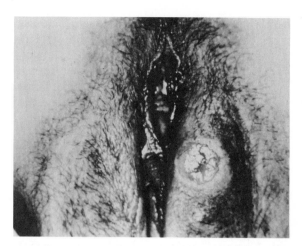

Fig. 4-4. Chancre of vulva.

adequately, no fetal stigmata will result, since the fetus is rarely infected before that time. Prompt treatment of the gravida even after 16 weeks' gestation will minimize the effects of the disease on the fetus, since most drugs used for treatment cross the placenta with ease.

The disease is increasingly common in young adults, at least partially because the condom is used infrequently for contraception today. The primary lesion, the chancre (Fig. 4-4), develops after an incubation period of 10 to 90 days and may appear on the labia, vagina, or cervix, as well as in the mouth or on the breast. The chancre is a painless ulcer that heals slowly with scar formation. In many cases, the primary lesion is missed, and the first evidence of the disease is a secondary lesion two to twelve weeks after the appearance of the chancre. Secondary manifestations of the disease include a generalized skin eruption that may mimic many other skin diseases, or condyloma latum of the genitalia, a lesion consisting of broad, flat, wartlike growths. If the patient is not treated, the myriad of manifestations of late syphilis develop.

Diagnosis of the primary lesion is best made by dark-field identification of the *Treponema pallidum* from material collected from the lesion. The dark-field examination may also be positive with the skin lesions of secondary lues, but serologic testing is usually more dependable at this stage. The diagnosis of late syphilis is dependent on serologic testing. The Venereal Disease Research Laboratory (VDRL) test is the test most often used for this purpose, although it is relatively nonspecific for syphilis and may be reactive to other diseases. Specific antibodies to *Treponema* may be identified by using the fluorescent treponemal antibody absorption test (FTA-ABS).

Since the disease so often fails to produce symptoms that become evident to the patient, it is best to screen *all* gravidas with the VDRL early in pregnancy (before the sixteenth week) and again in late pregnancy, since infection may occur at any time during pregnancy as well as before pregnancy. Confirmation of a positive VDRL with the FTA-ABS will make the diagnosis. Examination of spinal fluid is necessary before treatment is instituted for secondary or late syphilis, since the treatment of neurosyphilis requires larger doses of penicillin than does syphilis affecting other systems.

Treatment with 2.4 million units of benzathine penicillin G given simultaneously in two sites by the intramuscular route is preferred for primary or secondary disease. (Much larger doses of penicillin are required for late syphilis.) Most authorities recommend a similar dose one to two weeks later to assure a cure. A rise in the VDRL titer indicates the need for retreatment. When penicillin is contraindicated, erythromycin in a dose of 500 mg. orally four times a day for twenty days may be given before 16 weeks' gestation. Since erythromycin may not cross the placenta in effective dose levels, cephaloridine (1 gm. intramuscularly daily for 10 days) should be used after 16 weeks. Tetracycline, while effective, should be avoided because of the risk of fetal dental staining.

Gonorrhea

Exposure to gonorrhea is not limited to nonpregnant women. Pregnancy, however, at least after the first trimester, provides relative protection against ascending gonorrheal infection, perhaps because of the close approximation of the chorion laeve to the decidua parietalis. Infection in the lower genital tract (cervix, vagina, periurethral glands, or Bar-

tholin's glands) is just as prevalent as in the nonpregnant population and has been found in 5 percent of patients attending some prenatal clinics.

Gonorrhea may have devastating effects on the gravida and her offspring. Untreated disease often leads to gonococcal ophthalmia neonatorum in the newborn child. The disease in the mother can be expected to ascend to the fallopian tubes and other adnexal structures after delivery has occurred. Gonococcal arthritis can and does occur during pregnancy.

The diagnosis is made by smear and culture of the cervix and the rectum. The smear may reveal gram-negative diplococci, but a negative smear does not rule out disease. A culture is rolled onto a Thayer-Martin medium from a cotton-tipped application. The culture is kept in a 10 percent carbon dioxide atmosphere by placing it in a candle jar before transfer to the laboratory. Repeat cultures are needed in 6 to 8 percent of gravidas to make the diagnosis.

Treatment is with aqueous procaine penicillin G, 4.8 million units intramuscularly injected simultaneously in divided doses in two sites. The medication is preceded by an oral dose of 1 gm. of probenecid just before injection. If penicillin is contraindicated, erythromycin or spectinomycin may be substituted. Erythromycin is given orally in an initial dose of 1.5 gm., followed by 0.5 gm. four times a day for five days. Spectinomycin is effective in a single intramuscular dose of 2 gm., but its effect on the fetus has not been established. Effective treatment is demonstrated by negative cultures 7 to 14 days after therapy. Most "recurrences" are probably due to reinfection, but when true treatment failure occurs, spectinomycin can be used.

MISCELLANEOUS INFECTIONS

Malaria

Malaria, while not common in the United States, complicates pregnancy with some frequency in some parts of the world. Pregnancy aggravates the disease by increasing the severity of acute attacks and by causing exacerbation of a chronic process. Abortion and premature labor are increased with the disease, and infestation of the placenta—and less often, of the fetus—is well recognized. The commonly administered antimalarial drugs may be used during pregnancy. Quinine crosses the placenta and in larger doses may cause congenital deafness in the newborn. Pyrimethamine is a highly teratogenic drug.

Toxoplasmosis

Toxoplasmosis complicates pregnancy occasionally and may cause congenital disease by transplacental infection, especially if the disease occurs in the third trimester. The immediate manifestations include low birth weight, microcephaly, and hydrocephalus. Delayed manifestations of mental retardation and seizure activity may also be noted. The reservoir of the disease is the feces of the house cat as well as uncooked pork, lamb, and occasionally beef.

Coccidioidomycosis

Coccidioidomycosis is a fungal disease endemic to the southwestern United States. The disease is spread by inhalation of spores from infected soil. Although it usually runs a benign course, the disease can be overwhelming and fatal within a short period of time. Pregnancy appears to increase the risk of dissemination of the disease, with a resulting exacerbation. Surgical therapy (lobectomy) or medical therapy (amphotericin B) may be indicated. The drug is highly toxic to the mother and is used only with severe disease. The fetal effects of the drug are uncertain.

Disorders of the Nervous System

SUBARACHNOID HEMORRHAGE

Subarachnoid hemorrhage secondary to rupture of a congenital aneurysm is a common cause of maternal death. The potential frequency of this complication has been emphasized by Hunt et al. [29], who estimate that between 20,000 and 40,000 women with an intact congenital aneurysm of the brain deliver annually in the United States. Few of these aneurysms rupture during pregnancy. However, if it should occur, treatment of the patient

should be aggressive, according to Pool [30]. He reported a maternal mortality greater than 70 percent from recurrent hemorrhage among patients managed by observation alone, while less than 8 percent of gravidas treated surgically died. In the latter group, the fetal mortality was only 4 percent.

Delivery of the patient who has recovered from a previous ruptured aneurysm before pregnancy should be by the vaginal route unless there is an obstetrical indication for section. An abbreviated second stage of labor to avoid excessive bearing-down efforts is recommended by most, but not all, authorities.

EPILEPSY

Pregnancy has no predictable effect on epilepsy, and exacerbation of the disease may be on the basis of forgotten or missed medication. Good medical control of the disease is usually attained with diphenylhydantoin (Dilantin) and phenobarbital, and these drugs may be continued throughout pregnancy.

The hereditary effect of the disease will depend primarily on whether the cause of the convulsions is known (e.g., trauma) or unknown (idiopathic). An increase in the incidence of epilepsy in the offspring of a patient with idiopathic disease can be expected. Speidel and Madden [31] have demonstrated a doubling in the incidence of major congenital malformations among children born of epileptic mothers. These same authors also reported a doubling in the perinatal mortality that was apparently unrelated to the use of anticonvulsant drugs. Certain anticonvulsant drugs (diphenylhydantoin, trimethadione) used during pregnancy in patients with epilepsy are associated with an increased risk of congenital malformation. Whether the increase is due entirely to the drug or to the epilepsy as well as the drug remains controversial [32].

The decision for therapeutic abortion in the epileptic patient should be based primarily on the effect of the disease on the ability of the woman to care for the child after delivery, not on the effect of pregnancy on the disease. If the mother is uncertain that she can cope with child rearing because of her disease and desires abortion for this reason, the request seems reasonable.

MULTIPLE SCLEROSIS

Multiple sclerosis, a disseminated disease of the central nervous system of unknown etiology, has its peak incidence during the reproductive years. It is characterized by remissions and exacerbations during pregnancy, just as in nonpregnant patients. Predominant opinion is that pregnancy exerts no consistent effect on the disease process. The disease has little influence on the pregnancy unless the patient is severely debilitated. In this case, the bearing-down efforts of the second stage of labor may be absent, although the first stage usually progresses uneventfully. Therapeutic abortion is reserved for the patient who does not want the responsibility of child care.

OTHER DISEASES

Patients with *myasthenia gravis* usually do well during pregnancy, although the prostigmine dosage may have to be either increased or decreased; which will be necessary is not predictable. While labor is usually uneventful, the choice of analgesic and anesthetic agents assumes great importance. The neonate may be affected with the disease, and careful drug control during the newborn nursery period is necessary. The disease in the neonate usually lasts only two to four weeks after birth.

The importance of *Huntington's chorea* during pregnancy lies in the 50:50 chance of genetic transmission of the disease, which is inherited as a dominant autosomal trait. Therapeutic abortion seems wise. *Brain tumors* may enlarge rapidly during pregnancy, probably because of engorgement of cerebral vessels. The hearing loss of *otosclerosis* may accelerate during pregnancy, and, in this case, therapeutic abortion may be offered.

Diseases of the Skin and Connective Tissue

SKIN CHANGES

Certain changes in the skin or its appendages occur with some frequency during pregnancy and the puerperium.

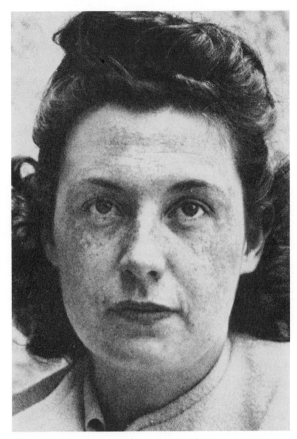

Fig. 4-5. Chloasma, also known as the "mask of pregnancy," is recognized by a typical increased pigmentation in a butterfly pattern across the upper cheeks, bridge of the nose, and forehead. (From M. M. Bookmiller et al. Textbook of Obstetrics and Obstetric Nursing. Philadelphia: Saunders, 1967.)

Hyperpigmentation of the skin during pregnancy is probably due to the presence of increased amounts of circulating estrogen, progesterone, and melanocyte-stimulating hormone. The pigmentation usually disappears after pregnancy, although areas that are especially darkened, namely, the areolae, linea nigra, and genitalia, usually do not return to the prepregnant color. Chloasma, a hyperpigmentation of the forehead, malar eminences, and cheeks is common and is similar to that seen with the use of oral contraceptive medication (Fig. 4-5). If the pigmentation is severe, it may not disappear entirely following pregnancy. Common nevi may darken or enlarge. An unusual change in a mole is reason for excisional biopsy to rule out melanoma.

Striae distensae (atrophicae) gravidarum (commonly called stretch marks), a disruption and clumping of the elastic fibers in the dermis, develop over the breasts, abdomen, and hips in some pregnant women. No topical remedies are helpful.

Spider angiomas commonly noted during pregnancy are more dense on the face, chest, and upper extremities. High levels of estrogen are thought to be the cause. Most of the lesions can be expected to disappear after delivery.

Palmar erythema may develop in the first trimester of pregnancy in over one-third of women. Higher percentages are reported in lightly pigmented races. The erythema may be limited to the thenar or hypothenar eminences, or it may develop in a blotchy pattern on the palms and fingers. No treatment other than reassurance is needed, since it disappears after delivery.

Hair loss is noted infrequently during pregnancy. Loss usually occurs during the postpartum period, starting about three months after delivery and persisting for several months. An increased percentage of hairs enter the resting phase and are shed. While regrowth of the hair may not occur for as long as a year, it is usually complete by the time the woman returns to the prepregnant state.

Pruritus associated with pregnancy, while rare, usually develops during the last trimester. In some cases it may be associated with subclinical jaundice. In most cases, however, the etiology is not well understood, but the symptom abates after delivery.

DISEASES OF THE SKIN

Some diseases with cutaneous or mucocutaneous manifestations may be worsened by pregnancy, are unique to pregnancy, or may threaten the fetus, or the mother, or both. The diagnosis and treatment of these diseases may require consultation with a dermatologist. Routine and specific laboratory studies may be needed to delineate the status of the mother and fetus. Smears and cultures from the skin for bacterial, viral, and fungal invaders are helpful when there is a possibility of infection. A punch biopsy taken from a typical skin lesion may be necessary when the diagnosis is not obvious clinically.

Candidiasis

An increased incidence of candidiasis is noted during pregnancy. Vaginitis or vulvovaginitis responds to nystatin (Mycostatin), either as a vaginal suppository or as an ointment, or to gentian violet in various forms.

Herpes Simplex

Infection of the birth canal by herpes simplex late in pregnancy is an indication for cesarean section to protect the fetus (see Infections). Supportive therapy is sufficient for the gravida, keeping in mind the possibility of secondary bacterial infection.

Neurofibromatosis

Neurofibromatosis usually worsens during pregnancy. Axillary freckling, café au lait spots, and soft cutaneous papules and nodules are present in typical cases. The papules and nodules occasionally develop for the first time during pregnancy. These persist but may decrease in size after delivery. Since the disease is transmitted as an autosomal dominant, genetic counseling of the mother is advised.

Papular Dermatitis

Papular dermatitis of pregnancy, though rare, may occur in any trimester. Widespread, random excoriated papules are noted. The eruption clears after pregnancy. Some investigators suggest that systemic corticosteroid therapy may prevent the fetal death that otherwise occurs in some cases [33].

Other papular skin eruptions may occur in pregnancy. They are poorly understood and not well defined.

Acute Intermittent Porphyria

Acute intermittent porphyria may be aggravated by pregnancy. Abdominal pain and neurologic symptoms are usually present, together with dark, occasionally fluorescent, urine.

Impetigo Herpetiformis

Impetigo herpetiformis is a rare disorder that resembles widespread pustular psoriasis. The patient is severely ill and febrile, and the areas of skin involved are erythematous and studded with sterile pustules. Body creases are usually severely involved. Hypoparathyroidism and hypocalcemia may be present, requiring treatment. Systemic corticosteroids are the treatment of choice, together with systemic antibiotics for secondary infection. Both the mother and fetus are at risk, and pregnancy interruption may be advisable.

Herpes Gestationis

Herpes gestationis, which is not related to the viral herpetic diseases, is a rare complication of pregnancy in which the skin, notably of the trunk and extremities, is involved with a multiform erythematous vesiculobullous eruption. Eosinophilia may be marked. The patient experiences severe burning and itching, and secondary infection may develop. The disease develops in any trimester, but usually the second, and persists until shortly after delivery. Occasional postpartum flare-ups have been noted. Treatment with corticosteroids is usually successful. An increased risk of fetal abnormalities has been suggested. Recurrence is possible during a subsequent pregnancy.

Erythema Multiforme

Erythema multiforme presents with erythematous macules, wheals, papules, target lesions, and, in severe cases, vesicles or bullae. Aside from pregnancy, drugs, collagen disease, infections, and a neoplasm should be considered as causative. There may be fetal disease or death in some cases. Corticosteroids are the treatment of choice in severe cases.

COLLAGEN DISEASES

Diseases of connective tissue are of unknown etiology, but their pathogenesis appears to involve an autoimmune response. They represent rare, but sometimes critically serious, complications of pregnancy.

Lupus Erythematosus

Although rare, systemic lupus erythematosus during pregnancy may present a serious problem in some patients. Since both remissions and exacerbations can occur without apparent explanation even in nonpregnant patients, it is little wonder that the effect of pregnancy on the disease continues to be the source of controversy. While many pregnant patients will exhibit little change in the clinical course of the disease, there are apparently about the same number of exacerbations as remissions, and the exacerbations tend to occur during the first 20 weeks of pregnancy and in the postpartum period. Since severe hypertension may occur with the disease, differentiation from acute toxemia is required. McGee and Makowski [34] have suggested that with corticosteroid therapy, pregnancy appears to have no ill effects on the disease in the absence of lupus glomerulonephritis. Fetal wastage (abortion, fetal death, premature labor) continues to be high in spite of corticosteroid therapy. The prevalence of postpartum exacerbation can be reduced by high-dose corticosteroid medication [34]. Sharon et al. [35] have recently recorded successful pregnancies in 5 patients with lupus erythematosus treated throughout pregnancy with an immunosuppressant (azathioprine).

Rheumatoid Arthritis

Since rheumatoid arthritis is relatively common in the young female, its association with pregnancy should not be surprising. A marked improvement in the symptoms of the disease during pregnancy has been recognized, although this relief from symptoms is not universal. Elevation of serum corticosteroid levels during pregnancy may account for the improvement. Systemic corticosteroid therapy is not recommended currently by most rheumatologists because the disease is not life-threatening; however, intra-articular corticosteroids are used. In an unreported series, we infused blood collected from normal postpartum patients into non-pregnant patients with rheumatoid arthritis. No clinical improvement was regularly observed.

Progressive Systemic Sclerosis
(Systemic Scleroderma)
Pregnancy may have no adverse effect on progressive systemic sclerosis. Fetal loss may be increased, however. A decrease in renal function with development of acute toxemia is a reason for termination of the pregnancy according to some investigators. Malignant hypertension occasionally complicates scleroderma, with maternal death within weeks a near certainty.

References

1. Ueland, K. Cardiovascular diseases complicating pregnancy. *Clin Obstet Gynecol* 21:429, 1978.
2. Burwell, C., and Metcalfe, J. *Heart Disease and Pregnancy.* Boston: Little, Brown, 1958.
3. Niswander, K., and Berendes, H. Effect of maternal cardiac disease in the infant. *Clin Obstet Gynecol* 11:1026, 1968.
4. Szekely, T. *Heart Disease in Pregnancy.* London: Churchill Livingstone, 1974.
5. Mengert, W., Goodson, J., Campbell, R., and Haynes, D. Observations on the pathogenesis of premature separation of the normally implanted placenta. *Am J Obstet Gynecol* 66:1104, 1953.
6. Pritchard, J., and Scott, D. Iron Demands during Pregnancy. In L. Hallberg, H. Harworth, and A. Vannotti (Eds.), *Iron Deficiency: Pathogenesis, Clinical Aspects, Therapy.* New York: Academic, 1970.
7. Laros, R., and Sweet, R. Management of idiopathic thrombocytopenic purpura during pregnancy. *Am J Obstet Gynecol* 122:182, 1975.
8. Harrington, W., Sprague, C., Minnich, V., Moore, C., Aulvin, R., and Dubach, R. Immunologic mechanism in idiopathic and neonatal thrombocytopenia. *Ann Intern Med* 38:433, 1953.
9. Heys, R. Child bearing and idiopathic thrombocytopenic purpura. *J Obstet Gynaecol Br Commonw* 73:205, 1966.
10. Gordon, M., Niswander, K., Berendes, H., and Kantor, A. G. Fetal morbidity following potentially anoxigenic obstetric conditions: Bronchial asthma. *Am J Obstet Gynecol* 106:421, 1970.
11. Kass, E. The Role of Asymptomatic Bacteriuria in the Pathogenesis of Pyelonephritis. In E. Quinn and E. Kass (Eds.), *Biology of Pyelonephritis.* Boston: Little, Brown, 1960. P. 399.
12. Whalley, P. Bacteriuria of pregnancy. *Am J Obstet Gynecol* 94:723, 1967.
13. Brumfitt, W., Davis, B., and Rosser, E. Urethral catheter as a cause of urinary tract infection in pregnancy and puerperium. *Lancet* 2:1059, 1961.
14. Sciarra, J., Toledo-Pereyra, L., Bendel, R., and Simmons, R. Pregnancy following renal transplantation. *Am J Obstet Gynecol* 123:411, 1975.
15. Davison, J., and Lindheimer, M. Renal disease in pregnant women. *Clin Obstet Gynecol* 24:411, 1978.
16. Felig, P. Diabetes Mellitus. In D. Burrow and T. Ferris (Eds.), *Medical Complications During Pregnancy.* Philadelphia: Saunders, 1975. P. 170.
17. White, P. Pregnancy and diabetes—medical aspects. *Med Clin North Am* 49:1015, 1965.
18. Delaney, J., and Ptacek, J. Three decades of experience with diabetic pregnancies. *Am J Obstet Gynecol* 106:550, 1970.
19. Reis, R., DeCosta, E., and Allweiss, M. The management of the pregnant diabetic woman and her newborn infant. *Am J Obstet Gynecol* 60:1023, 1950.
20. Ayromlooi, J., Zervoudakis, I., and Sadaghat, A. Thyrotoxicosis in pregnancy. *Am J Obstet Gynecol* 117:818, 1974.
21. Black, W. Acute appendicitis in pregnancy. *Brit Med J* 1:1938, 1960.
22. Cunningham, F., and McCubbin, J. Appendicitis complicating pregnancy. *Obstet Gynecol* 45:415, 1975.
23. D'Cruz, I., Balani, S., and Iyer, L. Infectious hepatitis and pregnancy. *Obstet Gynecol* 31:449, 1968.
24. Reid, R., Ivery, K., Rencoret, R., et al. Fetal complications of obstetric cholestasis. *Brit Med J* 1:870, 1976.
25. Gregg, N. Congenital cataract following German measles in the mother. *Trans Ophthal Soc Anesth* 3:35, 1942.
26. Hardy, J., McCracken, G., Gilkeson, M., and Sever, J. Adverse fetal outcome following maternal rubella after the first trimester of pregnancy. *JAMA* 207:2414, 1969.
27. Sever, J. Viral teratogens: A status report. *Hosp Pract* April, 1970. Pg. 75.
28. Freeman, D., and Barno, A. Deaths from Asian influenza associated with pregnancy. *Am J Obstet Gynecol* 78:1172, 1959.
29. Hunt, H., Schifrin, B., and Suzuki, K. Ruptured berry aneurysms and pregnancy. *Obstet Gynecol* 43:827, 1974.
30. Pool, J. Treatment of intracranial aneurysms during pregnancy. *JAMA* 192:209, 1965.

31. Speidel, B., and Madden, S.   Maternal epilepsy and abnormalities of the fetus and newborn. *Lancet* 2:839, 1972.

32. Shapiro, S., Slone, D., Hartz, S., et al.   Are hydantoins (phenytoins) human teratogens? *J Pediatrics* 20:673, 1977.

33. Spangler, A., Reddy, W., Wadi, A., et al.   Papular dermatitis of pregnancy. *JAMA* 181:577, 1962.

34. McGee, C., and Makowski, E.   Systemic lupus erythematosus in pregnancy. *Am J Obstet Gynecol* 107:1008, 1970.

35. Sharon, E., Jones, J., Diamond, H., and Kaplan, D.   Pregnancy and azathioprine in systemic lupus erythematosus. *Am J Obstet Gynecol* 118:25, 1974.

Additional Readings

Amstey, M., Monif, G., Nahmias, A., and Josey, W.   Cesarean section and genital herpes virus infection. *Obstet Gynecol* 53:541, 1979.

Chesley, L.   The remote prognosis for pregnant women with rheumatic cardiac disease. *Am J Obstet Gynecol* 100:732, 1968.

Crosby, W. M.   Trauma during pregnancy: Maternal and fetal injury. *Obstet Gynecol Surv* 29:683, 1974.

Cumming, D., and Taylor, P.   Urologic and obstetric significance of urinary calculi in pregnancy. *Obstet Gynecol* 53:505, 1979.

Drake, T., Kaplan, R., and Lewis, T.   The physiologic hyperparathyroidism of pregnancy. *Obstet Gynecol* 53:746, 1979.

Finn, W.   The outcome of pregnancy following vaginal operations. *Am J Obstet Gynecol* 56:291, 1948.

Fishburne, J.   Physiology and disease of the respiratory system in pregnancy: A review. *J Reprod Med* 22:177, 1979.

Hall, J., Boyce, J., and Nelson, J.   Carcinoma in situ of the cervix uteri. *Obstet Gynecol* 34:221, 1969.

Harris, R., and Dunnihou, D.   The incidence and significance of urinary calculi in pregnancy. *Am J Obstet Gynecol* 99:237, 1967.

Harris, R., and Gilstrap, L.   Prevention of recurrent pyelonephritis during pregnancy. *Obstet Gynecol* 44:637, 1974.

Harrison, K.   Maternal anaemia and fetal birth weight. *J Obstet Gynaecol Br Commw* 80:798, 1973.

Johnstone, R., II, Kreindler, T., and Johnstone, R.   Hyperparathyroidism during pregnancy. *Obstet Gynecol* 40:580, 1972.

McFee, J.   Anemia in pregnancy: A reappraisal. *Obstet Gynecol Surv* 28:769, 1973.

Monif, G.   Maternal mumps infection during gestation: Observations in the progeny. *Am J Obstet Gynecol* 119:549, 1974.

O'Sullivan, J., Mahan, C., Charles, D., and Dandrow, R.   Screening criteria for high-risk gestational diabetic patients. *Am J Obstet Gynecol* 116:895, 1973.

Perlmutter, J. F.   Heroin addiction and pregnancy. *Obstet Gynecol Surv* 29:439, 1974.

Pritchard, J., Scott, D., Whalley, P., Cunningham, F., and Mason, R.   The effects of maternal sickle-cell hemoglobinopathies and sickle-cell trait on reproductive performance. *Am J Obstet Gynecol* 117:662, 1974.

Schenker, J., and Chavers, I.   Pheochromocytoma and pregnancy: A review of 89 cases. *Obstet Gynecol Surv* 26:739, 1971.

Schenker, J., and Polishuk, W.   Pregnancy following mitral valvulotomy. *Obstet Gynecol* 32:214, 1968.

Talbert, L., Thomas, C., Holt, W., and Rankin, P.   Hyperthyroidism during pregnancy. *Obstet Gynecol* 36:779, 1970.

Waldrop, G., and Palmer, J.   Carcinoma of the cervix associated with pregnancy. *Am J Obstet Gynecol* 86:202, 1963.

Weis, J., Silberman, S., and Cohen, L.   Recurring oral pregnancy tumors. *Obstet Gynecol* 54:358, 1979.

Whalley, P.   Bacteriuria of pregnancy. *Am J Obstet Gynecol* 97:723, 1967.

Wilkinson, E.   Acute pancreatitis in pregnancy: A review of 98 cases. *Obstet Gynecol Surv* 28:281, 1973.

Wilson, B., and Haverkamp, A.   Cholestatic jaundice of pregnancy: New perspectives. *Obstet Gynecol* 54:650, 1979.

5

Abortion is a common event, yet it is rarely accepted with equanimity by the patient or her family. Viewed as a frustrating obstruction to acquiring a family by some, it may be welcomed with great relief by others.

Abortion is defined as the termination of pregnancy before 20 weeks' gestation, counting from the first day of the last menstrual period. A fetal weight criterion to define abortion has been suggested as a substitute for the sometimes indefinite 20-week gestational interval. If the expelled fetus, whether liveborn or stillborn, weighs less than 500 gm., abortion is said to have occurred. Fetal survival below this weight is extremely unlikely, although such an event may be reported with greater frequency in the future. Since the weight of the fetus is so frequently unknown in the clinical situation, we will use the 20-week limit in the ensuing discussion. In most states this is also the legal limit dividing an abortion from a birth. It should be remembered that *abortion* is a medical and legal term that to a patient may imply a purposeful attempt to interrupt a pregnancy. Thus, the term *miscarriage,* which is of uncertain scientific meaning, should be used when discussing abortion with a patient.

Classification

Abortions can be classified in various ways, each method satisfying a medical or legal need.

An *early abortion* is one that occurs before 12 weeks' gestation. A *late abortion* is one that occurs between 12 and 20 weeks. This division is a useful one clinically, since the etiology of each of these types of abortion is unique, although there is, of course, an overlap. Similarly, the treatment of early abortion is different from the treatment of late abortion.

Abortion may also be defined in terms of the symptoms experienced by the patient or the signs observed by the physician. Such a classification is of clinical usefulness. It allows the physician to arrive at a prognosis for the patient and defines the type of treatment that is the most appropriate in a particular case.

Threatened abortion is diagnosed when vaginal bleeding occurs during the first 20 weeks of pregnancy. Bleeding may be minimal or very heavy. Abdominal cramps may or may not be experienced, but, if present, they negatively alter the prognosis for continuation of the pregnancy. By this definition, at least 20 percent of pregnant patients threaten to abort. Of those who bleed, perhaps 25 to 50 percent will actually abort, while the others will successfully continue the pregnancy. In the latter group, the cause of bleeding usually remains unknown, but bleeding from a benign cervical condition or other local cause may explain some cases; in others, the bleeding is probably from placental disruption of such a minor degree that the pregnancy is not damaged. It is possible to assure the alarmed patient who asks if the pregnancy can be normal after an episode of bleeding that this is nearly always the case.

Inevitable abortion is diagnosed when cervical dilation of some degree is added to the symptoms of threatened abortion. In some cases, the products of conception can be felt to be present at the cervical os; in others, the cervix is empty.

Incomplete abortion is diagnosed when part of the products of conception are known to have passed from the uterus. Confusion with the diagnosis of inevitable abortion may exist. Fortunately, such differentiation is usually not of great clinical import, since the treatment may be the same in both instances.

Complete abortion is diagnosed when both the fetus and all of the placenta have been successfully expelled from the uterus. From a clinical point of view, we prefer not to make this diagnosis on any patient who aborts before 16 weeks. Too often, subsequent events show that such a patient has aborted incompletely, and the wrong diagnosis may have led to delay in treatment.

A *missed abortion* can be diagnosed when it becomes evident that the products of conception have been retained in the uterus after the fetus is known to have died. Missing from this definition is the element of time. How long must the products of conception be retained to justify the term *missed abortion*? Authorities do not agree. Four weeks is suggested as a reasonable time, since the major complication associated with missed abortion (a blood coagulopathy) rarely occurs before at least four weeks have passed. Symptoms are uncommon during the elapsed time before the expected abortion occurs. The American College of Obstetricians and Gynecologists, however, prefers an 8-week interval. Rarely, a fetus may be retained for months or years, with a resultant macerated mass of tissue that may become calcified. The etiology of missed abortion is unknown.

Septic abortion is diagnosed when evidence of intrauterine infection is superimposed on any other type of abortion. The sepsis nearly always results from a procedure designed to interrupt the pregnancy.

Habitual abortion is diagnosed when three or more consecutive abortions have occurred. Speculation on the etiology of this condition has occupied investigators for many years.

Induced abortion is an abortion that results from a procedure intended to interrupt a pregnancy. The terms *therapeutic abortion* (abortion for medical reasons) and *criminal abortion* (induced abortion without legal sanction) should probably be abandoned as no longer useful. Certainly, few induced abortions are performed for therapeutic "medical" reasons as the term has been used in the past. Advocates of liberalized availability of abortion maintain that there is no necessity for such a medical indication, a view shared by the author. It seems better to define the abortion in medical terms, that is, as incomplete, complete, or septic, as the case may be.

Etiology of Abortion

The cause of a particular abortion is rarely ascertainable by the physician. The patient will frequently explain the abortion on the basis of a fall or some other physical accident; the physician may shrug his shoulders and suggest that "nature knows best." Indeed, in at least half of abortions competently and exhaustively studied by experienced investigators, no explanation for the abortion will be found. Increasingly, however, a cause can be ascribed in a particular case. This is a fact with strong clinical implications, since it may provide both the patient and the physician with important information. On rare occasions, a correctable defect will be found, e.g., an intramural leiomyoma. In other cases, a chromosomal explanation can be offered, with the possibility of subsequent genetic advice on the likelihood of an abortion repetition. Certainly, at least patients who experience repeated abortion should be thoroughly investigated. Delineation of etiologic factors for abortion has been hampered by the fact that fetal death almost always occurs two to six weeks before expulsion of the fetus. The material for study is therefore macerated, and its usefulness is limited.

ABNORMALITY OF DEVELOPMENT

The classic study of abortion material by Hertig and Sheldon in 1943 [1], showed that an abnormality of development incompatible with fetal life occurred in 61.7 percent of cases. In most of these cases (48.9 percent), the ova were pathologic; in 3.2 percent, the embryo exhibited a localized anomaly; and in 9.6 percent, the placenta was found to be abnormal. It is of interest, especially in considering the etiology of hydatidiform mole, that hydropic degeneration of villi was noted in 63 percent of spontaneous abortions but in only 4 percent of induced abortions. Subsequent studies of chromosomal patterns have confirmed, clarified, and amplified the observations of Hertig and Sheldon.

While the precise number is in dispute, it is clear that chromosomal aberrations are present in a large percentage of spontaneous abortions and evident in a much lower percentage of induced abortions. McConnell and Carr [2] reported a figure of 59 percent with spontaneous abortions; Thiede and Salm [4] found chromosomal defects in 60 percent of their cases. Among 16 couples who had experienced 3 or more spontaneous abortions, Stenchever et al. [3] found balanced chromosomal translocations in 31.2 percent. Sasaki et al. [5] detected a chromosomal defect in only 2.8 percent of induced abortions. The most commonly reported anomalies are autosomal trisomy, X monosomy, and triploidy. It is of interest that the vast majority of fetuses with X monosomy (XO) are aborted, thus effectively reducing the number of infants born with Turner's syndrome. One can easily agree that "nature knows best" in this group of patients, since neither the physician nor the patient would wish to increase the number of chromosomally defective births.

Defective Uterine Environment

Another possible cause of abortion, not so easily identified or proved, is a defective uterine environment, due perhaps to poor endocrine preparation of the endometrium for nidation. In a series of papers Hughes and co-workers [6] have suggested that deficient endocrine preparation of the endometrium for implantation may be a major cause of habitual abortion. Their argument is further strengthened by the therapeutic success that followed exogenous hormonal stimulation of endometria previously identified histologically as "deficient." Successful pregnancy occurred among these patients with much greater frequency than one would have expected. The lack of a control group for judging the outcome without therapy, however, makes the validity of this work questionable.

External Factors

Externally applied factors certainly can cause congenital malformations, and, if the factor exerts its action at an appropriate time, probably abortion as well. Aminopterin, a folic acid antagonist, is an obvious example of this class of abortifacients. In a classic experiment, Thiersch [7] showed that if aminopterin is given in early pregnancy, abortion usually occurs. If abortion fails, the retained fetuses frequently exhibit a major congenital anomaly. Although other factors have not been so precisely identified, specific viruses and chemicals, as well as radiation, probably act in a similar manner.

Maternal Factors

Certain maternal factors may be etiologically related to abortion, although proof is frequently lacking. Severe systemic *acute infection* is one such agent, notably pneumonia, pyelonephritis, and influenza. However, it remains unclear whether the infectious disease exerts a specific infectious effect on the fetus, or whether the generalized maternal reaction, if severe enough, is the mechanism of abortion. Rubella, well known for its teratogenic effects, may also be associated with an increase in the abortion rate. *Chronic infections* of sufficiently severe degree (e.g., chronic tuberculosis) are also said to increase the risk of abortion, probably due simply to maternal wasting. Infectious agents recently reported as possibly associated with abortion include *Listeria monocytogenes* and *Toxoplasma gondii*, although these organisms seem to exert their effects more frequently on the incidence of late abortion rather than of early abortion. *Nutritional deficiencies* and *immunologic factors* may be capable of acting as abortifacients, although specific proof is lacking. The possibility of poor *endocrine preparation* of the endometrium has been mentioned as a cause of abortion.

Surgical Procedures

Certain surgical procedures apparently increase the risk of abortion. Excision of the corpus luteum will produce abortion in many species and probably also in the human, although, as suggested by the experiment of Tulsky and Koff [8], the surgery must be performed very early in human pregnancy to cause abortion. Laparotomy for surgical disase (e.g., appendicitis) increases the risk of abortion slightly if performed early in pregnancy, but failure to perform necessary surgery is a far graver hazard. Peritonitis seems especially prone to cause abortion. Amputation of the cervix, done as an integral step in certain pelvic repair operations, may cause midtrimester abortion, and overvigorous dilation of the cervix has been suggested as the cause for cervical incompetence (see p. 126).

Uterine Malformations or Tumors

Uterine malformations or tumors certainly increase the risk of premature labor, but their effect in producing abortion is less certain. A bicornuate uterus, for example, may permit adequate nutrition for the developing embryo, but when the fetus attains a certain size, it can no longer accommodate to the decrease in uterine capacity, and premature labor results. Uterine submucous myomas may exert a similar effect, perhaps by the same mechanism.

Miscellaneous Factors

Trauma plays a minor role in the production of abortion, with only one clear-cut example in the 1000 abortions analyzed by Hertig and Sheldon [1]. It seems logical to assume a *male factor,* perhaps a defective sperm, to account for many abortions, but proof is lacking. Although a psychogenic cause of abortion seems equally logical, again, proof is lacking.

Pathology of Abortion

For many reasons, the pathogenesis of abortion has not been fully described in the scientific literature. A major disadvantage to the study of abortion material is the long period of time that intervenes between death of the fetus and clinical abortion, which typically is about two weeks according to most authorities. Among pathologic fetuses, however, Hertig and Sheldon [1] estimated the average interval to be about six weeks. Clearly, pathologic study of material from a fetus that has been dead for many days or for weeks will leave many questions unanswered.

The fetus may appear relatively normal, although the delay between fetal death and abortion may have resulted in a size smaller than the gestational age might have suggested. Normal fetuses are more likely to be recovered from abortion occurring 10 or more weeks after the last menstrual period. Early abortion material is more likely to contain an obvi-

ously abnormal fetus, only a remnant of a fetus, or sometimes no fetal remains at all.

A description of the various types of pathologic ova may prove useful to the pathologist trying to assign a cause to a specific abortion. Benirschke favors the classification of pathologic ova suggested by Fujikura et al. [9], based on a study of 327 abortions:

Group   I: Incomplete specimen (22 percent).
Group II: Ruptured empty sac:
      a. With cord stump (4 percent).
      b. Without cord stump (23.5 percent).
Group III: Intact empty sac (5.5 percent).
Group IV: Specimens containing an embryo:
      a. Normal embryo (35.8 percent).
      b. Deformed embryo (4 percent).
      c. Embryo with specific anomaly (1.8 percent).
      d. Embryo so macerated as to preclude determination of normalcy (3.4 percent).

Specimens from groups I, II, and III were encountered more frequently earlier in pregnancy (the so-called blighted ovum), while the Group IV specimens containing a recognized fetus were more prevalent with later abortions.

Certain pathologic changes develop in the placenta with abortion. Hemorrhage into the decidua basalis usually occurs after the death of the fetus rather than preceding the event. Necrosis in the implantation site follows the hemorrhage, with subsequent infiltration of the entire area by inflammatory cells. The placenta detaches, and uterine contractions are initiated by the presence of a foreign body. Hydropic degeneration of the villi is a frequent finding.

Vaginal bleeding results from changes in the decidua, while uterine contractions and expulsion follow detachment of the placenta. This detachment is frequently incomplete, however, especially with early abortion, and the base of the placenta or the entire placenta may be retained after expulsion of the embryo. Various clinical pictures result, depending on the pathologic changes that occur.

The fate of a threatened abortion is determined pathologically long before the clinical outcome is known, since the vaginal bleeding observed may result from a slight detachment of the placenta or may follow complete disruption of the site. Cramps suggest a process much farther advanced, while cervical dilatation will not occur unless the abortion is inevitable. If abortion is long delayed (missed abortion), the embryo may be surrounded by a capsule of clotted blood and be gradually compressed. The capsule of clotted blood becomes organized, and a *blood,* or *carneous, mole* results.

Clinical Picture and Treatment

THREATENED ABORTION

Many pregnant patients bleed to some degree during early pregnancy. Because the precise cause of the bleeding usually cannot be ascertained, all such cases are diagnosed as threatened abortion. A large percentage will not progress to abortion (50 to 80 percent, depending on the criteria used to make the diagnosis), while the others will progress toward it at widely varying speeds.

Symptoms

The vaginal bleeding may be as little as "staining" when the patient first reports her symptom. The amount of bleeding may increase rapidly, or it may disappear completely, only to reappear later. There is wide variation in the amount of bleeding, as well as in the total length of time during which bleeding occurs. While abortion is more likely to follow heavy bleeding and bleeding for a prolonged time, exceptions are frequent enough to make prediction of the outcome hazardous. The added symptom of cramps indicates the onset of uterine contractions; the prognosis for abortion changes adversely, and abortion usually follows within a matter of hours, occasionally days.

Differential Diagnosis

When a patient reports vaginal bleeding, especially if cramps are absent, a differential diagnosis becomes important. Other causes of early pregnancy bleeding include local lesions of the cervix (cer-

vicitis, cervical polyp, carcinoma), an ectopic pregnancy with decidual bleeding, or trophoblastic disease. A large number of cases remain unexplained. Pelvic examination may reveal a local lesion, but demonstration of such a lesion does not rule out the additional presence of bleeding from an impending abortion. Ectopic pregnancy is usually accompanied by other more serious or severe symptoms (see Chap. 6). Trophoblastic disease may present a clinical picture suggestive of threatened abortion, but sooner or later, additional diagnostic evidence can be gathered (see Chap. 15). Frequently only time will differentiate the patient with unexplained causes of vaginal bleeding from the patient destined to abort.

Treatment

Treatment of threatened abortion must be based on the known clinical facts. Benign causes of bleeding must first be excluded. Significant bleeding from disruption of the decidua usually indicates that the abortion process has already progressed too far to allow reversal. Minimal bleeding with no placental disruption requires no treatment. The logic of a "do-nothing" approach is evident.

The use of exogenous progesterone in large doses has been suggested as a treatment for threatened abortion. The treatment is based on the theory that lack of progesterone may allow the uterus to contract and thus produce abortion. Both on theoretical and practical grounds, such treatment is not recommended. Klopper [10] has theorized that only therapeutically inadequate doses of progesterone can be delivered even if the theory is a correct one. In a carefully controlled double-blind study, Goldzeiher [11] has shown a lack of effect of progesterone in preventing abortion. There is evidence that progesterone may turn an inevitable abortion into a missed abortion, with greatly delayed extrusion of the products of conception. An additional argument against the use of progesterone to prevent abortion, if one is needed, is the possibility of the development of virilization in female fetuses whose mothers have been so treated. A recent report also suggests a relationship between progesterone administered during pregnancy and anomalies of the limbs, although the association is certainly a rare one [12]. The discussion is now academic since the FDA no longer supports the use of progesterone for any reason during pregnancy.

While a do-nothing approach seems realistic, a blunt refusal to prescribe for the patient is certainly not warranted. Bed rest is a long-used treatment and may be appropriate for some patients; mild sedation may make the bed rest more tolerable. Frequent communication with the patient not only permits early reporting of new symptoms that may require reappraisal of the therapeutic regimen but will also reassure the patient that someone is concerned about the outcome of her pregnancy. Some patients experience vaginal bleeding for many days or even weeks before the outcome becomes evident, and depression may become a major problem in the interim. The lack of effective therapeutic agents does not change the need for physician concern.

INEVITABLE AND INCOMPLETE ABORTION

With incomplete abortion, placental tissue has been passed and recognized; with inevitable abortion, the cervix is dilated, but no tissue has been seen. Clinical confusion between these two types of abortion is common. For this reason, they are considered together.

After uterine contractions have been added to the symptom of vaginal bleeding, threatened abortion usually progresses rapidly to either an inevitable abortion or an incomplete abortion. The patient may bleed very heavily, or she may be so uncomfortable from uterine cramps as to require analgesia. Clearly, an aggressive therapeutic approach is indicated.

While many hospital units prefer to admit all patients with inevitable or incomplete abortion, many clinicians feel that such patients can be managed in an outpatient setting. Admission is reserved for patients with severe bleeding or evidence of sepsis, or for those patients whose uterine size suggests a pregnancy of 12 weeks or more. If the outpatient setting is used, definitive treatment can usually be delayed long enough to evaluate the patient's condition fully by history and physical examination, to obtain a hematocrit determination, and to type and cross-match blood. A dilute solution of intravenous oxytocin may be started before proceeding with uterine evacuation.

With the patient in the lithotomy position and well sedated with 5 to 10 mg. of intravenous diazepam (Valium), a paracervical anesthesia block is performed. In some patients, the placental material will be seen exuding from the cervical os. With the tenaculum on the anterior lip of the cervix for countertraction, the cervix is carefully dilated unless it is already sufficiently dilated. An ovum forceps is introduced into the uterus, and the necrotic conceptus is removed. The oxytocin previously started will help prevent uterine perforation by causing the uterus to contract. Removal of all available material is followed by careful sharp curettage with a large curette. The curettage brings the uterine bleeding under control rapidly. Some physicians prefer to use a suction curette for the evacuation. We see no advantage to its use in this instance, because sharp curettage is usually required to assure complete evacuation of the uterus following suction. If the gestation is longer than 12 weeks, suction may prove more effective, however, since bleeding is minimized by its use. Following uterine evacuation, the outpatient is observed for 2 to 6 hours, and if no complication ensues, she is allowed to go home.

If the patient is hospitalized either as a routine measure or because of a specific problem, much the same procedure is employed, except that the use of general anesthesia is preferred by many physicians. If shock is present, whole blood in an amount sufficient to correct the shock should be transfused before performing the curettage. Recovery even in this instance is usually rapid, and the patient can return home within 24 to 48 hours in most cases. If the patient is believed to have an infection, as indicated by fever, the timing of the curettage may be more crucial. This circumstance will be discussed in a subsequent section on septic abortion.

If cervical dilation has occurred in midpregnancy without the passage of fetal or placental tissue, a diagnosis of incompetent cervix may be justified. An entirely different therapy is required, and this is discussed on page 126.

While the risk of sensitization of the Rh-negative patient to the Rh factor as a result of early or mid-trimester abortion is probably small, most authorities recommend the administration of Rh immune globulin to a previously unsensitized Rh-negative patient following abortion. With a gestation of 12 weeks or less, 50 μcg. of Rh immune globulin is used; after 12 weeks, a full 300 μcg. is recommended. The use of Rh immune globulin in patients delivering at term is discussed in Chapter 12.

COMPLETE ABORTION

Occasionally, a clinician may note the passage of the products of conception apparently in toto. This is a complete abortion. The management of such a patient continues to be a source of disagreement. If the uterus is well contracted and if the cervix is tightly closed, some clinicians choose simply to observe such patients and reserve curettage for recurrent bleeding or cramps. Others feel that it is better to perform curettage on all such patients, since it is a relatively innocuous operation and may spare the patient a subsequent hemorrhage or infection. It is our opinion that curettage should be performed routinely on all such patients if the abortion occurs before the thirteenth or fourteenth week. The chances for a subsequent bleeding episode, frequently a severe one, seem great enough to warrant curettage. If the gestational length of the pregnancy so terminated is greater than 14 weeks, curettage may be delayed, since abortion is more likely to be truly complete with longer gestations. Hospital observation for a minimum of 24 hours is necessary if curettage is to be postposed.

MISSED ABORTION

The major hazard associated with missed abortion is the development of a maternal blood coagulopathy, an event that rarely occurs if the fetus has been dead in the uterus less than a month. Delay in emptying the uterus for one month following fetal death does no harm. While the patient may press for earlier action, active treatment is better delayed to be certain that the fetus is indeed dead. If movement of the fetal heart is not observed with the real-time scanner, a diagnosis of fetal death is justified, especially if a similar finding is noted on 2 consecutive examinations. A flat radiographic film of the abdomen may also provide laboratory support for the diagnosis. With intrauterine death, edema of the fetal scalp may become sufficiently pronounced to create a "halo" sign, in which the outer limit of the fetal scalp is seen at a much greater distance than normal from the bony cranium.

When a decision to empty the uterus is made, the technique to be used will vary with the size of the uterus. If the uterus is smaller than that of a 12 weeks' gestation (an unusual occurrence), suction curettage may be successful. With a uterus up to 16 weeks size, dilatation and extraction of the fetal and placental material may be recommended if an operator experienced with the technique is available. Other therapeutic choices include intravenous oxytocin in large doses, intra-amniotic injection of hypertonic saline solution or prostaglandin $F_{2\alpha}$, or prostaglandin E_2 vaginal suppositories.

Intravenous oxytocin in high dosage may be successful, but it is not always so in our experience. The possibility of water intoxication from the antidiuretic effect of oxytocin and the administration of large amounts of intravenous fluid must be kept in mind. This complication may be more closely related to the amount of infused intravenous fluid than to the dose of oxytocin. The intra-amniotic technique is the one we favor, but in some cases of missed abortion, the amount of amniotic fluid is so scanty that the sac cannot be identified. In the past, hypertonic saline was injected into the sac, and labor began after a prolonged latent period. More recently, we have used intra-amniotic prostaglandin $F_{2\alpha}$ to produce abortion, greatly reducing the time from injection to abortion. We initially insert a laminaria tent the evening before the prostaglandin injection. Vaginal prostaglandin E_2 suppositories are also usually successful in securing abortion although side effects of nausea, vomiting, diarrhea, and hyperpyrexia occur with some frequency. There is a danger of bronchospasm in a patient sensitive to prostaglandin (see Chapter 15 for details of technique, hazards, and so on). Hysterotomy is needed on rare occasions for failed abortion following intra-amniotic injection, but this operative approach has been otherwise largely abandoned.

Weekly plasma fibrinogen determinations should be performed on all patients with a missed abortion of three or more weeks to recognize the onset of disseminated intravascular coagulopathy (DIC). While a drop in fibrinogen below a normal value of about 350 mg. per 100 ml. is unusual, immediate treatment is indicated with a drop to 150 mg. per 100 ml. or lower. The uterus must be emptied by the most expeditious route, with appropriate treatment of the blood coagulopathy if bleeding occurs. Delivery corrects the coagulopathy by terminating the release of thromboplastic material into the maternal circulation.

SEPTIC ABORTION

Septic abortion is diagnosed when fever complicates abortion. In nearly all cases of septic abortion, an active attempt to abort the pregnancy has been made. A precise history of the type of attempt should be obtained from the patient if at all possible. Certain chemical agents (Lysol, soap, detergents) may produce extensive pathologic changes, including necrosis of the myometrium and damage to the liver or kidneys. A history of their use mandates immediate hysterectomy to avert a fatal outcome and alerts the clinician to early signs of disruption of kidney or liver function.

A patient with septic abortion may be only mildly ill, with little evidence of the sepsis except an elevated temperature and perhaps moderate abdominal tenderness. Such minimal findings may be misleading, however, since rapid progression of the infection is common. The infection spreads to the parametrial tissues (parametritis) and beyond, involving the peritoneum (peritonitis) and the pelvic veins (pelvic thrombophlebitis). In many cases of severe infection, the bloodstream is also involved (septicemia). The effects of the infection may be devastating. Locally, the parametrial and peritoneal involvement may lead to pelvic abscess for-

mation. The infected pelvic veins may throw off septic emboli to the lungs and other organs. With a gram-negative infection (and also occasionally with gram-positive cocci), septic shock may occur with alarming rapidity. When septic shock supervenes, damage to vital organs (notably the kidney) can be expected.

Diagnosis

A history of interference with the pregnancy may or may not be elicited. Physical examination will usually reveal a patient with a temperature of 100° to 105°F. (37.8° to 40.3°C.), and tachycardia is prominent. The skin is hot and dry and the patient is apprehensive. The abdomen is tender, sometimes markedly so, with rebound tenderness suggesting peritonitis. Pelvic examination may be so painful as to preclude satisfactory palpation of the pelvic organs. At least some blood can usually be seen coming from the cervical os. The uterus is enlarged to a size appropriate for the gestation, and marked pain is elicited on motion of the cervix. The parametrial areas are thickened and tender, and a pelvic mass suggesting abscess formation may be felt if the disease has been present for some time.

Certain laboratory results may aid in the diagnosis or provide prognostic information.

BLOOD. A low hematocrit may be the result of blood loss, or it may be evidence of hemolysis due to a *Clostridium perfringens* infection. A blood urea nitrogen (BUN) determination will allow estimation of kidney function. The hematocrit, BUN, and a platelet count and plasma fibrinogen level will provide useful baseline values if septic shock, kidney failure, or DIC complicate the subsequent clinical course.

CULTURES. Ultimately, the information provided by cultures may prove the most important of all. Both aerobic and anaerobic cultures should be taken. The cervix (or better, the lower uterine segment) should be cultured and part of the material smeared on a slide and stained with Gram stain for a preliminary diagnosis of the causative organism. Of particular importance on the smear is the presence of gram-positive, encapsulated rods, which probably represent *C. perfringens* infection. With this report, an immediate hysterectomy is indicated, since delay will result in death. Gram-negative bacilli or gram-positive cocci may be evident on the smear. A blood culture should be taken and repeated with spikes of fever. The causative organism of septic abortion is likely to be a gram-negative bacillus of the coliform group or an anaerobic streptococcus, although one of many other organisms may be responsible. Gram stain is of particular use in identifying the deadly *C. perfringens*.

ROENTGENOGRAMS. An upright abdominal x-ray film of the abdomen may reveal either the presence of an intraperitoneal foreign body (catheter) or free air under the diaphragm if uterine perforation has complicated the abortion attempt. Such a circumstance demands immediate hysterectomy, since uterine perforation frequently leads to a fatal outcome. A typical gas pattern may be present with *C. perfringens* infection.

Management of Septic Abortion Without Complications

VITAL SIGNS. Measurement of vital signs at frequent intervals is of extreme importance if septic shock is to be recognized in an incipient stage. Temperature, pulse, respiratory rate, and blood pressure should be recorded at half-hour intervals until the danger has passed.

ANTIBIOTICS. Appropriate antibiotic medication should be prescribed. The choice of initial medication may be based on the organism seen on the Gram stain of the cervix, or on the desire to provide broad coverage (e.g., penicillin and tetracycline, or penicillin and gentamicin). Whatever drug or drugs are chosen, they should be given in very large doses, preferably by the intravenous route. When culture and sensitivity reports are available, or if good clinical response has not occurred with the initial choice, the drugs may be changed. Consultation with a bacteriologist should be sought in

selecting the best drug, since the choice may be a vital one.

TRANSFUSION. Whole blood should be transfused if anemia is evident or if bleeding from the interrupted pregnancy is severe or continuing. Hypovolemia may be due either to blood loss or to septic shock. The differentiation of these two causes may be of extreme importance; rapid administration of a liter of Ringer's lactate solution will correct the shock of hypovolemia but not that of sepsis and thus allow differentiation.

OXYTOCIN. Intravenous oxytocin in dilute solution will encourage abortion if it has not already occurred, and it will discourage bleeding by causing uterine contractions if the abortion is incomplete. Good contractility of the uterus will also decrease the risk of uterine perforation during the subsequent curettage.

CURETTAGE. Curettage should be performed 6 to 12 hours following admission and the administration of antibiotics in the absence of septic shock and with a uterus less than 12 weeks size. Impending shock or a large amount of necrotic material in the uterus may demand an earlier curettage. Earlier curettage is also indicated if hemorrhage is of concern. The procedure is performed not only to decrease the risk of subsequent hemorrhage but also to remove necrotic material that may be the source of a bacterial endotoxin. A diagnosis of complete abortion does not obviate the necessity for the curettage. Curettage should be avoided completely if *C. perfringens* is noted on the Gram stain, since immediate hysterectomy is the treatment most likely to result in patient survival.

TETANUS PREVENTION. Tetanus antitoxin or a booster tetanus toxoid injection is given by many clinicians because of the risk of tetanus.

Complications of Septic Abortion

SEPTIC SHOCK. *Pathogenesis.* The pathogenesis of septic shock remains in dispute, which explains the variation in treatment. An endotoxin present in the cell walls of gram-negative bacteria floods the circulation, causing intense vasoconstriction, especially in the capillary beds. The vasoconstriction may be caused by a direct action of the endotoxin, or it may be mediated through endotoxin-induced release of catecholamines, either in the capillary beds or in the adrenal medulla. The vasospasm leads to decrease in tissue perfusion, with damage to vital structures. If the vasoconstriction is not relieved, death results from destruction of vital organs, notably the kidney and the liver. Terminal vasodilatation is recognized.

Diagnosis. If hypotension develops in a patient who has had a septic abortion, septic shock should be suspected. As previously indicated, rapid infusion of intravenous fluid will differentiate the shock of hypovolemia from septic shock.

Some clinicians recognize an early warm, hypotensive phase, when the patient is alert but apprehensive. This is quickly succeeded by a phase in which the patient is pale, the skin is cold and clammy, and the alertness has disappeared. The temperature, which was markedly elevated earlier, may now be subnormal. The pulse is very rapid, and the blood pressure is extremely low. The effect of the shock on various organs, notably the kidney, is evident. The degree of oliguria is a useful prognostic sign, and a careful measurement of hourly urinary output is essential. If untreated, or if treatment is ineffective, shock becomes irreversible, and metabolic acidosis, anuria, cardiac and respiratory pathologic changes, and coma ensue, followed by death.

Treatment. In addition to the treatment previously suggested for septic abortion, the shock must be vigorously treated. The following guidelines for the management of septic abortion may be helpful.

Monitoring. Careful monitoring of the patient is necessary. In addition to the other laboratory tests that have been mentioned, serum electrolytes must be obtained, since electrolyte balance is essential in the treatment of septic shock. A central venous pressure (CVP) catheter is inserted, and periodic observations are recorded. The normal CVP is between 8 and 12 cm. H_2O; a reading below 5 cm.

H_2O suggests hypovolemia, while a reading over 15 cm. H_2O predicts circulatory overloading or impending pulmonary edema. However, other factors may alter this interpretation of CVP readings. Urine output per hour is recorded. A volume less than 25 to 30 ml. per hour is alarming.

Fluid Therapy. Fluid therapy is critical. Whole blood may be used to correct a low hematocrit, but overloading of the circulation must be avoided. Appropriate intravenous solutions should be used to correct electrolyte imbalance, including lactated Ringer's solution and sodium bicarbonate. The rate of fluid administration is controlled by the CVP reading and the urinary output. A good flow of urine is an excellent prognostic sign.

Adrenocorticosteroids. Adrenocorticosteroids are administered in high dosage. While the precise mechanism of action of this class of drugs is uncertain, most authorities recommend their use. If used for more than three to five days, a gradual tapering off of the amount of medication is necessary to avoid adrenal failure.

Vasoactive Drugs. Vasoactive drugs are recommended for use by all authorities, but there is no general agreement regarding which group of drugs to use. Earlier authorities found that vasoconstrictor drugs successfully controlled the hypotension and presumably also the pathophysiology of the disease, but according to current opinion, their effectiveness in most patients is doubtful [13]. Indeed, if vasoconstriction is the basic pathologic process of the syndrome, vasorelaxing drugs would seem more appropriate. The truth, though not evident at the present time, may lie somewhere between these two extremes. Dopamine is a frequently used drug since it seems to increase mesenteric flow with some increase in urinary output.

Oxygenation. Adequate oxygenation should be maintained by constant oxygen administration, either by tent or by intermittent positive pressure. Tracheostomy may be necessary in some patients. Digitalization should be prescribed if cardiac failure or pulmonary edema develops or is incipient.

If DIC complicates the syndrome, appropriate treatment should be instituted to prevent fatal hemorrhage. Fresh blood or fresh frozen plasma will replace the clotting factors. Fibrinogen is used in some patients.

Hysterectomy is indicated in certain situations and may be lifesaving. Although the decision will depend heavily on individual patient factors, the operation may be necessary in the following situations:

1. When the diagnosis of *C. perfringens* has been made.
2. When the uterus is perforated during the abortive attempt.
3. When the clinical condition of the patient, especially her renal function, fails to improve within a few hours following curettage.

Prophylactic vena caval ligation may be done at the time of the hysterectomy if evidence of septic emboli is present.

ACUTE RENAL FAILURE. Acute renal failure may complicate septic abortion, particularly when septic shock supervenes. The pathologic condition in the kidney is usually tubular necrosis, and recovery depends on the number of tubules permanently destroyed. The tubular necrosis may develop from the effects of infection or of shock, or it may follow the escape into the circulation of certain abortifacients (soap, Lysol, detergents). The treatment in any case is similar. Careful monitoring of urine flow in any patient with septic abortion should begin on admission. Oliguria or even anuria may be noted for a brief period following severe shock, but prolongation of the oliguria beyond a few hours suggests renal damage. The treatment consists of careful restriction of fluids and electrolytes to maintain electrolyte balance, and early peritoneal dialysis followed by hemodialysis if the peritoneal dialysis is unsatisfactory. Recovery will depend on the pathologic condition present (the less common bilateral cortical necrosis is more likely to be irreversible than is tubular necrosis) and the extent of the pathologic changes.

SURGICAL PERFORATION. Surgical perforation of the noninfected uterus is less damaging than is perforation during abortion performed under septic conditions. Should perforation occur with septic abortion, laparotomy and repair of the hole are indicated unless the infection has responded well to treatment. If the patient is in good condition, and if the hole is a small one and there is little fear of bowel injury, laparotomy may, in certain instances, be delayed until the clinical picture demands it.

HABITUAL ABORTION

By definition, a patient who experiences three or more consecutive abortions has suffered habitual abortion. Whether these repeated abortions are due to chance or to a repetitive cause has concerned obstetricians for many years. Contrary to the findings of earlier investigations, the evidence now suggests that abortion is about twice as likely to occur in a woman who has experienced a previous early abortion than in a woman with no previous abortion [14]. However, the incidence of early abortion does not increase with successively greater numbers of prior abortions. In a woman who has suffered repeated early abortions, an attempt should be made to discover a possible repetitive factor. Although such an investigation is not often fruitful, and therapy based on any findings is not always satisfactory, the occasional positive findings make the effort worthwhile.

ETIOLOGY

Earlier in this chapter, the possible causes of spontaneous abortion were discussed. These same factors also account for habitual abortion. With the addition of one other factor, they are briefly repeated here.

1. Defective germ cell or chromosomal abnormality.
2. Defective uterine environment.
3. Defective endocrine support for the pregnancy.
4. Nutritional factors.
5. Immunologic factors.
6. Uterine malformations or tumors.
7. Psychogenic influences.
8. Cervical incompetence.

It is worthwhile to discover a chromosomal cause for repeated abortion, since it will affect the patient's decision regarding subsequent pregnancy attempts. Chromosomal studies of the mother and father and of the abortion material may be necessary to identify a factor. While it is not possible to reverse a chromosomal defect, it is possible in certain cases to offer the patient the option of a genetic amniocentesis in a subsequent pregnancy and abortion if the defect is found to be present.

A defective uterine environment and a defective endocrine support for the pregnancy are related, if not identical, factors. Very little information of therapeutic value is available concerning these factors. The diagnostic plan for identification of these causes of abortion might include investigation of thyroid function and studies of human chorionic gonadotropin, estrogen, and progesterone levels either during early pregnancy or during the luteal phase of the cycle. More will be said of the usefulness of such measurements when therapy is discussed.

Although it is suspected that certain nutritional deficiencies can produce abortion, no irrefutable scientific data are available to support this contention. A poor general nutritional state may very well increase the risk of abortion.

An intriguing possibility in the study of the etiology of abortion is an immunologic rejection factor. At the present time, however, no definite information on such a factor is available. Some work suggests that a maternal antibody to sperm may cause infertility, but a causal relationship to abortion has not been proved.

Uterine malformations and submucosal myomas probably cause premature labor in some patients. The relationship between these factors and abortion before 20 weeks' gestation is less certain. If no other factor can be discovered, a therapeutic trial to remove the abnormality (myomectomy) may be useful.

A psychogenic cause for abortion is suspected by many physicians. The proof is difficult to secure. Some obstetricians are convinced that strong emotional support has reduced the likelihood of abortion in some patients, but such clinical impressions must be viewed with skepticism.

Cervical incompetence is the inability of the cervix to support the pregnancy. Painless cervical dilatation typically occurs in mid-pregnancy, apparently when the uterine contents attain sufficient size to necessitate support of the lower uterine segment. The diagnosis can be made with some degree of assurance only if repeated painless interruptions have occurred during the mid-trimester. The diagnosis is greatly strengthened if therapy directed at correction of the defect is successful. While a number of tests have been devised to allow a diagnosis of cervical incompetence to be made between pregnancies, none has proved of value. The diagnosis may be suspected if the nonpregnancy cervix of a patient with a typical history accepts an 8-mm. or larger Hegar dilator.

The cause of cervical incompetence is a subject of disagreement. Some feel that a congenital weakness of the cervix is involved. Others trace the development of the lesion to a damaging dilatation and curettage or to a difficult delivery. Others have suggested a psychogenic cause. This contention is supported by the claim that special emotional support alone has "cured" the condition and permitted pregnancies to progress to term.

It should be noted that an abortion due apparently to cervical incompetence is different from an early abortion due to other factors. The gestational interval at which abortion occurs is the most obvious difference, but other differences also exist. An early abortion is rarely complete, but late abortions due to cervical incompetence infrequently require curettage to remove the entire conceptus. Early abortions are usually painful, but abortion due to cervical incompetence is painless in most cases. Although the therapy of early abortion is unsatisfactory, cervical incompetence may be successfully treated.

THERAPY

Medical Treatment

No method of preventing chromosomal abberrations that cause abortion is currently available. A defective uterine environment or defective endocrine support of the pregnancy can be treated in some cases. If hypothyroidism can be detected, thyroid extract or thyroxine in an appropriate dosage may be effective. Although human chorionic gonadotropin has been administered in large doses to support placentation in a patient suspected of a deficient secretion of this hormone, the efficacy of the therapy remains unproved. The administration of progesterone to patients presumed to be deficient in progesterone production has been shown to be worthless and cannot be recommended. A possible exception to this rule is the therapy recommended by Hughes and co-workers [6] when a "deficient" endometrium for implantation accounts for the reproductive failure. Hughes and his group stained endometrial biopsies for glycogen and alkaline phosphatase from patients who had suffered repeated abortions. When a "deficient" endometrium could be diagnosed, the next few menstrual cycles were "supported" with tiny doses of estrogen, frequently with the addition of progesterone late in the cycle. When the treatment "improved" the endometrium, the chance of a successful pregnancy was greatly increased. While these results have not been confirmed, the recommended treatment may be worthwhile and is probably harmless at worst.

No treatment for presumed nutritional or immunologic factors in abortion is known at the present time.

Surgical Treatment

If, after investigation, uterine malformation or a submucosal myoma remains the only possible explanation of repeated abortions in a given patient, surgical treatment may be recommended, provided the patient is informed of the uncertainty of the relationship between the disease and the abortions. A unification operation is used for various uterine abnormalities, while myomectomy may be used for the myomas. The patient should be told that the operation entails a subsequent risk of uterine rupture during pregnancy.

The treatment for cervical incompetence is surgical and should be reserved for the patient with a reliable and typical history if an operation is to be performed between pregnancies. During pregnancy, surgery may be performed before actual cervical dilatation occurs if the past history of cervical incompetence is convincing; or it may be done after the cervix has dilated, but before the membranes have ruptured.

Three types of surgery have been described, with many variations of the techniques described by individual surgeons. The most popular technique is the one devised by Shirodkar and modified by Barter et al. [15], in which a ligature of one of various materials is placed around the internal os during pregnancy. The vagina overlying the anterior cervix is incised and the bladder advanced upward. A similar incision is made overlying the posterior cervix. With an aneurysm needle, the ligature (of Mersilene, for example) is passed around the cervix at the level of the internal os and tied through the anterior vaginal incision. The suture is attached posteriorly to the cervix by a ligature. The vagina is closed with interrupted absorbable sutures.

With the simpler McDonald technique [16], also used during pregnancy, a needle with braided silk is passed through the anterior cervix at its junction with the looser vaginal mucosa and then twice through the posterior cervix in a comparable location. Another bite through the anterior cervix completes the suture placement. The tying of the sutures is performed anteriorly.

Lash and Lash [17] have recommended surgery in the interval between pregnancies and have proposed the following technique: The anterior vagina is incised, and the bladder is advanced. An elliptical piece of tissue is excised longitudinally from the anterior cervix between the internal and external os. The edges of the cervix are reapproximated, and the vagina is closed. This operation has the advantage of permitting vaginal delivery without subsequent repair.

The Shirodkar-Barter and McDonald procedures during pregnancy result in a success rate approaching 60 to 80 percent. The results of the Lash and Lash procedure have not been reliably reported in the recent literature. Should the procedure during pregnancy fail, the ligature should be cut immediately to avoid uterine or cervical rupture as labor supervenes. If the pregnancy proceeds uneventfully, the ligature in the McDonald procedure should be cut before the onset of labor. With the Shirodkar-Barter operation, the ligature may be cut or cesarean section may be performed to allow preservation of the ligature for another pregnancy.

References

1. Hertig, A., and Sheldon, W.   Minimal criteria required to prove prima facie case of traumatic abortion or miscarriage: An analysis of 1,000 spontaneous abortions. *Ann Surg* 117:596, 1943.
2. McConnell, H., and Carr, D.   Recent advances in the cytogenic study of human spontaneous abortions. *Obstet Gynecol* 45:547, 1975.
3. Stenchever, M., Parks, K., Daines, T., et al.   Cytogenetics of habitual abortion and other reproductive wastage. *Am J Obstet Gynec* 127:143, 1977.
4. Thiede, H., and Salm, S.   Chromosome studies of human spontaneous abortions. *Am J Obstet Gynecol* 90:205, 1964.
5. Sasaki, M., Makino, S., Muramato, J., Ikeuchi, T., and Shumba, H.   A chromosome survey of induced abortuses in a Japanese population. *Obstet Gynecol Surv* 22:612, 1967.
6. Hughes, E., Lloyd, C., VanNess, A., and Ellis, W.   The Role of the Endometrium in Implantation and Fetal Growth. In E. Engle (Ed.), *Pregnancy Wastage*. Springfield, Ill.: Thomas, 1953, P. 51.
7. Thiersch, J.   Therapeutic abortions with a folic acid antagonist, 4-aminopteroylglutamic acid (4-amino PGA) administered by the oral route. *Am J Obstet Gynecol* 63:1298, 1952.
8. Tulsky, A., and Koff, A.   Some observations on the role of the corpus luteum in early human pregnancy. *Fertil Steril* 8:118, 1957.
9. Fujikura, T., Froehlich, L., and Driscoll, S.   A simplified anatomic classification of abortions. *Am J Obstet Gynecol* 95:902, 1966.
10. Klopper, A.   Endocrine Factors in Abortion and Premature Labor. In F. Fuchs, and A. Klopper (Eds.), *Endocrinology of Pregnancy*. New York: Harper & Row, 1971. P. 328.
11. Goldzieher, J.   Double-blind trial of a progestin in habitual abortion. *JAMA* 188:651, 1964.
12. Janerich, D., Piper, J., and Glebatis, D.   Oral contraceptives and congenital limb reduction defects. *N Engl J Med* 291:697, 1974.
13. Kitzmiller, J.   Septic shock: An eclectic view. *Obstet Gynecol Surv* 26:105, 1971.
14. Warburton, D., and Fraser, F.   Spontaneous abortion risks in man: Data from reproductive histories collected in a medical genetics unit. *Am J Hum Genet* 16:1, 1964.
15. Barter, R., Dustabek, J., Riva, H., and Park, J.   Surgical closure of incompetent cervix during pregnancy. *Am J Obstet Gynecol* 75:511, 1958.
16. McDonald, J.   Suture of the cervix for inevitable miscarriage. *J Obstet Gynaecol Br Commonw* 64:346, 1957.
17. Lash, A., and Lash, S.   Habitual abortion: The incompetent internal os of the cervix. *Am J Obstet Gynecol* 59:68, 1950.

Additional Readings

Atienza, M., Burkman, R., King, T., Burnett, L., Lau, H., Parmley, T., and Woodruff, J.   Menstrual extraction. *Am J Obstet Gynecol* 121:490, 1975.
Berger, G., Tietze, C., Pakter, J., and Katz, S. Maternal mortality associated with legal abortion in New York State: July 1, 1970–June 30, 1972. *Obstet Gynecol* 43:315, 1974.
Edwards, L., and Hakanson, E. Changing status of tubal sterilization: An evaluation of fourteen years' experience. *Am J Obstet Gynecol* 115:347, 1973.
Reid, D.   Assessment and management of the seriously ill patient following abortion. *JAMA* 199:805, 1967.
Reid, D. E., and Benirschke, K.   Abortion. In D. E. Reid, K. J. Ryan, and K. Benirschke (Eds.), *Principles and Management of Human Reproduction*. Philadelphia: Saunders, 1972.
Seward, P., Ballard, C., and Ulene, A.   The effect of legal abortion on the rate of septic abortion at a large county hospital. *Am J Obstet Gynecol* 115:335, 1973.
Studdiford, W., and Douglas, G.   Placental bacteremia: A significant finding in septic abortion accompanied by vascular collapse. *Am J Obstet Gynecol* 71:842, 1956.
Tietze, C.   Ranking of contraceptive methods by levels of effectiveness. *Adv Plann Parent* 6:117, 1970.
Wheeless, C., and Thompson, B.   Laparoscopic sterilization: Review of 3600 cases. *Obstet Gynecol* 42:751, 1973.

6   Ectopic Pregnancy

Ectopic pregnancy is the term used to designate the implantation of the zygote in a location other than the uterine corpus. Although tubal pregnancy accounts for about 95 percent of ectopic pregnancies, other locations include both intrauterine and extrauterine nidation sites (Fig. 6-1). The ectopic pregnancy may implant in the cervix, in the interstitial portion of the tube, or in the cornu of the uterus. It may attach itself to the ovary or to other abdominal sites. It may locate ultimately in the broad ligament, probably as a result of extrusion of a tubal gestation between the leaves of peritoneum.

Ectopic pregnancy occurs in about 1 in every 125 to 300 pregnancies, depending on the type of institution reporting its experience. The disease is more prevalent among blacks than among the white population, due perhaps to the higher incidence of gonorrheal salpingitis in blacks. It is seen more often in lower socioeconomic groups than in private patients. There is evidence that the frequency of the disease has been on the increase over the past few years.

Tubal Pregnancy

ETIOLOGY

An etiologic factor can be detected in no more than 50 percent of patients with ectopic pregnancy. Factors that block or delay passage of the fertilized ovum through the tube can be recognized in certain cases. Factors that increase the receptivity of the tubal mucosa to a zygote are also postulated as etiologic influences.

Gonorrheal salpingitis, which usually involves the endosalpinx, is more likely to precede tubal pregnancy than is a postabortal or postpartum salpingitis in which the infection is limited primarily to the peritubal tissue. A preceding chronic salpingitis may explain 25 to 30 percent of observed tubal pregnancies.

Other factors that obstruct the passage of the fertilized ovum probably account for many fewer cases of tubal pregnancy than does chronic salpingitis. Among such factors are diverticula or other congenital defects in the tubal mucosa, tubal cysts or tumors, peritubal adhesions that may cause kinking of the tube, and uterine myomas at the uterotubal junction. The risk of subsequent ectopic pregnancy is greatly increased by prior tubal surgery, particularly by any attempt to repair tubal damage or occlusion caused either by prior infection or by a tubal ligation. The theoretical possibility that the delay associated with transmigration of a fertilized ovum from one ovary to the contralateral tube could be a cause for tubal pregnancy should also be considered. The transmigration may occur through the peritoneal cavity (external), or it may occur by passage down one tube, through the uterus, and up the opposite tube (internal).

While endometriosis in the tubal mucosa can be considered a theoretical attraction for tubal implantation, the case has not been proved and is dismissed as an infrequent etiologic factor by most authorities.

Among tubal pregnancies unexplained by any of the preceding possibilities, a disruption of tubal physiologic processes seems the most likely etiologic factor. While hard to prove, such an explanation seems entirely possible when the intricacies of the physiologic processes necessary to proper tubal function are considered. Peristalsis, cilial action, and tubal mucosal secretions are all highly dependent on precise relationships between estrogen and progesterone and perhaps other hormone secretions. A minor disruption of one or more of the tubal functions may prevent conception. One of the

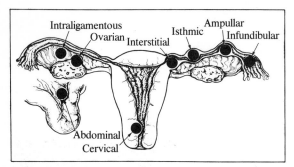

Fig. 6-1. Anatomic variance of ectopic pregnancy. (After T. McElin. In D. Danforth [Ed.], Textbook of Obstetrics and Gynecology [3rd ed.]. New York: Harper & Row, 1977. P. 357.)

bases for the contraceptive action of progesterone is its effect on tubal physiology. With these facts in mind, it is not difficult to imagine a slight dysfunction in tubal physiology sufficient to delay the pickup of a fertilized ovum or the passage of the zygote through the tube long enough to allow tubal implantation.

A change in tubal physiology might also result from emotional factors. Most physicians have seen infertility patients whose tubes simply would not allow the passage of a dye used at salpingography yet who become pregnant. "Tubal spasm" is the diagnosis usually made in such a patient, and the spasm is presumed to be emotionally induced. Tubal spasm mild enough to allow the entrance of the zygote but strong enough to retard its passage through the tube seems a reasonable etiologic explanation.

PATHOLOGY

The pathologic sequelae of tubal pregnancy result from the maternal reaction to the misplaced zygote; the implanting ovum is identical microscopically to one implanting in the endometrium. Most important in determining the type of pathologic reaction to the invading zygote is the location of the implantation (see Fig. 6-1). If the pregnancy site is the relatively voluminous ampullary portion of the tube, the pregnancy may enlarge into the tubal lumen and thus survive for some time. If the ovum has become implanted in the narrow isthmic por-

tion of the tube, tubal rupture is likely to occur early. In any case, the fetus is usually represented as a blighted ovum.

Implantation in the tube, as in the endometrium, is characterized by almost immediate penetration of the epithelium by the invading trophoblast and lodgment in the tissue beneath the epithelium. Little decidual reaction occurs, and the ovum begins growing in the thin myometrium of the tube, which is ill equipped to accommodate the pregnancy. Very little muscle hypertrophy occurs as the trophoblast continues its burrowing, invading activity in its search for nutrition. Very soon, maternal blood vessels are entered and bleeding ensues. If the vessel is a large one, the ovum may be surrounded by expanding clots. Rupture either into the tubal lumen or through the tubal wall results from expansion of the clot or from the invasion of the trophoblast itself.

Whether luminal or serosal rupture occurs is dependent primarily on the location of the conceptus. With a pregnancy in the narrow isthmus, rupture is likely to occur through the external wall, either into the peritoneal cavity or, if the initial implantation is on the mesosalpingeal side of the tube, between the leaves of the broad ligament. If the pregnancy implanted in the ampulla near the fimbria, rupture is more likely through the fimbriated end of the tube (tubal abortion) (Fig. 6-2). With a pregnancy in the ampulla, a longer distance from the fimbria, rupture through the tubal wall is the more likely termination.

Tubal abortion usually occurs between the sixth and twelfth weeks. Various pathologic outcomes may follow intratubal rupture. The pregnancy may have been separated completely from the tubal mucosa by bleeding, and the abortus is then forced out through the tubal lumen and into the peritoneal cavity. Bleeding may cease, and it is likely that some patients who experience this outcome recover without operative interference and with the true diagnosis frequently unrecognized. If some placental tissue remains attached to the tube following tubal rupture, or if extrusion fails to occur, the tube may become distended with blood, forming a hematosalpinx; or the exuding blood may

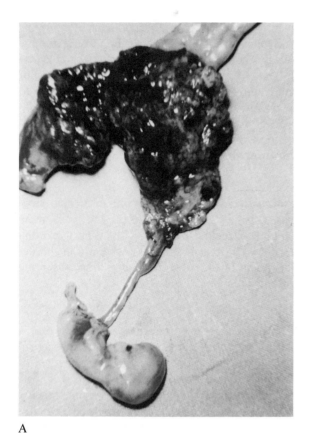

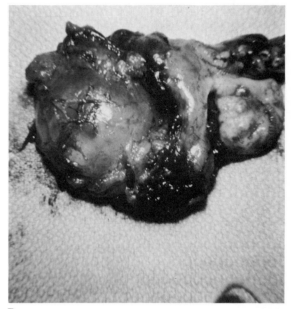

A

B

Fig. 6-2. A. Ruptured tubal pregnancy with fetus extruded. B. Unruptured tubal pregnancy. Ovary on right.

collect in the cul-de-sac, forming a pelvic hematocele. In rare instances, the partially extruded placenta may become attached to surrounding organs, thus forming an abdominal pregnancy.

Tubal rupture into the peritoneal cavity is to be expected with an isthmic location, in many instances of ampullary ectopic pregnancy, and with interstitial or cornual pregnancy. A rupture usually occurs early with an isthmic or ampullary location, but with interstitial pregnancy, the catastrophe may not occur until the third or fourth month. Following rupture, intra-abdominal bleeding is usually of sufficient severity to demand laparotomy. Death may occur before medical help can be obtained. In some instances, the bleeding may be milder, occa-

sionally allowing the placenta to attach to an abdominal organ and form an abdominal pregnancy. With an interstitial pregnancy, the amount of bleeding is usually very large, producing real danger of death before treatment can be instituted.

If the tubal rupture occurs between the leaves of the broad ligament, a hematoma develops. Acute symptoms may subside, since the closed space provides hemostasis. A "chronic" ectopic pregnancy may thus develop. In some cases, subsequent rupture of the hematoma may occur; in others, only palpation of a broad ligament "tumor" will reveal the pathologic condition.

Changes in the uterus occur with regularity with an ectopic pregnancy, although the degree of change is related to the amount of steroid hormone secreted by the chorionic villi. A decidual reaction is seen in the endometrium in less than half the cases. In some cases, a proliferative or a secretory endometrium is identified. An atypical endometrial reaction, the Arias-Stella phenomenon, is seen with some frequency. With this pathologic reaction, the epithelial cells contain hypertrophied, hyperchromatic, irregularly shaped nuclei, with plentiful vacuolated cytoplasm. The cells may be piled up and even wrongly suggest a malignant process. Their pathologic appearance is thought to be a peculiar reaction to overstimulation of the endometrium with steroids. Withdrawal of steroids is thought to account for the vaginal bleeding seen so regularly with ectopic pregnancy.

CLINICAL PICTURE

Only a small minority of patients with tubal pregnancy present with a classic history and physical findings, namely, abdominal pain, amenorrhea followed by slight vaginal bleeding, and an adnexal mass, shock, and other evidences of intraperitoneal bleeding. The diagnostic acumen of the physician may be sorely tried in making the diagnosis early enough to spare the patient the hazards of continued intraperitoneal bleeding.

Although the diagnosis of an unruptured tubal pregnancy is not often made with certainty, the physician will have considered the diagnosis in many cases because of certain factors in the history and physical findings. The reproductive history may be helpful, since a long period of infertility frequently precedes the development of a tubal pregnancy. A reliable history of an episode of acute salpingitis, of a plastic surgical procedure on the fallopian tubes, or of appendicitis with rupture will further support such a diagnosis. Of particular importance is a history of abnormal vaginal bleeding combined with the complaint of crampy lower abdominal pain, even of a minor degree. While other diagnoses, such as a threatened abortion, will need to be considered, the astute clinician will seriously consider a tubal pregnancy in such patients.

Abdominal Pain

Abdominal pain is the most reliable symptom of tubal pregnancy. Before rupture, the pain is frequently of a colicky variety and in one of the lower abdominal quadrants. It is usually not severe, may be intermittent, and may be associated with bladder or bowel irritability. It frequently disappears for some hours or days before rupture occurs, only to reappear. When the tube ruptures, the pain increases markedly in severity for a short time, following which it becomes more diffuse throughout the lower abdomen.

Amenorrhea

Amenorrhea is a classic symptom of ectopic pregnancy, but this history is not elicited from many patients. Decidual bleeding with vaginal spotting occurs with great frequency very early in the development of the tubal pregnancy, thus obscuring the expected amenorrhea.

Vaginal Bleeding

Vaginal bleeding is present in most patients and is usually scanty in amount. Indeed, heavy vaginal bleeding, although present in perhaps 5 percent of patients with tubal pregnancy, suggests a diagnosis of threatened abortion of an intrauterine pregnancy rather than ectopic gestation. The bleeding is frequently intermittent, although it may be persistent, and, on occasion, it has been observed for days before the appearance of other symptoms.

Pelvic Mass

A pelvic mass is discovered in only about half of the patients with a tubal gestation. The absence of the expected mass on pelvic examination should not negate other evidence suggestive of the diagnosis. On the other hand, it must be remembered that the presence of a pelvic mass without other confirming evidence of tubal pregnancy is not a reliable physical sign.

Pain on Motion of the Cervix

Pain on motion of the cervix is an extremely reliable sign of an adnexal abnormality. To elicit this sign, the utmost gentleness is vital, since most patients will complain of pain during a clumsy pelvic examination. If other adnexal disease, such as salpingitis or a twisted ovarian cyst, can be ruled out, this sign is of great importance in arriving at the diagnosis of ectopic pregnancy.

Other Symptoms

Certain other symptoms or signs are of occasional value in approaching the diagnosis of ectopic pregnancy. *Cullen's sign,* a bluish discoloration of the skin in the periumbilical area, is a rare observation and may be useful. The sign results from a leakage of intraperitoneal blood into the tissue underlying the skin. *Shoulder pain* is observed on occasion as intraperitoneal blood comes into contact with the subdiaphragmatic peritoneum. *A pregnancy test* is positive in about 50 percent of patients, depending on the amount of human chorionic gonadotropin (HCG) secreted by the trophoblast, but the test is not often of diagnostic use. *Hemoglobin and hematocrit readings* may drop as intraperitoneal bleeding persists. A mild *leukocytosis* (15,000 cells) is frequently noted; higher readings are unusual. The patient is usually *afebrile,* although progressive dehydration or a "chronic" ectopic pregnancy may cause a mild fever of 100°F. Higher temperatures suggest a diagnosis of salpingitis.

Clinical History

While the clinical history in some patients seems to begin acutely with immediate evidence of massive intraperitoneal bleeding and shock, in most patients, an antecedent illness will have been noted. Frequently, the earliest sign is abnormal vaginal bleeding, with or without a period of amenorrhea. Bleeding is usually minimal and is frequently noted for a few days or a week or two before the onset of lower abdominal pain. The abdominal pain is typically crampy and not too severe. It may be associated with frequency of urination and the urge to defecate. Other symptoms of pregnancy, such as breast soreness, nausea, and vomiting, are usually absent.

Physical Findings

Abdominal examination may reveal lower abdominal tenderness, especially in one quadrant, but this may not be marked. The pelvic examination is an especially useful diagnostic tool; even at this early stage of the disease, marked pain may be elicited on motion of the cervix. The uterus is often slightly enlarged and slightly softened, a normal response to the hormones of pregnancy, but these signs may not be observable. A pelvic mass may be palpated in half of the patients.

A useful triad in the diagnosis of an early unruptured tubal pregnancy is abnormal vaginal bleeding, abdominal pain, and pain on motion of the cervix in the absence of evidence of infection. With this triad to suggest tubal pregnancy, further diagnostic investigation is in order. We prefer to admit the patient to the hospital for a work-up.

Diagnostic Techniques

While many patients with an unruptured tubal pregnancy improve clinically after the initial symptoms, the clinician is obliged to rule out the disease before allowing the patient to go home. Various time-consuming measures used in the past to arrive at a diagnosis are rarely applicable since newer diagnostic tools have become available. While a progressive decrease in the hematocrit and the hemoglobin readings has been of diagnostic importance in the past, many hours are lost while waiting for this evidence. A more aggressive diagnostic plan is indicated in patients with an uncertain diagnosis.

A cul-de-sac puncture can be performed without anesthesia (Fig. 6-3). With a tenaculum on the posterior cervical lip, the posterior fornix is cleansed with an antiseptic. With or without local vaginal-wall infiltration with a local anesthetic, the cul-de-sac is punctured sharply in the midline with a No. 18 or 19 spinal needle. Aspiration of nonclotting blood strongly suggests the diagnosis of intraperitoneal bleeding. Blood from a vein will usually clot. The absence of any blood is a negative test. While both false-positive and false-negative tests occur, they are infrequent (Table 6-1).

In some cases it may be preferable to examine the patient under general anesthesia and to open the cul-de-sac surgically for direct inspection. The

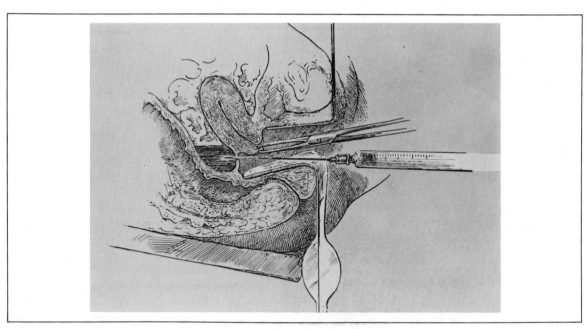

Fig. 6-3. Technique of cul-de-sac aspiration. (From V. Capraro, J. Chuang, and C. Randall. Cul-de-sac aspiration and other diagnostic aids for ectopic pregnancy. Int Surg 53:254, 1970.)

technique is as follows: The vaginal mucosa posterior to the cervix is incised transversely and dissected off the underlying peritoneum for a short distance. The peritoneum can usually be opened without difficulty. If blood is present in the cul-de-sac, it can be seen. The approach also allows visualization and palpation of both ovaries and tubes. While some surgeons excise an obvious tubal pregnancy through this approach, most prefer to postpone definitive surgery until the laparotomy incision is made.

A third diagnostic tool of increasing importance is visualization through a laparoscope. Except in the presence of a large amount of intraperitoneal blood, when the laparoscope is not needed to make the diagnosis, great diagnostic accuracy attends its use. We feel that the instrument should be used in all doubtful cases of tubal pregnancy in which the cul-de-sac puncture has been unsatisfactory for some reason. Ultrasound has been of only minimal help of our experience.

On occasion, abnormal vaginal bleeding is the primary symptom, with abdominal pain a minimal complaint. A dilatation and curettage may be per-

formed with a preoperative diagnosis of incomplete abortion. If the pathologist reports microscopic evidence of decidua (maternal tissue) with no chorionic villi (fetal tissue) seen, a diagnosis of tubal pregnancy must be seriously entertained. Similarly, the presence of the Arias-Stella phenomenon described earlier should arouse suspicion. A further diagnostic work-up in such a patient will usually include a laparoscopic examination.

Rupture

When the tubal pregnancy ruptures, the clinical picture is usually more characteristic. While a history suggestive of an unruptured pregnancy will usually be elicited, occasionally the history is a very short one. The patient will complain that the severe abdominal pain began in one of the lower quadrants but became subsequently more generalized. It may have become severe immedi-

Table 6-1. Correct Preoperative Diagnosis Based on Cul-de-Sac Aspiration

Results of Aspiration	Number of Patients	Number of Correct Diagnoses	Number of Incorrect Diagnoses	Percent Correct Diagnosis
Cul-de-sac aspiration positive[a]	256	227	29	88.7
Cul-de-sac aspiration negative	435	432	4	99.3
No cul-de-sac aspiration	51	33	18	64.7
Total	742	692	51	93.2

[a]Of 691 cul-de-sac aspirations, 29 (4.2%) were false-positive and 4 (0.67%) were false-negative.
Source: V. Capraro, J. Chuang, and C. Randall. Cul-de-sac aspiration and other diagnostic aids for ectopic pregnancy. *Int. Surg.* 53:247, 1970.

ately following straining at stool or coitus. Examination of the abdomen will reveal muscle spasm and frequently rebound tenderness. It may be possible to detect a fluid wave or other evidence of intraperitoneal blood. Pelvic examination will now show generalized tenderness with marked pain on motion of the cervix. The cul-de-sac may have the "doughy" feeling that indicates the presence of intraperitoneal blood, and an adnexal mass may be palpated. Shock will either be present or should be expected. Sometimes, the shock is so profound that the depressed sensorium obscures many of the physical findings. Dizziness and fainting are frequent symptoms.

DIFFERENTIAL DIAGNOSIS

A ruptured tubal pregnancy with intraperitoneal bleeding and shock is usually an obvious diagnosis. Unruptured tubal pregnancy, however, presents such a varied clinical picture that a differential diagnosis of tubal pregnancy and a number of other disease states is essential. The more commonly confused conditions and the factors that usually allow a differentiation are as follows:

1. Intrauterine pregnancy with threatened abortion:
   a. The amount of vaginal bleeding is usually much greater with threatened abortion.
   b. The abdominal pain may be more in the midline with threatened abortion, and it may be less severe. Differentiation by this symptom may be difficult.
   c. Findings on physical examination are different from those in threatened abortion. In threatened abortion, abdominal and pelvic tenderness is usually absent, the uterus is substantially larger, and the usual pregnancy signs of uterine and cervical softness are more evident. An adnexal mass is usually not felt.

2. Pelvic inflammatory disease:
   a. A typical history of acute attacks can usually be elicited, frequently at the time of the menses.
   b. The symptom complex of amenorrhea and abnormal vaginal bleeding is much less frequent with pelvic inflammatory disease.
   c. Both the abdominal symptoms and the pelvic findings are more likely to be bilateral with pelvic inflammatory disease.
   d. A temperature elevation above 100° to 101°F. is usual with pelvic inflammatory disease but rare with tubal pregnancy.

3. Acute appendicitis:
   a. The "typical" history of appendicitis is usually present: epigastric pain moving to the right lower quadrant, accompanied by nausea and vomiting. The physical findings may be similar, with tenderness and muscle spasm usually greater with appendicitis.
   b. Data from the history suggesting pregnancy (amenorrhea, abnormal vaginal bleeding) are absent.
   c. Pelvic examination rarely elicits positive findings. The uterus is usually not enlarged;

pain on motion of the cervix is usually not elicited; tenderness is unusual and, if present, is high in the pelvis.

4. Other adnexal pathology:
   a. A *corpus luteum cyst* develops when the corpus luteum fails to regress at the expected time. Amenorrhea, mild lower quadrant pain, and an adnexal mass may all suggest a diagnosis of tubal pregnancy. The symptoms of a corpus luteum cyst, however, are less severe, and pain is seldom elicited on motion of the cervix. Frequent reexamination will confirm the correct diagnosis.
   b. A *twisted ovarian cyst* of any variety may simulate the pain of tubal pregnancy. Amenorrhea and abnormal vaginal bleeding are rarely present. No evidence of intraperitoneal bleeding or shock is apparent. While there will be pain on motion of the cervix, the adnexal mass will be firmer and usually larger than with tubal pregnancy. A rare cause of a clinical picture like that of tubal pregnancy is a twisted hydatid cyst of Morgagni. A ruptured endometrial cyst of the ovary will cause similar abdominopelvic findings, but no amenorrhea or vaginal bleeding is noted.

TREATMENT

The treatment of tubal pregnancy is surgical, whether the tube is ruptured or intact. An unruptured tubal pregnancy has not often been diagnosed preoperatively in the past, but the use of a laparoscope should make earlier diagnosis possible today. Clearly, the earlier the diagnosis is made, the greater the surgical options once the peritoneal cavity has been entered.

The operative procedure chosen will depend on: (1) the patient's general condition, (2) her wishes concerning future childbearing, (3) the location of the tubal pregnancy, and (4) the degree of tissue destruction that has resulted from the disease. The major possible surgical choices include (1) milking of the conceptus out the fimbriated end of the tube, (2) salpingectomy, (3) removal of the ipsolateral ovary, together with the affected tube, and (4) salpingostomy.

If the patient is in shock, the easiest and quickest procedure is obviously the best. As soon as adequate amounts of blood have become available, the abdominal incision is made. Attempts to transfuse blood to achieve a normal circulatory volume before beginning surgery are usually futile, since raising the blood pressure simply increases the intraperitoneal bleeding. After entering the abdomen, with minimal maneuvering, the uterus is grasped with the hand, and the involved adnexal structures are visualized. A clamp across the broad ligament below the tube will usually stop the bleeding, and transfused blood should now quickly reestablish blood volume. In cases of severe shock, central venous pressure monitoring before and during surgery may be essential to control the amount and type of intravenous fluid to be administered. Subsequent surgery, if indicated, can be done with the shock under control.

If the patient's general condition will allow it, an assessment of both tubes and ovaries should be made before performing definitive surgery. Contralateral disease or a missing tube will influence the type of surgical attack on the affected tube. Similarly, a severely damaged or infected tube will exclude all possible surgical choices except excision.

If the involved tube is unruptured or is minimally damaged from rupture, especially if the uninvolved tube is abnormal, a simple salpingostomy may be performed (Fig. 6-4). The tube overlying the conceptus is incised longitudinally, and the conceptus is removed. Hemostasis is achieved with delicate ligatures; the surgical rent in the tube is not sutured, since tubal constriction may result. Some authors recommend primary closure of the incision [1]. For more extensive disease with severe tubal damage, a simple salpingectomy will be necessary. If the ovary is involved in the disease process, a salpingo-oophorectomy may be required.

If the patient is particularly anxious to preserve her fertility even in the face of an added risk of a repeat tubal pregnancy, tubal reconstruction of an

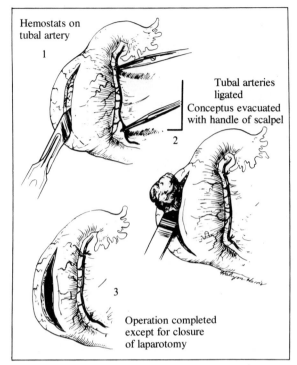

Hemostats on
tubal artery

1

Tubal arteries
ligated
Conceptus evacuated
with handle of scalpel

2

3

Operation completed
except for closure
of laparotomy

Fig. 6-4. Conservative management of unruptured tubal pregnancy by salpingostomy. (From P. Tompkins. Preservation of fertility by conservative surgery for ectopic pregnancy. Fertil Steril *7:448, 1956.)*

abnormal contralateral tube may be attempted. If the patient does not wish to have any future pregnancies, tubal ligation of the contralateral tube, or a total hysterectomy, may be desirable at the time of the surgical treatment of the tubal pregnancy, assuming the patient's general condition warrants the additional surgery. Appendectomy may safely be performed following the treatment of a tubal pregnancy.

In a few instances, simple milking of the tubal pregnancy past the fimbria may be possible. Similarly, if tubal abortion has occurred without significant tubal damage, no further surgery except for hemostasis may be necessary. In all cases, the clotted blood in the peritoneal cavity should be removed to help prevent the development of peritoneal adhesions.

INTERSTITIAL PREGNANCY

Pregnancy in the portion of the fallopian tube that lies within the myometrium is termed an *interstitial tubal pregnancy*, or a *cornual pregnancy* (Fig. 6-5), and accounts for less than 1 percent of tubal pregnancies. This variety of tubal gestation deserves special attention since most of the deaths associated with tubal pregnancy occur with this lesion. Because of its location, the pregnancy can expand into the uterine fundus, and the resulting placenta is much more luxuriant than with other varieties of tubal gestation. A large placenta produces adequate steroids, and the decidual bleeding so often noted with the other varieties of tubal pregnancy is frequently absent. The location also permits the pregnancy to progress much further before rupture, and the pain associated with enlargement of the tube is frequently absent. There is little to suggest the diagnosis until rupture occurs, frequently as late as the fourth month and usually after 8 to 10 weeks. The rupture occurs in a highly vascular area, where bleeding is brisk. It is among this group of patients that death may occur before hospitalization can be arranged. If the necessary hysterectomy is performed very early in the course of the disease, however, the prognosis should be good. When reviewing in retrospect why the diagnosis was not made earlier, the physician will usually uncover no evidence that would have led him to suspect the disease before the catastrophic rupture.

Ovarian Pregnancy

To qualify as an ovarian pregnancy, the fetal sac must be surrounded by ovarian tissue and the ipsilateral fallopian tube must be normal. In such cases, fertilization probably occurred in the ovary itself, although subsequent implantation following tubal fertilization and abortion cannot be excluded. The disease accounts for about 1 percent of ectopic gestations and is of interest pathologically because of the peculiar location of the pregnancy.

Clinically, the disease usually cannot be distinguished from a tubal pregnancy, although ovarian pregnancy has been reported to go to term in some

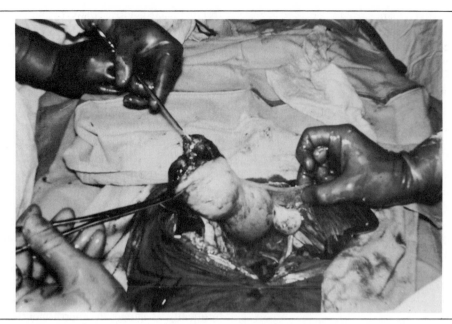

Fig. 6-5. Cornual angle pregnancy, which has been surgically opened, can be seen on the left. The normal uterus can be seen below the conceptus, and a normal ovary lies next to the uterus.

cases. In other cases, ovarian tumor will have been the preoperative diagnosis, and the true diagnosis is not appreciated until the pathology report is completed.

Cervical Pregnancy

Cervical pregnancy, a very rare and serious form of ectopic pregnancy, results from implantation in the cervical mucosa. The pregnancy invades the fibrous cervix and quickly forms a palpable tumor that can usually be distinguished from the uterine fundus above it. Bleeding is an early symptom and demands termination of the pregnancy before midgestation. Since excision of the pregnancy by the vaginal approach is apt to be bloody, this procedure should be reserved for the patient willing to take the surgical risk to preserve her fertility. A better treatment is abdominal hysterectomy, and even this procedure may be technically difficult because of the greatly enlarged cervix [2].

Abdominal Pregnancy

Abdominal pregnancy is a very rare condition that is probably more prevalent among the medically indigent, since it nearly always follows neglected tubal pregnancy. The pregnancy may implant anywhere on the peritoneal surface and frequently involves several organs. In most cases, a tubal abortion has resulted in reattachment of the placenta to the organs surrounding the fimbria of the tube, although occasionally a far-distant implantation site is found. There is evidence that the abdominal pregnancy is "primary" in some cases, i.e., there was no prior tubal gestation. A number of cases have appeared in the literature in which an initial intrauterine implantation was followed by extrusion of the conceptus through a defect in the uterine wall resulting from a previous cesarean section.

Unlike pregnancies in other extrauterine gestation sites, pregnancy in the abdominal cavity can, and frequently does, progress to late pregnancy and even to term. This is not to suggest a good fetal prognosis, however, since many accidents may befall the fetus during its precarious existence. If fetal death occurs, and if the fetus is not removed surgically, one of several terminations can be expected. (1) Pyogenic bacteria may gain access to the amniotic sac, resulting in formation of an abscess that usually ruptures intraperitoneally, with high maternal risk. (2) The fetus may become calcified and remain for years as a lithopedion. (3) The fetal bones may extrude through the maternal abdominal wall, intestines, or bladder. (4) The fetus may simply degenerate to form adipocere, a greasy mass of tissue.

Maternal risk is apparent from the chain of events that follows untreated fetal death. Also, at any time during the pregnancy, the placenta may become detached from its bed and produce life-threatening hemorrhage. Even when exploratory laparotomy is performed early enough to avoid this hazard during pregnancy, the placenta may become detached and produce a fatal hemorrhage even during meticulously careful surgery. Of great importance to the mother is the site of placental attachment, since adherence to a nonvital structure may allow removal of the organ, a treatment that is not possible with some attachments.

DIAGNOSIS
The diagnosis is a difficult one to make. The history will usually include an episode of vaginal bleeding and abdominal pain at six to eight weeks' gestation when the tubal abortion occurred. After reattachment to abdominal viscera the pregnancy thereafter may have continued in a normal fashion, except perhaps for more bladder and bowel complaints than usual. In the absence of an accident to the fetus or to the placenta, the diagnosis may be first suspected by the physician when the fetus is palpated "too easily" on abdominal examination. A separate uterus, slightly larger than normal, may be palpated but is usually not felt. It is said that the maternal souffle, the soft swishing sound heard normally over the area of the placenta, is much louder with abdominal pregnancy. This sign, however, is not present following fetal death. While in such pregnancies the fetus is usually in a transverse

lie or breech presentation, this finding is only suggestive of the diagnosis.

Confirmation of the diagnosis can be attempted in several ways. All types of x-ray examinations have been tried. The most useful has been found to be a direct lateral film, which may show a fetal skeleton overlying the maternal vertebrae—an almost certain sign of abdominal pregnancy. Interest is increasing in the use of hysterography to outline the empty uterus or the use of retrograde femoral aortography. The oxytocin test suggest by Cross et al. [3] is of great usefulness if the results are positive. If the abdominal mass contracts after the administration of 1 unit of oxytocin given intramuscularly, an abdominal pregnancy can be ruled out with certainty. A negative test result is less useful.

TREATMENT
The treatment of abdominal pregnancy is immediate surgical intervention. Delay to allow fetal maturation is not recommended because of the possibility of a placental accident at any time and because the fetal survival rate is low (perhaps 20 percent) under the best of circumstances.

With a large amount of cross-matched blood available, and with an expert anesthesiologist prepared to handle a sudden massive hemorrhage, the abdomen is opened. The fetus is delivered with great care and with as little trauma as possible. All efforts should be directed toward avoiding placental detachment. If, and only if, the placenta is obviously attached to nonvital and removable structures (uterus, broad ligament) may an attempt be made to remove it, usually also with removal of the attached organs. In most instances, particularly when the placenta is known to be attached to an unremovable peritoneal surface, it is best to leave the placenta in situ and close the abdomen without drainage. Even with this procedure, the risk is not over, since a placental detachment may occur in the postoperative period, before the placental vessels are thrombosed. Subsequent intraperitoneal infection, abscess formation, development of bowel adhesions, and other unhappy events can be expected, and subsequent surgery is the rule. The risk of these complications is less, however, than the risk of fatal hemorrhage from attempting to remove the placenta.

References

1. DeCherney, A., and Kase, N. The conservative surgical management of unruptured ectopic pregnancy. *Obstet Gynecol* 54:451, 1979.
2. Ranade, V., Palermino, D., and Tronik, B. Cervical pregnancy. *Obstet Gynecol* 51:502, 1978.
3. Cross, J., Lester, W., and McCain, J. The diagnosis and management of abdominal pregnancy with a review of 19 cases. *Am J Obstet Gynecol* 62:303, 1951.

Additional Readings

Boronow, R., McElin, T., West, R., and Buckingham, M. Ovarian pregnancy. *Am J Obstet Gynecol* 91:1095, 1965.

Breen, J. A 21-year survey of 654 ectopic pregnancies. *Am J Obstet Gynecol* 106:1004, 1970.

Franklin, E., and Zeiderman, A. Tubal ectopic pregnancy: Etiology and obstetric and gynecologic sequelae. *Am J Obstet Gynecol* 117:220, 1974.

Stander, R. Abdominal pregnancy. *Clin Obstet Gynecol* 5:1065, 1962.

Stromme, W. Conservative surgery for ectopic pregnancy: A twenty-year review. *Obstet Gynecol* 41:215, 1973.

Placenta Previa

When the site of placental development and attachment is at a point lower in the uterus than usual, so that all or a portion of the placenta will precede the fetus during expulsion, *placenta previa* is said to be present.

If the placenta totally covers the internal cervical os, placenta previa is said to be *complete* or total. *Partial* placenta previa is diagnosed if only a portion of the internal cervical os is covered. *Marginal* placenta previa is a subdivision of partial placenta previa and is present if the placenta extends to the margin of the internal cervical os but does not protrude into the os (Fig. 7-1). While this terminology seems clear enough pathologically, in the clinical setting, precision in identifying the degree of placenta previa may not be possible. Thus, a complete placenta previa at 2-cm. dilatation of the cervix may be of the partial variety at 6-cm. dilatation. The extent of the placental encroachment on the cervix is best recognized at the time of cesarean section, when a good view of the location of placental attachment can be made after delivery of the fetus. Gentle vaginal examination is less satisfactory in this regard. Fortunately, the precise location of the placenta is less important than the severity of the clinical symptoms. However, the observation that the lower the placental attachment (i.e., the greater the degree of previa), the greater the amount of bleeding is generally valid.

Placenta previa occurs in about 1 percent of deliveries, is more common in the multipara than in the primipara, and increases in frequency with the age of the gravida and the shortness of the interval between pregnancies. Indeed, the decreasing incidence of placenta previa in the United States is probably related to the lower parity of the obstetri-

cal population or, more likely, to the lower average age of the population.

The etiology of placenta previa is unknown, but a number of possible causative factors may be considered. Damage to the endometrium from previous pregnancies or from inadequate blood supply to the endometrium caused by the aging process may necessitate a wider area of attachment and subsequent extension of the attachment to the lower uterine pole to provide adequate placental perfusion. The commonly noted thinner, larger placenta associated with placenta previa supports this concept. Placenta accreta (see Chap. 12) may coexist with placenta previa. Late fertilization of the ovum occurring in the portion of the tube near the uterus may permit a longer journey before implantation occurs. The increased frequency with which placenta previa is noted with abnormal presentation of the fetus, notably transverse lie and breech presentation, is probably the cause, rather than the result, of the abnormal presentation. The fetus tries to accommodate itself to an altered intrauterine shape. A markedly increased risk of recurrence of placenta previa in a patient previously affected has been noted, a fact which suggests an etiologic predisposition to the disease. The factor or factors responsible, however, remain obscure.

DIAGNOSIS

Clinical History

As pregnancy progresses, the lower uterine segment thins, and the cervix begins to efface and eventually to dilate. A placental attachment in the lower pole of the uterus during this process will be damaged. The resultant separation of the margin of the placenta causes painless vaginal bleeding. The

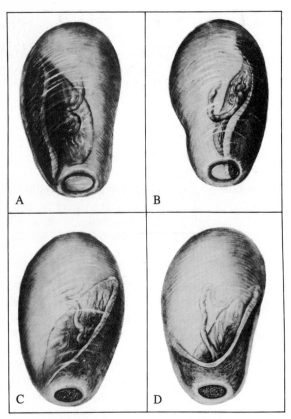

Fig. 7-1. Types of placenta previa. A. Low-lying placenta. B. Marginal placenta previa. C and D. Variations of complete placenta previa. (From J. Willson. Atlas of Obstetric Technic [2nd ed.]. St. Louis: Mosby, 1969. Daisy Stilwell, medical illustrator.)

lower the placental attachment, the earlier the vaginal bleeding. A clot usually forms over the damaged placental edge, and bleeding stops for a variable time—sometimes a few weeks; occasionally only for a few hours. Subsequent marginal separation is the rule, however, and a second or third bleeding episode will occur. During one of these episodes, the bleeding does not stop, and the time for active interference will have arrived.

About 50 percent of patients will experience the first bleeding episode after the thirty-fourth week of pregnancy, but in some patients the first bleeding may be noted as early as mid-pregnancy. If there is no maternal shock, the fetus usually is not jeopar-

dized in utero. The major danger to the fetus is prematurity, and prolongation of the pregnancy to the thirty-sixth week or longer is highly desirable if the mother's life is not at risk from continued bleeding and shock from blood loss. Shock, of course, is also a hazard to the fetus. Vaginal bleeding from placenta previa is painless unless labor supervenes, and this fact usually permits differentiation of placenta previa from premature separation of the normally implanted placenta.

Physical Examination

Before initiating any examination, blood is drawn for an immediate hematocrit, blood typing, and cross matching. A balanced electrolyte solution infusion must be instituted if bleeding is excessive, and a central venous catheter is also necessary in this instance. Physical examination of the patient must *not* include rectal or vaginal examination, since any palpation of the placenta may induce uncontrollable bleeding. In the absence of maternal shock, evaluation of the patient's clinical status will include repeated measurements of vital signs, hematocrit determinations, and estimations of blood loss. Johnson [1] and Macafee [2] independently reported that the first vaginal bleeding episode is rarely, if ever, fatal if no local examination is performed, and that the effect of a subsequent bleeding episode is determined largely by the hematocrit of the patient. The fetal heart tones are usually audible and normal. In the absence of continued vaginal bleeding, certain special tests for placental localization may be employed (see Special Tests).

In the presence of maternal shock, or if significant vaginal bleeding continues, it may be necessary to determine quickly and accurately the cause for the bleeding by performing a pelvic examination. Since any palpation of the placenta may induce hemorrhage, the examination should be performed only in the operating theater with the equipment and personnel necessary to effect immediate abdominal delivery if that becomes necessary; this is the so-called double setup examination. The patient should have an intravenous infusion of balanced electrolyte solution running, with at least

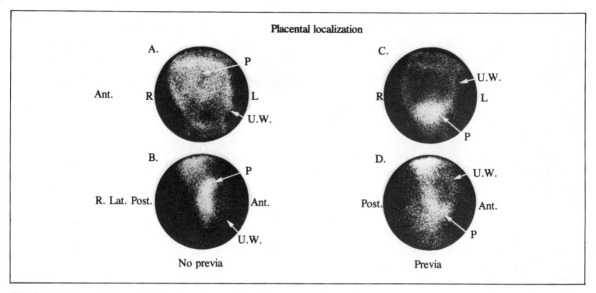

Placental localization

A. P · R · L · U.W. · Ant.

B. P · R. Lat. Post. · Ant. · U.W.

No previa

C. U.W. · R · L · P

D. U.W. · Post. · Ant. · P

Previa

Fig. 7-2. Radionuclidic study for placenta previa using indium 113m and the scintillation camera. A and C. Anterior views. B and D. Right lateral views. Left column shows images from a patient with a high posterior placenta. Right column shows images from a patient with central placenta previa. (P = placenta; U.W. = uterine wall; R = right; L = left; Ant. = anterior; Post. = posterior.) (Courtesy of Dr. Daniel Berman.)

three pints of blood cross-matched and present in the operating room before the examination is attempted. The indications for the procedure as well as the differential diagnosis of placenta previa will be discussed subsequently.

Special Tests

In certain instances, when the clinical situation permits, it may be desirable to localize the placenta by an indirect method to differentiate a placenta previa from other causes of late hemorrhage of pregnancy. Many tests have been devised for this purpose, with varying success rates. Radiographic examinations have included soft-tissue techniques, the injection of a contrast material into the bladder, and amniography. A substantial risk of misdiagnosis is present with any of these techniques. Retrograde femoral angiography with the injection of a dye above the level of the hypogastric artery will

outline the placenta with great accuracy, but the procedure entails some risk both for the mother and the fetus and no longer seems justified.

The injection of an isotope into the maternal circulation results in concentration of the isotope in the markedly vascular placenta, since the amount of isotope localized is directly proportional to the amount of blood in any particular organ (Fig. 7-2). Accurate localization of the placenta is usual. Technetium 99–tagged albuminate or indium 113m are safe and commonly used isotopes. Radioisotopic study is nearly as accurate and is performed with much less radiation exposure than the conventional radiographic techniques. Localization of the placenta using ultrasonography (Fig. 7-3) is increasingly used and is the most accurate and safest technique available today. The equipment for this test and personnel trained in its use and interpretation are presently available in most centers and are becoming increasingly available in the community hospital. In the final analysis, the clinician should consult his laboratory support team about the best method at his institution.

Differential Diagnosis

Local causes of third-trimester bleeding include carcinoma of the cervix as well as other more benign

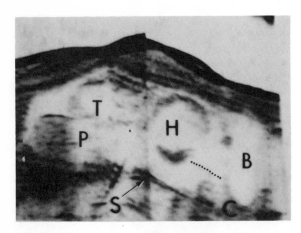

Fig. 7-3. Placenta previa: Sagittal B-scan. Note that the distance between the fetal head and the maternal spine is 3 cm. (normal distance is 1.5 cm. or less) due to the interposition of a posterior placenta previa. A dotted line has been added to the sonogram to illustrate the approximate anterior edge of the placenta. (P = placenta; S = [maternal] spine; B = [maternal] bladder; H = fetal head; T = fetal trunk; C = cervix.)

conditions such as cervical polyp, and these diseases must be ruled out if the expectant management to be described is to be instituted. Less easily excluded from the differential diagnosis are intrauterine causes of bleeding, such as abruptio placentae and velamentous insertion of the cord (resulting sometimes in vasa previa). In the latter case, bleeding usually occurs coincidental to rupture of the membranes and may be associated with significant fetal bradycardia on auscultation or via physical monitoring. In a suspected case, the diagnosis can be made by examination of a stained smear of the blood (see Chap. 12). Premature separation of the normally implanted placenta most frequently requires differentiation from placenta previa. The methods used for this differentiation are described under Abruptio Placentae.

TREATMENT

A major change in the treatment of placenta previa occurred in 1927 when Bill [3] recommended adequate transfusion and immediate cesarean section in place of the Braxton Hicks' version (extraction of a fetal leg through the cervix to tamponade bleeding) and various other techniques previously used. The maternal mortality rate was lowered, but perinatal mortality remained distressingly high. In 1945, Macafee [2] and Johnson [1] independently suggested delay in the definitive treatment of placenta previa in certain cases, thus allowing further maturation of the fetus. They showed that the first episode of bleeding was rarely, if ever, fatal if rectal and vaginal examinations were avoided. Risk of a subsequent hemorrhage was found to be extremely small if the patient was not permitted to become anemic. A recent study reported the use of expectant management in about two-thirds of patients compared to less than one-half a decade ago [4]. Expectant management, when appropriate, and cesarean section for delivery have become the cornerstones of the treatment of placenta previa.

Expectant Management

Expectant management may be indicated (1) when the first bleeding episode occurs at less than 35 weeks' gestation; (2) when the bleeding quickly stops; and (3) when a rectal or vaginal examination is avoided. Expectant management allows time for the employment of an indirect technique of localization of the placenta. Subsequent management of the patient is determined by the results of this localization, since definite identification of placenta previa as a cuase for the bleeding necessitates continued hospitalization until delivery occurs, or at least careful observation at home throughout the remaining pregnancy. If the placenta is found not to be in the lower uterine segment, a local condition or a minor degree of abruptio placentae is the likely cause of the bleeding.

Expectant management is *not* indicated if (1) the bleeding persists and demands intervention; (2) the bleeding episode has occurred at 35 weeks' gestation or later; or (3) the bleeding has been severe enough to jeopardize the mother. Since half the patients with placenta previa have the first bleeding episode after 35 weeks' gestation, and since many such patients experience heavy bleeding or continue to bleed, expectant management is applicable to only about one-third of the patients. The use of the L/S ratio to determine fetal maturity before an elective termination of pregnancy has significantly lowered the risk of neonatal mortality and morbidity [4].

If the gestation is at 35 weeks or more, or if the bleeding persists or is severe, a definitive diagnosis should be made unless maternal shock dictates immediate delivery. As soon after admission as possible, the patient is taken to the operating room, where a double-setup examination is performed. After careful speculum visualization of the cervix, the index finger is inserted carefully into the vagina, and the vaginal fornices are palpated. The finger is then gently inserted through the os. The gritty, spongelike placenta may be felt overlying the internal os. Minimal examination should be done to establish the diagnosis, since the danger of producing life-threatening hemorrhage is always present. If the placenta is not immediately felt, the internal os is palpated throughout its circumference. If the placenta is still not felt, the membranes should be carefully stripped from the lower uterine segment and a marginal or low-lying placenta sought. With a presumed diagnosis of low-lying placenta, or of abruptio placentae established by the absence of placenta previa, amniotomy is indicated. Tamponade of bleeding by the fetal head pressing on a low-lying placenta will result, and the desired labor should begin.

Cesarean Section

Diagnosis of a central or partial placenta previa by pelvic examination dictates immediate cesarean section. All but the most minor degrees of marginal placenta previa also demand section. The uterine incision is best made in a longitudinal direction because of the underlying placenta. Incision may be made in the anterior wall of the fundus or in the lower uterine segment. Following extraction of the infant, immediate removal of the placenta is essential. Oxytocic drugs and massage of the uterus will usually stop bleeding from the placental site, but bleeding may occasionally continue. An immediate

hysterectomy (frequently a supracervical hysterectomy is safer and will suffice) or ligation of the hypogastric arteries may be necessary in this instance and may be lifesaving.

PROGNOSIS FOR MOTHER AND CHILD
Until the introduction of transfusion and cesarean section into the treatment of placenta previa, maternal mortality was as high as 1 in 10, with perinatal mortality approaching 50 percent. Today, many clinics report no maternal mortality from placenta previa in large series of cases. Perinatal mortality remains distressingly high—about 10 percent among mature infants and 30 to 35 percent among low-birth-weight infants. Cotton et al. [4] experienced a perinatal mortality rate of only 12.6 percent overall, a reduction of about one-half from a decade earlier. Early delivery can be shown to decrease the fetal death rate but only at the cost of an increase in the neonatal mortality [5]. Expectant treatment lowers the risk of neonatal death, but a higher fetal mortality results.

Is the infant who survives the insult of placenta previa likely to be neurologically damaged from the hypoxia he may experience? A recent study suggests that the infant born following placenta previa is no more likely to be neurologically abnormal than is an infant of the same birth weight born without the complication [6]. Low birth weight continues to be the major factor accounting for infant mortality and for neurologic damage in the surviving child.

COMPLICATIONS
Intrauterine infection may complicate the clinical picture because of the close proximity of the placenta to the vaginal flora. Infection is a grave complication and should be treated vigorously with a broad-spectrum antibiotic until a more specific drug can be identified from a culture report. Delivery should be accomplished either by induction with amniotomy with the lesser degrees of placenta previa or by early cesarean section followed by hysterectomy.

It is not surprising that a placenta that attaches

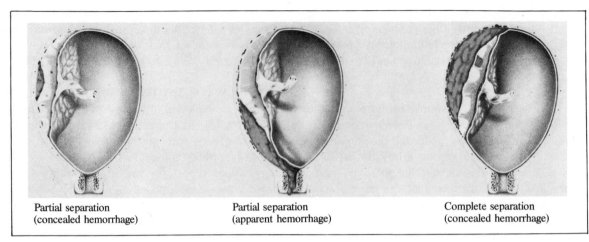

Partial separation
(concealed hemorrhage)

Partial separation
(apparent hemorrhage)

Complete separation
(concealed hemorrhage)

Fig. 7-4. Types of abruptio placentae (premature separation of the normally implanted placenta). (From Abnormalities of the Placenta. *Clinical Education Aid No. 12. Columbus, Ohio: Ross Laboratories, 1972.)*

itself to an area with relatively poor decidua may grow into the uterine muscle, resulting in placenta accreta or one of its more serious forms, placenta increta or placenta percreta. These rare complications are discussed in Chapter 15. It is important that the clinician recognize the possibility of these abnormalities, since hysterectomy in such cases is usually preferable to piecemeal removal of the placenta, with the risk of uncontrollable bleeding.

Abruptio Placentae

Detachment from the uterine wall of a portion, or all, of the normally implanted placenta before delivery of the baby is known as premature separation of the normally implanted placenta, or, synonymously, abruptio placentae. In its severe form, premature separation is one of the most serious abnormalities encountered in obstetrics, with almost inevitable fetal loss and a substantial risk of maternal mortality. About 1 percent of viable pregnancies show some degree of placental separation, with the severe form occurring in only about 10 percent of separations. Classification of cases can be made according to clinical condition (severe, moderate, or mild premature separation). In general, there tends to be agreement between the pathologic findings and the clinical severity of disease.

If the placental separation is *complete,* the ma-

ternal symptoms are usually severe, and the fetus is nearly always dead. With *partial* abruptio placentae, the clinical manifestations are characteristically mild to moderate, although the patient may exhibit symptoms and clinical findings as disturbing and severe as does the patient with complete separation (Fig. 7-4). *Marginal* placental separation (sometimes referred to as marginal sinus rupture) usually presents with mild signs and symptoms, and unless progression to a more severe form occurs, the prognosis for both mother and infant is good.

ETIOLOGY

The etiology of premature separation remains unknown, but a number of factors are recognized or suspected to be associated with the abnormality. The disease is much more common in women with high parity than in primigravidas, and an increase with maternal age has been reported by some observers. Since the incidence of chronic hypertension also increases with maternal age and with in-

[handwritten margin note: most typically ass w/ clotting defect but not in Pl. Previa !]

creasing parity, a possible explanation for the reported relationship between chronic hypertensive disease and premature separation of the placenta is evident.

Some investigators have observed a relationship between dietary folic acid deficiency and an increased risk of placental abruption [7]. Recent studies have failed to confirm this finding. Mengert and his group [8] caused premature separation of the placenta simply by compression of the vena cava above the level of the renal veins in two patients undergoing repeat cesarean section. The possibility must be considered that spontaneously occurring vena caval compression may be an etiologic factor in abruptio placentae, but the absence of placental separation following vena caval ligation for thrombophlebitis in a number of reported cases must also be noted.

Extremely rare causes of the disease are occasionally recognized. A direct blow to the abdomen may precede the appearance of abruptio placentae, but the infrequency of the relationship is noteworthy. An extremely short umbilical cord may exert tension on the placenta as the fetus descends through the pelvis and cause placental separation. Amniocentesis is a modern, but a rare, cause for the disease.

The relationship between placental separation and acute or chronic hypertensive disease is of special importance because of the high incidence of hypertensive disease in patients with placental separation reported by some investigators (40 to 60 percent). Among 199 cases of abruptio placentae reported from the Collaborative Perinatal Project, toxemia of pregnancy was noted in 15.0 percent of patients with placental abruption but in only 8.5 percent of patients who did not have the placental accident [9]. The incidence of toxemia was higher in younger gravidas (in 30 percent under the age of 16) and in older gravidas (in 19.6 percent over the age of 29). Pritchard [10] noted hypertension in 47 percent of gravidas suffering placental abruption of a degree sufficient to kill the baby but a much lower incidence with less severe abruption. It is evident that hypertension and placental abruption fre-quently coexist, but an etiologic relationship remains unestablished.

PATHOPHYSIOLOGY

Decidual degeneration may be caused by an arteriolitis. Whatever the cause of the decidual degeneration, whether it be vascular disease, trauma, or other factors, rupture of blood vessels in the decidua occurs, with bleeding into the retroplacental space. The blood quickly clots because the decidual tissue is rich in thromboplastic material, and the clot expands as bleeding continues. The uterine musculature, already stretched by the pregnancy, is unable to contract to control the bleeding. The clot compresses a portion of the placenta and distorts the contour of the placenta, which is useful in identifying premature separation in the specimen following delivery of the placenta. As the bleeding continues, the blood usually dissects the membranes free from the decidua, and external bleeding is seen as blood escapes from the external cervical os. Occasionally, no external bleeding is noted, and these cases are frequently the more severe. Blood may infiltrate into the myometrium, causing the uterus to assume a mottled blue or purple color (Couvelaire uterus). This is a development of some clinical importance, since such a uterus contracts poorly during the postpartum period, leading to postpartum hemorrhage. The blood may also break through the fetal membranes and enter the amniotic sac.

The retroplacental hemorrhage may be sudden and massive and cause a complete separation of the placenta, with the dramatic clinical picture of severe abdominal pain and uterine tenderness, hypovolemic shock, and absence of fetal heart sounds, followed quickly by renal complications or a blood coagulopathy (Fig. 7-5). The bleeding, however, may develop at a slower rate, with less dramatic clinical signs. One should always expect the pathologic picture to become progressively worse, and treatment should not be delayed because the disease appears mild. The frequency of the development of a complication of placental separation, notably a blood coagulopathy or a renal

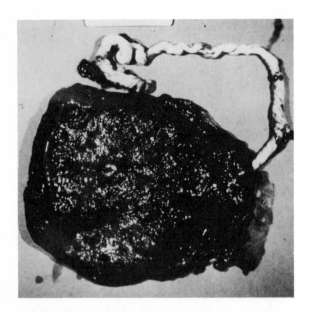

Fig. 7-5. Placenta with partial abruptio placentae. There is adherent clot throughout most of the periphery of the placenta. Note particularly the adherent clot over 25 percent of the surface of the placenta on the right of the illustration.

lesion, is time-related; i.e., it is less likely to develop if the uterus is emptied within a reasonable period of time, usually said to be 6 hours following the onset of the disease.

DIAGNOSIS AND CLINICAL COURSE

Severe Abruptio Placentae

Severe abruptio placentae is easily diagnosed when a patient presents with severe unremitting abdominal pain, a boardlike uterus that fails to relax and is exquisitely tender and irritable, and varying degrees of shock, frequently severe. Dark vaginal bleeding is noted in most cases, and the fetal heart sounds are usually absent or hard to hear because of the poor uterine relaxation. The fetal heart rate (FHR) may reflect fetal distress due to hypoxia. A renal complication—either the usually fatal acute cortical necrosis or the possibly reversible acute tubular necrosis—or a blood coagulopathy is likely to occur. Treatment of the disease must be prompt and vigorous if the risk of a serious complication is to be minimized.

Moderate Abruptio Placentae

Moderate abruptio placentae is usually easy to differentiate from placenta previa, but the signs and symptoms are less pronounced than with the severe variety. Shock may be present but is easily treated; the fetal heart sounds are usually present, although evidence of fetal distress may be noted; and the abdominal pain and uterine irritability and tenderness are less pronounced than with severe disease. Although the patient may initially appear to have only a moderately severe abruption, rapid progression of the disease may occur. Treatment should be instituted immediately.

Mild Abruptio Placentae

Mild abruptio placentae presents few obvious signs other than vaginal bleeding. While the uterus may be slightly irritable, the sign may not be an easy one to recognize; indeed, obvious uterine irritability suggests progression of the disease. In many instances, the vaginal bleeding may suggest placenta previa, and a double-setup examination may be required for differentiation. Treatment of the disease will depend on the severity of the symptoms. Many instances of mild vaginal bleeding in the third trimester with no recurrence or further complications go undiagnosed. In all likelihood, these are cases of mild abruption or marginal sinus rupture.

The differential diagnosis between mild abruption and placenta previa depends ultimately on indirect placentography, as described under Placenta Previa, or on the results of a double-setup examination (Table 7-1); if the clinical picture is progressive and a differentiation cannot be made any other way, a double-setup pelvic examination should be employed.

MANAGEMENT OF MODERATE AND SEVERE ABRUPTIO PLACENTAE

In all but the mildest cases, the management of premature separation of the placenta is directed toward correction and maintenance of the mother's cardiovascular status and emptying of the uterus.

Table 7-1. Differential Diagnosis of Placenta Previa and Abruptio Placentae

Sign	Placenta Previa	Premature Separation of Placenta
Vaginal bleeding	Frequently bright red	May be dark
Uterine irritability	Absent	Present in many cases
Uterine tenderness	Absent	Frequently present, at least in small circumscribed areas
Fetal heart sounds	Normal	May be evidence of fetal distress
Associated hypertension	Rare	May be present

Since many of the complications of the disease are time-related, emptying the uterus is a matter of some urgency, and it should be accomplished within a few hours of the onset of symptoms in most instances.

Monitoring of the Vital Functions

In severe or moderate placental abruption, monitoring of the vital functions of the mother and of the fetus is essential, since deterioration of both patients' clinical status must be recognized early and the results of therapeutic measures assessed. Monitoring should include: (1) central venous pressure (CVP) measurements on a continuing basis; (2) hourly measurement of urinary output through catheter drainage; (3) periodic determination of the status of the blood coagulation mechanism; and (4) continuous FHR monitoring. Adequate blood must be cross-matched for possible transfusion, and other measures to prevent or combat shock must be taken. Steps to empty the uterus must be initiated, including amniotomy or the administration of oxytocin to induce labor, or cesarean section unless labor is expected to be rapid. The possibility of uncontrollable bleeding at cesarean section or during the postpartum period must be kept constantly in mind, since a myometrium that has been infiltrated with blood may not contract appropriately to prevent hemorrhage.

CENTRAL VENOUS PRESSURE MONITORING. Monitoring the CVP is necessary if the patient is in shock or if shock is anticipated. Large amounts of intravenous fluid and blood may be necessary in the treatment of shock and hypovolemia, and care must be exercised if circulatory overload is to be avoided. If the CVP exceeds 12 cm. H_2O, incipient heart failure or pulmonary edema can be anticipated. Monitoring of the CVP provides useful information concerning the patient's functional cardiac capacity to manage the fluid load being presented. It is not a measure of the sufficiency of intravascular fluid volume, which is best determined by the arterial blood pressure, urinary output, state of the peripheral vasculature, and other clinical signs.

KIDNEY FUNCTION MONITORING. A catheter should be inserted into the bladder on the patient's admission to the hospital. The kidney is very sensitive to lack of perfusion from hypovolemic shock, and kidney function should be constantly assessed by measurement of urinary output. A urinary flow of 60 to 100 ml. per hour suggests normal kidney function. If urinary output falls below this level, a rapid intravenous infusion of 150 ml. of normal saline will result in an increase of urinary output if kidney function is adequate; absence of this effect suggests kidney failure.

BLOOD COAGULATION MONITORING. Measurement of the ability of the maternal blood to clot is essential in all patients, since hypofibrinogenemia occurs in about 10 percent of cases, more commonly in the severe form of abruptio placentae. Conventional laboratory tests for measuring fibrinogen are too time-consuming to help clinical management. Of more use is observation of a 5-ml. sample of the patient's venous blood placed in a clean, dry test tube at her bedside. Failure of the blood to clot within 5 to 10 minutes, or dissolution of the clot as it stands at room temperature for half an hour or more, suggests that fibrinogen is below a crucial level, probably about 100 mg. per 100 ml. A normal test result, however, does not assure a continued normal level of fibrinogen. The test should be repeated hourly until the patient delivers, and even after delivery if bleeding persists.

Treatment of hypofibrinogenemia (or increased fibrinolysis) remains controversial. The standard infusion of 4 gm. of fibrinogen intravenously has recently been called into question not only because of the significant danger of subsequent hepatitis but also because continued consumption of fibrinogen produces fibrin split products that are in themselves fibrinolytic. The use of heparin to stop the consumption of fibrinogen has been recommended. Consultation with a hematologist is essential.

Fetal Heart Rate Monitoring

Continuous FHR monitoring is the best method of fetal assessment currently available. With complete placental abruption, fetuses are nearly always dead or so severely damaged as to be beyond salvage. With lesser degrees of abruption, abnormal FHR patterns may be recognized early enough to allow rapid delivery by forceps if full dilatation of the cervix has occurred—or by cesarean section if it has not.

Delivery

While the monitoring of these various physiologic parameters proceeds and while necessary intravenous fluid or blood and other measures to combat shock are being taken, a decision should be made regarding the method of delivery. In the absence of evidence of fetal distress, amniotomy will usually quickly induce rapid labor. Careful intravenous administration of dilute oxytocin may be added, if necessary (see Induction of Labor). Cesarean section is indicated (1) if the amniotomy and oxytocin fail to induce effective labor; (2) if delivery cannot

be anticipated within a few hours; (3) if the treatment for shock is unsuccessful and the mother's condition is not improving; or (4) if fetal distress can be diagnosed from the FHR tracing. In many instances, vaginal delivery can be anticipated. With severe shock, however, cesarean section may be the safest method of delivery because it is the only rapid way of stopping the hemorrhage.

Postpartum Care

If bleeding persists after cesarean section or during the postpartum period, and if a blood coagulopathy can be ruled out, it is likely that poor contractility of the uterus is the cause, and supracervical hysterectomy or hypogastric artery ligation may be necessary.

Sheehan's syndrome (pituitary necrosis) occasionally follows the shock associated with premature separation, and this disease must be suspected in the postpartum period. Lactation at the appropriate time suggests that the pituitary has escaped damage, but subsequent management of gonadal, thyroid, and adrenal function may be required.

MANAGEMENT OF MILD ABRUPTIO PLACENTAE

Management of mild abruptio placentae consists primarily of the differentiation of placenta previa from abruption as previously described, and observation, in the absence of uterine irritability or continued vaginal bleeding. If the vaginal bleeding occurs before 36 weeks' gestation, tests of placental localization should be ordered. If the bleeding occurs after 36 weeks, a double-setup pelvic examination is indicated, with an amniotomy performed if placenta previa can be ruled out. If the uterus is irritable or if the patient experiences pain, the disease should no longer be considered mild and should be managed in the same manner as described for moderate degrees of placental separation.

PROGNOSIS

Maternal mortality from premature separation of the placenta should be very low. Many clinics report no deaths from this disease over a period of many years. Death may be the direct result of hemorrhage, i.e., shock; or it may be due indirectly to the effect of hemorrhage, i.e., renal failure secondary to acute cortical necrosis. A good fetal outcome is much less certain, because the fetus usually dies with complete abruption and because even mild disease frequently occurs at an early gestational interval, thus exposing the fetus to the additional hazard of immaturity. If the fetus survives the accident and lives, there is evidence that he is likely to develop normally for the gestational interval in which delivery occurs.

References

1. Johnson, H. The conservative management of some varieties of placenta previa. *Am J Obstet Gynecol* 50:248, 1945.
2. Macafee, C. Placenta praevia: Study of 174 cases. *J Obstet Gynaecol Br Emp* 52:4, 1945.
3. Bill, A. The treatment of placenta previa by prophylactic blood transfusion and cesarean section. *Am J Obstet Gynecol* 14:523, 1927.
4. Cotton, D., Read, J., Paul, R., and Quilligan, E. The conservative aggressive management of placenta previa. *Am J Obstet Gynecol* 137:687, 1980.
5. Nesbitt, R., Yanhauer, A., Schlesinger, E., and Allaway, N. Investigation of perinatal mortality rates associated with placenta previa in upstate New York, 1942–1958. *N Engl J Med* 267:381, 1962.
6. Niswander, K., Friedman, E., Hoover, D., Pietrowski, H., and Westphal, M. Fetal morbidity following potentially anoxigenic obstetric conditions. II. Placenta previa. *Am J Obstet Gynecol* 95:853, 1966.
7. Hibbard, B. The role of folic acid in pregnancy with particular reference to anaemia, abruption and abortion. *J Obstet Gynaecol Br Commonw* 71:529, 1964.
8. Mengert, W., Goodson, J., Campbell, R., and Haynes, D. Observations on pathogenesis of normally implanted placenta. *Am J Obstet Gynecol* 66:1104, 1953.
9. Niswander, K., Friedman, E., Hoover, D., Pietrowski, H., and Westphal, M. Fetal morbidity following potentially anoxigenic obstetric conditions. I. Abruptio placentae. *Am J Obstet Gynecol* 95:838, 1966.
10. Pritchard, J. Genesis of severe placental abruption. *Am J Obstet Gynecol* 108:22, 1970.

Additional Readings

Benirschke, K. A review of the pathologic anatomy of the human placenta. *Am J Obstet Gynecol* 84:1595, 1962.

Crenshaw, C. Placenta previa: A survey of twenty years' experience with improved perinatal survival by expectant therapy and cesarean delivery. *Obstet Gynecol Surv* 28:461, 1973.

Kobayashi, M., Hellman, L., and Fillisti, L. Placental localization by ultrasound. *Am J Obstet Gynecol* 106:279, 1970.

Malkasian, G., and Welch, J. Placenta previa percreta. *Obstet Gynecol* 24:298, 1964.

Sher, G. A rational basis for the management of abruptio placentae. *J Reprod Med* 21:123, 1978.

Studer, H., and Lock, F. Sudden maternal death associated with amniotic fluid embolism. *Am J Obstet Gynecol* 64:118, 1952.

Tatum, H., and Mule, J. Placenta previa: A functional classification and a report on 408 cases. *Am J Obstet Gynecol* 93:767, 1965.

Weiner, A., Reid, D., and Roby, C., II. Incoagulable blood in severe premature separation of the placenta: A method of management. *Am J Obstet Gynecol* 66:475, 1953.

Baca Post Partum Bleeding suelas Prodih an Trimess he - 3 mi

Hypertensive Disorders During Pregnancy

Hypertensive disease complicates pregnancy in 5 to 10 percent of gravidas. With hemorrhage and infection, it ranks as one of the three major causes of maternal mortality and accounts for a large proportion of perinatal deaths. About two-thirds of patients suffering from hypertensive disease have a *chronic* disorder, which is etiologically unrelated to pregnancy. About one-third experience a disease peculiar to pregnancy, which has its onset during late gestation and subsides completely following delivery. This disease is called *preeclampsia-eclampsia* and in previous years *toxemia of pregnancy*. Chesley [1] has pointed out that the term *toxemia* is confusing, since no toxin has been discovered in connection with this disorder. By long usage, the term has achieved respectability, but we will identify the disease as preeclampsia-eclampsia.

The differentiation of chronic hypertension from preeclampsia-eclampsia is important, since both maternal and fetal prognoses are markedly different for the two disease states. In some cases, the differentiation can be made during pregnancy, but in all too many cases, a precise diagnosis must await termination of the pregnancy. To confuse the differentiation further, chronic hypertension can be complicated by an exacerbation during pregnancy (chronic hypertension with superimposed preeclampsia-eclampsia). The criteria used to identify this complication will be discussed under Chronic Hypertensive Disease.

Classification

The classification of the hypertensive disorders of pregnancy has recently been revised by the American College of Obstetricians and Gynecologists [2]. The old classification of the American Committee on Maternal Welfare proposed in 1940 and still in wide use has many shortcomings. The new classification is as follows:

1. Transient hypertension.
2. Diseases peculiar to pregnancy.
   a. Preeclampsia.
   b. Eclampsia.
3. Diseases independent of pregnancy.
   a. Chronic hypertension of whatever cause.
4. Preeclampsia or eclampsia superimposed on chronic hypertension.
5. Unclassified hypertensive disorders.

Transient Hypertension

Transient hypertension is a newly recognized entity in which hypertension without proteinuria or edema develops during pregnancy but disappears within a few days following delivery. The diagnosis may be considered a catchall, since it probably includes patients suffering from mild preeclampsia as well as others who have chronic hypertension that is manifested only under the stress of pregnancy. In the Collaborative Perinatal Project [3] 1 to 2 percent of patients were classified as having transient hypertension.

Acute Preeclampsia-Eclampsia

The two forms of the hypertensive diseases peculiar to pregnancy are preeclampsia and eclampsia, differentiated by the presence of generalized convulsions or coma in eclampsia. Preeclampsia-eclampsia is recognized by the appearance of hypertension with proteinuria, or edema, or both after the twentieth week of pregnancy. Hypertension, by definition, is said to be present when the systolic reading is 140 mm. Hg or greater, or when the diastolic reading is 90 mm. Hg or greater, or when there has been an increase of 30 mm. Hg or more systolic or 15 mm. Hg or more diastolic. The abnormal reading must be present on two or more occasions at least 6 hours apart. Proteinuria is best measured in a 24-hour sample of urine, and for the purpose of diagnosis is defined as 500 mg. or more of protein per 24 hours; 1 gm. of protein per liter in two or more random clean samples of urine collected 6 hours or more apart will also satisfy the definition of proteinuria. A third acceptable method for identifying proteinuria is a 1+ or 2+ dipstick reading that is confirmed 6 hours later. Lesser amounts of proteinuria are not uncommon during normal pregnancy. Edema is less easily defined, but swelling of the legs and ankles only may be due merely to a dependent position of the extremities. Swelling of the hands and face can be labeled edema and is usually preceded by excessive weight gain.

Differentiation of *mild* preeclampsia from *severe* preeclampsia is desirable but not always easy. Chesley [1] identifies five factors, any one of which justifies a label of *severe* for the disease:

1. Systolic blood pressure of 160 mm. Hg or more or diastolic blood pressure of 110 mm. Hg or more on at least two occasions 6 hours apart with the patient at bed rest.
2. Proteinuria of 5 gm. or more in 24 hours (3+ or 4+).
3. Oliguria (400 ml. or less for 24 hours).
4. Cerebral or visual disturbances.
5. Pulmonary edema or cyanosis.

It should be remembered, however, that preeclampsia need not be severe to progress to eclampsia. A patient with mild preeclampsia may convulse before the attendant recognizes the seriousness of her disease. Since the addition of convulsions or coma to the preeclamptic state sharply increases both maternal and fetal mortality, it is important to institute therapy as soon as the diagnosis of preeclampsia has been made.

ETIOLOGY

The cause of preeclampsia (and of eclampsia, since the two conditions can be considered different manifestations of the same disease state) remains obscure, which explains why all treatment of the disease is symptomatic and empirical. Although many causes have been suggested, none has gained general acceptance, and most are unsupported by sufficient evidence.

Certain environmental factors have been proposed to account for differences in the incidence of preeclampsia-eclampsia. Because the disease is so prevalent in the southeastern United States, which has a large black population, race has been considered a possible etiologic factor. However, Chesley [1] notes that from 1931 through 1951, 9 percent of the obstetric population at one institution, the Margaret Hague Hospital, was black and 8.5 percent of the patients with eclampsia were black. Low socioeconomic status is thought by some to predispose to preeclampsia-eclampsia. However, Baird [4], in a study in Aberdeen, Scotland, found preeclampsia equally prevalent in the upper socioeconomic groups.

It has been suggested that preeclampsia-eclampsia may result from an immune reaction in the mother to fetal protein or to placental endotoxins. Renal disease has been thought by some to be the initiating factor in the development of the disease. There is some evidence that the syndrome may result from the liberation of thromboplastic material from the placenta into the general circulation, with a resultant disseminated intravascular coagulation. Certainly, in preeclampsia-eclampsia, there is a deposition of fibrinoid material in many organs.

Abnormalities in the renin-angiotensin system and in aldosterone secretion have been postulated as etiologic in preeclampsia-eclampsia. Renin plasma activity is lower in preeclampsia than in normal pregnancy, but angiotensin may increase arteriolar reaction. Aldosterone secretion is subnormal with preeclampsia-eclampsia and apparently does not explain the sodium retention so characteristic of the syndrome.

Dietary change is a commonly proposed cause of preeclampsia-eclampsia. The incidence of eclampsia decreased remarkably in Germany during World War I, when poor nutrition in Germany was the rule. A theory attributing this observed decrease in eclampsia to a low dietary intake of protein was later shown to be wrong, and the explanation for the phenomenon seems to have been a sharp decrease in the number of primigravidas; since the disease is primarily a disorder of primigravidas, a decrease in preeclampsia-eclampsia should have been expected. More recently, a lack of protein in the diet has again been suggested as the cause of the disease [5], but proof is lacking.

The best contemporary explanation for the onset of acute toxemia is the uterine ischemia theory. This idea is not a new one, but recent experimental evidence has provided strong support for it. Proponents of the theory point to the relationship between uterine overdistention and the incidence of preeclampsia-eclampsia, analogous to the relationship between multiple gestation and hydatidiform mole; or to the relationship between uterine vascular damage and acute or chronic hypertensive disease. In all of these illustrations, the blood flow to the uterus is decreased. A number of investigators have reported that experimental diminution in the uterine circulation in animals produces hypertension and proteinuria when abortion does not occur. Hodari [6], for example, ligated the ovarian arteries and banded the uterine arteries in nonpregnant dogs to prevent their dilatation during pregnancy. Hypertension and proteinuria developed in the few dogs who achieved a pregnancy that did not abort.

No theory, however, is generally accepted, and the cause of preeclampsia-eclampsia remains obscure. Much more is known about the pathophysiology of the disease resulting after the exciting factor or factors has had its effect, and these processes are discussed later (see Pathophysiology of Preeclampsia-Eclampsia).

PREECLAMPSIA

Clinical Course

Preeclampsia is a disease of the last 20 weeks of pregnancy. However, if a hydatidiform mole is present, the preeclampsia may occur much earlier and be very severe. McCartney [7] performed renal bi-opsies on 62 primigravidas whose condition had been diagnosed as preeclamptic. In only 43 of the patients were the typical microscopic kidney findings associated with preeclampsia noted; in 16, there were changes consistent with chronic renal disease, and 3 showed no abnormality. Among multiparas, the typical renal lesion was present in only 21 of 152 patients in whom the clinical diagnosis was preeclampsia. McCartney's study illustrates the uncertainty of the clinical diagnosis of preeclampsia even in the primigravid patient and the likelihood that the diagnosis will be incorrect when made in the multiparous patient.

Since all the early indications of preeclampsia fail to alert the patient, the importance of prenatal care can be recognized. Gant et al. [8] described a "roll-over" test that they found could identify the patient in whom preeclampsia-eclampsia is ultimately destined to develop. The "normal" primigravida at between 28 and 32 weeks' gestation was rotated from the lateral recumbent to the supine position. A rise in diastolic pressure of 20 mm. Hg or more was considered a positive test. Preeclampsia-eclampsia failed to develop in 91 percent of patients with a negative test. These results have been confirmed by others. Marx et al., for example, found that 33 percent of patients with a positive test develop preeclampsia while only 6 percent of those with a negative test subsequently develop the syndrome [9].

Frequently, the first clinical evidence that preeclampsia may be developing is excessive weight gain, especially if it occurs in a short period of time. A gain of 3 pounds (1.36 kg.) or more in a single week should certainly arouse suspicion in the clinician. The weight gain may reflect edema, which will be evident to the patient. Hypertension then develops, or hypertension may be the first evidence of the disease. A rise in blood pressure is more significant than an absolute high value; a rise in the diastolic reading should be viewed with special alarm. Proteinuria is a later finding and does not consistently occur with early preeclampsia. If the disease is well established, however, proteinuria nearly always will be found. The amount of protein spillage will vary remarkably from hour to hour, necessitating a 24-hour urine sample or multiple random samplings for its identification.

If the preeclampsia is very early and very mild, treatment may cause the disease to subside. Perhaps more exactly, the diagnosis may have been in error in this circumstance. More characteristically, the disease progresses and the signs become more obvious, necessitating hospitalization for observation and therapy. All but the mildest forms of the disease demand hospitalization.

Symptoms of preeclampsia eventually develop, but they usually occur late in the course of the disease and may be ominous. Blurring of vision is experienced because of retinal changes. Headache or nervous irritability suggests that a convulsive episode may be imminent. Epigastric pain, frequently severe and possibly the result of stretching of the liver capsule, is a particularly disturbing symptom, since a convulsion often follows this symptom within a short time. ∨ Scotomata,

Physical Findings

Physical examination of the preeclamptic patient will usually reveal edema, although a "dry" form of preeclampsia is recognized and is especially fulminating. The edema will usually involve the hands and face, as well as the lower extremities. The presacral area should be examined for edema if the patient has been kept in bed. Hyperactivity and apprehension in the preeclamptic patient suggest that she may be about to convulse. Hyperreflexia, and even ankle clonus, will usually be present in this circumstance; it is wise to monitor reflexes in all preeclamptic patients. Examination of the retina may show varying degrees of arteriolar spasm, and progression of this spasm usually heralds progression of the disease. The presence of hemorrhages or exudates in the ocular fundi suggests a diagnosis of chronic hypertension rather than acute preeclamptic toxemia, although the retinal changes with eclampsia may be less easily distinguished from those of chronic hypertension. With severe preeclampsia or eclampsia, detachment of the retina may occur. With recovery from the syndrome prognosis for a complete reattachment of the retina is good.

Treatment

PREVENTION. Prevention of preeclampsia may not be possible, but identification of the disease in its very early stage is the major objective of prenatal care. Since most of the early evidences of preeclampsia are not apparent to the patient, careful evaluation of the patient in the prenatal period is the only method of identifying these early signs. The goal of prenatal care is to avoid the disease altogether, or at least to limit its severity or terminate its effect by early delivery. Pregnant patients should be seen at least every other week in the seventh and eighth months of pregnancy and weekly during the final month. Abnormalities may necessitate more frequent examinations.

WEIGHT GAIN. A rapid gain in weight almost inevitably occurs with preeclampsia-eclampsia. Excessive weight gain should alert the physician to the possible development of the disease, but in most instances the weight gain will *not* be followed by other evidence of the syndrome. Thus, Fish et al. [10] found weight gains of 25 pounds (11.35 kg.) or more in 58 percent of patients in whom preeclampsia-eclampsia subsequently developed, while 44.7 percent of normal patients displayed similar weight gains. Indeed, Chesley [1] thinks there may be two distinct types of water retention, one benign and one identifying preeclampsia-eclampsia. He feels, however, that they are clinically indistinguishable. There is no evidence that the classic restriction of weight gain imposed tyrannically on pregnant women, primarily by American obstetricians, will decrease the risk of preeclampsia. Rather, weight gain should be recognized as an early sign of incipient disease and investigated as such.

EDEMA. Treatment of edema or excessive weight gain in pregnant women by a diuretic drug is no longer considered desirable by most authorities. There is no evidence that saluretic drugs either decrease the risk of preeclampsia when given routinely to all pregnant patients or minimize the progression of the disease when it appears. Indeed, thiazide diuretics have been associated with maternal death in a few cases, due apparently to electrolyte depletion and pancreatitis. Thrombocytopenia in the newborns of mothers who received thiazides has also been reported.

It is unsettled whether or not sodium ingestion should be restricted in patients with incipient preeclampsia-eclampsia. Since sodium and water retention are known to occur with the syndrome, sodium restriction would seem logical, and the practice is certainly widespread. Chesley [11] feels that salt ingestion may be a good test for the diagnosis of preeclampsia. If the disease progresses with salt ingestion, the diagnosis is confirmed. If, on the other hand, the salt seems to have no effect on the symptomatology, the diagnosis of preeclampsia is probably wrong.

AMBULATORY TREATMENT. If the diagnosis of preeclampsia is definitely established, hospitalization is essential. If the patient exhibits only excessive weight gain with perhaps a slight increase in blood pressure, management at home may be permissible, with more frequent office visits to detect any deterioration in the patient's condition. Such cases might be called incipient preeclampsia or perhaps mild preeclampsia. The weight gain and slight hypertension may disappear if the patient rests in bed much of the time, limits her sodium intake, and takes a mild sedative primarily to enforce the bed rest. Any progression of the disease demands hospitalization.

HOSPITAL THERAPY. Appraisal of the severity of the disease for a few hours is essential before therapy is started in most instances. Obviously, severe preeclampsia may progress rapidly to the eclamptic stage, however, and the observation in this case should be brief but thorough. The objectives of the therapy of preeclampsia-eclampsia are: (1) to prevent a convulsion, (2) to improve the patient's status, and (3) to empty the uterus at a time most likely to preserve the life of the mother and baby.

Admissions Procedures. The most pressing immediate need is to prevent a convulsion, and the following procedures are indicated on admission:

1. Taking of a careful history to elicit disturbing symptoms such as headache, blurring of vision, or epigastric pain.
2. Physical examination, including blood pressure reading, evaluation of edema, checking of neurologic reflexes, and assessment of fetal size and condition. The retina should also be examined.
3. Urinalysis for immediate determination of the degree of albuminuria, with institution of 24-hour urine collection for a more accurate record.
4. Baseline renal function tests (creatinine, creatinine clearance, blood urea nitrogen [BUN], and electrolytes). Other useful laboratory tests include liver function tests, fibrinogen level, and a complete blood count.
5. Repeat blood pressure determinations every 4 hours or more often if indicated.
6. Recording of fluid intake and output.
7. Daily weighing of patient before breakfast.
8. Fetoplacental function tests if indicated (e.g., 24-hour urinary estriol excretion, oxytocin challenge test) (see Chap. 12).

General Measures. Bed rest should be enforced. Dietary restriction of sodium has been practiced traditionally, but the effectiveness of the treatment has recently been seriously questioned. Fluid intake needs little regulation unless oliguria is present, when more stringent requirements are prescribed (see pp. 160–161). If the patient exhibits evidence of an impending convulsion, or if the preeclampsia is not mild, parenteral magnesium sulfate should be administered in an attempt to forestall a convulsion (see below). If the clinician is in doubt about the severity of the disease, it is probably best to begin magnesium sulfate therapy, since the medication has a wide range of safety if its effects are monitored properly.

In a few instances, evidence of the preeclamptic state will disappear completely, and the clinician may consider the possibility of discharging the patient to her home for close ambulatory supervision. Whether or not this is wise remains unclear. Many patients of this type will suffer a resurgence of the preeclampsia, with increased hazard. It may be wiser to treat such patients in the same way as

*because at this time, the risk of
Seizures is still significantly increase.*

those with more persistent disease, that is, by continued medical suppression of the pathologic changes of the disease and by termination of the pregnancy at the earliest date consistent with high perinatal survival and continued good maternal health (see Timing of Delivery).

Prevention of Convulsions. If the mild preeclampsia becomes progressively more severe, or if the initial disease seems severe or fulminating, more aggressive medical management is necessary. To help forestall a convulsion, the patient should be kept in a darkened room, with few visitors and minimal nursing disturbance. Magnesium sulfate [$MgSO_4 \cdot 7H_2O(USP)$] is generally felt to be the safest and most effective anticonvulsant agent available and should be prescribed in adequate amounts. The medication may be given intravenously or intramuscularly. The intravenous dose used by Zuspan [12] is 3 to 4 gm. as a loading dose, with constant infusion of 1 gm. per hour thereafter. The initial intramuscular dose is 10 gm. of a 50% solution given in divided doses in each buttock. Subsequent doses of 5 gm. intramuscularly may be given at 4-hour intervals. Some authorities prefer that an intravenous loading dose of 3 to 4 gm. precede the intramuscular maintenance medication. Since magnesium may reach toxic levels in the maternal blood, careful monitoring of its effects on the mother are necessary at frequent intervals, certainly before each subsequent intramuscular dose is injected (see below). It is essential to keep a syringe filled with 10 ml. of a solution containing 1 gm. of calcium lactate at the bedside, since calcium is an immediate antagonist of magnesium, and its use may forestall a cardiac arrest.

Magnesium sulfate has been thought to act by depressing the activity of the neuromuscular junction. New evidence suggests that the anticonvulsant effect of the drug may occur centrally [13]. It is known that at plasma levels of 10 mEq per liter, the knee jerk reflex disappears. At about 15 mEq per liter, respirations may cease and at 30 mEq per liter cardiac arrest will occur. Dosage is regulated by periodic checking of the knee jerk reflex and counting the respiratory rate. An absent or near-absent knee jerk reflex or a respiratory rate below

12 per minute contraindicate the next dose of the drug. Similarly, if the urine output has been less than 30 milliliters per hr., the next dose should be omitted. The drug, however, enjoys a wide range of safety and should be used in effective doses. With poor maternal kidney function, more careful monitoring is indicated. Toxicity in the fetus is apparently rare.

The duration of magnesium therapy is usually no longer than about 24 hours. The drug is used to prevent convulsions in the preeclamptic patient or to control convulsions in the woman with eclampsia. In any case, the patient is usually sufficiently ill to require early delivery after control of the convulsions is assured. The drug is continued throughout labor and the immediate puerperium. *for 24 hours* *

We do not use thiazide diuretics in the management of either preeclampsia or eclampsia. Bed rest is in itself a good diuretic. Sedation other than that provided by the magnesium sulfate may be desirable, especially with very mild preeclampsia. Phenobarbital in a dosage of 0.3 to 0.6 gm. three times a day may be tried.

Severe preeclampsia is treated as described above, with the objectives of preventing convulsions and improving, or at least stabilizing, the patient's medical status, so that a safe termination of the pregnancy becomes possible. If the magnesium sulfate fails to sedate the patient appropriately, paraldehyde administered rectally may be tried. The drug has been a standard treatment for many years. The dosage is 10 to 15 ml. in oil, repeated at 8- to 10-hour intervals as necessary.

Timing of Delivery. A patient at less than 35 weeks' gestation with mild preeclampsia may be managed by bed rest and sedation in an attempt to allow the fetus to gain maturity before delivery. Determination of the lecithin-sphingomyelin ratio in fluid obtained by amniocentesis will allow precise determination of fetal maturity (see Chap. 12). In most cases of preeclampsia, however, such conservative therapy will not be desirable, not only because prolonged preeclampsia may increase the risk of permanent vascular damage to the mother, but also because the infant usually does better in the nursery than in the uterus. Delayed intrauterine growth is the rule with preeclampsia, and a hypoxic episode may prove fatal. With most preeclampsia, therefore, delivery should be accomplished as soon as the disease is brought under control and the patient seems in optimal condition. If the treatment of preeclampsia is unsuccessful and if the condition of the patient deteriorates, early delivery is also indicated.

Induction of labor with amniotomy and oxytocin is frequently successful even when the cervix is unripe, and this technique should be tried in most cases. Careful fetal monitoring is essential to permit recognition of fetal hypoxia. If induction fails, if fetal hypoxia develops, or if the preeclampsia is very severe and not improving, cesarean section is indicated. Immaturity of the fetus is an ever-present hazard, but immaturity augmented by poor intrauterine environment is even more deadly.

ECLAMPSIA

Eclampsia may occur before delivery, during delivery, or in the early postpartum period. The appearance of convulsions or coma due to eclampsia usually means medical failure, either because the patient has not sought medical attention during pregnancy or the physician has not recognized the seriousness of the preeclamptic stage of the disease or has not treated preeclampsia with sufficient vigor. Even in the best clinics, however, convulsions will complicate a preeclamptic syndrome that has appeared mild by all measurable criteria; such a development is to all intents and purposes non-preventable in this circumstance. Fortunately, the incidence of eclampsia has been decreasing for a number of years in the United States.

Pathophysiological Factors in Preeclampsia-Eclampsia

Although the initiating factor in preeclampsia-eclampsia is unknown, much has been learned about the pathophysiologic results of this unknown factor or factors. The primary (or at least the very early) pathologic effect is vascular spasm, which has been well documented and can explain many of the pathologic findings associated with the disease. Preeclamptic patients have a hyperreactive vaso-

motor system, as shown by a hyperreactivity of the blood pressure to a dose of vasopressin, norepinephrine, or angiotensin. Arteriolar vasospasm in the retina as well as in other locations has been observed with very early preeclampsia, and hypertension results from the vasospasm. Blood flow to the uterus (and possibly the liver) is decreased, although there is no decrease in blood flow to most other organs. The vasospasm apparently interferes with the circulation in the vasa vasorum, resulting in hypoxia of the vessel wall and consequent damage. This action may explain the necrosis seen in various organs in the late or end stage of eclampsia.

The cause of the edema associated with preeclampsia-eclampsia is unknown. However, the edema may be due to an imbalance of changes that occur in the glomerular filtration rate (decrease) and in tubular reabsorption rate (increase). It is known that water and sodium are excreted poorly in patients with acute toxemia, but the exact mechanism of this effect is unknown.

Hemoconcentration (decrease in plasma volume) and an increase in total serum proteins as a result of the hemoconcentration is a regular finding with severe preeclampsia-eclampsia, probably due to a shift of fluid to the extravascular compartment. Indeed, hemodilution is usually correlated with an improving clinical picture. Some authorities have recommended expansion of the intravascular fluid compartment by the administration of albumin, thus causing hemodilution [14]. Chesley [1] doubts the wisdom of this treatment.

Pathologic findings have been described almost exclusively in patients with fatal eclampsia, but it is presumed that lesser degrees of the same changes are present in patients with nonfatal eclampsia and preeclampsia. The characteristic hepatic lesion is periportal hemorrhage and necrosis, although the necrosis may extend well into the liver parenchyma. The brain has usually been described as edematous and hyperemic, with small hemorrhagic lesions and often with fibrinoid changes in many of the small vessels. Brain hemorrhage accounts for about one-fourth of deaths from eclampsia. The heart may show hemorrhages with necrosis or hyaline changes in the myometrium. Myocarditis has been described. The lungs also have multiple hemorrhages, and pulmonary edema may occur in fatal cases. The adrenal glands may undergo cortical necrosis, with adrenal insufficiency a possible clinical correlate.

The kidney shows the most characteristic pathologic features. Microscopic changes in this organ have been described even with early preeclampsia, since transcutaneous kidney biopsies have been performed in large numbers of patients. The primary change is in the capillaries of the glomerular tuft. The capillary wall shows thickening of the basement membrane and, more particularly, enormous swelling of the endothelial cells, probably producing complete occlusion of many of the capillaries. There is fibrinoid deposition in the capillaries. The endothelial cell and basement membrane changes have been considered diagnostic of preeclampsia-eclampsia and apparently are totally reversible, as shown by serial biopsy specimens taken from patients who have recovered from the severe form of the disease.

Clinical Course

Although a convulsive episode of eclampsia may occur in a patient previously unsuspected of having preeclampsia, this is the exception and not the rule. Furthermore, the preceding preeclampsia need not have been "severe"; eclampsia may develop in a patient thought to be experiencing only mild preeclampsia. The convulsion is usually heralded by apprehension, or excitability, or hyperreflexia in the patient, and epigastric pain is also said to be a premonitory sign. These evidences of impending convulsion may go unnoticed or may not be present at all.

The initial convulsion may occur before labor, during labor, or in the early postpartum period. The first evidence of a convulsion is a fixed, glassy stare, with evident loss of consciousness. This is quickly followed by a tonic contraction of all the muscles of the body as the body is held in a taut, rigid, hyperextended position. After 15 seconds or so, the clonic phase supervenes, and for the next 30 to 60 seconds or longer, the muscles of the body alternately contract and relax, giving the appearance of a typical grand mal seizure. During the clonic phase, the jaws open and close tightly, and the tongue will be severely damaged if the jaws are not prevented from closing completely by inserting a very firm rubber tube or other appropriate protection between the teeth. As the convulsion ends, the patient relaxes completely, and respiratory activity, which may have nearly ceased during the convulsion, begins again. Loss of consciousness will persist for a variable time after the convulsion, and if appropriate therapy is not initiated, another convulsive episode will occur. The patient may die from brain hemorrhage shortly after or during a convulsive episode.

During and following the convulsive episode, the blood pressure reading usually becomes markedly elevated. Proteinuria is a constant finding and frequently increases in amount. Oliguria or anuria may develop. With repeated convulsions or coma, the body temperature increases to as high as 100° to 103°F. (37.8° to 39.4°C.), which is probably a central nervous system phenomenon. Without clinical improvement, pulmonary edema and heart failure may ensue. Deaths from eclampsia are usually due to pulmonary edema or cerebral hemorrhage; if death appears after long-standing eclampsia, bronchopneumonia or renal failure may be responsible.

If the eclampsia develops before the onset of labor contractions, labor may begin spontaneously. Rapid labor and delivery frequently follows intrapartum eclampsia. If labor does not ensue spontaneously, therapy must be instituted to prevent further convulsions and to empty the uterus at the most advantageous time.

Treatment

GENERAL MEASURES. Since eclampsia is nearly always preceded by preeclampsia, the appearance of convulsions must in many instances be considered a treatment failure of preeclampsia. Prophylaxis against eclampsia is of obvious importance.

When eclampsia does occur, the objectives of treatment are to (1) prevent further convulsions, (2) improve the clinical status of the patient, if possible, and (3) empty the uterus at the most advantageous time. Monitoring of the patient's condition will include (1) evaluation of the patient's sensorium and the tendon reflexes, (2) urinary output and fluid intake measurements, and (3) repeated hematocrit determination, since clinical improvement usually coincides with hemodilution. The patient should be kept in a quiet darkened room with catheter drainage of the bladder; frequent blood pressure readings and pulse and respiratory rates should be recorded. Fluid intake, usually by slow intravenous infusion of 10% dextrose in water, should be 1000 ml. plus the volume of urine output over a 24-hour period. Sedation and protection from further convulsive episodes are probably best provided by magnesium sulfate as described earlier in the section on preeclampsia, although paraldehyde and barbiturates are preferred by some therapists. Many authorities recommend that an initial dose of 15 mg. of morphine sulfate be given at the time of the first convulsion. Oxygen should be administered to all eclamptic patients, and digitalization may be indicated with incipient or actual heart failure.

Antihypertensive therapy is favored by a number of eminent authorities, including Assali and Brinkman [15]. Such therapy should be reserved for those patients with severe hypertension (above 170/120 mm. Hg). Assali and Brinkman prefer hydralazine (Apresoline) because it increases renal blood flow. The drug relieves vasospasm and may be useful in the prevention of vascular damage and cerebral hemorrhage. Other antihypertensive drugs that have been recommended include cryptenamine (Unitensen) (derived from *Veratrum viride*), reserpine, and chlorpromazine.

TIMING OF DELIVERY. Some patients will be in labor at the time of the first convulsion, and a number of others will begin labor spontaneously soon thereafter. The labor will usually be rapid because of the uterine irritability associated with eclampsia, and vaginal delivery can be anticipated. If labor does not begin spontaneously, the choice of method and timing of delivery may be crucial both to mother and baby. Induction of labor or cesarean section should usually be postponed until therapy has been instituted and further convulsions seem unlikely. In older textbooks, a period of 24 hours free from convulsions was usually recommended, but this seems unduly long with improved anesthesia and better methods of monitoring fluid balance. Perhaps 3 to 8 hours is a more appropriate recommendation.

If the cervix is ripe, amniotomy and dilute intravenous oxytocin may initiate good labor. Indeed, even with an unripe cervix, labor may progress rapidly. Cesarean section as an alternative to induction or with failed induction offers certain advantages over induced labor, notably a lack of labor stimulus for further convulsive episodes and perhaps a better perinatal survival. Fetal heart rate monitoring techniques during labor will usually identify the hypoxic fetus who should be delivered by immediate section.

With repeated convulsions or with other deterioration of maternal status, no method of delivery will prove universally satisfactory. Meticulous physiologic monitoring of these patients, with correction of acid-base imbalance, may permit delivery by either route.

Prognosis in Preeclampsia-Eclampsia
Maternal mortality should be near zero for preeclampsia, but when eclampsia develops maternal mortality increases. If therapy is instituted immediately after the first convulsion, particularly if the patient has had good prenatal care, maternal mortality should be low. Without immediate therapy, or if repeated convulsions occur, the prognosis is much more serious, with a maternal mortality of about 5 percent. Perinatal mortality is greatly increased over that for infants of nonhypertensive patients, both as a result of the effects of prematurity and the effects of the disease itself. Chesley [1] reports a perinatal mortality of 5.7 percent among preeclamptic patients and 17.7 percent among eclamptic patients at the Kings County Hospital from 1958 to 1967. Using results from the 11 hospitals of the Obstetric Statistical Cooperative, Chesley [1] reported that 12.5 percent of all perinatal deaths occurred in association with maternal hypo-

tension which, in turn, was diagnosed in 5.8 percent of all deliveries.

With the improvement in nursing care over the past decade, earlier delivery is increasingly attractive, especially since the preeclamptic mother also benefits from this therapy. The increase in neonatal death rate that may result from the shorter gestation of early delivery is usually more than balanced by the lower fetal death rate that may result from removal of the fetus from a deleterious intrauterine environment.

The persistence of residual hypertension following preeclampsia-eclampsia apparently depends almost entirely on whether the disease is truly preeclampsia-eclampsia or whether a misdiagnosis of chronic hypertensive disease has been made. Long-term follow-up of women who had eclampsia *in the first pregnancy* has revealed no evidence of increased risk of hypertensive disease. Among multiparas, the incidence of residual hypertensive disease is greater than expected, suggesting that many of these women had chronic hypertension preceding the acute disease. The pathologic findings in McCartney's study of kidney biopsies [7] confirm that true preeclampsia-eclampsia is overwhelmingly a disease of the first pregnancy.

Chronic Hypertensive Disease

Chronic hypertensive disease in pregnancy is usually due to essential hypertension, less often to chronic glomerulonephritis. However, many other diseases are rare causes of the hypertension. Of special interest are certain collagen diseases (lupus erythematosus, scleroderma, periarteritis nodosa) in which renal involvement is part of the clinical picture. Diabetic nephropathy or severe chronic pyelonephritis may occasionally be found. Pheochromocytoma is a very rare but especially dangerous etiologic possibility, and wide variations in the degree of hypertension should suggest this possibility.

When pregnancy occurs in a patient with chronic hypertension, the outcome depends primarily on the extent of the original pathologic changes, notably in the kidney, and to the superimposition of

preeclampsia-eclampsia in certain patients. While many patients with chronic hypertension progress through pregnancy without difficulty, some will require therapeutic abortion or heroic measures (dialysis) to survive, and in many other cases there will be fetal or neonatal death. Careful evaluation and monitoring of all hypertensive patients is clearly necessary.

DIAGNOSIS
Most chronic hypertension in pregnancy is mild, and most hypertensive patients tolerate pregnancy well. The diagnosis is made by eliciting a history (preferably substantiated by medical records) of hypertension before pregnancy, or by observing hypertension during pregnancy before the twentieth week. Symptoms are usually absent, and hypertension is frequently the only abnormality noted on physical examination. Edema is usually absent. Retinopathy is an early manifestation of the disease and is noted in some patients. Albuminuria is frequently absent and is usually minimal when present. Evidences for cardiac disease or kidney disease are regularly sought. Delayed intrauterine growth occurs in some cases, and regular assessment of fetal growth is essential in all hypertensive gravidas (see below). Intrauterine growth retardation may be noted by estimation of fetal size during examination, or, more precisely, laboratory evidences of the syndrome should be regularly measured as described in Chapter 12.

Superimposed preeclampsia-eclampsia is the most serious complication of chronic hypertension and immediately increases maternal mortality to about 1 to 2 percent and perinatal mortality to about 20 percent [1]. The diagnosis of superimposed preeclampsia is inexact and may be made in some clinics with minimal increase in blood pressure reading. The diagnosis should be restricted to cases in which the blood pressure rises 30 mm. Hg systolic or 15 mm. Hg diastolic or more, or albuminuria appears or increases, or edema, usually absent with uncomplicated hypertension, appears. With obvious superimposed preeclampsia-eclampsia, early delivery will certainly safeguard the mother and may be the preferred treatment for the fetus, even with the usually observed immaturity.

TREATMENT

All patients with significant hypertensive disease should have evaluation of kidney and heart status early in pregnancy. Absence of kidney or heart involvement by the disease is reassuring. Antihypertensive drugs (methyldopa, hydralazine) should be used to protect the mother from the complications of hypertension, but the drugs have not been shown to lower perinatal mortality.

With mild or uncomplicated moderate hypertension, prenatal care is routine except for a constant diligent search for the appearance of superimposed preeclampsia and for frequent assessment of fetal condition and maturity. With all but the mildest hypertension, delayed intrauterine growth and fetal death remain possibilities. Ultrasonic measurement of the biparietal diameter should be obtained at 16 to 20 weeks gestation and at 4 to 6 week intervals thereafter. These determinations may allow recognition of intrauterine growth retardation. The fetal head to abdominal circumference ratio, as determined by ultrasound, is said to be a more sensitive indicator of intrauterine growth retardation than the biparietal diameter [16]. A history of decreased fetal movements suggests deteriorating fetal condition and demands the initiation of other tests of fetoplacental function. The nonstress test and the oxytocin challenge test described in Chapter 12 may be useful. Repeated human placental lactogen levels and serum or urinary estriol levels are used by some clinics to measure fetoplacental function. Premature delivery, either by induction of labor with meticulous fetal heart rate monitoring or by cesarean section, may be necessary. The degree of fetal maturity can be evaluated before undertaking early delivery by appropriate sampling of amniotic fluid by amniocentesis as described in Chapter 12.

Chesley [1] has identified five groups of chronic hypertensive patients whose prognosis may be especially bad:

1. Patients with cardiac enlargement.
2. Patients with markedly impaired renal function.
3. Patients with old retinal exudates or fresh hemorrhage.
4. Patients with an initial systolic pressure of 200 mm. Hg or higher or with a diastolic pressure of 120 mm. Hg or higher.
5. Patients with a history of acute toxemia superimposed on chronic hypertension during a prior pregnancy.

Indeed, therapeutic abortion with sterilization is probably indicated in any patient with one or more of these manifestations of her disease.

References
1. Chesley, L. *Hypertensive Disorders in Pregnancy.* New York: Appleton-Century-Crofts, 1978.
2. Hughes, E. C. (Ed.). *Obstetric-Gynecologic Terminology.* Philadelphia: Davis, 1972. P. 422.
3. Niswander, K. Unpublished data, 1973.
4. Baird, D. *Combined Textbook of Obstetrics and Gynecology for Students and Practitioners.* Edinburgh and London: Livingstone, 1969. P. 631.
5. Brewer, T. *Metabolic Toxemia of Late Pregnancy: A Disease of Malnutrition.* Springfield, Ill.: Thomas, 1966.
6. Hodari, A. Chronic uterine ischemia and reversible experimental "toxemia of pregnancy." *Am J Obstet Gynecol* 97:597, 1967.
7. McCartney, C. Pathological anatomy of acute hypertension of pregnancy. *Circulation* 30 (Suppl. 2):66, 1964.
8. Gant, H., Chand, S., Worley, R., Whalley, P., Crosby, U., and MacDonald, P. A clinical test useful for predicting the development of acute hypertension in pregnancy. *Am J Obstet Gynecol* 120:1, 1974.
9. Marx, G., Husain, F., and Shiau, H. Brachial and femoral blood pressures during the prenatal period. *Am J Obstet Gynecol* 136:11, 1980.
10. Fish, J., Bartholomew, R., Colvin, E., Grimes, W., Lester, W., and Galloway, W. The relationship of pregnancy weight gain to toxemia. *Am J Obstet Gynecol* 78:743, 1959.
11. Chesley, L. Personal communication, 1971.
12. Zuspan, F. Treatment of severe preeclampsia and eclampsia. *Clin Obstet Gynecol* 9:954, 1966.
13. Shelley, W., and Gutsche, B. Magnesium and seizure control (Letter to the Editor). *Am J Obstet Gynecol* 136:146, 1980.
14. Goodlin, R. *Care of the Fetus.* New York: Masson, 1978.
15. Assali, N., and Brinkman, C. Disorders of Mater-

nal Circulatory and Respiratory Adjustments. In N. Assali (Ed.), *Pathophysiology of Gestation*. New York and London: Academic, 1972, Vol. 1, p. 269.

16. Campbell, S., and Thomas, A. Ultrasound measurement of fetal head to abdomen ratio in the assessment of growth retardation. *Brit J Obstet Gynaecol* 84:165, 1977.

Additional Readings

Chesley, L., Annitto, J., and Cosgrove, R. Long term follow-up study of eclamptic women. *Am J Obstet Gynecol* 101:886, 1968.

Cibils, L. The placenta and newborn infant in hypertensive conditions. *Am J Obstet Gynecol* 118:256, 1974.

Roberts, J., Hill, C., and Riopelle, A. Maternal protein deprivation and toxemia of pregnancy: Studies in the rhesus monkey (*Macaca mulatta*). *Am J Obstet Gynecol* 118:14, 1974.

Thompson, H. Evaluation of the obstetric and gynecologic patient by the use of diagnostic ultrasound. *Clin Obstet Gynecol* 17:1, 1974.

Tillman, A. The effect of normal and toxemic pregnancy on blood pressure. *Am J Obstet Gynecol* 70:589, 1965.

9   Normal Labor

Labor is the process by which the uterus expels the mature or nearly mature products of conception at a time appropriate, or nearly so, for the newborn child to exist semi-independently from the mother. The factor or factors initiating labor remain one of the major unsolved mysteries of biology. Equally baffling and obscure is why the uterus so efficiently houses the fetus for nine months without expelling it.

The uterus contracts throughout the reproductive phase of a woman's life, and pregnancy is no exception to this rule. Early in pregnancy, the contractions are sporadic and involve only a portion of the uterine musculature. They gradually increase in frequency as pregnancy progresses, involving larger numbers of muscle fibers, and they culminate in the regular contractions of labor, which spread throughout the uterus and occur at precise and increasingly frequent intervals. The contractions during early pregnancy are usually not sensed by the gravida. The prelabor contractions, known as Braxton Hicks contractions, are felt but usually without pain. As labor begins, contractions occur at regular intervals and are usually described as painful by the gravida.

Why Does Labor Begin?

Perhaps the oldest theory thought to explain the onset of labor is the *uterine stretch theory*. The advocates of this theory point to the premature labor usually associated with multiple gestation or other conditions in which the uterus is distended. But how can this theory explain the onset of labor with a dead fetus, a labor that usually occurs before the full gestational interval and before the uterus is fully distended?

A second theory suggests that *withdrawal of progesterone* allows the uterine musculature to contract and begin labor. It is known that exogenous progesterone prolongs gestation in the rabbit, but a direct transfer of this information to the human is not possible. There is little evidence to support progesterone withdrawal as the factor initiating labor in the human. Indeed, exogenous progesterone in the human has been shown *not* to stop labor once it has begun.

Oxytocin, secreted by the posterior pituitary gland, is known to be an effective uterine stimulant, a fact that has led to various theories that oxytocin initiates labor in some fashion. There is no evidence to suggest an increase in oxytocin secretion as pregnancy progresses. It is known, however, that the uterus can be stimulated to contract with smaller and smaller doses of exogenous oxytocin as term is approached; i.e., the sensitivity of the uterus to oxytocin is greatly enhanced. The theory that oxytocin activity is increased because oxytocinase, an enzyme known to inactivate oxytocin, may be secreted in decreasing amounts during pregnancy is unacceptable because most investigators have measured no such decrease. The oxytocin theory has been most seriously challenged by the observation that labor occurs both in the human and in animals even after destruction of the posterior pituitary gland.

A more recent theory is that the *fetus* itself in some way regulates the onset of labor. The evidence to support this theory comes both from animal work and from clinical observations. In certain breeds of cattle, prolonged gestation occurs because the fetus has congenital aplasia of the adenohypophysis, with resultant hypoplasia of the fetal adrenal gland. Destruction of the fetal pituitary gland or the fetal adrenal gland in sheep markedly prolongs gestation. The secretions of the fetal adrenal gland are thought to be essential in initiating labor. In the human, anencephaly is associated with aplasia or poor development of the fetal pituitary gland, with a resultant adrenal hypoplasia. Prolonged gestation has been reported to occur in a large percentage of women carrying an anencephalic monster.

Certain *prostaglandins* are known to be potent uterine musculature stimulants, and the suggestion that a prostaglandin may account in some way for the onset of labor has been offered. Liggins thinks that a disturbance in the relationship between the decidua and the fetal membranes will release prostaglandins [1]. Prostaglandins probably "ripen" the cervix as well as causing uterine contractility. A variety of mechanisms known to induce labor do disturb the interaction between fetal membranes and decidua (e.g., amniotomy, placement of cervical tents, passage of catheters into the extra-amniotic space). The release of prostaglandins may well be the major mechanism controlling the onset of labor.

Catecholamines similarly stimulate uterine contractility, but whether or not this activity provides an adequate explanation for the onset of labor is uncertain.

No single theory seems to explain in a satisfactory and universal manner why labor begins. It is altogether likely that a combination of factors, a culmination of physiologic events, leads to labor. Even with incomplete information on the cause of the onset of labor, however, the initiation of labor can be regularly accomplished in the human with various drugs or maneuvers when the clinical situation demands it. Less success has followed efforts to halt labor once it has begun.

Prelabor Changes

Before describing the labor process, it is necessary to study the anatomic and physiologic changes of pregnancy that prepare the uterus for the labor process.

UTERINE FUNDUS

Up to about the end of the fourth month, the fundus of the uterus enlarges by hypertrophy and hyperplasia of the muscle cells. The uterine musculature increases in thickness and is about 1 cm. thick at this time. The individual muscle cell increases in size to a volume about 100 times greater than in the nonpregnant state. The fetus has grown at a much slower rate than the uterus, and the placenta occupies most of the intrauterine space.

At the end of the fourth month, uterine hypertrophy ceases, and further enlargement of the uterus is due to stretching as the fetus begins a period of rapid growth. The uterine musculature thins as stretching progresses and the wall of the uterus thins to about 5 mm. at term.

LOWER UTERINE SEGMENT

The lower uterine segment is the part of the uterine fundus just above the cervix that does not participate actively in the uterine contractility that causes the fetus to be extruded. More will be said of the lower uterine segment when the labor process is described. The lower uterine segment cannot be distinguished from the fundus during the first half of pregnancy. Indeed, the musculature in the contractile portion of the fundus looks exactly the same as the noncontractile lower segment. In late pregnancy, a line of demarcation develops between the dominant fundus and the passive lower uterine segment and identifies the upper limit of the lower uterine segment. As labor begins, this line is called the physiologic retraction ring.

CERVIX

The cervix is composed almost entirely of connective tissue, and there are few cervical changes in early pregnancy during the period when the fundus hypertrophies and stretches. As labor approaches, however, the cervix becomes softened, probably by engorgement with blood. Effacement, a decrease in the length of the cervix (see Cervical Effacement), and dilatation of the cervix then begin in preparation for labor (Fig. 9-1). The biochemical change that permits stretching of the cervix is an alteration in the "cement" holding the collagen fibers together. This biochemical change permits sliding of the collagen fibers one on the other, and

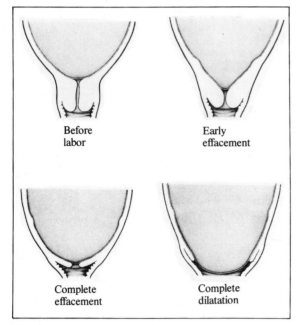

Before labor

Early effacement

Complete effacement

Complete dilatation

Fig. 9-1. Cervical effacement and dilatation in the primigravida. (From Mechanism of Normal Labor, *Ross Clinical Education Aid No. 13. Columbus, Ohio: Ross Laboratories, 1975.)*

cervical dilatation sufficient to permit passage of the fetus then occurs—a remarkably rapid physiologic accommodation.

UTERINE CONTRACTIONS

While more quiescent in the first half of pregnancy than later, the uterus does exhibit contractions early, but they are sporadic, infrequent, and usually of low amplitude. The resting tonus (intrauterine pressure) of the uterus at this time is 5 to 10 mm. Hg. The contractions become increasingly frequent as pregnancy progresses, and the occasional contractions of higher amplitude that occurred in early pregnancy begin to recur with more regularity. Most of these contractions are not sensed by the patient, but as term approaches, their amplitude increases, and the patient may experience them as Braxton Hicks contractions. On occasion, they are sufficiently uncomfortable to

suggest to the patient—and sometimes to the physician—that labor has begun.

With the onset of labor, the larger contractions occur with regularity and at shorter and shorter intervals. Contractions that result in an intrauterine pressure of 30 mm. Hg are sufficient to initiate cervical dilatation, although pressures of 50 mm. Hg quickly become common. The contractions begin in the uterine fundus, which contains the bulk of the myometrial cells. A pacemaker in one cornual angle, or in both, has been postulated as the point of onset of the contraction, with the sweep of the contraction downward toward the lower uterine segment and the cervix.

The individual uterine muscle cells display a remarkable property that suits them ideally to the task they must accomplish, namely, retraction of the lower uterine segment and cervix upward to permit extrusion of the fetus. This property is called brachystasis (Fig. 9-2). Following the contraction (shortening) of the muscle cell, the cell fails to recover all its prior length during the relaxation phase. With each subsequent contraction, further shortening of the cell occurs, with an overall effect of broadening of the individual cell, thickening of the fundal musculature, and decreasing the intrauterine volume.

The lower uterine segment is passive while the dominant upper segment is contracting, both during the prelabor period and during labor. The result is a gradual thinning and retraction of the lower segment (Fig. 9-3). The point of juncture of the upper uterine segment with the lower segment (the physiologic retraction ring) gradually moves upward as the lower uterine segment is retracted (Fig. 9-4). The physiologic retraction ring thus formed can be felt abdominally during labor in some patients and can usually be seen at the time of cesarean section.

The cervix softens during the prelabor period, and the prelabor contractions of the fundus gradually cause some dilatation of the cervical os—up to a little less than 2 cm. in the primigravida and a little more than 2 cm. in the multigravida. If labor starts before this prelabor preparation of the cervix, a prolonged labor is the likely result.

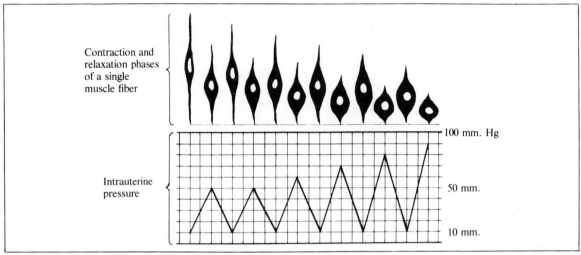

Fig. 9-2. Brachystasis. Progressive shortening of muscle fiber and fixation at new shorter length are shown. Intrauterine pressures that accompany first stage contractions are also shown. The early first stage is on the left and the late first stage, on the right. (From D. Danforth. Textbook of Obstetrics and Gynecology *[2nd ed.]. New York: Harper & Row, 1971.)*

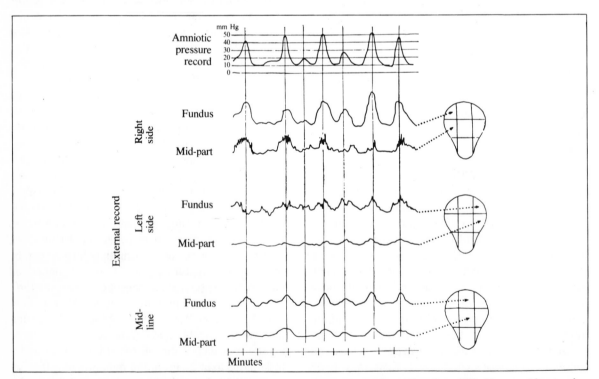

Fig. 9-3. Normal first stage of labor. Simultaneous record of amniotic pressure and local contractility (by external receptors) in six different parts of the uterus.

(From R. Caldeyro-Barcia and H. Alvarez. Abnormal uterine action in labour. J Obstet Gynaecol Br Emp *59:646, 1952.)*

2 A term
1 Premature
1 Abortus
3 Live.

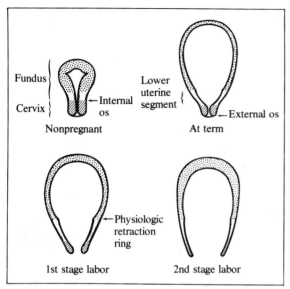

Fig. 9-4. Changes induced in the fundus, lower uterine segment, and cervix by pregnancy and labor. (From K. Niswander. Obstetric and Gynecologic Disorders: A Practitioner's Guide. Flushing, N.Y.: Medical Examination Publishing Co., 1975.)

Labor

Labor is the process by which the mother expels the fetus after 20 weeks of gestation. Expulsion of the products of conception before that time is termed *abortion*. Abortion is *early* if it occurs before three months; mid-trimester or *late* if it occurs thereafter. Labor may be *immature* if it occurs after 20 weeks but before 28 weeks, the gestational interval at which fetal survival is a possibility. *Premature* labor is labor occurring after 27 weeks but before 37 weeks. Labor at *term* encompasses gestations of 37 to 42 weeks. Labor occurring after 42 weeks is called *post-term* labor and may in some cases be associated with a higher perinatal risk than birth at term.

A *parturient*, a woman in labor, can be described in terms of her previous reproductive history. *Gravidity* refers to the number of prior pregnancies (including abortion, ectopic pregnancy, and hydaditiform mole) of any gestational interval, and *parity* describes the number of pregnancies (not of infants—twins constitute an increase of one

in parity) that have been carried for 20 weeks or more. Some clinics, including our own, prefer to describe reproductive history in terms of a four-digit number, e.g., 2113. The first digit indicates the number of term infants delivered; the second indicates the number of prematures delivered; the third indicates the number of abortions; and the fourth indicates the number of children currently living. Thus, in the example (2113), the patient has delivered 2 term infants and 1 premature infant; she has experienced 1 abortion and she has 3 children currently living.

Labor consists of three stages: the *first stage* begins with the onset of labor and ends when the cervix is fully dilated; the *second stage* begins with full dilatation of the cervix and ends with complete expulsion of the fetus; and the *third stage* begins with complete expulsion of the fetus and ends with expulsion of the placenta. Friedman [2] has further divided the first stage of labor into a latent phase and an active phase. Friedman's description of the first stage of labor has proved to be a useful clinical tool, and more will be said of it later.

LABOR CHANGES

The upper uterine segment has been stretched for the five months preceding labor until it is now about 5 mm. thick. As labor approaches, the musculature becomes more "irritable," with many more contractions of greater amplitude than previously. Although these are not usually experienced by the patient as labor, they nevertheless are effective in bringing about necessary cervical changes as the uterus prepares for labor.

As labor begins, the sporadic contractions become regular, and they now involve the upper segment in toto. The muscle fibers do not stretch out to their previous length after a contraction but gradually shorten, as previously described. This effect on the upper segment gradually diminishes the size of the uterine cavity, causing the fetus to assume a more erect position at right angles to the pelvic inlet. The decrease in uterine capacity also causes a gradual retraction of the passive lower uterine segment, with gradual thinning of the wall of this segment. The cervix has been partially ef-

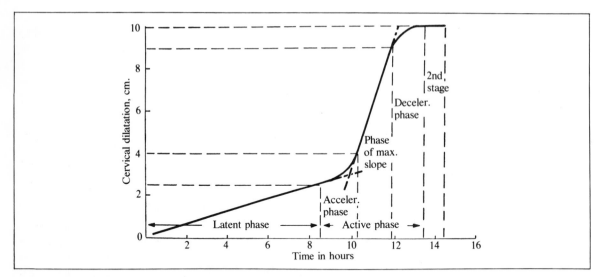

Fig. 9-5. A composite Friedman labor curve based on 500 nulliparas. (From E. Friedman. Primigravid labor. Obstet Gynecol 6:569, 1955.)

faced by the gradual retraction of the lower uterine segment and by the descent of the presenting part.

At this time, dilatation of the cervix begins as retraction on the lower uterine segment puts tension on the cervix. The cervix, too, is retracted upward by the fundal contractions. With full dilatation of the cervix, no further upward pull on the cervix is possible because of the attachment of the cervix to the uterine ligaments, especially the cardinal ligaments, the pubocervical fascia, and the uterosacral ligaments (see Fig. 9-4). Thus, excursion of the cervix upward is stopped at about the plane of the pelvic inlet. Subsequent uterine contractions and the resultant diminution in the size of the uterine cavity push the fetus downward through the pelvis. Any obstruction to the descent of the fetus will result in more than the usual thinning of the lower uterine segment, since the cervix will retract no higher. It is therefore in the lower uterine segment that uterine rupture from obstructed labor is likely to occur. It is this fact that resulted in the establishment of the "2-hour second stage" rule that will be described.

It has been shown by many investigators that the uterine contractions occur primarily in the upper uterine segment. The lower segment can be considered a passageway that must be opened by the downward thrust of the upper segment, which ac-

complishes expulsion of the fetus. When this physiologic mechanism breaks down, as with inadequate contractile effort or reversal of the contraction wave, uterine dysfunction results. This complication of the labor process will be described in Chapter 11.

The average length of labor in the primigravida is about 14 hours according to Friedman [2], although others have reported a substantially shorter mean time. Certainly, there is wide variation in the length of normal labor. The first stage of labor occupies most of the 14 hours; the second stage lasts an average of about 1¼ hours; and the third stage lasts a few minutes. In the multipara, the mean total labor length is about 8 hours, with the second stage averaging about a half hour.

As recommended by Friedman [2], it is useful to plot dilatation of the cervix against time on a graph to gauge whether labor is normal or abnormal (Fig. 9-5). The graphing of the dilatation-time curve can be made on any piece of graph paper and will allow the physician to recognize labor abnormalities early. Friedman has pointed out that the curve normally assumes a sigmoid shape in both primigravid and multigravid patients, although the curve is somewhat more definitely sigmoid in the primigravida because of the longer time intervals involved. Hendricks and others [3] have not recognized the S shape of the graph but note a straight-line relationship. The data of all authorities, however, are in general agreement except for highly technical differences that will not be discussed here.

Friedman has described (1) a latent phase of the first stage of labor that begins with the onset of labor and ends when the cervical dilatation pattern assumes a more vertical inclination and (2) an active phase of the first stage. The active phase consists of an acceleration phase, a phase of maximum slope, and a deceleration phase. The brief acceleration phase precedes the phase of maximum slope that ends when the dilatation pattern again changes, this time toward a slower rate until full dilatation in the second stage of labor is reached (deceleration phase). The acceleration and deceleration phases are of technical interest only and will be discussed no further here.

Friedman recognizes certain abnormalities of the cervical dilatation-time curve that will be described in some detail in Chapter 11. At this point it is important merely to recognize that the plotting of cervical dilatation against time has provided an important clinical tool to "describe" labor and to allow recognition of its abnormalities.

LABOR IN VERTEX PRESENTATION

The mechanism of labor, that is, the accommodation in attitude and relationships to the pelvis assumed by the fetus as it traverses the birth canal, is determined by the following: (1) the amount and the direction of the uterine force exerted on the fetus; (2) the particular pelvis to which the fetus must accommodate itself; and (3) the fetus's size and ability to accommodate physically to the pelvic restrictions and to the particular presentation it assumes. Before discussing the mechanism of labor with various presentations, it is necessary to describe the maternal pelvis in some detail and to point out some of the anatomic and physiologic features of the fetus.

Maternal Pelvis

The true pelvis is a cylindrically shaped, curved, tubular, largely bony structure through which the fetus must pass for delivery. To judge the adequacy of the pelvis for the passage of the fetus, certain anatomic features must be recognized and evaluated. The position of the fetus at crucial times during the labor process in relation to certain of these anatomic features provides an excellent means of predicting the likelihood for success of labor. Thus, knowledge of the clinical anatomy of the pelvis is a useful diagnostic tool.

The sacrum and coccyx form the posterior boundary of the pelvis. The lateral and anterior walls are composed of portions of the innominate bone, in itself formed from the ilium, the ischium, and the pubis. The pelvis is much longer posteriorly than anteriorly, and the result is a gentle curvature of the pelvic axis, which is first directed inferiorly and posteriorly and then curved anteriorly and inferiorly. The upper limit of the true pelvis, the pelvic inlet, is formed by the posterosuperior border of the symphysis pubis anteriorly, a point just below the promontory of the sacrum posteriorly, and the linea terminalis laterally. The lower limit of the pelvis, the outlet, is formed by the inferior border of the symphysis pubis and the pubic rami anteriorly, the ischial tuberosities laterally, and the tip of the sacrum and the coccyx posteriorly. The sacrosciatic ligament helps form the lateral boundary of the outlet and, indeed, of much of the pelvis. In the mid-pelvis, the ischial spines form the lateral margins and are of special clinical importance since they are so easily palpated.

For convenience in describing anatomic features of the pelvis that are of clinical importance, certain planes that transect the pelvis have been identified. The borders of the planes of (1) the pelvic inlet and (2) the pelvic outlet have been previously described. The plane of (3) the mid-pelvis is bordered anteriorly by the posterior wall of the symphysis pubis, posteriorly by the anterior surface of the S-3 or S-4 vertebral bodies, and laterally by the ischial spines. Measurements or estimates of the various diameters of these three planes can be made either by physical examination or by radiographic tech-

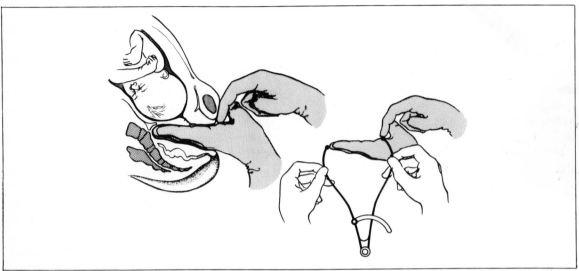

Fig. 9-6. Estimation of diagonal conjugate measurement. Vaginal fingers reach for the promontory of the sacrum, with note taken of the point at which the symphysis pubis touches the metacarpal bone (left). This distance is measured with a calipers (right).

niques. On the basis of these measurements, the adequacy of the pelvis can be ascertained.

Certain pelvic measurements can be made with relative accuracy by vaginal examination. An estimate of the pelvic features that defy precise clinical measurement is also possible. Careful vaginal examination is a necessary step in evaluation of the bony pelvis. If the clinical situation demands greater accuracy than that provided by physical examination, x-ray pelvimetry may be used.

PELVIC EXAMINATION FOR EVALUATION OF THE BONY PELVIS. Of perhaps greatest importance is the measurement of the anteroposterior (AP) diameter of the *pelvic inlet*. The transverse diameter cannot be measured clinically. The anterior surface of the sacrum is palpated with the index and middle fingers, which have been inserted into the vagina. With gradual movement of the fingers upward on the sacrum, the sacral promontory is sought. The hand is gently pressed against the undersurface of the symphysis pubis while the middle finger simultaneously touches the sacral promontory (Fig. 9-6). The point where the anterior surface of the index finger touches the symphysis pubis is carefully marked, and the distance between this point and the tip of the middle finger is measured with calipers. In this manner the *diagonal conjugate* mea-

surement is recorded. (If the promontory cannot be reached, the diagonal conjugate is known to be greater than this measurement.) The diameter of greater clinical importance is the obstetrical conjugate measurement, which is the distance from the sacral promontory to a point on the posterior surface of the symphysis pubis just below its upper margin. The obstetrical conjugate cannot be measured directly but can be calculated by subtracting 1.5 to 2.0 cm. from the diagonal conjugate measurement; this is admittedly an estimate but the only method possible by clinical examination. An obstetrical conjugate of greater than 10 cm. usually denotes an adequate pelvic inlet.

A sacrum with a gently curving shape is usual and provides the maximal pelvic room. A flat sacrum or one that juts anteriorly diminishes the pelvic capacity, especially the AP diameter of the *mid-pelvis*. The width of the sacrosciatic notch can also be estimated; a width smaller than normal suggests a mid-pelvic AP diameter less than normal. Of major importance is palpation of the ischial spines

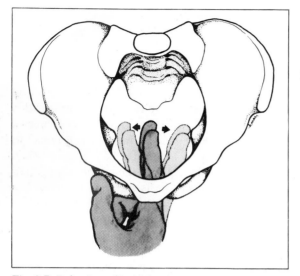

Fig. 9-7. Palpation of ischial spines to estimate interspinous diameter.

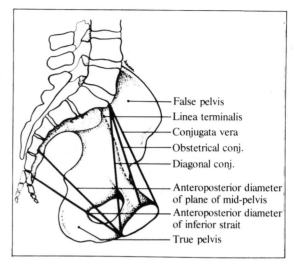

False pelvis
Linea terminalis
Conjugata vera
Obstetrical conj.
Diagonal conj.
Anteroposterior diameter of plane of mid-pelvis
Anteroposterior diameter of inferior strait
True pelvis

Fig. 9-8. Anteroposterior pelvic measurements. (From Mechanism of Normal Labor, *Ross Clinical Education Aid No. 13. Columbus, Ohio: Ross Laboratories, 1975.*)

and estimation of the interspinous diameter (Fig. 9-7). Although there is no practical tool for making this measurement with precision, a clinical impression of the closeness of the spines to one another suffices. This completes the estimate of mid-pelvic capacity.

The *pelvic outlet* can be estimated by measuring the distance between the ischial tuberosities with the Thom's pelvimeter. An easier method is to determine if the clenched fist of the examiner will fit between the tuberosities, thus assuring a minimal intertuberous diameter of 8 cm. for most examiners. The angle of the pubic arch should be described as wide or narrow; a narrow arch diminishes the area of the pelvic outlet, especially of the forepelvis (Fig. 9-8).

Of great importance clinically, but not measurable, is the degree to which the pelvic joints will mobilize and stretch during passage of the fetus through the pelvis. Neither the symphysis pubis nor the sacroiliac joints allow appreciable movement in the nonpregnant patient. During pregnancy, a significant loosening of the joints can be observed, which is apparently an effect of pregnancy hormones (relaxin?). While this "stretching"

of the pelvis is of great advantage to the fetus, the pelvic instability that results is probably the cause of the pelvic aching many patients complain of.

TYPES OF BONY PELVES. The shape of the pelvis will determine to a great degree how the fetus will pass through it. A pelvis that is longer in an anteroposterior direction than in a transverse direction will encourage the accommodation of the widest diameter of the fetal head (the AP diameter) in the anteroposterior plane. A flat pelvis with a diminished AP diameter will accommodate the fetus best in the transverse plane.

For many years, the shape of the pelvis has been recognized as an important clinical fact in managing the labor of the parturient. A classification of pelves formulated many years ago by Caldwell and Moloy [4] was based on the general configuration of the pelvis. This classification is still in wide use today. Caldwell and Moloy identified four types of normal pelves that are seen often in the human population (Fig. 9-9).

Gynecoid. The gynecoid or normal female pelvis has a pelvic inlet with an AP diameter only slightly less than the transverse diameter. The inlet is

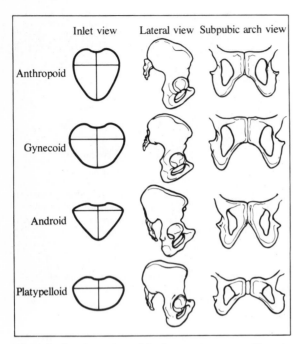

Inlet view   Lateral view Subpubic arch view

Anthropoid

Gynecoid

Android

Platypelloid

Fig. 9-9. Configuration of the four major types of female pelves.

gently rounded, with a generous forepelvis. The pelvic walls are straight, the pubic arch is wide, and the interspinous diameter is not diminished. The sacrum is curved neither anteriorly nor posteriorly, and the sacrosciatic notch is wide. This type of pelvis is the most common variety in women.

Android. While the transverse and AP diameters of the android pelvis inlet may be the same as in the gynecoid pelvis, the forepelvis is narrowed and the inlet area diminished. The area of the mid-pelvis is diminished by a shortened interspinous diameter, converging of the pelvic walls, and a jutting sacrum with a narrow sacrosciatic notch.

Anthropoid. The AP diameter of the anthropoid pelvis inlet is substantially greater than the narrow transverse diameter. The sacrum is straight and inclined posteriorly. The ischial spines may be prominent.

Platypelloid. Except for a markedly decreased AP diameter throughout the pelvis, the platypelloid pelvis is similar to the gynecoid. It is noted in 1 to 2 percent of patients.

When the mechanism of labor is discussed, the importance of the type of pelvis will be stressed.

The Fetus

LIE OF THE FETUS. The fetus can be described in terms of its spacial relationship to the mother; this is called the *lie* of the fetus. If the fetus occupies a position in the long axis of the mother, it is said to lie *longitudinally.* A *transverse* lie is present when the fetus is at right angles to the mother's longitudinal axis. An *oblique* lie is rare and occupies the position midway between the longitudinal and transverse lies, always converting during labor to one or the other of these lies.

PRESENTATION OF THE FETUS. The *presentation* of the fetus is determined by the part of the fetus that is lowermost in the pelvis—or nearest to it if the fetus has not entered the pelvis. A cephalic, breech, or shoulder presentation may be recognized. Subdivision of these categories more accurately describes the *presenting part.* The cephalic presentation may be (1) an occiput if the parietal bones are foremost; (2) a face (mentum) if the chin is presenting; or (3) a brow (bregma) if the forehead of the fetus is lowermost in the pelvis. In a *frank breech* presentation, the thighs and legs are flexed on the abdominal wall. In a *complete breech,* the thighs are flexed on the abdominal wall, but the knees are flexed on the thighs. In a *footling breech,* one foot (single footling) or both feet (double footling) are lowermost in the pelvis. These differentiations are often important ones to make clinically because they carry widely varying prognoses for the infant.

POSITION OF THE FETUS. The position of the fetus is a description of the relationship of the presenting part to one of the four quadrants of the maternal pelvic outlet, namely, the right anterior, right posterior, left anterior, or left posterior. Thus, if the presenting part is the parietal bone (occiput), and if the occiput is presenting in the left anterior quadrant of the mother's pelvis, the position is said to be left occiput anterior (LOA). (See Fig. 9-16 for other possible occiput presentations.) Note, then, that an occiput presenting directly anteriorly or directly posteriorly is designated an OA or an OP, and an occiput presenting directly laterally is called an LOT or an ROT. Presentations other than occiput have similar designations. Thus, the face presentation will be left mentum anterior (LMA) if the chin is presenting in the mother's left anterior quadrant. A breech presentation is identified by the position of the fetal sacrum; thus a left sacrum anterior (LSA) position is diagnosed if the sacrum is in the mother's left anterior pelvic quadrant. With transverse lie, the scapula (Sc) is the presenting part (LScA, or example).

FETAL HEAD. The bony anatomy of the fetal head is important to the obstetrician because certain anatomic landmarks are useful in helping him identify its position before delivery and because certain anatomic features of the head help to explain its ability to traverse even the small pelvis during the labor process.

The fetal skull bones are not fused as in the adult but are separated and joined by areas of cartilage. The skull bones of major interest to the obstetrician are the two parietal bones, the frontal bone, and the occipital bone. The suture lines of interest are the sagittal suture between the two parietal bones, the lambdoidal suture between the occipital bone and the parietal bones, and the frontal suture between the frontal bone and the two parietal bones. Of even greater interest are the points where these sutures meet, since a fontanelle is formed at each of these locations, a three-pronged structure in the posterior fontanelle and a four-pronged one in the anterior fontanelle. Palpation of the suture lines and the fontanelles permits the obstetrician to label the position of the occiput appropriately. (The vaginal touch findings of the various positions are illustrated in Fig. 9-16.)

Of obstetrical importance, too, is the fact that the fetal head may change shape to accommodate itself to the anatomy of the pelvis it must traverse. The skull bones may be pushed closer together, with a decrease in fetal skull diameter ("molding" of the fetal head), even to the point of overriding of the

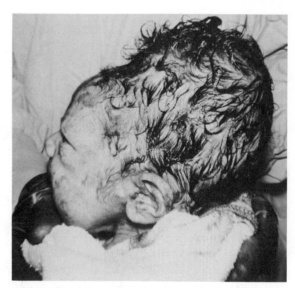

Fig. 9-10. Typical molding of fetal head.

fetal skull bones on occasion (Fig. 9-10). While this accommodation to the pelvis is of great physiologic advantage, on occasion the molding may be greater than the fetus can tolerate, since the molding may put undue stress on certain of the dural sinuses, resulting in tearing and rupture of the sinuses with bleeding.

The various diameters of the fetal head are also of obstetrical importance (Fig. 9-11). The transverse diameter of the head (the biparietal diameter), is the narrowest part of the head. In a 7-pound (3.2 kg.) baby, this diameter is about 9.5 cm. The degree of flexion of the fetal head on the chest will determine the length of the AP diameter that must negotiate the pelvis. A poorly flexed head will cause the occipitofrontal diameter (about 12.5 cm.) to present; an even more extended head will present the occipitomental diameter (13.5 cm). If the head is well flexed on the chest, the suboccipitobregmatic diameter will be the widest diameter (about 9.5 cm. in a normal-sized baby). (Extreme extension of the head, as in a face presentation, will result in presentation of a diameter little greater than the suboccipitobregmatic; this explains the frequently short labor noted with face presentation.)

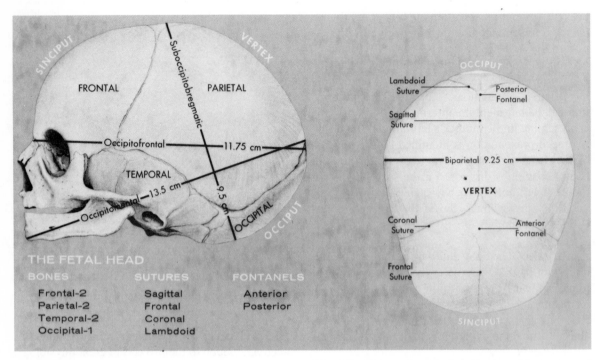

The fetal head illustration shows:

FRONTAL   PARIETAL

Suboccipitobregmatic

Occipitofrontal — 11.75 cm

TEMPORAL

13.5 cm

9.5 cm

Occipitomental

OCCIPITAL

SINCIPUT   VERTEX   OCCIPUT

THE FETAL HEAD

BONES	SUTURES	FONTANELS
Frontal-2	Sagittal	Anterior
Parietal-2	Frontal	Posterior
Temporal-2	Coronal	
Occipital-1	Lambdoid	

Right diagram:

OCCIPUT

Lambdoid Suture — Posterior Fontanel

Sagittal Suture

Biparietal 9.25 cm

VERTEX

Coronal Suture — Anterior Fontanel

Frontal Suture

SINCIPUT

Fig. 9-11. Diameters of fetal skull. (From Mechanism of Normal Labor, *Ross Clinical Education Aid No. 13. Columbus, Ohio: Ross Laboratories, 1975.)*

Mechanism of Labor in Vertex Presentation

The position the fetus assumes at the onset of labor, the variations in position as the pelvis is traversed, and the position of the fetus just before delivery are all determined by a number of important factors. These are (1) the size and shape of the bony pelvis, (2) the resiliency of the soft tissue, (3) the size of the fetal head and the degree to which it can mold, and (4) the strength of the uterine contractions as well as the direction of their force. In nearly two-thirds of occiput presentations, labor begins with the fetus's head in the transverse diameter, i.e., LOT or ROT. In most cases, the fetus ultimately delivers in an anterior position. The mechanism of labor in this instance can be described.

Engagement of the fetal head (e.g., when the widest of the diameters of the skull has passed the plane of the inlet [see Lightening, or Engagement]) usually occurs in the transverse position because the transverse diameter of the pelvis is usually greater than the AP diameter (Fig. 9-12). The fetal head at this point is usually not well flexed, and the

occipitofrontal diameter (12.5 cm.) can be best accommodated in the wider transverse diameter of the pelvis. As the head descends, *flexion* occurs due to the pressure of the soft tissue of the pelvis. The smaller suboccipitobregmatic diameter now becomes the greatest diameter. As the head continues its *descent, internal rotation* from the transverse position to an anterior position results because of the shape of the levator sling and because the narrowest diameter of the mid-pelvis is the transverse one, i.e., the interspinous diameter. As the head reaches the pelvic floor, the occiput impinges on the symphysis pubis, and the subsequent uterine force causes the head to *extend*, with birth of the head by this maneuver. With extrusion of the head complete, the head rotates back to a transverse position (*restitution and external rotation*) as the fetal shoulders enter the mid-pelvis and the bisacromial diameter accommodates to the AP di-

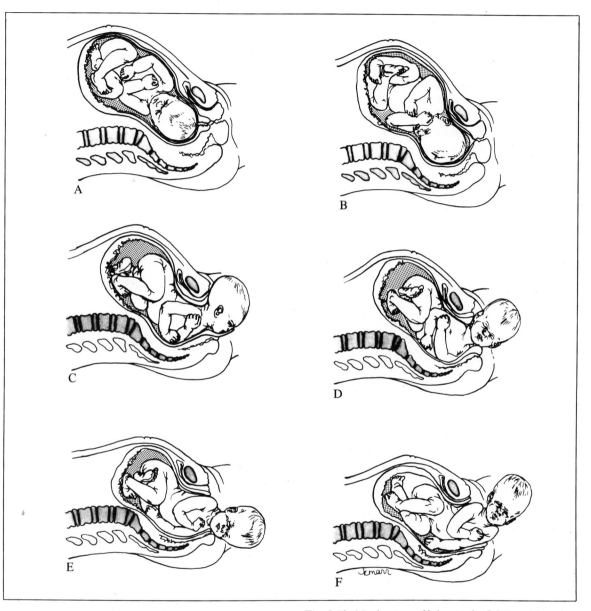

Fig. 9-12. Mechanism of labor in the LOA position. A. Engagement and flexion of the head. B. Internal rotation. C. Delivery by extension of the head. D. External rotation. E. Delivery of the anterior shoulder. F. Delivery of the posterior shoulder. (From K. Niswander. Obstetric and Gynecologic Disorders: A Practitioner's Guide. *Flushing, N.Y.: Medical Examination Publishing Co., 1975.)*

ameter of the mother's mid-pelvis. With further descent, the anterior shoulder is born, followed quickly by birth of the posterior shoulder. The body is born by lateral flexion of the fetus.

Variations of this mechanism occur as individual pelvic, fetal, or uterine factors are exerted. The same factors will determine the length of any particular phase of the mechanism. Molding of the fetal head or the development of edema of the head (caput succadaneum) are regular features in all but the most rapid vertex labors. These accommodations of the head are more extreme in primiparous labor.

Engagement of the fetal head in the pelvis is an important concept, since it implies that the pelvic inlet, at least, is adequate for the fetus. Unfortunately, there is no way of determining with precision by clinical examination whether or not engagement has occurred, but it can be determined radiologically. Experience has shown that engagement has usually occurred when the lowest part of the presenting vertex has reached the level of the maternal ischial spines. This fact is therefore used in determining engagement clinically. Furthermore, the degree of descent of the head can be described in terms of the relationship of the presenting part to the level of the spines. When the head is at the level of the spines, a descent to station *zero* (0) can be described (Fig. 9-13). If the head is 1 cm. below this level, a position of +1 can be diagnosed, or +2 or +3 for lower positions. Above the spines (i.e., an unengaged head) the head can be described as being in a −1, −2, or −3 position, depending on the level of the head above the level of the spines.

* When the head is 2 cm above the plane of the pelvic inlet → It's called: FLOATING !

CLINICAL COURSE OF LABOR

Prodromata

In many gravidas, certain symptoms or signs appear that are useful in predicting impending labor. Although very few of them are precise in pinpointing the exact moment when labor will begin, they are reassuring to the patient and useful to the physician in certain clinical situations. If elective induction is anticipated, for example, some evidence that labor will soon ensue spontaneously is

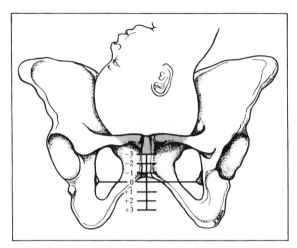

Fig. 9-13. Estimation of descent of fetal head into the pelvis. Station 0 is diagnosed when the fetal vertex has reached the level of the ischial spines.

essential for patient selection. Similarly, repeat cesarean section is best delayed until labor is imminent.

LIGHTENING, OR ENGAGEMENT. Lightening is experienced by the primigravid patient when the fetus enters the pelvis as term approaches. The mother senses a decrease in upper abdominal pressure as this occurs. This added comfort, however, is more than offset by the increased bladder pressure and the increased difficulty in moving the pelvic joints as fetal pressure is exerted on certain features of the pelvic anatomy. The physician can recognize fetal descent into the pelvis by abdominal examination of the area just above the symphysis and by pelvic examination. The fetal head, which previously could be moved back and forth easily just above the symphysis pubis, is now "fixed" and immovable. Pelvic examination will show the presenting part to be in the pelvis, perhaps even as low as station 0 or station +1. Fetal descent occurs with regularity in the primigravid patient two to four weeks before the onset of labor but rarely in the multigravid patient before labor actually begins. Indeed, lack of descent in the primigravid patient should alert the physician to possible cephalopelvic disproportion, although the majority of primigravidas without engagement before labor progress through labor without difficulty.

PELVIC CHANGES. Repeat pelvic examinations at weekly intervals during the last few weeks of pregnancy will show cervical changes that suggest the imminent onset of labor. The lower uterine segment gradually develops during this period of time as the fetus descends to obliterate the area. The cervix shows increasing degrees of effacement (see Cervical Effacement) and softening, and by the time of onset of labor, the cervix is typically dilated to about 2 cm. on the average. Occasionally, much greater degrees of cervical dilatation are achieved before labor ensues.

PASSAGE OF MUCUS AND BLOOD. When the gravid patient passes mucus or blood, labor can usually be expected within a few hours. The "bloody show" and the "mucus plug" are caused by increased dilatation and effacement of the cervix, with the extrusion of cervical mucus as the cervical glands are obliterated. While not universally present, these signs are seen often enough to provide clinically useful information.

Diagnosis of Labor

In some patients, labor starts abruptly and there is no doubt about the diagnosis. In others, the evidence for the diagnosis is less convincing, and the expertise of the physician is sought. False labor must be excluded.

Labor contractions usually begin at regular intervals. The regularity of the contractions is important, since false labor contractions are rarely regular; nor are they increasingly severe, as is true with labor pains. True labor contractions are usually experienced initially in the low lumbar area. Only later do they radiate around to the lower abdominal region. False labor is experienced in the lower abdomen. True labor is usually associated with the passage of mucus or blood, false labor rarely so. In many instances, the differentiation between false and true labor can be made on the basis of these points, but occasionally only hospital observation will clarify the issue. Labor is associ-

ated with progressive changes in the cervix, while false labor causes no such changes. Sedation will stop false labor in the majority of cases, but there is no evidence that true labor can be terminated in this fashion.

FIRST STAGE. The first stage of labor begins with the onset of regular, progressive contractions that result in cervical dilatation. The precise time of the onset of labor is usually recognized retrospectively and is frequently preceded by prelabor contractions or false labor. When labor starts, it is progressive unless an abnormality intervenes. The nature of labor is well illustrated by the cervical dilatation-time curves described previously under Labor Changes.

The precise limits of normalcy of the latent phase of the first stage of labor as illustrated by the cervical dilatation-time curve have been arbitrarily established by Friedman [2] as less than 20 hours in the primigravida and less than 14 hours in the multiparous patient. The maximal slope phase should show a speed of cervical dilatation of at least 1.2 cm. per hour in the primigravida and 1.5 cm. per hour in the multigravida. After the phase of maximal slope has been entered, dilatation must continue to progress until near full dilatation if the labor is to be considered normal. Variations from these criteria are considered abnormal. Specific abnormalities described by Friedman are discussed in a later section.

SECOND STAGE. Full dilatation of the cervix marks the onset of the second stage of labor. While descent of the presenting part has occurred to some degree in the first stage of labor and even before labor, most of the essential fetal descent occurs in this stage. Progressive fetal descent caused by the uterine contractions is as much a part of this stage of labor as cervical dilatation is of the first stage.

As the second stage begins, the cervix has been fully retracted, and the attachment of the cervix to the pelvic ligaments will allow it to rise no further cephalad. The uterine contractions must either propel the fetus toward the perineum or continue thinning of the already thinned lower uterine segment. This physiologic fact is the basis of the "2-hour second stage" rule, which has been a part of good obstetrical practice for the past 75 years. If the fetus of a primigravid patient is not extruded in a maximum of 2 hours following full cervical dilatation, the physician should consider terminating the labor either by a forceps operation, if that is appropriate, or by cesarean section. Slightly less time should be allowed in the multipara. A prolonged second stage will be discussed under abnormalities of labor in a later section.

THIRD STAGE. With the delivery of the child, the third stage of labor begins. Immediately following delivery of the fetus, the uterus is flaccid and discoid in shape. Within 1 or 2 minutes, however, the first postpartum uterine contraction occurs. These contractions, as well as the preceding diminution in uterine size from expulsion of the fetus, shrink the size of the uterine attachment of the placenta, usually causing the placenta to shear off the uterine wall. Retroplacental bleeding occurs, and further separation is accomplished. With a few contractions, the placenta will be expelled spontaneously.

The bleeding during this stage of labor, when spontaneous expulsion of the placenta is awaited, may be copious, however. It is good practice to terminate the third stage of labor prematurely to minimize maternal blood loss. The maneuvers to accomplish delivery of the placenta are discussed under Clinical Management of Labor.

Fetal Condition During Labor
Methods used to appraise fetal health and vigor may identify *chronic fetal distress* or a fetus who is in *acute* jeopardy. Chronic stress is best evaluated by tests of placental or fetoplacental function, which are described in Chapter 12. Acute distress may be recognized during labor by observing certain clinical signs (fetal tachycardia or bradycardia, meconium in the amniotic fluid), by identifying certain abnormal heart rate patterns during continuous electronic fetal heart rate monitoring (EFM), or by measuring certain ominous changes in the fetal acid-base balance by sampling of the fetal scalp blood.

By long tradition, frequent determinations of the fetal heart rate (FHR) by auscultation remain an important element of fetal care during labor. Although electronic equipment for measuring FHR has come into wide use in the past few years, the stethoscope remains a prevalent method of observing FHR changes. It is unfortunate that stethoscopic sampling of the FHR will not always identify the fetus in acute distress. Continuous EFM approaches this goal more closely. The major diagnostic problem rests in the interpretation of observed FHR pattern changes. Experts, however, are in general agreement on what constitutes an abnormality of the FHR pattern in most cases.

Bradycardia recognized with the stethoscope seems to correlate well with poor fetal condition, especially if the bradycardic episode extends beyond the disappearance of the uterine contraction. Tachycardia seems more innocuous but sometimes presages the development of bradycardia. Staining of the amniotic fluid with meconium also correlates to some degree with fetal distress and is a sign that should always be looked for. A combination of fetal bradycardia with meconium staining of the fluid, especially if the staining is heavy, correlates best with a compromised fetal condition. Yet at least two-thirds of babies with both these signs survive, and many of these do not appear to have suffered intrauterine hypoxia at all, as judged by condition at birth. Clearly, a more precise method of recognizing fetal distress is needed.

EFM, together with simultaneous recording of uterine contractions, provides a better method of recognizing fetal distress than do the clinical tools of FHR sampling and observation for meconium staining. EFM is now available in most hospitals and has almost replaced stethoscopic observation of FHR in some institutions, at least for high-risk pregnancies. Certainly, it is more reliable than other methods of observing FHR changes and has the additional advantage of being "automatic" once it is initiated. Criteria for interpreting the FHR patterns have been developed primarily by Hon [5] and by Caldeyro-Barcia over the past few years and a fair correlation between abnormal FHR patterns and abnormalities in fetal condition has been observed.

The FHR may be recorded in one of three ways,

by phonocardiography, electrocardiography, or ultrasonic techniques. The latter two methods are in widespread use. The fetal electrocardiograph is obtained through a metal lead attached directly to the fetus, nearly always to the fetal scalp (or buttocks with breech presentations). This technique requires a ruptured amniotic sac. Increasingly simple electrodes have become available, and with the recent introduction of a spiral electrode, the technique now requires a minimum of skill. However, electrocardiographic monitoring requires that the membranes be ruptured. This disadvantage has been overcome by the introduction of ultrasonic equipment that can identify the fetal heart rate transabdominally. The technique uses the Doppler principle. An ultrasonic beam is directed toward the fetal heart, and the reflected waves are recovered and recorded. Since the frequency of the waves varies with heart movement, the FHR can be determined from these waves. Ultrasonic measurement of FHR has the advantage of not requiring invasion of the uterus, but, a satisfactory recording cannot always be obtained, and direct fetal scalp electronic monitoring may have to be substituted.

The most important FHR abnormalities can be recognized only when they are time-related to the uterine contractions. Thus, the uterine contractions are always measured and displayed on the recording paper. They may be recorded by measuring intrauterine pressure directly through a plastic catheter inserted transcervically into the amniotic sac. They may also be recorded without uterine invasion by external devices placed on the abdomen overlying the fundus. This method depends on changes in fundal shape during contractions. While the former method is more precise in measuring the exact intra-amniotic pressure, the latter is frequently adequate for clinical monitoring.

The FHR is under the control of accelerator (sympathetic) and decelerator (parasympathetic) centers of the midbrain. The parasympathetic (vagal) effects are dominant during fetal life, especially as term is approached. The vagal stimulation also accounts for beat-to-beat variability of the FHR, which is thought to be an important sign of good fetal health. Certain factors (e.g., fetal move-

ment) stimulate the midbrain of the fetus to evoke short tachycardic episodes. This effect is the end point of the nonstress test (NST) described in Chapter 12 and is usually considered a sign of good fetal health. If the fetus experiences a stressful situation, however, he evokes selective vasoconstriction with a resultant bradycardia. The "stress" may be harmful (hypoxia) or it may be relatively innocuous (head compression, fetal grunting). While interpretation of FHR deceleration patterns is now precise enough to justify clinical decisions based on these patterns, much remains to be learned.

The normal instantaneous FHR pattern is one in which the baseline FHR is between 120 and 160 beats per minute with beat-to-beat variability of 6 to 10 beats per minute (Fig. 9-14). The baseline FHR is identified between uterine contractions, but the normal FHR does not vary with a contraction. Bradycardia (a baseline rate below 120) usually is not pathologic; however, it may be due to congenital heart block in the fetus. Tachycardia (a baseline rate above 160) may be due to maternal fever or maternal hyperthyroidism; or it may follow the mother's use of certain drugs (atropine is the best example). On occasion, tachycardia may also be an early sign of fetal hypoxia.

The baseline FHR does not trace a smooth line, since beat-to-beat variability is normal and expected. A decrease or disappearance of the normal baseline variability can be caused by drugs (e.g., central nervous system depressants, atropine), miscellaneous factors (immaturity, "sleep"), and —of greatest importance—by fetal cerebral hypoxia. Periodic accelerations or decelerations in FHR may occur. Accelerations occur frequently and are usually interpreted as evidence that the fetus is reactive and in good condition. Decelerations are of greater clinical significance and may be ominous. These patterns, as well as other abnormal FHR patterns, are discussed in Chapter 11.

Continuous FHR monitoring is performed routinely on all pregnant patients in some hospitals. This may or may not prove to be wise since the disadvantages (e.g., fetal infection) may prove to be of greater magnitude than the advantages (better diagnosis of fetal distress?). In a hospital unit where

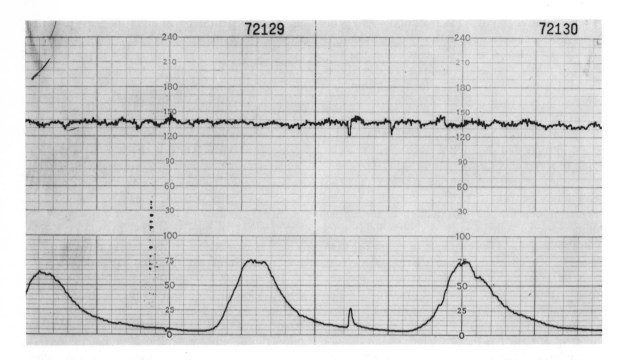

Fig. 9-14. Normal fetal heart rate pattern. (From K. Niswander. Obstetric and Gynecologic Disorders: A Practitioner's Guide. Flushing, N.Y.: Medical Examination Publishing Co., 1975.)

it is logistically impossible to monitor all patients in labor, there are certain high-risk patients that should be selected for monitoring according to the following criteria:

1. Oxytocin induction or augmentation.
2. Suspected fetal distress (abnormal ausculatory FHR or meconium in the amniotic fluid).
3. Any other patient who has been identified as at high risk, e.g., with acute toxemia, diabetes mellitus, prolonged gestation, poor reproductive history (see section on high-risk pregnancy in Chap. 3).

Fetal scalp sampling to determine the acid-base status of the fetus is the most recently developed method of diagnosing hypoxia and acidosis in the intrauterine patient. The technique requires (1) a ruptured amniotic sac and sufficient dilatation of the cervix to allow the introduction of an endoscope and (2) a fetus low enough in the pelvic canal to be reached. The procedure is carried out as follows: An endoscope is introduced through the cer-

vix while an assistant exerts pressure on the uterine fundus to keep the presenting part low in the pelvis. After cleansing of the fetal scalp, a premeasured puncture wound is made in the skin of the scalp, and a blood sample is obtained in a capillary tube.

The most important measurement to be made is the blood pH. If the pH is below 7.25, fetal asphyxia is suspected and repetition of sampling within 10 to 30 minutes is indicated. If the pH is below 7.20, significant fetal acidosis is probably present and immediate delivery is indicated. The maternal pH should be checked since maternal acidosis will be reflected in the fetal pH and result in a falsely low pH.

The exact role of fetal blood scalp sampling in the assessment of the fetus is not yet clear. False-positive readings have been reported to occur in 4 to 26 percent of cases [6]. False-negative rates between 10.4 and 55 percent have also been reported. Most clinics now reserve the use of fetal scalp blood sampling for fetuses whose EFM patterns suggest a distressed condition.

Other methods of diagnosing fetal distress and potential fetal distress include both amnioscopy and amniotic fluid sampling to detect meconium. Amnioscopy is performed by inserting an endoscope through the cervix and observing the color of the amniotic fluid through intact membranes. Meconium staining can be recognized in this fashion. While good results have been reported by Saling and others with the method, it has not been used to a significant degree in the United States. Transabdominal amniotic fluid sampling is occasionally performed for the sole purpose of detecting meconium staining, and the sign is sometimes useful when the puncture has been performed for other reasons (e.g., to determine fetal age by lecithin-sphingomyelin ratio).

CLINICAL MANAGEMENT OF LABOR

Admission to the hospital should, if possible, be delayed until labor is established, but not so long that there is a risk of delivery outside the hospital. While early labor may be more comfortable for the patient in familiar home surroundings, the increased perinatal risk associated with delivery outside the aseptic hospital setting cannot be disregarded. The primigravid patient should be admitted when her contractions are regular, progressively hard and closer, and occurring at about 5-minute intervals. The multigravid patient should be admitted as soon as her contractions are regular and the diagnosis of labor seems likely. These generalizations should be ignored for specific patients, such as the highly tense primigravida who needs the reassurance of hospital care with early contractions; or the multigravid patient who gives a history of a short labor with a previous pregnancy. What is most important is that the patient feel free to consult with her physician, either by telephone or in person, about early labor. She should be encouraged to report the earliest evidence of labor so that she and her physician can jointly make the decision regarding the time of admission. The patient's attitudes and, indeed, her knowledge and intuition must not be ignored in making plans regarding her care.

Admission Procedures

The condition of the patient at the time of admission will determine the thoroughness of the admission procedures. While certain elements cannot be eliminated, many can, if necessary, wait until after delivery. A rapid evaluation of the patient's appearance, her degree of discomfort, and evidence suggesting the second stage of labor, as well as a brief history of the severity and frequency of contractions will allow the person admitting the patient to determine the appropriate steps to be taken.

Unless delivery appears imminent or the patient appears extremely uncomfortable, the temperature, pulse, and respirations are measured. A history of time of onset of contractions, the contraction interval, and the severity of the contractions is taken. Evidences of abnormal bleeding are sought both by history and by examination of the vulva. The blood pressure is recorded at the earliest opportunity, preferably between contractions. The FHR is recorded, and the contractions are observed by fundal palpation and timing. Blood may be drawn for a hematocrit determination and for possible cross matching if this procedure is indicated. A clean catch urine sample should be tested immediately for albumin and glucose and the remainder sent to the laboratory for routine urinalysis.

The lower abdominal and vulvar areas are prepared with soap and the hair is shaved. While some clinics find shaving unnecessary, most authorities feel that a better aseptic technique is possible with shaving. A plain water enema is usually given to empty the lower bowel and reduce the risk of fecal contamination during delivery. The enema is omitted or delayed if (1) the labor seems very active, with delivery a likely possibility within 1 to 2 hours; (2) the labor is premature, especially if the diagnosis of labor is uncertain; and (3) there is a history of abnormal vaginal bleeding.

While the nurse is performing these initial admitting procedures, the physician should be reviewing the history and physical examination previously performed during the prenatal period. He should bring the history up to date briefly, with as few questions as possible, taking special note of the history of contractions and evidences of abnormality, i.e., bleeding, symptoms of hypertension, premature rupture of the membranes. A brief general physical examination is performed, with emphasis on the blood pressure, heart, and lungs. Pallor, cyanosis, and jaundice should be noted. The abdomen is examined with particular care to note the lie and position of the fetus (Fig. 9-15), its estimated size, and its condition as measured by the FHR. The contractions are timed and evaluated by fundal palpation. Of utmost importance is that the physician take a reassuring, kindly attitude toward the patient. The degree of rapport that he can establish with her will frequently determine the degree of comfort with which labor is experienced and perhaps also the length of labor.

PELVIC EXAMINATION. Pelvic examination is always performed unless there is a history of abnormal vaginal bleeding or of prolonged rupture of the membranes. While pelvic examination may be indicated even under these circumstances, special precautions must be taken as described elsewhere (see Chap. 7).

Pelvic examination should provide the following information: the station of the presenting part, the degree of cervical effacement and consistency of the cervix, and the amount of cervical dilatation. At times, the presentation of the fetus may be diagnosed or abnormalities may be recognized, e.g., prolapse of the umbilical cord. The appearance of the amniotic fluid should be noted if the membranes have ruptured. Rectal examination is performed in preference to pelvic examination in some clinics, but we usually choose the pelvic approach. Care should be exercised to use a sterile glove and to avoid contamination by the vulvar skin during insertion of the fingers into the vagina.

Station of the Presenting Part. Details of the determination of the degree of the descent of the fetus through the pelvis have been described previously. The ischial spines are palpated, and the level of the

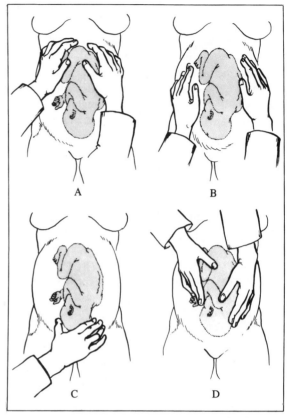

Fig. 9-15. Leopold's maneuvers to diagnose fetal presentation and position of the fetus. A. Palpation of the upper pole. B. Determining the side of the small parts. C. Palpation of the lower pole. The vertex is freely movable, and the breech moves with the body. D. Is the prominence of the presenting part on the side opposite the small parts, as with vertex presentation? Or is it on the same side, as with face presentation? (From K. Niswander. Obstetric and Gynecologic Disorders: A Practitioner's Guide. *Flushing, N.Y.: Medical Examination Publishing Co., 1975.)*

presenting part in relation to the level of the spines is described. If the presenting part is exactly at the level of the interspinous diameter, the fetus is said to be at station 0. If it is judged to be 1 cm. below this level, it is at station +1, or +2, or +3 at correspondingly lower levels. Above the spines, the fetus is "unengaged"; it is at level −1 if 1 cm. above the spines and level −2 or −3 if 2 or 3 cm.

above the spines. The importance of determining the station of the presenting part is that (1) a fetus presenting by the vertex at station 0 is known to have entered the pelvis (except with extreme molding of the fetal head or with asynclitism as described below) and (2) progress of labor can be assessed by repeated determination of this level.

Cervical Effacement. Cervical effacement is estimated by determining the degree to which the length of the cervical canal has been reduced by compression of the presenting part on the cervix and by retraction upward of the cervix by the contractions of the fundus. An uneffaced cervix is about 2 cm. long, while a cervix 1 cm. long can be described as 50 percent effaced. Ultimately, the cervix becomes paper-thin and can then be described as being 100 percent effaced.

Cervical Dilatation. Dilatation of the cervix proceeds with cervical effacement, although cervical effacement is usually well underway before rapid dilatation of the cervix is observed. All degrees of cervical dilatation may be present before the onset of labor, from none to many centimeters; the average is about 2 cm. The amount of cervical dilatation is best expressed in centimeters, with 10 cm. (the approximate width of the widest fetal vertex diameter) considered full dilatation. The estimation of cervical dilatation should be made with repeated examinations at a consistent time, preferably at the height of a contraction. Cervical dilatation can be plotted against time on an appropriate graph as described by Friedman [2]. Such a practice allows early recognition of labor abnormalities. Friedman has also reported that plotting of the station of the presenting part against time is a useful clinical tool, although observations of station will vary more from examiner to examiner than does cervical dilatation. The graph of fetal station is therefore subject to wider variations from the normal or expected curve.

First Stage

Once the diagnosis of labor has been made, the patient should be observed in the hospital. The admitting examination previously described is performed. The pelvic examination is repeated as necessary, usually at the time the patient appears to need analgesic medication, when her symptoms suggest full dilatation has occurred, or when delivery seems imminent. A longer labor will obviously require more examinations than a shorter one.

In addition to determining the station of the presenting part and cervical dilatation and effacement with the first pelvic examination, an appraisal of pelvic measurements can be made. A special effort should be directed toward determining the status of the fetal membranes by examination as well as by history. If the membranes are not ruptured, the bulging forewaters can often be felt through the dilated cervix. If the membranes are ruptured, amniotic fluid will usually be observed, especially if the presenting part is pushed up slightly, allowing escape of fluid. Care should be exercised with this maneuver, however, since severe upward displacement may allow the cord to prolapse.

If the status of the membranes remains uncertain, certain tests should be performed to clarify the matter. The most widely used test is the determination of the pH of the fluid presumed to be amniotic; or the pH of the upper vagina if no fluid is observed. The pH of the vagina is normally about 5.0, while the amniotic fluid is more alkaline (pH 7.0 or 7.5). Nitrazine paper is placed against the upper vaginal mucosa, preferably in the posterior fornix, through a speculum, and the resulting color of the paper is compared to a standard. A yellowish color results from an acid pH; a bluish green or blue, from a pH of 7.0 to 7.5. This is not a completely reliable test, but no more accurate or simpler method is currently available.

To diagnose fetal membrane rupture, some physicians look for "ferning" in the vaginal material placed on a glass slide and allowed to dry. The presence of "ferns" is caused by the sodium chloride present in the amniotic fluid and suggests a diagnosis of membrane rupture. Blood interferes with the ferning, probably to a greater degree than it interferes with the determination of the vaginal pH. No test, however, is universally reliable.

The patient may request or may obviously require analgesic medication during the first stage of labor. The types of medication available are described in Chapter 10. The medication usually should not be given until the diagnosis of labor seems certain or before definite progress in cervical dilatation has been observed. Exceptions to this rule include the treatment of a prolonged latent phase as described in Chapter 11. Most analgesics will exert some effect on the fetus, and the amount, as well as the timing, of the medication should be considered with this fact in mind. In general, medication should be avoided if delivery is judged to be less than 1½ hours away.

Second Stage

In the majority of instances, evidence that the second stage of labor may have been reached is apparent from the patient's symptoms or from certain readily observable signs. There may be slightly more bloody show than has previously been noted. The patient may begin to experience an urge to bear down for the first time. The sounds emitted by the patient during a contraction may change, and the experienced ear will hear the difference. Confirmation of the suspicion should be made by pelvic examination, not only to allow transfer of the patient to the delivery room for further care but also to provide a baseline of time to determine length of the second stage should delivery be delayed. While the primigravida will usually be transported to the delivery room at this time, the onset of the second stage in the multigravida should have been anticipated, since the second stage may be very brief in this case. Our description of the early second stage therefore relates to the typical primigravid patient.

The contractions increase in severity, and a definite urge to bear down or defecate is experienced with each contraction, especially as the fetal head approaches closer to the pelvic floor. Bradycardia is a frequent accompaniment of the fetal head pressure that occurs especially in this state of labor. EFM allows the clearest differentiation of FHR dips due to head compression from those due to uteroplacental insufficiency or other causes.

The passage of maternal feces frequently precedes vulvar spreading by the fetal head. The feces should be disposed of without contaminating the vulva. Gradually, more and more distention of the vulva and perineum occurs, and this part of the second stage should be managed by an appropriately scrubbed and gowned attendant. The vulvar and perineal areas are scrubbed with soap, taking care to move the soapy sponge from anterior to posterior. The perineal area is scrubbed last, and the sponge is immediately discarded thereafter.

SPONTANEOUS DELIVERY. Determination of fetal position, previously assessed by abdominal palpation of the fetus (Leopold's maneuvers) (see Fig. 9-15), is now determined by vaginal palpation of the various fetal head sutures and fontanelles (Fig. 9-16). If, for example, the small, three-pronged posterior fontanelle is palpated in the mother's left anterior quadrant, the position is known to be left occiput anterior (LOA) (Fig. 9-17). Rarely, the fetal head landmarks will be obscured by molding of the head or for some other reason, and it may be necessary to palpate a fetal ear to determine position. Care not to dislodge the head from the pelvis is essential.

With each contraction, the head distends the perineum more. The attendant should prevent the sudden expulsion of the fetal head by gentle pressure on the vertex. As the perineum is distended, an episiotomy may be performed to prevent it from tearing. The head is gradually allowed to deliver, and, following this, the anterior shoulder comes into view. With the combination of maternal pushing or the fundal pressure of an assistant and gentle traction in a posterior direction by the obstetrician, the anterior shoulder is delivered. With similar fundal pressure and with the traction by the attendant now provided in an upward direction, the posterior shoulder is delivered. Lateral traction on the fetal body quickly allows the remainder of the fetus to be delivered.

The baby is held head downward to encourage drainage of pharyngeal and tracheal fluid. The cord is clamped, tied, and cut about ½ inch (12 mm.) from the baby's abdomen, and the baby is quickly transferred to an assistant for necessary attention. Management of the normal baby as well as of the baby with respiratory difficulty is described in

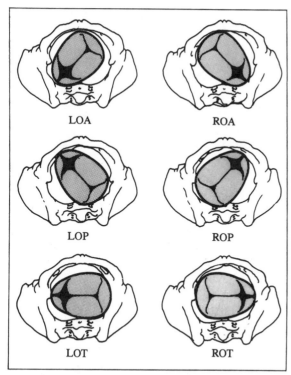

Fig. 9-16. Vaginal palpation of the large and small fontanelles and the frontal, sagittal, and lambdoidal sutures determine the position of the vertex. (LOA = left occiput anterior; ROA = right occiput anterior; LOP = left occiput posterior; ROP = right occiput posterior; LOT = left occiput transverse; ROT = right occiput transverse.) (From K. Niswander. Obstetric and Gynecologic Disorders: A Practitioner's Guide. *Flushing, N.Y.: Medical Examination Publishing Co., 1975.)*

Chapter 13. While the time of clamping of the cord remains in dispute after many years of investigation, our preference is for early clamping at the first convenient time without undue speed and yet without delay. Delay will indeed increase the fetal blood volume by as much as 80 to 100 ml., but this may be offset by increased hemolysis during the first few days of life. We prefer earlier clamping, although others will disagree.

PROPHYLACTIC OUTLET FORCEPS DELIVERY. An alternative method of delivery of the normal obstetrical patient is by outlet forceps, described by DeLee [7] in 1920 as the "prophylactic forceps operation." DeLee contended that the slow dilatation of the vulva by the fetal head during spontaneous delivery, especially in the primigravid patient, caused undue head compression, with an increased possibility of brain hemorrhage. He felt that an outlet forceps operation combined with a well-timed episiotomy when the fetal head reaches the outlet will spare the fetal brain and lower the perinatal mortality of spontaneous delivery. It can be said with certainty that the outlet forceps operation in competent hands provides a method of delivery at least as safe for the baby as spontaneous delivery and perhaps safer [8]. It is good obstetrical practice to perform the outlet forceps operation if desired.

Under pudendal block anesthesia (or alternatively a conduction anesthetic or a general anesthetic), the fetal head is noted to be on the pelvic floor. The exact position is determined by vaginal palpation. If the position is found to be LOA, the forceps are applied as follows (a direct OA or an ROA position will vary the procedure slightly): The left blade (the blade is labeled according to the side of the mother's pelvis in which it is to be placed) is inserted with the operator's left hand. (Simpson forceps are illustrated, although a number of other instruments are equally good.) The right hand gently distends the vagina in the path of the blade and is used to ensure that the blade slips easily between the head and the vagina. The right blade is inserted in a similar manner with the right hand. The English lock is engaged, and the application of the blades is checked.

Three conditions must be met for good application: (1) the blades should be equidistant from the lambdoidal sutures; (2) the fenestrations of the blades should be barely if at all palpable (if the fenestration is felt, the blade probably overlies the face); and (3) the posterior fontanelle should be no more than 1 cm. above the level of the handles of the blades (a greater distance suggests a poorly flexed head). If these criteria are not met, the blades must be readjusted until the application is considered satisfactory.

The downward force exerted by the forceps

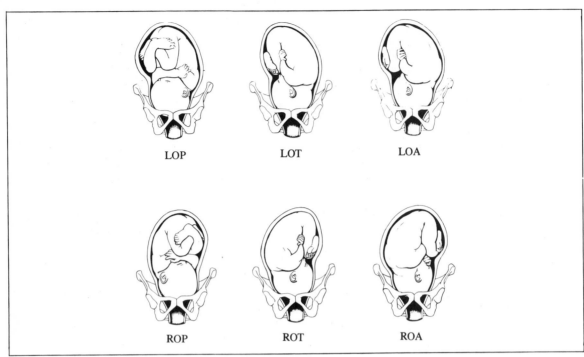

LOP   LOT   LOA

ROP   ROT   ROA

Fig. 9-17. Various vertex presentations. (LOA = left occiput anterior; ROA = right occiput anterior; LOP = left occiput posterior; ROP = right occiput posterior; LOT = left occiput transverse; ROT = right occiput transverse.) (From Obstetrical Presentation and Position, Ross Clinical Education Aid No. 18. Columbus, Ohio: Ross Laboratories, 1975.)

should pull the head in the axis of the pelvis (Fig. 9-18). Thus, with the patient on her back, the initial pull will be at a 45-degree angle posteriorly between the horizontal and the vertical. Force in this direction is provided by pulling in a horizontal plane with the right hand and pushing downward on the shank of the blade in the vertical direction with the left hand. The resultant force will be between these two forces. As the head slides under the symphysis pubis, the pull is changed to a more horizontal direction and then a slightly more vertical direction. Care should be exercised not to lift the forceps too high, since periurethral lacerations will result. As the head is delivered, the blades are removed, and the remainder of the delivery is accomplished as in spontaneous delivery.

Third Stage

A few minutes after delivery of the fetus and the clamping of the umbilical cord, the relaxed uterus usually contracts. This contraction, together with the diminution of uterine size from expulsion of the fetus, causes the placenta to become de-

tached from the uterus. At this time, the uterus changes its shape from a soft flat organ to a somewhat smaller, firm, globular shape. There may be a gush of blood, and the umbilical cord may protrude from the vagina more than previously as the placenta enters the lower uterine segment. Within a short time, the placenta will usually be extruded by uterine contractions.

Most obstetricians, however, prefer not to wait for these events to occur spontaneously, since doing so may allow a substantial amount of bleeding in some patients. Rather, immediately after delivery, the fundus is gently massaged to speed up the first contraction. When the uterus becomes firm—and not until it becomes firm—attempts at

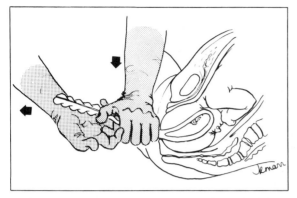

Fig. 9-18. Pajot's maneuver for forceps delivery of the fetal head. The force of the left arm is toward the floor; the force of the right arm is in the horizontal plane. The resulting force follows the curve of the pelvis. (From K. Niswander. Obstetric and Gynecologic Disorders: A Practitioner's Guide. Flushing, N.Y.: Medical Examination Publishing Co., 1975.)

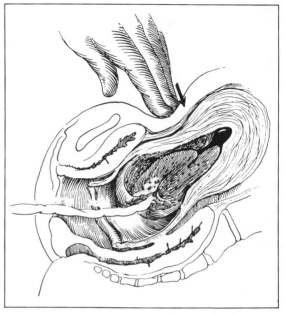

Fig. 9-19. Brandt delivery of the placenta. After the fundus is firm, moderate tension is exerted on the umbilical cord while the other hand "shears off" the placenta from the uterine wall by upward kneading pressure on the anterior uterine wall. (From J. R. Willson. Atlas of Obstetric Technic [2nd ed.]. St. Louis: Mosby, 1969. Daisy Stilwell, medical illustrator.)

hurrying its expulsion are in order. We believe that Brandt's maneuver is the one most likely to cause complete and rapid expulsion of all the membranes as well as the placenta. Others have used Credé's or the modified Credé's maneuver, i.e., fundal pressure in a downward direction until the placenta is delivered.

With Brandt's maneuver (Fig. 9-19), a well-contracted fundus is essential. With gentle traction on the transected umbilical cord with the right hand, the left hand exerts moderate pressure first on the anterior wall of the uterus and then in a kneading fashion on the anterior uterus and up toward the fundus. This maneuver shears the uterus off the placenta, and traction on the cord helps the expulsion. The maneuver must be performed soon after delivery of the fetus, but only when the fundus is well contracted.

Should the placenta be difficult to deliver or if significant bleeding ensues, manual removal of the placenta is indicated. It is unwise to wait more than a few minutes for delivery of the placenta. With general or conduction anesthesia, the left hand holds the fundus downward by fundal pressure. The right hand is introduced through the cervix and into the fundus to palpate the placenta. Occasion-

ally, the placenta will be found free in the lower uterine segment, and delivery of the organ is easily accomplished. More characteristically, the placenta is still attached or partially attached to the uterus, and manual separation with the fingers is necessary. Care not to rupture the uterine musculature is most important. Usually, the placenta can be detached in toto; occasionally, it must be removed piecemeal. If a line of cleavage cannot be recognized, placenta accreta should be suspected and appropriate treatment instituted, frequently hysterectomy. Placenta accreta is a rare condition, however, and many never be encountered in an obstetrician's lifetime, at least in full-blown form.

With expulsion of the placenta, the fundus should be gently massaged to keep it firm and thus minimize bleeding. It is usually wise to use an oxytoxic drug, either Methergine, 0.2 mg. intramuscularly, or an intravenous drip containing 10 units of oxytocin in 500 ml. of 5 percent D/W at a rapid rate (100 drops per minute). If bleeding persists, postpartum hemorrhage is present and should be treated as described in Chapter 11.

Membrane Rupture

THE QUESTION OF AMNIOTOMY

The fetal membranes usually rupture spontaneously during the first or second stage of labor. Artificial rupture of the membranes (amniotomy) may be used to "speed labor" in instances when the membranes fail to rupture spontaneously. Whether or not amniotomy actually speeds labor is uncertain and will be discussed in Chapter 11. What is certain is that amniotomy performed before the fetal vertex is well engaged distinctly increases the risk of prolapse of the umbilical cord.

To perform elective amniotomy, the vertex should be well engaged. During pelvic examination, the membranes are punctured with a pointed instrument, either with a sharp pointed clamp or with an instrument specifically designed for amniotomy. Some obstetricians prefer to puncture the amniotic sac at the height of a contraction, when the fluid is tense and the distance between the fetal head and membranes is at a maximum. Others prefer to perform the procedure between contractions to prevent a sudden gush of fluid under high pressure that may carry an umbilical cord with it. This accident should not occur if the fetal vertex is well engaged.

PREMATURE RUPTURE OF MEMBRANES

The time sequence between rupture of the fetal membranes and the onset of labor is of diagnostic and therapeutic importance. Premature rupture of the membranes (PROM), i.e., rupture before the onset of labor, is of potential serious clinical significance. The therapy of PROM is discussed in Chapter 11. The diagnosis is discussed here.

Many patients will give a history of a gush of a large amount of fluid, and if the fluid is found by the examiner to exude from the vagina, the diagnosis is obvious. Frequently, however, the patient will give a history of the passage of a small amount of fluid from the vagina, and the diagnosis may be less certain. Certain tests will allow amniotic fluid to be differentiated from other vaginal secretions or from urine. The vagina has an acid pH while the endocervix and amniotic fluid are basic. Thus, nitrazine paper applied to the vagina with care to avoid the cervix will turn blue (basic) in the presence of amniotic fluid. Blood will also cause a basic pH reading and should be avoided. A drop of amniotic fluid placed on a clean glass slide and allowed to dry will reveal a fernlike pattern that is not seen with vaginal secretions (Fig. 9-20). A careful history supplemented by these two tests will allow a diagnosis of rupture of the membranes in most instances.

Lacerations of the Birth Canal

TYPES OF LACERATIONS

Lacerations of the vagina and the perineum are described as follows:

First degree: The perineal skin, or the vaginal mucosa, or both are involved.

Second degree: The perineal musculature is included in the laceration.

Third degree: The tear involves all or part of the anal spincter.

Fourth degree: The rectal mucosa is involved. The anal spincter is almost always also torn with fourth-degree laceration, although occasionally the rectal mucosa is lacerated and the anal spincter is intact.

Various types of lacerations have been described under these major headings; e.g., vaginal vault laceration, which extends into the upper half of the vagina; sulcus laceration, which involves the posterolateral aspect of the vagina; and periurethral laceration. Lacerations may be caused by a normal spontaneous delivery, but the likelihood that a laceration will occur is increased under the following conditions: (1) when a wide diameter of the head is emerging (posterior presentation, poorly flexed head); (2) when the pelvic bony architecture is un-

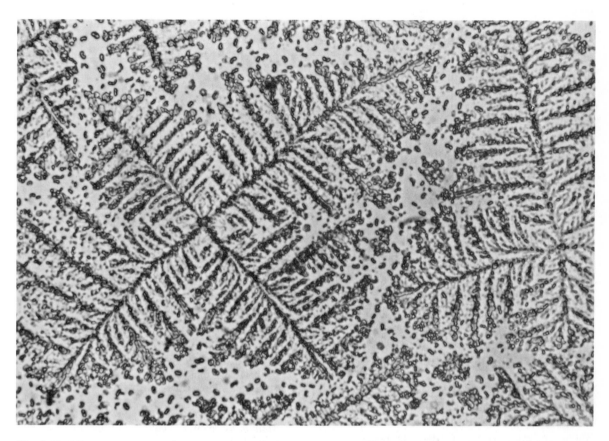

Fig. 9-20. "Ferning" in smear from vagina suggests that amniotic fluid is present in the vagina.

usual (narrow pelvic arch that decreases the area of the anterior portion of the pelvic outlet); or (3) when an obstetrical operation (difficult forceps delivery) is needed. Repair of the laceration is performed as is any surgical repair, with careful approximation of tissue planes in separate fashion, much as described under Episiotomy. Lacerations of the cervix or lower uterine segment are discussed in Chapter 11.

EPISIOTOMY

Episiotomy is the term used to describe a surgical incision of the perineum, usually performed just before the birth of the presenting part. A surgical incision is preferable to a laceration for the following reasons: (1) the straight edges of the episiotomy are easier to repair than the frequently jagged edges of the laceration; (2) a judiciously timed episiotomy may prevent injuries to the perineal musculature and vaginal lacerations high in the vault of the vagina; and (3) the fetal head is spared a battering against the perineum as it dilates the vaginal outlet (see Prophylactic Outlet Forceps Delivery). The episiotomy may be used when spontaneous delivery is planned, especially in the primigravida, and it is used almost routinely with any forceps operation. Indeed, DeLee's prophylactic forceps operation included an episiotomy as an integral part of the procedure.

The episiotomy may be made in the midline directly toward the anus (midline), or it may be started at the midpoint of the vaginal perineal junction but extended in a mediolateral direction at about a 45-degree angle either to the left or to the right (mediolateral episiotomy). The skin of the perineum, the vaginal mucosa, and the underlying perineal musculature are incised, usually with large scissors. The incision is made early enough to prevent injuries to the perineal musculature caused by the extruding head but late enough to minimize the sometimes significant blood loss from the episiotomy. With spontaneous delivery, the episiotomy may be made as the vertex distends the perineum slightly. With forceps delivery, we prefer to make the episiotomy after the forceps have been applied, but before the perineum has been distended by the pulling of the forceps.

The median episiotomy has a number of advantages over the mediolateral type: (1) it provides more space per centimeter of incision; (2) it heals well and is easier to repair; (3) there is less blood loss; (4) the incidence of immediate postpartum discomfort as well as subsequent dyspareunia is reduced. The major drawback to midline episiotomy is that it is more likely to result in perineal laceration through the anal spincter (third-degree) or even through the rectal mucosa (fourth-degree) than is a mediolateral incision. This accident, however, is not a serious one, since adequate repair of the episiotomy extension under hospital conditions almost always prevents the only complication worth noting, namely, rectovaginal fistula. Studies have shown that a rectovaginal fistula that requires surgical repair (two-thirds heal spontaneously) occurs only once in every 3000 median episiotomies.

We prefer to deliver the placenta routinely before beginning repair of the episiotomy. Many techniques of repair have been described and we will not detail any particular one. In all repairs, however, the perineal musculature, the vaginal mucosa, and the perineal skin are each approximated in separate steps, usually with very fine chromic catgut (2-0 or 3-0). The purpose of the repair is to secure a functional result, not an anatomic one, although the two needs usually coincide. Should a third- or fourth-degree laceration complicate the episiotomy, the rectal mucosa is repaired with small interrupted sutures (3-0 chromic catgut), with careful placement of two rows of interrupted sutures over the rectal mucosal repair to approximate the perirectal tissue. The ends of the cut anal spincter are approximated with two or three interrupted sutures, and the remainder of the repair is that of an uncomplicated episiotomy. During the puerperium following a third- or fourth-degree laceration, enemas should be avoided, and stool softeners by mouth should be prescribed to protect the repair.

References

1. Liggins, G. What factors initiate human labor? *Contemp Obstet Gynecol* 13:147, 1979.
2. Friedman, E. *Labor: Clinical Evaluation and Management* (2nd ed.). New York: Appleton-Century-Crofts, 1978.
3. Hendricks, C. H., Brenner, W. E., and Kraus, G. Normal cervical dilatation pattern in late pregnancy and labor. *Am J. Obstet Gynecol* 106: 1065, 1970.
4. Caldwell, W., and Moloy, H. Anatomical variations in the female pelvis and their effect in labor with a suggested classification. *Am J Obstet Gynecol* 26:479, 1933.
5. Hon, E. *An Introduction to Fetal Heart Rate Monitoring.* New Haven: Yale Cooperative Corporation, 1971.
6. *Antenatal Diagnosis.* NIH Publication Number 79-1973, April, 1979.
7. DeLee, J. The prophylactic forceps operation. *Am J Obstet Gynecol* 1:34, 1920.
8. Niswander, K., and Gordon, M. Safety of the low-forceps operation. *Am J Obstet Gynecol* 117:619, 1973.

Additional Readings

Brenner, W., Bruce, R., and Hendricks, C. The characteristics and perils of breech presentation. *Am J Obstet Gynecol* 118:700, 1974.

MacDonald, P., Schultz, F., Duenhoelter, J., Gant, N., Jimenez, J., Pritchard, J., Porter, J., and Johnston, J. Initiation of human parturition. I. Mechanism factor of arachidonic acid. *Obstet Gynecol* 44:629, 1974.

Reynolds, S. *Physiology of the Uterus with Clinical Correlations* (2nd ed.). New York: Hoeber Med. Div., Harper & Row, 1949.

10

Obstetrical Analgesia and Anesthesia

Analgesia and anesthesia for labor and delivery are developments of the last century. The introduction of pain relief for the laboring woman was opposed by the clergy and medical practitioners, who thought the pain of childbirth was "physiologic" and that attempts to provide relief from this pain were immoral. With the discovery in the mid-nineteenth century that ether, and later that chloroform, could relieve the pain of childbirth, "those piercing cries—those inexpressible agonies, and those pains apparently intolerable" of vaginal delivery described by Velpeau were relieved by anesthesia [1]. The opponents of obstetrical anesthesia were doomed to failure from the beginning, because the demands from patients for pain relief would become irresistible. The question that remained was not *if* obstetrical anesthesia would become commonplace, but *what* anesthetic agent would prove to be the most effective and the safest. The search for this agent continues to the present day.

The perfect analgesic or anesthetic agent would provide complete pain relief during both labor and delivery without hazard to mother or fetus. With the introduction of each new analgesic or anesthetic drug, the enthusiastic initial reports suggest that the perfect agent has been discovered. Subsequent investigation always reveals certain shortcomings of the treatment. This is not to suggest that no progress has been made; on the contrary, analgesia and anesthesia become more effective and safer with each passing year. The progress is made primarily by capitalizing on the advantages and minimizing the shortcomings of the agent, rather than by discovering an agent without fault. A wide variety of techniques are available to the modern practitioner, most of which are safe *if used with care and with due precaution for minimizing shortcomings*. It is probably best for the student of medicine to select two or three such techniques and become thoroughly familiar with them rather than to try to master all the techniques.

The question of whether analgesia or anesthesia should be used in obstetrics stubbornly persists. The opponents point out that most labors will progress without complication to an easy and uneventful vaginal delivery whether or not pain relief is used. The same, however, could be said of many surgical procedures if the patient were to be vigorously and appropriately restrained, but few would suggest surgery without at least local anesthesia. The pain of labor and delivery is hard to quantitate for many reasons—the variation in pain tolerance among individual patients and the lack of adequate testing devices, to mention two. There is evidence to suggest, however, that the pain of delivery is the most intense that the human being can experience. Certainly, the woman in labor deserves safe pain relief as much as the surgical patient who is experiencing a leg amputation or other operation. Indeed, when one considers that two lives are at stake with obstetrical delivery, one might conclude that the woman in labor needs a safe anesthetic more than does the surgical patient.

The disadvantages of analgesia and anesthesia for labor and delivery must be known so that they can be minimized. Anesthesia continues to be a major contributant to maternal mortality, usually ranking fourth after acute toxemia, bleeding, and infection. This fact emphasizes the never-ending need to improve the technique of administration of the agent and particularly to secure the services of a truly skilled physician for this practice. It is no longer acceptable to encourage the expert anesthesia support enjoyed by most American surgical suites at the expense of poor obstetrical anesthesia.

More expert anesthesia support of obstetrical units will decrease maternal mortality from anesthesia to near zero.

A second disadvantage of obstetrical analgesia and anesthesia is the fetal and neonatal depression that results nearly universally from pain-relieving agents. With optimal dosage, expert timing in medication administration, and careful choice of agent, this hazard can be greatly minimized. It should be remembered, however, that almost every pharmacologic agent reaches the baby through the placental circulation, with a fetal effect that is not always predictable. The fetal effects of any new agent must therefore be studied with care before a recommendation for its widespread use is made.

Analgesia

Pain relief during labor can be produced by techniques of suggestion, by pharmacologic agents systemically administered, and by agents that block nerve impulses at various neural levels.

SUGGESTION

Natural childbirth is a term used by Dr. Grantley Dick-Read in his book *Childbirth Without Fear* [2], first published in 1942. Dick-Read suggested that labor is usually a pain-free experience unless the accoutrements of modern civilization interfere. Women in primitive societies do not experience pain during labor, he insisted. Most physicians, and probably also most patients, cannot accept this simplified dismissal of labor as pain-free. Dick-Read did, however, perform a valuable service for obstetrics; he emphasized psychological preparation for childbirth, so that analgesic drugs might be used in smaller amounts with augmented effectiveness. Most obstetricians find that patients prepared for childbirth through prenatal classes do better during the labor process, require less analgesia, and cooperate more fully with the labor attendants. Universal availability of prenatal classes is highly desirable.

Hypnosis is another variant of natural childbirth, but in this case the suggestion of a hypnotist rather than the individual herself is the medium through which pain relief is achieved. The technique has been successfully used in some clinics, and glowing reports of its effectiveness have been published. While widespread usage has not resulted from these reports, the technique must be considered an effective one in expert hands. Since suggestion is a potent psychological tool, however, hypnosis should not be performed by the novice. Psychological breakdown has been reported after its use, and consultation with a psychiatrist may be desirable before using it in the obstetrical patient.

SYSTEMIC ANALGESIA

While all systemic agents freely cross the placenta and may produce fetal and neonatal depression as well as maternal depression, these effects can be minimized by careful timing of the smallest effective dosage of a drug with the fewest side effects and the most analgesic potency in the mother. Various obstetricians will choose various drugs, suggesting that a number of choices are equally satisfactory. The choice of a drug depends primarily on the familiarity of the obstetrician with its pharmacologic effects and its undesirable side effects. Familiarity is the key to successful drug usage.

In general, the administration of drugs should be delayed until the labor pattern is well established, since most agents are presumed to slow labor to a varying degree, usually minimally. The drug should be used early enough in labor, however, to allow its maximal effect to be exerted *before delivery,* to minimize its effect in the newborn. While the maternal organism may compensate in various ways for undesirable drug effects in the fetus, the fetus itself must metabolize the drug. The drug should be given in a dosage that is safe for the fetus yet is effective in relieving maternal pain. Few drugs give complete relief of maternal pain, but most gravidas will be satisfied with partial pain relief if fetal well-being is simultaneously assured. Any drug should be given with care or avoided completely when fetal compromise has been or may be produced by other factors. Premature labor, prolonged labor, and fetal disease (e.g., hemolytic disease induced by an Rh incompatibility) are examples of such factors.

Analgesic drugs may be administered to the laboring patient in the following circumstances (variability of patient reaction to the drug must be considered when general rules are laid down, however):

1. Analgesic drugs may be given when labor is well established, as confirmed by changes in effacement and dilatation of the cervix, and when the patient feels she needs pain relief. She should be encouraged to tolerate modest pain but not to the point of desperation. In the primigravida, the time for medication may be reached at 3 to 4 cm. dilatation of the cervix, rarely earlier. In the multigravida, a cervical dilatation of 5 to 6 cm. is desirable. Lesser dilatation suggests the possibility of false labor, while greater dilatation may suggest impending delivery.
2. The medication should be given 2 to 3 hours before delivery is anticipated, the time depending on the agent. Maternal medication shortly before delivery will result in a high percentage of sleepy babies.
3. The medication may be repeated at 2- to 4-hour intervals, with longer intervals required for larger dosages. Repeat medication shortly before delivery should be avoided.
4. With certain types of uterine dysfunction (prolonged latent phase), or when false labor is suspected but undiagnosed, a systemic analgesic may be useful. The uterine dysfunction may quickly disappear following such medication. False labor may become evident by the absence of contractions following recovery from the analgesic effects of the drug.

While these rules apply to analgesic drugs, certain exceptions can be made for tranquilizing drugs. With a highly nervous primigravid patient in labor, for example, a tranquilizer may be prescribed even before labor is well established to help her relax. Reassurance may accomplish the same objective in some patients. There is little evidence that a tranquilizer will stop established labor.

Sedatives

Barbiturates are rarely used in contemporary practice in a laboring patient, but these drugs are still useful in a patient who is in early labor or in false labor without a certain diagnosis. An oral dose of secobarbital (Seconal), 100 mg., for example, will allow the patient to rest and relax for an hour or two. Thereafter, she will either awaken refreshed and in good active labor or find the contractions completely gone. In the latter case, the barbiturate did not stop true labor but made the diagnosis of false labor possible.

Analgesics

A major analgesic in current use is meperidine (Demerol). Other related drugs, notably alphaprodine (Nisentil), are also available but are used less widely. Morphine was used frequently in earlier years to relieve labor pain, which it does superbly. The fetal depression that follows the use of morphine has relegated this drug to only one use in the laboring patient, that is, for heavy sedation when certain types of uterine dysfunction require this type of pharmacologic action.

Meperidine is usually administered intramuscularly in a dose of 50 to 100 mg., with the higher doses reserved for larger women. The smaller doses may be repeated at 2- to 3-hour intervals, while the larger doses require 4-hour intervals. The drug also may be given very slowly by the intravenous route, usually in doses of 25 to 50 mg. This dose produces the same analgesic effect as 50 to 100 mg. given intramuscularly, but the time of peak action differs—a few minutes by the intravenous route and 30 to 60 minutes when the drug is given intramuscularly. While the intravenous route is safe and has been widely used, the medication should be given slowly to observe its pharmacologic effects in the individual patient, namely, drowsiness and decrease in pain. If the drug is administered during a time period that encompasses two or three contractions, its dramatic effect on labor pain can be noted. Such an effect indicates adequate drug dosage. Large intravenous doses have produced hypotension and even respiratory depression in the hypersensitive person.

Alphaprodine has similar pharmacologic effects but is more rapid and shorter-acting than meperidine. If given in doses of 20 to 30 mg. by the subcutaneous route, relief from pain is frequently dramatic and amazingly rapid. The drug may be given intravenously in a maximum dose of 20 mg., but respiratory depression is an inherent risk with this route of administration. The intramuscular route is not recommended because of limited clinical experience. We have had wide experience with alphaprodine and prefer it over meperidine because of its rapid action and the lower incidence of depressed newborns we have observed with its use.

Ataractics

Ataractic drugs are highly effective adjuncts to analgesic drugs during labor. While they do not in themselves relieve pain, they decrease nervousness and tension in the patient, and there is good experimental evidence to suggest that they potentiate analgesic action and permit lower doses of an analgesic to secure the same pharmacologic effects [3]. The ataractics in current use are promethazine (Phenergan), hydroxyzine (Vistaril), and diazepam (Valium). Promethazine may be given intramuscularly in a dose of 25 to 75 mg., or hydroxyzine in a dose of 50 to 100 mg., to potentiate meperidine. We have had extensive experience with diazepam by the intravenous route in a dose of 5 to 15 mg. Doses of 20 mg. have not produced significant untoward effects in our hands. Diazepam should be given when the patient first needs sedation and should be injected very slowly over a 7- to 10-minute time span; this length of time will permit an appraisal of the patient's reaction to the drug. The effect desired is slight to moderate drowsiness, with some slurring of speech. This effect may occur with only 5 to 10 mg. of the drug; it is then discontinued. A maximum dose of 10 mg. should be used. Frequently, no further sedation is necessary for some time; in some patients, no analgesia at all is needed. If meperidine or alphaprodine is given, the dosage can usually be cut by one-third or one-half to get the same pharmacologic action expected by a larger dosage without the diazepam. Unless it is given shortly before birth, diazepam has no apparent effect on the respiratory center of the newborn. Hypotonia of the newborn for the first 24 hours in the nursery is observed, but this apparently produces no ill effects. It should be noted, however, that diazepam has *not* been approved by the Fed-

eral Drug Administration for use in obstetrical patients and other drugs should therefore be used at the present time.

If analgesic drugs are given skillfully, depression of the newborn from overdose will be rare. If labor progresses much faster than expected, and if the infant is born during the period of maximal drug effect, respiratory depression may occur in the baby. This will rarely be of serious import, but in an infant already at risk (fetal distress from cord prolapse, for example), the effect may be disastrous. It is important to know that naloxone (Narcan) is an antagonist to morphine and its derivatives (meperidine, alphaprodine) and may be expected to reverse immediately the depression of the newborn's respiratory center if given to the infant through the umbilical vein. The drug has no agonist activity that might result in cardiorespiratory depression. The drug should *not* be given to the infant if the respiratory depression is due to any other drugs, notably barbiturates and certain anesthetics. The need for this drug is rare, but it may be lifesaving in certain instances. While it is also effective if given intravenously to the mother just before delivery, it is better to observe respiratory depression in the infant before giving the drug.

Inhalants

Nitrous oxide, if administered briefly and with at least 20 percent oxygen in the mixture, will produce some analgesia as well as amnesia. While the need for this drug is limited, it may be useful in the primigravid patient during the second stage of labor when previous narcosis has worn off, but before fetal descent is sufficient to allow the use of an anesthetic. The gas should be breathed at the very start of the contraction and discontinued as the pain eases. During the administration of the drug, loss of consciousness should be avoided because of the hazard of aspiration. The anesthesiologist should keep verbal contact with the patient by asking her to respond to simple commands.

Trichloroethylene (Trilene) is a self-administered volatile drug that will relieve the discomfort of early labor. While the drug enjoyed some popularity a number of years ago, it is no longer available in the

United States. Its use cannot be followed by other volatile anesthetics since the soda lime absorption device will transform the trichloroethylene to a neurotoxic substance. Methoxyflurane (Penthrane) can be used in a similar fashion and is now preferred. This drug, used in low concentrations, does not cause fetal "depression" [4].

REGIONAL ANALGESIA

Before detailing the various nerve block techniques used in relieving the pain of labor or delivery, the sensory nerve supply of the area involved should be described.

While the precise cause of labor pain is uncertain, it is known to be elicited by stimulation of nerves in the cervix or lower uterine segment or in the surrounding uterine ligaments. The sensory nerve supply of these structures is by way of either sympathetic or parasympathetic nerve fibers, the former traveling via the posterior cervical ganglia and entering the spinal cord at the level of T-11 and T-12 and the latter entering the cord at the S-2, S-3, and S-4 levels. Since the motor fibers to the uterus originate from the T-7 and T-8 levels, a nerve block below this level will not affect uterine contractions. The sensory nerve supply to the vulva and the vagina comes primarily through the pudendal nerve. Bilateral local anesthesia to these anatomic areas can be obtained by an anesthetic block of these nerves.

The block techniques used to relieve pain during labor (and in most cases pain during delivery) include pudendal block, paracervical block, and caudal or lumbar epidural block. While all these techniques are safe in expert hands, untoward reactions can occur and should be anticipated. Reactions may be allergic or related to excessive drug absorption into the maternal circulation, either from inadvertent intravenous injection, too large an initial dose, or for an unknown reason. Most reactions can be avoided if a careful history of allergies is taken and a meticulous technique is followed.

PUDENDAL BLOCK. Pudendal block may be used to relieve the pain of the early second stage of labor, although this block is usually reserved for the

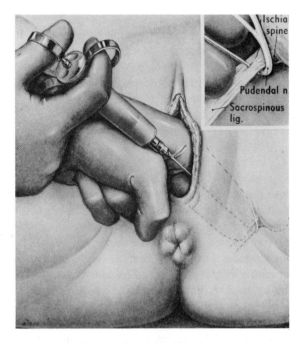

Fig. 10-1. Technique of pudendal block. (From J. Bonica. Principles and Practice of Obstetric Analgesia and Anesthesia. *Philadelphia: Davis, 1967.*)

actual vaginal delivery. While some prefer a transperineal insertion of the needle, we use a transvaginal approach, as follows (Fig. 10-1): With the patient in stirrups and in the lithotomy position, the perineum and vagina are prepared with an antiseptic solution. An Iowa trumpet needle is passed into the vagina, and with the tip of the needle retracted, the end of the tube is gently guided to the ischial spine. The needle is inserted to a predetermined depth, no greater than 1.5 cm., to a point just posterior and medial to the tip of the ischial spine, where half the anesthetic solution is deposited. The needle is advanced slightly to a point just beyond the spine, and the remainder of the solution is injected after withdrawal into the syringe to check for intravenous placement of the needle. The technique is repeated with the opposite ischial spine. A total dose for both sides of 20 ml. of a 2% solution of chloroprocaine or a 1% solution of lidocaine should not be exceeded and should give an adequate block for a minimum of 1 hour. While the failure rate even in expert hands is high (10 to 15 percent), the pudendal block provides excellent anesthesia for spontaneous vaginal delivery and usually also for outlet forceps. Uterine pain is not relieved, and a systemic analgesic agent may be used to supplement the pudendal block for delivery.

PARACERVICAL BLOCK. By blocking the sympathetic sensory pathway from the uterus, paracervical injection of a local anesthetic agent produces excellent relief of labor pain but does not provide vaginal or perineal anesthesia. The technique is usually carried out when the cervix has reached a dilatation of 4 to 5 cm. Using a tubular protection around a long 20-gauge needle that is preset to protrude 1.5 cm. from the tube, the needle is inserted into the cervix at 3 o'clock and at 9 o'clock (Fig. 10-2). After careful aspiration to assure that the needle tip is not in a vessel, a maximum of 10 ml. of a 1.5% solution of chloroprocaine (or an equivalent amount of another anesthetic) is injected into each side. The dose may be repeated at intervals of 1 to 2 hours. Continuous techniques with indwelling catheters have also been devised.

Recent reports of fetal bradycardia in about 10 percent of patients so injected have been alarming. The etiology of the bradycardia remains unclear but is thought to be due to a toxic effect of the anesthetic caused by high fetal blood levels of the agent, apparently because of rapid absorption at the site of injection or to decreased uterine blood flow from vasoconstriction. Care should be exercised to avoid injection into the fetal scalp, which may lie nearby, and total drug dosage should be kept as low as possible. The fetus already in jeopardy from other causes is especially likely to experience bradycardia. In most instances, the bradycardia has been transitory, but about 50 perinatal deaths have been reported. The technique should be used only when other procedures are contraindicated and certainly not with a distressed fetus.

CONTINUOUS CAUDAL BLOCK. Caudal analgesia and anesthesia constitute a safe, effective tech-

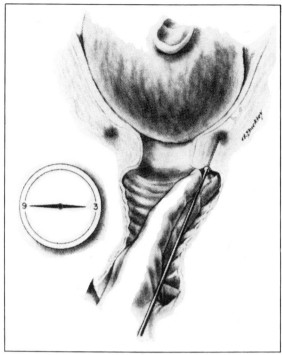

Fig. 10-2. Paracervical block. Injection immediately lateral to cervix (3 and 9 o'clock positions) with depth of 1.5 to 2.0 cm. (From R. Pitkin and W. Goddard. Obstet Gynecol 21:738, 1963.)

nique, but since more skill is required to place the needle than with other regional blocks, its use has not become widespread. The needle is inserted through the sacral hiatus into the caudal space, an area well below the level of the dura mater and thus lower than the subarachnoid space. Injection of anesthetic solution into this space successfully blocks the sacral nerves, thus providing caudal anesthesia. If the block is a good one, the ensuing labor may be completely painless.

Since the technique interferes with the bearing-down sensation of the second stage of labor, it may interfere with descent of the head. The resulting need for an increase in the number of forceps deliveries is not a major disadvantage, since the level of forceps application is nearly always on the perineum, a safe procedure. The major hazard to the technique is the inadvertent injection of anesthetic solution into the subarachnoid space, an accident that can be avoided if an appropriate test dose of the solution has been given before trying to produce anesthesia. Contraindications to the use of caudal analgesia and anesthesia include the following: (1) infection of the skin overlying the area of injection; (2) the presence of a bleeding complication of pregnancy (placenta previa, premature separation of the placenta), since hypotension follows caudal anesthesia in 20 percent of cases; and, (3) severe preeclampsia or eclampsia, also because of the possibility of a hypotensive episode.

The procedure is technically difficult and requires the presence of an anesthesiologist not only for its administration but also while the indwelling catheter is in situ. Mengert's shock syndrome, caused by uterine pressure on the vena cava, is especially likely to occur because of the chemical sympathectomy. The disadvantages of the technique seem to have outweighed its advantages for most American clinics, since it is being used less and less frequently.

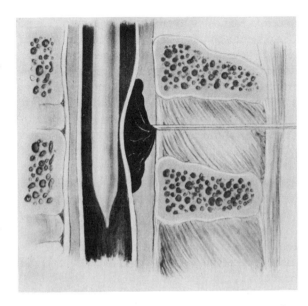

Fig. 10-3. Epidural anesthesia. The anesthetic agent has been introduced into the epidural space. (From D. Moore. Regional Block *[4th ed.]), 1967. Courtesy of Charles C Thomas, Publisher, Springfield, Illinois.)*

CONTINUOUS LUMBAR EPIDURAL ANALGESIA AND ANESTHESIA. As with caudal analgesia, continuous lumbar epidural analgesia and anesthesia achieves its effect by the injection of an anesthetic agent into the extradural space. Whereas caudal analgesia is decreasing in popularity, lumbar epidural analgesia is being used more and more commonly because the technique is easier to perform and because smaller doses of drug are effective. The caudal block provides slightly better anesthesia for the delivery itself. The lumbar block shares certain disadvantages with caudal analgesia, namely, the risk of perforation of the dura and the risk of subarachnoid injection if test doses are not given. The failure of this technique is lower than with the caudal technique, and inadequate anesthesia occurs in only about 3 percent of patients. The placement of the needle and injection of the drug require the services of an experienced operator, just as with the caudal approach.

The patient lies on her left side on a firm surface with her legs flexed and with her shoulders at a right angle to the surface. The lumbar area of the back is cleansed, and an antiseptic solution is applied. The lumbar vertebral spines are palpated. A wide interspace is chosen (L3 to L4 or L2 to L3), and the skin and interspinous ligament are anesthetized with the chosen anesthetic agent. With a 16-gauge Tuohy spinal needle, blunted on the end but with a sharp stylet, the lumbar interspace is entered to the level of the ligamentum flavum. This location is checked by an attempt to inject 2 ml. of air which should not be possible. With advancement of the needle 1 or 2 mm., the epidural space is entered (Fig. 10-3). The location is checked by noting the absence of cerebrospinal fluid in the needle and by experiencing ease of injection of 5 ml. of air.

When placement is considered adequate, a small-bore plastic catheter is passed through the needle and into the epidural space cephalad for a distance of 2 cm. beyond the needle point. The needle is removed, and the distal catheter is attached to a skin site distant from the point of injection. A test dose of bupivacaine is injected, followed in 5 minutes by a second similar test dose. The absence of spinal anesthesia indicates correct placement of the needle. Appropriate doses of the drug are given at intervals to produce excellent analgesia. If desired, somewhat larger doses can be administered to anesthetize the sacral segment just before delivery to provide adequate anesthesia for delivery. Bupivacaine is the most reliable and safest local anesthetic available for epidural analgesia in labor and delivery. Of great importance is the absence of neurobehavioral abnormalities in the newborn after three hours of epidural analgesia with bupivacaine [5].

While the technique of epidural analgesia is easier to learn than that for caudal analgesia, the side effects of the two techniques are similar. Dural puncture is more frequent with the lumbar block. Hypotension is an ever-present hazard and frequent blood pressure and pulse determinations should be made. The incidence and severity of hypotension can be reduced by (1) rapid hydration with 500 to 1000 ml. of a balanced electrolyte solution before the analgesia is initiated, (2) the use of ephedrine intramuscularly before the analgesic is injected, and (3) continuous left uterine displacement to minimize aorto-caval compression [6]. The technique is safe and provides most satisfactory analgesia, but its shortcomings must always be kept in mind.

Anesthesia for Delivery

VAGINAL DELIVERY

Anesthesia for vaginal delivery can be provided by nerve-block techniques or by general anesthesia. The nerve supply can be blocked peripherally, as with local infiltration of the perineum or a pudendal block, or at the level of exit of the nerves as they leave the spinal cord, as with caudal or lumbar epidural and spinal (subarachnoid) anesthesia. Many agents have been used for the induction of general anesthesia for delivery, and a few of the safer ones will be discussed. In general, the simpler the technique, the safer but the less effective it is. No single choice can be recommended for all cases,

and individual patient factors must be considered before the final selection is made.

Nerve-Block Techniques

LOCAL INFILTRATION. Local infiltration of the vulva with an anesthetic agent may suffice for an easy spontaneous delivery. The technique is simple and successful even in the hands of the inexperienced. However, minimal pain relief is achieved, and more elaborate methods may be necessary to satisfy the patient's needs. The technique is usually satisfactory for the performance and repair of an episiotomy.

PUDENDAL BLOCK ANESTHESIA. Pudendal block anesthesia provides greater patient comfort than local infiltration and will frequently suffice not only for spontaneous delivery but also for outlet forceps delivery. While the uterine pain of labor is not relieved, vaginal and perineal pain are largely abolished. A combination of pudendal block with a systemically administered analgesic or tranquilizing drug (e.g., intravenous meperidine) is a good technique in wide usage. Such a combination provides excellent relief from pain with great safety and can be used when expert anesthesiology consultation is not available. The technique of pudendal block has been discussed under analgesic agents.

EPIDURAL ANESTHESIA. Epidural techniques may be planned to provide anesthesia for delivery as well as analgesia for labor. The lumbar epidural block may be extended to cover the sacral roots to relieve perineal pain and the lumbar roots to relieve uterine pain. This is done by varying the medication dosage and by appropriate positioning of the patient.

SPINAL (SUBARACHNOID) BLOCK. Single-injection spinal anesthesia is one of the most popular techniques in the United States today. It is easy to administer and, if given properly, is safe. Thousands of patients have delivered in many centers under spinal anesthesia without maternal death due to the anesthetic. While there is a risk of subsequent neurologic impairment, the risk is of a very low magnitude, and complete recovery is the rule. The major drawbacks are the significant risk of hypotension and the small risk of "post-spinal" headaches. The hypotension can usually be reversed by elevating the legs in stirrups and displacing the uterus to the left to increase venous return to the heart. An intravenous drip of 5% D/W should always be started before attempting a spinal anesthetic, and rapid infusion of fluid will also combat the observed hypotension. Rarely, vasoconstrictor drugs are needed; ephedrine and mephentermine are the drugs of choice.

The incidence of headaches has been lowered by use of a very small-gauge needle (No. 26) in place of the needles previously used (No. 20 or 22). The cause of the headache is unknown, but it is presumed to result from subarachnoid fluid continually leaking around the needle puncture site. The headache typically develops on the first or second postpartum day and is usually relieved if the patient lies flat in bed. It uniformly disappears in two or three days but may be very severe while it is present.

Spinal block is performed when delivery is considered imminent, when the vertex is on or near the pelvic floor in the primigravida and just before full cervical dilatation occurs in the multigravida. The timing is crucial and may vary, depending on the rapidity with which labor is progressing. Outlet forceps are usually required and, indeed, planned, following the anesthetic. Because of poor uterine relaxation with its use, spinal anesthesia is not recommended if an intrauterine manipulation is planned.

With the patient sitting up on the edge of the operating table with her neck well flexed and with her back rounded as much as possible, the skin overlying the lumbar vertebrae is cleansed with an antiseptic solution. The No. 26 spinal needle is inserted in the third or fourth lumbar interspace; usually without skin anesthesia. When spinal fluid is noted in the needle shank, a syringe containing the anesthetic is attached. A small amount of spinal fluid is withdrawn into the syringe, and the syringe is emptied with due speed. The patient sits for a specified period of time (usually 30 seconds) to allow the glucose-weighted anesthetic solution to settle caudally in the subarachnoid space. She is then placed in a supine position with her head well flexed on a pillow. The spinal anesthetic level is checked and should extend to just above the T-10 or T-11 level. The table may be tilted to raise or lower the patient's head to control the anesthetic level. The anesthetic should be injected between contractions for better control of the anesthetic level; 3 to 5 mg. of a 1% solution of tetracaine (Pontocaine) weighted with 10% dextrose is an average dose. For greater detail, the reader is referred to a text on obstetrical anesthesia.

The anesthesia will last for 1 to 1½ hours, thus demanding precise timing in judging when the anesthetic should be administered. If a low spinal is achieved (block to S-1), the procedure has been called a "saddle block," since the area of the body that touches the saddle of a horse is the area anesthetized.

General Anesthesia

While general anesthesia may be the best choice in certain patients, the uniform passage of any agent presently in use across the placenta should be recognized. As the mother is sedated, so is the fetus. However, fetal depression can be minimized by early delivery before the anesthetic agent has fully narcotized the baby and by the avoidance of analgesic depressant drugs during labor. The second major hazard of general anesthesia in the labor patient is the prevalence of vomiting and aspiration, not only because the gastric emptying time is delayed in pregnancy, but also because labor may begin at any time, even immediately after a full meal. Two rules minimize these dangers: (1) use general anesthesia for delivery only if rapid delivery is anticipated, and (2) always insert an endotracheal tube.

Commonly used anesthetic agents include nitrous oxide and halothane. Ether is rarely used today and cyclopropane, while once popular, is now used in relatively few centers. Methoxyflurane (Penthrane) enjoys popularity in some major centers. Intravenous thiopental sodium (Pentothal) has been tried, but in large doses it severely depresses the fetus. In a dose of 4 mg. per kg. there is very little effect on Apgar scores and the agent is used by some anesthesiologists for induction. For many years chloroform was an extremely useful and apparently safe drug, but the shortcomings of this medication have nearly relegated it to history.

NITROUS OXIDE. Nitrous oxide may be used for analgesia as described earlier, but it also may be used to induce anesthesia if combined with other agents. Nitrous oxide must be given with a concentration of oxygen of at least 25% and it must be supplemented with another agent if deep anesthesia is to be achieved.

CYCLOPROPANE. Cyclopropane is still used in some clinics and has particular advantages for the patient in labor. Good uterine relaxation is achieved, and induction, which is very rapid, can be accomplished with high concentrations of oxygen. If delivery is delayed, however, the fetus is apt to be depressed. The agent is highly explosive and is known to produce cardiac irregularity, even ventricular fibrillation, when pituitary extracts containing vasopressin are administered simultaneously; synthetic oxytocin seems safer in this regard.

METHOXYFLURANE. Methoxyflurane (Penthrane) is nonexplosive and is said to be less depressive to the baby than are other agents. Because of nephrotoxicity, it should not be used in the presence of kidney disease.

HALOTHANE. Halothane (Fluothane) is a nonexplosive volatile agent that has achieved great popularity in surgical anesthesia. However, it is less safe for obstetrical anesthesia because of its propensity for markedly relaxing the uterus. This property might seem an advantage for intrauterine manipulation, but the extreme degree of postpartum relaxation that occurs following its use makes it unac-

ceptable to many obstetricians. In lower dosages, it is said to produce much less uterine relaxation.

CESAREAN SECTION

Spinal, epidural, and general anesthesia as described for vaginal delivery can be easily modified to provide excellent anesthesia for cesarean section. The choice between them should be made by an anesthesiologist well acquainted with the pharmacology of all the agents.

References

1. Speert, H. Historical Highlights. In D. Danforth (Ed.), *Textbook of Obstetrics and Gynecology* (3rd ed.). New York: Harper & Row, 1977.
2. Wessel, H., and Ellis, H. (Eds.). *Childbirth without Fear* (4th ed.). New York: Harper & Row, 1972.
3. Niswander, K. Effect of diazepam on meperidine requirements of patients during labor. *Obstet Gynecol* 34:62, 1969.
4. Clark, R., Cooper, J., Brown, W., et al. The effect of methoxyflurane on the foetus. *Brit J Anaesth* 42:286, 1970.
5. Scanlon, J. W., Ostheimer, G. W., Lurie, A. L., et al. Neurobehavioral responses and drug concentrations in newborns after maternal epidural anesthesia with bupivacaine. *Anesthesiology* 45:400, 1976.
6. Shnider, S., and Levinson, G. *Anesthesia for Obstetrics.* Baltimore: Williams & Wilkins, 1979. P. 282.

Additional Readings

Bonica, J. *Principles and Practice of Obstetric Analgesia and Anesthesia.* Philadelphia: Davis, 1967.
Fisher, D., and Paton, J. The effect of maternal anesthetic and analgesic drugs on the fetus and newborn. *Clin Obstet Gynecol* 17:275, 1974.
Javert, C., and Hardy, J. Influence of analgesics on pain intensity during labor. *Anesthesiology* 12:189, 1951.
McDonald, J., Bjorkman, L., and Reed, E. Epidural analgesia for obstetrics: A maternal, fetal, and neonatal study. *Am J Obstet Gynecol* 120:1055, 1974.
Petrie, R., Paul, W., Miller, F., Arce, J., Paul, R., Nakamura, R., and Hon, E. Placental transfer of lidocaine following paracervical block. *Am J Obstet Gynecol* 120:791, 1974.
Shnider, S., and Levinson, G. *Anesthesia for Obstetrics.* Baltimore: Williams & Wilkins, 1979.

11

Abnormal labor is recognized when the expected patterns of descent of the presenting part and cervical dilatation fail to occur in the appropriate time sequence. *Prolonged labor* is an older term of imprecise meaning that usually referred to a labor lasting more than 24, or 36, or 48 hours, depending on the observer's bias. In modern obstetrics, such a "prolonged" labor is no longer experienced, not only because the usual maternity patient cannot emotionally tolerate a labor of this length, but also—and more important—because the perinatal loss rises sharply when the labor lasts more than 15 to 20 hours. If good progress in labor has not occurred during the first 6 to 8 hours, suspicion of an abnormality should be aroused and a plan of management with a definite time limit outlined. Only with an early alarm system of this type operating in the labor suite will abnormalities of labor be recognized early enough to allow adequate treatment before the perinatal loss rate begins to mount.

Traditionally, three causes of abnormal labor have been recognized. These are: poor or inadequate uterine contractions, a fetus too large in size or in an unusual presentation, and a pelvis of inadequate size, shape, or consistency. An attempt is made to identify one or more of these causes for the abnormal labor pattern observed in the laboring patient and to treat the patient in such a way that the abnormality can be overcome by the forces of nature or compensated for by obstetrical intervention. Inherent in this clinical approach is the recognition that time is working against the best interest of the fetus and the mother. Judicious neglect has no place in the treatment of abnormal labor.

Unfortunately, clinical tools and skills are not always adequate to the task of determining with accuracy what is causing the abnormal labor. The pelvis can be appraised by pelvic examination or by x-ray studies if necessary, but the precise pelvic size needed to accommodate the particular fetus can only be estimated. Fetal size can be assessed by abdominal examination, x-ray examination, or ultrasonic measurement of the biparietal diameter of the head (the latter with a high degree of accuracy). A physician can only guess what degree of molding a particular fetal head will undergo. Poor uterine contractions can be recognized with sophisticated electronic gadgetry, if not with clinical skills. Yet uterine contractions of low amplitude and of infrequent occurrence are sometimes entirely adequate to effect successful delivery. Obvious anatomic abnormalities are easy to recognize (e.g., a severely rachitic pelvis or a hydrocephalic baby), but such clear-cut factors are often not found in practice. A better clinical approach to the problem of poor progress in labor is to take a more comprehensive view and to recognize clinical diagnoses for what they are, namely, speculation based on judgment and experience. A pragmatic therapeutic approach will lead to success more often than one that attempts to be etiologically precise.

To approach a diagnosis in a patient with abnormal labor, it is necessary to recall the physiology of labor. The upper uterine segment contracts with regularity to expel the fetus. The uterine musculature of the upper segment gradually thickens, since the individual muscle cells do not elongate to their precontraction length but maintain part of their contracted shape. The lower uterine segment and the cervix are passively dilated and retracted by contractions of the fundal musculature and by the descent of the fetus as the cavity of the upper segment decreases in size. The forces of the uterus must then act against the resistance of the lower uterine segment, cervix, and other soft parts, as well as that of the bony pelvis. The fetus assumes a position that will make best use of the uterine contraction, i.e., one at a right angle to the inlet of the pelvis, as well as one that will minimize the diameters of the presenting part that must traverse the pelvis, usually by flexion of the fetal head on the chest. The fetus must continually accommodate to the pelvic architecture as it descends through the birth canal.

The interrelatedness of these events is apparent. If the fetus assumes an unusual posture, or if the pelvis cannot accommodate the fetus with ease, the intensity of the uterine contractions may change. The contractions may increase to overcome the pelvic or fetal factor, or they may decrease as the uterus "recognizes" the futility of further effort. Alternatively, the initial fault may lie with uterine contractility inadequate to propel a well-positioned fetus through an adequate pelvis. The clinician must decide which of a number of factors is responsible for the lack of progress and act accordingly.

Friedman [1] has suggested that his two graphs (cervical dilatation versus time, and station of the presenting part versus time) of labor progress "summate" all the factors of labor. The pattern of cervical dilatation is dependent not only on how effectively the uterus contracts but also on the fit of the fetus to the pelvis and the resistance of the maternal soft parts. He maintains that an abnormal cervical dilatation–time pattern demands a careful evaluation of the fetus and the pelvis as well as of the frequency and effectiveness of the uterine contractions. This clinical approach seems entirely logical and we will pursue it in our discussion. For the sake of clarity, however, the factors that affect labor progress will be discussed separately to the degree that this approach seems helpful. The reader should recognize that this separation is a literary device that may not be useful when one is confronted with a real patient.

Uterine Dysfunction

EXPERIMENTAL APPROACHES TO RECOGNITION OF UTERINE DYSFUNCTION

Three experimental approaches have been utilized to describe the uterine contractions in the human patient: (1) intramyometrial sensors that measure actual myometrial pressure at various locations in the uterus; (2) external tokodynamometry, in which a change in the curvature of the fundus during a contraction is used to record the contraction; and (3) intra-amniotic pressure measurements that record pressure changes from the resting state to the contracted state.

Intramyometrial Approach

The intramyometrial approach is not clinically applicable because of the intricacy of the method and the potential hazard inherent in it. However, it has provided valuable physiologic information that suggests that the contraction begins in the fundus, where the intensity is the greatest, and progresses downward over the remainder of the upper uterine segment and to the lower uterine segment as the intensity decreases. Abnormalities may occur in this contraction wave (multiple foci of contraction, greater intensity in the lower uterine segment than in the fundus) but are not clinically measurable.

External Tokodynamometry

External tokodynamometry is easy to use in a clinical setting and is a widely utilized clinical tool. The method's chief shortcoming is that scientific accuracy in the recording of the intensity of the contraction is not achieved, although the timing of the contraction is readily apparent and can be measured accurately. When precision in recording of uterine contractions is necessary, a direct intra-amniotic measurement should be made.

Intra-Amniotic Pressure Recording

Various methods of recording intra-amniotic pressure have been devised, including the use of balloons or simply open-ended plastic catheters. A transcervical or transabdominal approach may be used. For use as a clinical tool, a semirigid plastic catheter is inserted through the cervix and the resulting fluid pressure recorded on paper. Great precision in recording is possible. During early labor, the resting tonus of the intra-amniotic pressure is 5 to 10 mm. Hg; it increases to 12 to 14 mm. Hg in late labor. Uterine contractions of an intensity of 30

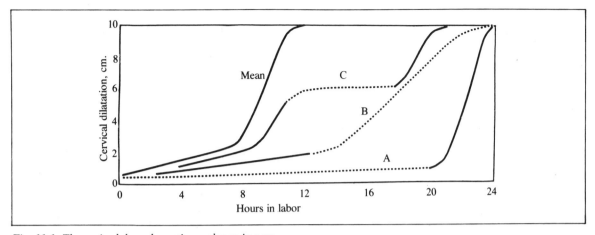

Fig. 11-1. The major labor aberrations, shown in comparison with the mean cervical dilatation–time curve for nulliparas. A. Prolonged latent phase. B. Protracted active phase dilatation. C. Secondary arrest of dilatation. (From Friedman, E. A.: Dysfunctional Labor. In Greenhill, J. P.: Obstetrics [13th ed.]. Philadelphia: W. B. Saunders Company, 1965. P. 833.)

mm. Hg or greater cause dilatation of the cervix (labor), while pressures of 50 to 80 mm. are usual during labor. Peaks of 80 to 100 mm. Hg may be recorded during the second stage. Contractions occur at 3- to 5-minute intervals during labor; their frequency increases to as often as every 2 minutes as delivery approaches. Interpretation of intra-amniotic pressure recordings will allow recognition of uterine dysfunction when the expected frequency or intensity of the contractions does not occur, or when the resting tonus is greater than expected.

A fourth method of describing progress during labor, which does not precisely reflect uterine contractions but in large measure does so, is a graphic portrayal of cervical dilatation progress. While we have described Friedman's normal cervical dilatation graph in some detail previously, we should also recognize that other investigators have described slightly different results. Hendricks et al. [2], for example, do not describe a latent phase, and they plot a continuously accelerating labor graph. The difference between the approaches of Friedman

and Hendricks et al. is not great, and to argue the fine points of whether the active phase assumes a straight line or an S-shaped curve is of little importance to the clinician.

We have found Friedman's description more in keeping with our own experience, and the abnormalities in the cervical dilatation pattern recognized by Friedman will therefore be described in some detail. The reader should realize that progress in this field is continuous, that new information, as it becomes available, should be synthesized with the old, and that oversimplification is necessary to reduce the confusion encountered in trying to transfer clinical experience in this inexact field to paper.

TYPES OF ABNORMALITIES

We will describe three abnormalities of the labor curve that constitute the major types of uterine dysfunction (Fig. 11-1). Prolonged latent phase, primary dysfunction of the active phase, and secondary arrest of dilatation may occur individually or two or more may occur in the same patient. Fortunately, more than one abnormality in any individual patient is unusual. Friedman has also plotted descent of the presenting part versus time (Fig. 11-2). We will also briefly discuss abnormalities of the descent curve.

Prolonged Latent Phase

The latent phase begins with the onset of labor and ends with the beginning of the active phase, when

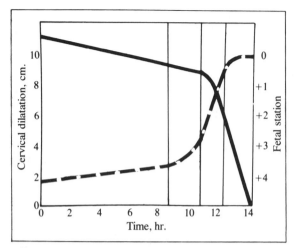

Fig. 11-2. Inter-relationship between descent curve (solid line) and concurrently developing dilatation pattern (broken line) for nulliparas. Active descent generally begins when the dilatation curve reaches its phase of maximum slope, reaching its maximum at the beginning of the deceleration phase of dilatation. (From E. A. Friedman, Labor: Clinical Evaluation and Management *[2nd. ed.]. New York: Appleton-Century-Crofts, 1978.)*

cervical dilatation proceeds at a substantially increased rate. Clearly, the identification of the point in time when labor begins is crucial to recognition of the latent phase or any abnormality of the latent phase. This determination can only be made with accuracy in retrospect, although it usually coincides with the onset of regular, progressively close, and progressively severe contractions. Cervical dilatation must occur after the onset of labor to confirm the diagnosis. With the uncertainty centered around identifying this event, it is little wonder that the diagnosis of a prolonged latent phase can be made with certainty only retrospectively. It is important to differentiate a prolonged latent phase from false labor, however, since attempts to stimulate the uterus of a patient who is in false labor may lead to prolonged labor with its attendant complications. Fortunately, the same treatment, sedation, allows correction of the prolonged latent phase and identification of the patient who is in false labor.

Friedman [1] has defined a prolonged latent phase as a period of 20 hours or more in the primigravida or 14 hours or more in the multigravida during which labor has not progressed to the active phase. In old parlance, this roughly corresponds to "hypertonic uterine inertia" or "primary inertia." Friedman has attempted to identify etiologic factors or, perhaps more accurately, related factors. He finds that too early and too heavy sedation is present in 30 to 40 percent of these patients. About 10 percent are later found to be in false labor. It is difficult to prove but highly likely that the causation of this abnormality is an emotional factor. A physiologic explanation for such a relationship is the observation that L-epinephrine decreases uterine contractility. It is possible that fear or pain or anxiety causes the adrenal medulla to secrete catecholamines that interfere with uterine contractility. What is certain is that sedation deep enough to cause the patient to sleep for a few hours is effective therapy, perhaps because the catecholamines are no longer secreted.

While it is necessary for purposes of data analysis to define a precise time limit for the diagnosis of dysfunction of the latent phase, in practice, a period of little progress in the latent phase much shorter than 20 hours should alert the obstetrician to the possibility of dysfunction. After 6 to 8 hours of little progress, both the patient and the obstetrician will be alarmed. A careful search for factors of fetopelvic disproportion should be made, although such a search is rarely productive. While some prefer to stimulate the labor of such a patient with oxytocin, Friedman [1] thinks it wiser to provide sedation (subcutaneous morphine sulfate, 10 to 15 mg., is a good drug for this purpose in our experience). The advantage of sedation is that the patient with false labor will be identified by the absence of contractions when she awakens, and the majority of the remaining patients will be well into the active phase when they awaken. The unusual patient whose contractions continue without appreciable progress will usually respond to a dilute solution of intravenous oxytocin, and she will be in a better condition to receive the medication after her rest.

We prefer to avoid an amniotomy in these patients for reasons to be indicated.

Primary Dysfunction of the Active Phase

Primary dysfunction of the active phase is identified when the slope of cervical dilatation is less than 1.2 cm. per hour in the primigravida or 1.5 cm. per hour in the multigravida. Etiologic factors suggested by Friedman [1] include fetal malpositions, fetopelvic disproportion, and excessive or premature analgesia or anesthesia. In about a third of these patients, fetopelvic disproportion will be present, but secondary arrest of dilatation usually develops (see the next section). Friedman finds that two-thirds of patients with primary dysfunction of the active phase will progress steadily through labor, if slowly, with ultimate uneventful vaginal delivery. He insists that the uterus with this type of dysfunction is highly sensitive to any manipulation and thus warns against heavy sedation, amniotomy, or oxytocin in these patients. Hydration should be maintained with appropriate intravenous fluids. The patient should be reassured about her steady, if slow, progress, and the efforts of nature should be maximized. If secondary arrest of dilatation occurs, or if failure of descent develops, this new abnormality should be treated appropriately.

Secondary Arrest of Dilatation

Secondary arrest of dilatation is diagnosed when no progress in dilatation occurs for a period of 2 hours or more in a patient who has entered the active phase. The arrest usually occurs at a cervical dilatation of 5 to 8 cm. This abnormality corresponds roughly to the old classification of "hypotonic uterine inertia" and may be the most ominous of the recognized types of dysfunction. Should this abnormality occur, the obstetrician should search carefully for factors causing fetopelvic disproportion. After clinical evaluation of the patient, the radiologist may be consulted; x-ray pelvimetry may be indicated, or the clinician may feel that his clinical evaluation of the pelvis is sufficient. The presentation of the fetus and the level of the presenting part of the fetus can be reported with accuracy by the radiologist. During the time needed for these x-ray examinations, the patient should be hydrated with intravenous fluids. If fetopelvic disproportion is diagnosed, as occurs in nearly half of these patients, immediate cesarean section is indicated. With fetopelvic disproportion ruled out, a dilute solution of intravenous oxytocin will quickly terminate labor in many of these patients; in this situation, it is likely that the uterus has simply become exhausted. Amniotomy at the time of the oxytocin administration may also be useful.

ABNORMALITIES OF DESCENT

Friedman has identified three abnormalities of the descent pattern of labor: protracted descent, failure of descent, and arrest of descent. Protracted descent is characterized by a rate of descent of less than 1 cm. per hour in nulliparas or 2 cm. per hour in multiparas. Most patients with this abnormality will deliver uneventfully, and since the adverse effects of this abnormality are related primarily to intervention with midforceps, the use of oxytocin is usually recommended. Arrest of descent (cessation of progressive descent for at least 1 hour after the beginning of the descent phase) and failure of descent are ominous abnormalities associated with a cesarean section rate of approximately 50 percent because of an associated fetopelvic disproportion. If fetopelvic disproportion cannot be documented, amniotomy and oxytocin stimulation can be used.

DIAGNOSIS

We have laid out a plan of management for each of the common types of uterine dysfunction and of failure to descend. In our experience, these therapeutic plans are effective. However, we glibly talked of ruling out fetopelvic disproportion before proceeding with the necessary therapy, and a few words of explanation are in order. Severe fetopelvic disproportion—or, more precisely, a very large or malpresenting baby or a small or deformed pelvis—may be an easy diagnosis to make, and the details are covered in the next section. Lesser degrees of fetopelvic disproportion are not easy to identify, however, and the novice should not be discouraged when he has difficulty doing so. Indeed, the diagnosis can frequently be made only by exclusion.

After ruling out disproportion by clinical examination and perhaps also with x-ray help, the clinician may experience lack of therapeutic success with oxytocin. The contractions may improve to the point where they are physiologically "good" as measured by intrauterine pressure determinations, but poor progress in cervical dilatation or descent of the presenting part may be noted. Thus, the diagnosis of fetopelvic disproportion may be arrived at by exclusion. This theoretical experience illustrates an important point about the use of oxytocin. A definite time limit should be set on its employment. Lack of progress may lead to rupture of the lower uterine segment, since this anatomic area thins from lack of progress in descent of the fetus. More will be said of this hazard later.

OXYTOCIN IN OBSTETRICS

Oxytocin is perhaps the most valuable therapeutic tool available to the modern obstetrician and is the treatment of choice in many clinical situations. However, the hazards of an idiosyncratic reaction or the effect of an overdose of the drug cannot be overstated. While the drug should and must be used in appropriate clinical situations, care must always be exercised in its use. The physician who uses it must by thoroughly familiar with the physiologic role of endogenous oxytocin, the expected effects of the drug when given exogenously, its untoward effects, and the therapy to be employed if an unexpected reaction to the drug occurs.

Oxytocin is known to be produced in the human posterior pituitary gland and is secreted throughout pregnancy. It probably does not play a major role in the initiation of labor, but this has not been proved. The uterus in early pregnancy is resistant to the effects of oxytocin, large doses being required to cause laborlike contractions. As pregnancy progresses, the uterus becomes increasingly sensitive to oxytocin. Near term, minute amounts of the drug can provoke contraction waves that appear in every detail identical to those of spontaneous labor. It is important to recognize this amplified effect of dosage so evident in late pregnancy.

When indicated, the drug may be given intramuscularly, intravenously, sublingually, and intranasally. Certainly, the intravenous route is the safest route of administration and the one by which the physiologic action of the drug can be most meticulously controlled. The interested reader is referred to more extensive publications on the use of oxytocin for details of other routes of administration [3].

The intravenous solution is prepared by mixing 10 units of oxytocin and 1000 ml. of 5% glucose in water. While drip sizes vary from one commercial intravenous administration set to another, a good estimate is that the typical intravenous set will deliver 1 ml. of solution per 15 drops. While it is much better to deliver the drug with a constant infusion pump, this apparatus is not available in all centers. The drug should be started at 1 milliunit per minute (approximately 3 drops per minute of the prepared solution). In some this dosage will be sufficient. Indeed, in a susceptible person, a tetanic contraction may develop, necessitating the immediate discontinuation of the drug. If the desired result is not achieved, the dose can be gradually increased at 15- to 20-minute intervals, recognizing that the initial effect of the intravenous drug will occur in 2 to 3 minutes and the maximal effect in 10 to 15 minutes. The dosage may be gradually increased to a maximal dosage of 20 to 30 milliunits per minute. This dosage should not be exceeded.

Uterine and fetal reactions to the drug should be constantly assessed. While it is best to monitor uterine contractions and the fetal heart rate (FHR) electronically, most clinics must still rely on abdominal palpation for uterine contractions and the stethoscope for the FHR. A tetanic contraction or a change in the FHR demands immediate cessation of the drug. The physiologic end point sought is uterine contractions that mimic labor precisely without causing fetal distress.

Certain precautions or contraindications to the use of oxytocin should be recognized and may be summarized as follows:

Use oxytocin to stimulate labor only for good clinical indications. The drug is safe, but untoward effects occur and must be anticipated. Indications include certain types of uterine dysfunction (see above) and necessary induction of labor such as for premature rupture of the membranes.

The patient receiving oxytocin must be constantly attended. Electronic monitoring of uterine contractions and the FHR is increasingly used and provides much more precise measurement of physiologic effects than older techniques.

The drug is relatively contraindicated in women with a parity of five or greater and of advanced reproductive age. Uterine rupture through the lower uterine segment is most likely to occur in these patients. Careful monitoring of intrauterine pressure greatly increases the safety of oxytocin in these patients.

A definite time limit should be placed on the use of the drug. With uterine dysfunction, lack of progress for 2 to 3 hours should be sufficient to suggest drug failure and the need for reliance on other therapy. The drug should be used with care when the uterus is overdistended, as with twins or a large baby.

Fetopelvic disproportion should be ruled out by the best means available before starting oxytocin. Should the diagnosis be missed (a not uncommon situation), a second line of defense against uterine rupture can be drawn by limiting the period during which the drug is used, as previously described.

It is wise to avoid the use of oxytocin in false labor. A prolonged latent phase is easily confused with false labor. A common clinical mistake is to diagnose lack of labor progress when the patient is not in labor at all. Sedation is better therapy for false labor or a prolonged latent phase and will avoid this hazard.

AMNIOTOMY AS A UTERINE STIMULANT

Opinions vary on the effectiveness of amniotomy as a uterine stimulant. While Friedman [1] believes that the effect of amniotomy varies unpredictably from effective stimulation, to no effect, to actual delay in labor, most others have reported an increase in work performed by the uterus following amniotomy. In one well-controlled study, a distinct shortening of labor subsequent to amniotomy was demonstrated [4].

Amniotomy should be used with secondary arrest of dilatation when fetopelvic disproportion has been excluded and vaginal delivery is expected. It should probably not be used with primary dysfunction of the active phase. Friedman [1] has shown clearly that the procedure exerts little favorable effect on the subsequent labor pattern of these patients and may actually delay labor. Amniotomy may effectively stimulate labor in a patient whose latent phase is prolonged, but its use is not recommended. If amniotomy is performed and if good labor does not ensue, the physician will ultimately be faced with a patient not in labor or in poor labor who is undelivered at 12 to 24 hours following the amniotomy. It is better to sedate such a patient to differentiate false labor from true early labor and allow a wider subsequent therapeutic choice.

PATHOLOGIC RETRACTION RINGS

With prolonged labor, the normal physiologic retraction ring that forms at the junction of the contractile upper uterine segment and the passive lower segment will rise higher and higher in the body of the uterus. The lower segment is retracted and becomes thinner and thinner. While the physiologic retraction ring is seldom palpated abdominally, a pathologic retraction ring (Bandl's ring) is felt during abdominal examination as an indentation between the upper segment and the rising lower segment. Bandl's ring is a sign of obstructed labor and evidence that rupture of the lower segment will occur if the obstructed labor is not relieved. It should never be seen in the modern obstetrical ward.

A constriction ring of the cervix that actually obstructs the progress of labor by grasping the neck of the fetus and preventing descent has been described in the older literature. This constriction ring is probably simply an extreme example of Bandl's ring and should be treated accordingly.

Abnormal Labor Due to Fetal and Pelvic Factors

Abnormal labor may be caused by fetal or pelvic factors as well as by dysfunction of the uterine contractions. Some factors (e.g., a poorly flexed vertex) are minor deterrents to the progress of labor and cause only a slight delay. Other factors (e.g., a severely contracted pelvis) produce insurmountable disproportion and demand abdominal delivery if tragedy is to be avoided.

The normal fetal and pelvic obstetrical anatomy has been discussed in Chapter 9, where abnormalities of the pelvis and fetal malpresentations were discussed together, since multiple factors frequently combine to cause abnormal labor. In the clinical situation, it is usually impossible to separate them. Therefore, in discussion, it seems wise not to try to separate them artificially.

PERSISTENT OCCIPITOPOSTERIOR POSITION

As was noted in the discussion on the mechanism of normal labor in Chapter 9, in most instances the fetal head engages in a transverse diameter but rotates early in its descent to an anterior position. Certain factors predispose to engagement, or descent, or both with the fetal head in an occipitoposterior position. This situation prevails in about 10 to 15 percent of labors. When the transverse diameter of the inlet is less than the anteroposterior (AP) diameter, as with the anthropoid pelvis, the fetal head engages in the AP diameter, frequently in an oblique or directly posterior position. If the midpelvis is narrow, the spontaneous rotation that usually develops as the fetal head reaches the level of the spines may not occur simply because there is no room for the maneuver. Flexion of the fetal head is also less likely to be present, and the much longer occipitofrontal diameter (11.5 cm.) is more likely to present than the smaller and more usual suboccipitobregmatic diameter (9.5 cm.). If internal rotation fails to occur in the mid-pelvis, this rotation will occur as the fetal head reaches the pelvic floor unless the outlet, too, is greatly narrowed. The rotation is usually toward an anterior position, but it may also occur toward a direct posterior position. It is variously estimated that 5 to 30 percent of

fetuses descending through the pelvis in the posterior position fail to rotate to an anterior position before delivery. The great variation in incidence is probably related to the amount of time that is allowed to elapse before obstetrical rotation of the head to an anterior position is attempted.

Diagnosis

The diagnosis of an occipitoposterior position will usually be first suspected when slowness in cervical dilatation or in descent of the fetal head is noted. In retrospect, an unusual amount of backache complained of by the patient may have been an early sign. While it has been said that the average length of labor is prolonged only slightly with posterior positions, considerable delay may be experienced as the head approaches the pelvic floor. At this time, the suspected diagnosis of posterior position can be confirmed by pelvic examination, since the cervix will be well dilated. The anterior fontanelle of the fetal head will be palpated in one of the maternal anterior quadrants, and there will probably be a good deal of molding of the fetal head. The posterior fontanelle usually cannot be reached since slight deflection of the head is the rule.

Management

Labor is managed as described above, except that uterine dysfunction may be a problem. Careful use of analgesia is necessary, since overdosage may favor the development of uterine dysfunction, while minimal dosage may be insufficient for this frequently uncomfortable labor. If fetopelvic disproportion of a major degree can be ruled out, and if progress of labor is slow, dilute intravenous oxytocin may be used to aid descent. Posterior position may cause the secondary arrest of dilatation previously described.

Delivery of the fetus presenting in the posterior position can be managed in several ways. In most instances, procrastination will allow the fetal head to rotate to the AP diameter, usually to an anterior position, with subsequent delivery. If the head delivers in a posterior position, more than the usual outlet space is required because of the greater AP diameter of the presenting part that must traverse the outlet. A deep episiotomy may be required. If an earlier delivery is desired, obstetrical rotation of the head may be used either by a manual maneuver or with use of forceps. Manual rotation is accomplished by grasping the fetal head in the operator's hand with the fingers well spread to provide maximal traction (Fig. 11-3). When the uterine contraction occurs, the hand rotates the head in the desired direction. The help of an assistant who provides appropriate abdominal pressure on the fetal shoulders to aid in rotation is useful. The manual rotation may be better performed between contractions when the fetal head can be elevated to a higher level in the pelvis where more pelvic room may be encountered. After rotation, forceps are applied as described below for a fetus in a left occipitoanterior (LOA), right occipitoanterior (ROA), or direct occipitoanterior (OA) position.

If forceps rotation is chosen, our personal preference, the Scanzoni maneuver, will be used. With good anesthesia, preferably a regional block, the forceps are applied for a right occipitoposterior (ROP) position for example, as if the fetus were in the LOA position. Simpson forceps are entirely satisfactory for the purpose, although the Tucker-McLean instrument is preferred by many. The head is flexed with the forceps, and the handles are swept in a wide arc to effect the rotation, avoiding or minimizing vaginal lacerations. The pelvic curve of the forceps demands the wide arc, since the use of a narrow arc with the handles produces an unacceptably wide arc of the toe of the blades. The rotation should be performed only if it can be done easily. Pushing the head to a higher pelvic level, or occasionally pulling it down to a slightly lower plane, may provide the needed room.

When the rotation has been completed, one blade is removed (toward the floor, since the blades are now upside down) and reapplied inside the remaining blade to accommodate the new anterior position of the fetal head. The second blade is similarly removed and reapplied. After checking for good forceps application, traction is applied as described in Chapter 9 under Prophylactic Outlet Forceps Delivery for an anterior position. Those who use the Tucker-McLean blades may switch to

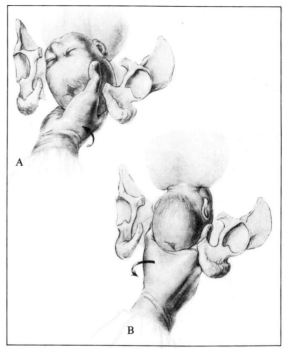

Fig. 11-3. Manual rotation of the head from LOP (A) to OA (B). (From J. R. Willson, Atlas of Obstetric Technic [2nd ed.]. St. Louis: Mosby, 1969. Daisy Stilwell, medical illustrator.)

a Simpson instrument for traction, since the Simpson forceps supply more effective traction. Kielland blades have also been used for this rotation, but they should be reserved for the fetal head in deep transverse arrest, as described in the next section.

TRANSVERSE ARREST OF THE HEAD
When the fetal head descends to the mid-pelvis and no further, transverse mid-pelvic arrest has occurred. This abnormality is usually seen in a pelvis with a decreased AP diameter of the mid-pelvis or outlet or both, although it may also be seen in an adequate gynecoid pelvis. The prognosis is entirely different in these two situations. If careful pelvic assessment assures the operator that the arrest has occurred in a gynecoid pelvis of adequate size, the major etiologic factor may be secondary arrest of dilatation, which will respond well to dilute intra-

venous oxytocin. Should further descent continue
to be slow and if full cervical dilatation has occurred, an obstetrician with the requisite skill may
apply mid-forceps, using the Kielland or Barton instruments as described subsequently. The outcome
is usually satisfactory unless the application has
been tried with the vertex higher than at station +2.

If the arrest is due to a pelvis flattened in the AP
diameter, the problem is different. In skilled hands,
the Kielland or Barton instruments may be tried
when cervical dilatation is full and the presenting
part is at +2 station or lower. Traction should be
applied with the vertex in the transverse diameter
until the pelvic floor is reached, when anterior rotation will usually occur. Alternatively, rotation
may be attempted by pushing the fetal head somewhat higher after forceps application before applying traction. At no time should rotation and traction
be simultaneously applied, since major damage to
the pelvis, and possibly also to the fetus, may result.

It is clear from what has been said that cesarean
section may prove the safest form of therapy for
transverse arrest of the head. When the patient's
pelvis is adequate, dilute intravenous oxytocin may
be tried for a brief interval before resorting to section. It should be remembered that there is a very
real risk of rupture of the lower uterine segment if
the second stage of labor is permitted to continue
for more than 2 hours with an obstructed labor, as
well illustrated by mid-pelvic arrest.

BROW PRESENTATION

With brow (bregma) presentation, the fetal head
presents in a position midway between the well-
flexed occiput and the extreme extension of face
presentation (Fig. 11-4). It is fortunately rare, occurring less than once in every 1000 deliveries,
since vaginal delivery usually cannot occur with
this presentation. The presentation has been reported by some, but not all, investigators to be associated with fetuses of premature size. Brow presentation is apt to occur when the uterine force is
directed obliquely on the fetus, as with the pendu-
lous abdomen of the multipara; or when a fetal neck

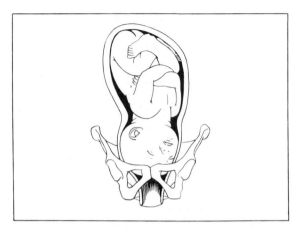

Fig. 11-4. Brow presentation. (From Obstetrical Presentation and Position, Ross Clinical Education Aid No.
18. Columbus, Ohio: Ross Laboratories, 1975.)

tumor or nuchal loops of cord prevent flexion of the
head on the chest.

Brow presentation is usually first suspected
when descent of the presenting part fails to occur or
occurs very slowly. Furthermore, the arrest is apt
to occur in the upper pelvis. Diagnosis by abdominal palpation is possible but uncertain. Vaginal palpation may reveal the anterior fontanelle and parts
of the eye sockets and nasal bone if sufficient cervical dilatation has occurred. An x-ray film may be
needed to confirm the diagnosis.

Since delivery of the brow rarely occurs, conversion by flexion to an occiput presentation or by
extension to a face presentation is usually necessary and usually occurs spontaneously. If the conversion fails to occur, the experienced obstetrician
may attempt manual conversion by vaginal digital
pressure on the presenting part, combined with appropriate abdominal pressure on the fetal chest by
an assistant. It is unwise to pursue this maneuver
too vigorously, since dislodgment of the vertex
may produce prolapse of the cord. For the same
reason, the maneuver should not be attempted if
the membranes have ruptured. Cesarean section is
the preferred method of treatment after a short trial
of labor has failed to produce the desired conversion.

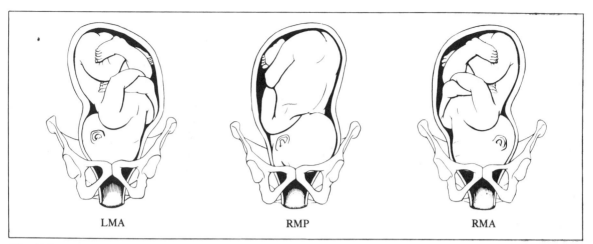

Fig. 11-5. Types of face presentation. (LMA = left mentum anterior; RMP = right mentum posterior; RMA = right mentum anterior.) (From Obstetrical Presentation and Position, *Ross Clinical Education Aid No. 18. Columbus, Ohio: Ross Laboratories, 1975.)*

FACE PRESENTATION

Face (mentum) presentation occurs about once in every 400 to 500 deliveries and probably results in most instances from an initial brow presentation that extended to a face presentation at the pelvic inlet (Fig. 11-5). The prognosis for this presentation is good unless the mentum presents in one of the posterior quadrants of the mother's pelvis, when vaginal delivery of a live fetus is impossible. Fortunately, even with posterior face presentation, rotation to an anterior face presentation occurs in two-thirds of cases. Posterior face delivery is impossible because the neck of the fetus is unable to extend further and to negotiate the long arc formed by the maternal sacrum. The patient with an anterior face presentation may experience a labor not unlike a normal occipital labor since the widest diameter presented (submentobregmatic) is little larger than the suboccipitobregmatic usual with an occiput position. Indeed, a rapid labor may occur and low forceps can be used with almost as great ease with face presentation as with occiput.

The diagnosis of face presentation is rarely made abdominally, largely because descent of the presenting part is typically not abnormal and because no special care is exerted in examining the fetus abdominally. Vaginal palpatory findings are quickly recognized as atypical, but the presentation may easily be confused with the breech presentation. The mouth of the fetus, however, forms a triangle with the malar eminences of the face, whereas the readily confused anal opening is on a straight line between the ischial spines of the breech. Palpation of the orbital ridges confirms the diagnosis of face presentation.

If the mentum is in the anterior quadrant, typical progress of labor and delivery should be anticipated. If the mentum is posterior, labor should usually be permitted to progress spontaneously until it is evident that internal rotation to an anterior position is not going to occur. Cesarean section is then mandatory. Since shortened gestation is common with face presentation, perinatal mortality is increased due to this factor. If attempts at conversion and other manipulative maneuvers are avoided, face presentation should otherwise not cause an increase in perinatal mortality.

(= letak belakang)

Breech Presentation

Breech presentation occurs in about 4 percent of deliveries, in somewhat fewer if only term births

the prolapse of umbilical cord in this presentation occurs More frequently than for a vertex presentation. (3 to 20×)

are included, and in substantially more if only babies of low birth weight are studied. The importance of the breech presentation stems from the high perinatal mortality with this unusual presentation. While much of the perinatal loss is due to the effects of prematurity, the perinatal death rate even in term breech presentations remains higher than with vertex presentations. The higher death rate can be accounted for by a number of factors, some preventable and others apparently unavoidable. Since the breech does not fit as snugly into the cervix as does the vertex, prolapse of the umbilical cord is more likely to occur with a breech, especially with a footling breech. Since the breech is a poor dilating wedge against the cervix, cervical dilatation may be more erratic, and uterine dysfunction is a common complication. While with the vertex presentation the fetal head has many hours to mold to accommodate itself to the maternal pelvis, the aftercoming head of the breech enjoys no similar period of accommodation. The delivery of the aftercoming head is not infrequently technically difficult, with a resultant increase in cerebral trauma.

Etiology

Breeches are said to occur with increased frequency when the fetus is small compared with the size of the uterine cavity because the fetus does not have to conform to the uterine shape. Certainly, many fetuses present by the breech in mid-pregnancy, with conversion to vertex occurring most frequently before the thirty-second week. The wider fetal buttocks usually accommodate best to the upper uterine segment instead of the narrower lower uterine segment, but with changes in intrauterine shape, this tendency may not be present. Examples of this change in accommodation include uterine anomalies, such as a septate uterus, hydramnios, multiple fetuses, and perhaps placenta previa. Multiparity with uterine relaxation may also predispose to breech presentation.

Types of Breech Presentation

The breech may present in a number of different ways as described on p. 174 and shown in Figure

11-6. Each type has its peculiar hazards and disadvantages. While the frank breech fits better against the cervix, the extended legs may interfere with the lateral flexion of the body required for delivery of the hips. The complete breech and footling breeches are not as effective cervical dilators as is the frank breech, and the footling breech is frequently complicated by prolapse of the cord. While abdominal diagnosis of a breech presentation may be easy to make, differentiation into the various types of breech presentation is usually not possible with this method. Abdominal examination usually reveals an absence of the hard, globular, movable head just above the symphysis and its replacement by a softer presenting part that cannot be moved separately from the body. The fetal head can usually be outlined in the fundus. The fetal heart sounds may be heard best in one of the upper quadrants, but this is not universally so. If necessary, the diagnosis can be confirmed by pelvic examination if cervical dilatation has begun, or by an x-ray film. The presence of a breech presentation beyond 36 weeks' gestation usually requires only one film to confirm the diagnosis. X-ray pelvimetry is advisable if the patient is a primigravida. Of great importance also is determination of the fetal size, which is virtually impossible to do accurately except with ultrasonic measurement of the fetal biparietal diameter, a technique available only in large medical centers at the present time.

Many authorities have recommended external version of all breech presentations to decrease the incidence of this presentation at the time of labor. Others suggest that this practice carries the significant hazard of cord complication and that it fails to decrease the number of breeches significantly because most of them revert after the version. We are of the latter school. Certainly, if an external version is to be done, it should be performed while the uterus is relaxed, before the membranes have ruptured, and in a gentle manner.

Mechanism of Labor

Engagement of the presenting part before labor is unusual. With the onset of labor, the hips engage, usually in the oblique diameter of the inlet, and de-

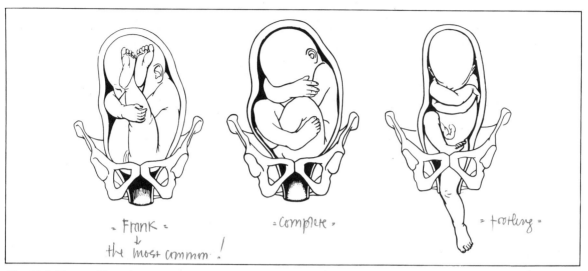

Fig. 11-6. Types of breech presentation: (left) *frank breech;* (middle) *complete breech;* (right) *footling breech. (From* Obstetrical Presentation and Position, *Ross Clinical Education Aid No. 18. Columbus, Ohio: Ross Laboratories, 1975.)*

scend through the pelvis until the levator sling is reached, when internal rotation occurs. The AP diameter assumed by the fetal hips at this time persists through delivery. The anterior hip impinges under the symphysis pubis, and the posterior hip descends as the fetal body undergoes lateral flexion. With the birth of the hips, rotation to a sacrum anterior position occurs as the shoulders accommodate to the inlet. The shoulders also internally rotate at the levator sling and deliver in an AP diameter. The fetal head usually has maintained a well-flexed position throughout labor, and it now engages with the face facing the sacrum. Near the outlet, the head is almost always in the AP diameter; and, as the suboccipital area impinges under the symphysis pubis, the face is born by further flexion on the chest.

Management of Labor and Delivery

Recently, increasing numbers of obstetricians are recommending and practicing cesarean section on virtually all patients with breech presentation. This

approach, while apparently a radical and extreme departure from tradition, is based on several established facts. Cesarean section has become very safe for the mother. Death from the operation is rare with modern medical techniques. Many of the factors leading to fetal death or damage with breech presentation (difficult delivery of the shoulders and head, brain damage, prolapse of the umbilical cord) are avoided, or at least minimized, by abdominal delivery.

Those opposed to routine cesarean section advocate vaginal delivery for the breech presentation with the following exceptions:

1. Footling presentations, because of the substantial risk of umbilical cord prolapse.
2. Fetuses with an estimated weight of 8 pounds (3600 gm.) or greater, because of potential fetopelvic disproportion.
3. A small maternal pelvis.
4. Fetuses with a gestation of less than 36 weeks, since immature fetuses are more prone to delivery trauma.
5. A breech that is in a poor attitude, e.g., extended fetal head.
6. Uterine dysfunction or poor fetal descent.

Under these circumstances, 25 to 50 percent of

breech presentations will be delivered abdominally. This approach statistically reduces the risk of uterine rupture in pregnancy subsequent to the cesarean section and avoids, for many patients, the higher maternal mortality and morbidity associated with cesarean section. Furthermore, family size is not limited by the traditional and wise practice of restricting to three the number of cesarean sections that can be done safely.

We prefer to deliver a fetus presenting by the breech per vaginam, if possible, and the subsequent discussion is based on that premise. The student should be alert to changing medical opinion, however, and the method of delivering in a breech presentation is a prime case in point.

The first stage of labor is managed much as with the vertex presentation, except that a prolapsed cord should be expected and excluded or confirmed by pelvic examination at the time of rupture of the membranes. The usual sedation can be given, taking due note of the possibility the infant may be premature. As long as the fetopelvic relationships have been judged adequate and steady progress is made, vaginal delivery can be anticipated. If progress ceases, either in cervical dilatation or in descent, cesarean section should be seriously considered.

Some clinicians are willing to administer oxytocin to encourage stronger uterine contractions and better progress of labor, but we prefer to use this drug infrequently in breech presentation. While a short trial of oxytocin is not likely to cause uterine rupture, the progress that ensues in cervical dilatation or descent may lull the obstetrician into thinking that the delivery will be an easy one. More often than not, the delay in labor progress is a red flag signaling that all is not well, that the delivery may not be easy.

METHODS OF DELIVERY. With the fetal buttocks at the introitus, one of three approaches may be taken:

1. The breech may be allowed to deliver completely spontaneously. This is unlikely to be advantageous except for a very small fetus.

2. The breech may be "decomposed and extracted." The details of this procedure are given on page 218. We do not favor this practice except in special clinical situations (see p. 218).
3. The breech may be allowed to deliver spontaneously, with little interference, to the level of the umbilicus, following which the obstetrician actively assists in the remaining delivery. Almost without exception, we favor assisted breech delivery, since this technique results in the lowest perinatal mortality possible and is least likely to damage the maternal soft parts.

Minimal assistance is needed as the mother's efforts deliver the hips. The delivery may be preceded by pudendal block anesthesia and a deep episiotomy, but general anesthesia is inappropriate, since maternal expulsive efforts are essential. When the fetus is delivered to the level of the umbilicus, rapid general anesthesia is helpful, since subsequent maneuvers are best performed by the obstetrician without maternal help. The fetal sacrum must be positioned so that it faces upward, a position usually assumed even with spontaneous delivery.

With a clean towel over the fetal hips to provide traction downward, deliberate but gentle pull is exerted by the obstetrician. As the thorax comes into view, the obstetrician's hands are moved upward so that further traction is exerted on this area. The traction now is continued downward, but a gentle spiral pull is added in the direction away from one of the fetal shoulders (Fig. 11-7). Shortly, the fetal scapula comes into view and is delivered. When this is accomplished, splinting of the fetal humerus with two fingers of the obstetrician's hands will deliver the arm and hand. Again, a downward spiral pull is exerted on the fetus in a direction away from the remaining undelivered shoulder. The shoulder and arm delivery maneuver is repeated for the other side. The head follows the shoulder delivery, and gentle suprapubic pressure can be exerted on the vertex if needed (Fig. 11-8). When the head is on the pelvic floor, we prefer to apply Piper forceps to complete the delivery. The assistance of an attendant to hold the fetal body up

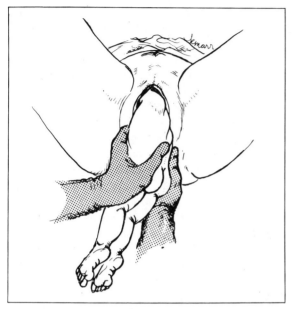

Fig. 11-7. Breech delivery of initial shoulder. Traction is exerted downward on the body simultaneously with rotation of the chest away from the shoulder to be delivered. (From K. Niswander. Obstetric and Gynecologic Disorders: A Practitioner's Guide. Flushing, N.Y.: Medical Examination Publishing Co., 1975.)

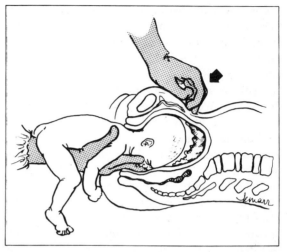

Fig. 11-8. Breech delivery of head. Engagement of the head by suprapubic pressure of the external hand and guidance of the head through the pelvis with the internal hand. (From K. Niswander. Obstetric and Gynecologic Disorders: A Practitioner's Guide. Flushing, N.Y.: Medical Examination Publishing Co., 1975.)

while the forceps are being applied is essential. If delivery of the head appears to require little effort, the Mauriceau-Smellie-Veit maneuver can be used. In this maneuver, the baby is laid astraddle the obstetrician's left hand while his left index finger is placed in the baby's mouth to provide direction. The head is delivered with the right hand, however, as it exerts pressure over the fetal occiput behind the symphysis pubis.

Our description of the management of delivery has suggested that all will go smoothly. This, unfortunately, is not always so. The fetal arms may not be easy to deliver; indeed, extension of the arm alongside the fetal head or nuchal entrapment of an arm may occur, especially if delivery of the body has been too rapid. If an extended or nuchal arm is recognized, it can usually be released and delivered by rotating the body 180 degrees away from the nuchal arm while downward traction continues to be employed on the thorax. The arm or hand will

lag behind the shoulder as it encounters the resistance of the cervical and vaginal tissues and dislodges from its position behind the neck. It will now be possible to deliver the arm as it lies in a posterior position overlying the perineum. Some operators prefer always to deliver the posterior shoulder first, rather than the anterior shoulder underlying the symphysis pubis.

Forceps cannot be applied to the aftercoming head until the head is on the perineum. A higher application will seriously injure maternal structures and damage the fetus. Fetopelvic disproportion in a breech can therefore not be tolerated and must be anticipated by a careful prelabor and early labor evaluation of the pelvis and the fetus that must pass through it. This fact helps to explain the increasingly high rate of cesarean section deliveries being used for breech presentations.

We advise against routine or even frequent use of total breech extraction, or, as it is sometimes called, breech decomposition and extraction. While this operation is spectacular to watch, the higher perinatal mortality rate that results from such a major maneuver does not justify its frequent use. Certain situations, however, may require it: for example, prolapse of the umbilical cord with the cervix fully dilated and the breech well descended into the pelvis; fetal hypoxia from another cause but with the same cervical dilatation and position of the breech. We advise against its use simply for a delay in descent even with a fully dilated cervix.

Decomposition and extraction is carried out as follows: with deep general anesthesia, the hand of the obstetrician is introduced through the vagina and into the uterine cavity, where one or preferably both fetal legs are grasped after dislodging them from their extended position. The legs are withdrawn, and slow traction is exerted on them to effect delivery. The remainder of the delivery is as previously described. Single or double footling breeches may be delivered in a similar manner, but care must be taken that delivery is not effected before full cervical dilatation has occurred. A prolapsed foot presenting through the introitus presents a tempting target for the overzealous obstetrician. Delay is recommended. Cesarean section should be used in most instances when a footling breech presentation is recognized.

Tentorial tear and subsequent subdural brain hemorrhage is a major cause of fetal death in breech delivery. Hemorrhage into the upper spinal cord has also recently been emphasized as a cause of fetal death with breech presentation [5]. Most of these accidents probably occur at the time of delivery of the head and should be assiduously avoided. Excess traction on the cervical spine certainly accounts for a major proportion of the hazard and can be avoided to a large extent by forceps delivery of the aftercoming head. Sudden extrusion of the head may also put undue stress on the delicate brain structures, and this, too, should be guarded against. As emphasized previously, cesarean section should not be thought of as a last resort in breech presentation but as a primary method of delivery when it seems indicated. While some have suggested routine abdominal delivery for breech presentation, we cannot agree. Lack of progress in labor, however, should demand a reassessment of

the plan of management, and cesarean section will frequently be chosen in this situation.

ANESTHESIA FOR DELIVERY. Deep general anesthesia is required for total breech extraction. Assisted delivery is best accomplished with minimal anesthesia until the breech delivers to the umbilicus, then an anesthetic that produces total muscle relaxation should be used for the remainder of the delivery. No single agent fulfills these requirements perfectly. One possible choice is a pudendal block followed by a rapid-acting general anesthetic at the appropriate time. Most inhalation agents become effective too slowly to be useful, although cyclopropane partially satisfies the peculiar needs of the situation. The final choice should be made by an experienced anesthesiologist—who must always be present for breech delivery—in consultation with the obstetrician.

A second possible anesthetic choice is lumbar epidural anesthesia or caudal anesthesia. While pain relief and good muscle relaxation are secure with these methods, the patient may still be able to bear down on command even though she may have no urge to do so. A spinal anesthetic given at a low enough level may provide the same advantages.

Breech Delivery Summary

Breech presentation should be considered abnormal and deserving of special attention because of the high perinatal risk attending it. Careful prelabor or early labor study of pelvic size, pelvic architecture, and fetal size will identify which patients are likely to deliver successfully by the vaginal route. The remaining patients should be delivered by cesarean section as soon as labor begins. Should progress in cervical dilatation or descent of the presenting part be delayed when vaginal delivery is planned, cesarean section is usually indicated.

Vaginal delivery should be attempted only by an experienced obstetrician who has assistance with the delivery and who has an experienced anesthesiologist to provide appropriate anesthesia. Under these circumstances, the perinatal death rate in term breech births should approach that of vertex presentation. The low-birth-weight baby so commonly associated with the breech presentation should be delivered in a hospital where expert neonatal care is available.

TRANSVERSE LIE

A transverse lie is present when the part of the fetus presenting over the cervix is the shoulder or arm (Fig. 11-9). The fetal head occupies one iliac fossa and the breech the other. This abnormal presentation occurs about once in every 400 deliveries and is especially associated with multiparity. An oblique lie is a variation of transverse lie. Predisposing causes include the presence of something in the lower uterine segment that blocks the entrance of the fetus into the pelvis (placenta previa, uterine myoma), a contracted pelvis, and a relaxed abdominal musculature that fails to keep the fetus in a position where uterine contractions can force it into the pelvis.

Diagnosis

The diagnosis is usually made during abdominal examination, when the abdomen appears much wider than expected. Absence of both the vertex and breech from the inferior strait and palpation of the vertex in one of the iliac fossae confirm the diagnosis. If transverse lie occurs in the primigravid patient, a contracted pelvis should be suspected. The multipara is the more typical patient, and placenta previa as a coincidental complication should be kept constantly in mind. Bleeding from the placenta previa may precede the diagnosis of transverse lie.

Management

Management of the patient with transverse lie may include external attempts to convert the fetus to a longitudinal lie, usually the vertex position. The conversion should not be attempted in the primigravid patient and should be reserved for early labor or very late pregnancy, even in the multigravida. The uterus must be relaxed, and the fetus should be of sufficient size to permit immediate delivery should a cord complication occur or to anticipate

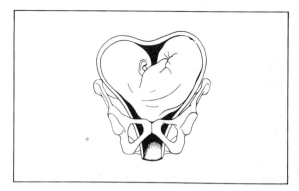

Fig. 11-9. Shoulder presentation. (From Obstetrical Presentation and Position. *Ross Clinical Education Aid No. 18. Columbus, Ohio: Ross Laboratories, 1975.)*

the onset of labor if the maneuver is successful. A cord complication demands immediate cesarean section. A successful external version should usually be followed by immediate amniotomy, with the longitudinal position of the fetus maintained by an assistant. Labor will ensue, and vaginal delivery should be possible.

If the lie is not recognized until the patient is in labor, and if the uterus is insufficiently relaxed to attempt external version, an immediate cesarean section is usually the best management. Indeed, a patient with a transverse lie near term and not in labor should be delivered by an early cesarean section unless version appears easy. Thus, cesarean section will be used in most patients with a transverse lie. One possible exception may be the case in which transverse lie is recognized in a patient with a small fetus, a fully dilated cervix, and intact membranes. Version and extraction may be chosen by an obstetrician thoroughly familiar with this operation, which is performed as follows: With the patient under deep general anesthesia, the left hand is introduced into the uterus. The feet are grasped and pulled through the vaginal canal as the vertex is dislodged abdominally with the right hand. The operation is not feasible if the fetus's back is closer to the introitus than is the ventral surface. The procedure is mentioned primarily to be condemned in all but the most experienced hands. Carrying a significant maternal mortality from ruptured uterus and a high perinatal mortality, it is rarely justified simply to avoid cesarean section.

The transverse lie before 36 weeks' gestation frequently converts spontaneously to longitudinal lie. Indeed, transverse lie at any gestation may do the same. Thus, expectancy is the best treatment for transverse lie before term gestation is reached. At term, more active interference is justified because of the high maternal and perinatal risk associated with a neglected transverse lie. If the abnormality is ignored for long, a prolapsed cord and fetal death can be expected, followed by fetal impaction. Such an event should never occur in a technologically advanced society, but if it does occur, it may require abdominal delivery to empty the uterus, followed by hysterectomy because of intrauterine infection.

COMPOUND PRESENTATION

When a fetal extremity presents with a breech or a vertex, a compound presentation is recognized. The most common combination is a hand prolapse with vertex presentation. However, a leg with the vertex presentation or a hand alongside the breech is also occasionally recognized. A poorly fitting presenting part, as with a small fetus, is a predisposing factor. Compound presentation is frequently recognized with prematurity.

It is important to diagnose compound presentation, since prolapse of the umbilical cord remains an ever-present threat because of the poor fit between the fetus and the pelvis. The extremity rarely interferes with the progress of labor, and in the absence of cord prolapse, the extremity can usually be ignored and the presentation managed in the same fashion as a simple one. Occasionally, with a term-sized baby and with a severely prolapsed arm, labor will be obstructed. In this instance, an attempt at replacement of the arm should be made, although the effort may be fruitless. Special care in the application of forceps is indicated to avoid injury to the extremity.

When cord prolapse occurs, emergency cesarean section is usually necessary. Section may also occasionally be needed when fetopelvic disproportion

develops. Under the most unusual circumstances, a version and extraction may be employed if the cord prolapses after full cervical dilatation has occurred.

HYDROCEPHALUS

Hydrocephalus, which is enlargement of the cranium from an excessive accumulation of cerebrospinal fluid, is an occasionally encountered cause of fetopelvic dystocia. The diagnosis should be suspected when the lower uterine segment remains empty in spite of good labor and continuing cervical dilatation. Abdominal examination is frequently diagnostic, since the enlarged fetal head can usually be felt. X-ray may be used to establish the diagnosis in a doubtful case. When the breech presents, as it often does, the diagnosis is less easily established, since the radiographic film may be read as negative due to distortion of the size of the head. In this instance, a misdiagnosis may be made when the head is actually of normal size.

When the diagnosis is made with a vertex presentation, the fluid should be drained through a large-bore spinal needle or a trochar after the cervix has dilated sufficiently. Little hazard to the mother results from this procedure, and the fetus is usually delivered uneventfully. With breech presentation, the abnormality may not be recognized until after the body is delivered and the head is found to be undeliverable. Again, drainage of the fluid will permit easy delivery, but care should be exercised in this case to avoid maternal injury during the drainage.

It is important to recognize and treat fetal hydrocephalus. Delay has been costly in the past. Uterine rupture from an overdistended lower uterine segment has occurred, and maternal mortality has been significant. The fetal prognosis is poor when the head is enlarged enough to cause dystocia.

SHOULDER DYSTOCIA

The unexpected misfortune of being unable to deliver the shoulders of a fetus after the head has been successfully extracted is one of the most disconcerting events experienced by an obstetrician.

While the complication usually appears "out of the blue," warning signs have often been present but unfortunately not always. The infant is almost universally a large one, with a birth weight usually greater than 4000 gm. The labor has frequently been dysfunctional, and the delivery of the head may have been difficult. Following the expulsion of the head, the vertex remains unusually close to the perineum, and attempts to deliver the anterior shoulder are of no avail.

Panic must not be allowed to set in, since the unusual tension on the fetal head and neck may result in brachial plexus injury. If fundal pressure from above, with guidance from below for fetal direction, is unsuccessful, delivery of the anterior shoulder should be abandoned and attention directed to the posterior shoulder. It is usually possible, although difficult, for the operator to insert his hand between the perineum and the fetal shoulder. The humerus can be splinted and the arm swept over the chest to deliver the shoulder. Once this has been accomplished, the anterior shoulder usually can be delivered with relative ease. Other maneuvers to deliver an impacted shoulder are described in books on obstetric operations.

This unfortunate complication can occur in the multigravida just as readily as in the primigravida. In our present state of knowledge, we are not able to avoid it in every instance.

Trial of Labor

There is little place for trial of labor when fetopelvic disproportion is suspected with breech presentation. When the vertex presents, the problem is different. Since a trial of labor of a limited number of hours rarely does harm either to the mother or to the fetus, a trial may be indicated to avoid a cesarean section. We advocate a trial of labor in all vertex presentations unless a disproportion is clearly insurmountable or unless other complicating factors are present.

Usually, pelvic diameters can be measured radiographically with great accuracy. Fetal head diameters, notably the biparietal diameter, can also be measured with accuracy by ultrasonography. What cannot be measured, however, is how much the fetal head will mold, how a particular fetus will fit into a particular pelvis, how effectively a particular uterus will contract, and how determined a particular patient is to experience vaginal delivery. Except with extremely large babies or extremely small or deformed pelves, it is impossible to know with certainty whether vaginal delivery will succeed or fail. A trial of labor is clearly in order in most instances.

When a trial is planned, labor should be awaited. The long-held idea that fetopelvic disproportion can be avoided by premature delivery of the infant no longer is valid. The labor should be observed with unusual care if the pelvis seems small or if the fetus seems large. Continuous progress should be expected. A specific type of uterine dysfunction should be treated as described previously. Oxytocin should not be used if the diagnosis of fetopelvic disproportion becomes increasingly evident. If the pelvis appears adequate for the fetus, an oxytocin trial may be employed for a limited number of hours—no more than 2 hours without progress.

Cervical dilatation should assume the expected S-shaped curve when graphed against time. Any aberrant shape should be managed as described earlier. Descent particularly, and especially in the second stage, should be progressive, and, as with any labor, a second stage no longer than 2 hours should be permitted lest the lower uterine segment rupture or the fetus become distressed. A forceps delivery or cesarean section, as indicated, should be performed at the end of this time.

Special note should be taken of the multigravid patient who fails to make the expected progress during labor. There is a tendency to believe that a previously successful vaginal delivery guarantees subsequent successful vaginal deliveries. This is totally unfounded. Fetopelvic disproportion in the multigravida is more hazardous than in the primigravida because it is unexpected, and the multigravida is just as suspect as the primigravida.

Forceps Delivery

The use of forceps to effect delivery of a child constitutes one of the most interesting and important chapters in the history of medicine. The instruments were first used to deliver a live child in the late sixteenth or early seventeenth century by a member of the famous Chamberlen family of British obstetricians. Their use was a carefully guarded Chamberlen family secret for about a century, but in the early part of the eighteenth century, knowledge regarding the usefulness of forceps became widespread. The medical literature since that time has contained hundreds of articles either extolling their use or suggesting that they are agents of the devil. Today, they are in common use in modern obstetrical units, since they provide a safer, more comfortable delivery for many women than would otherwise be possible.

Although forceps are capable of exerting enormous pressure and inflicting major damage, in competent hands they are not only safe but also are frequently essential for the successful termination of delivery. If the prerequisites for use are observed, if the forceps are applied so as to fit the fetal head properly (cephalic application), and if undue pressure is not exerted, only good can come from their use.

Types of Forceps
The obstetrical forcep has a blade, a shank, and a handle. Variations in the construction of these three components identify particular forceps (Fig. 11-10). The blade always has a cephalic curve to fit the fetal head, but the pelvic curve to fit the shape of the pelvis is absent in certain instruments (Kielland, Barton) to allow specific maneuvers. The blade may be fenestrated (Simpson) or it may be solid (Tucker-McLean). Some instruments have a separated shank (Simpson), and some have a sliding lock (Kielland), or a French lock (DeWees), or an English lock (Simpson) at the junction of the shank and the handle. In the Barton forceps, the junction of the blade and the shank has a hinge to allow motion. The Piper instrument has a greatly elongated and curved shank to permit its use with delivery of the aftercoming head of the breech. The choice of instrument is technical and highly individualistic and will not be discussed here. The technique for the use of forceps is described briefly

both in Chapter 9 and in the section on Forceps Application.

CLASSIFICATION OF FORCEPS DELIVERIES
Outlet forceps is the designated term when the forceps are applied to a fetal skull that has reached the pelvic floor and is visible at the introitus and when the sagittal suture of the head is in the AP diameter of the mother's pelvis. This operation may be indicated or elected.

Mid-forceps is the term used to describe a forceps application after the fetal head is engaged and when the other criteria for outlet forceps are not met. This designation includes a large spectrum of possibilities, from delivery with the vertex high in the pelvis, but engaged, to a forceps delivery with the fetal skull on the pelvic floor but not in the AP diameter. Some have subdivided this group into low mid-forceps and mid-forceps deliveries in an attempt to modify this shortcoming. All forceps rotations at any pelvic level are included in this grouping.

High forceps are applied with the fetal skull unengaged, a procedure *never* justified in modern obstetrics.

OUTLET FORCEPS DELIVERY
The procedure for outlet forceps delivery has been described in detail in Chapter 9 under Prophylactic Outlet Forceps Delivery. Elective or prophylactic forceps are commonly used as an alternative to a spontaneous delivery, not only because the operator thinks the operation is safe or safer for the baby than spontaneous delivery, but also because the mother is spared the severe pain of perineal stretching. Elective forceps deliveries represent the major use of forceps operations in this country. Outlet forceps may also be applied for most of the indications listed under the mid-forceps operation, including fetal distress, second stage of 2 hours or more, and so forth. The prerequisites described for the mid-forceps operation must also be met. A major distinction is that the outlet forceps operation is usually easier than the mid-forceps procedure.

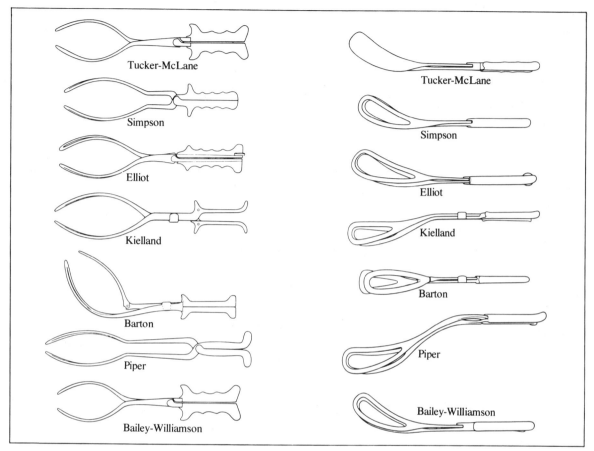

Fig. 11-10. Commonly used forceps. (From R. Douglas and W. Stromme. Operative Obstetrics *[2nd ed.]. New York: Appleton, 1957. Courtesy of the authors and Prentice-Hall, Inc.)*

Episiotomy is nearly always done routinely with any forceps application.

MID-FORCEPS OPERATION

The mid-forceps operation, while justifiably becoming less common in favor of an increasing cesarean section rate, is still of great value in the management of certain obstetrical problems. The traumatic heroic extraction of former years is no longer justified or prevalent, yet the operation, skillfully performed, will spare the woman the def-

inite, if small, hazard of section and a uterine scar that may rupture during a subsequent pregnancy. Of overriding importance in the use of mid-forceps is the skill and experience of the operator. Mid-forceps delivery is not an operation for the novice.

Indications

Fetal indications include a variety of factors that may be included under the term *fetal distress*. Fetal distress may be evidenced by the passage of meconium or by bradycardia. A somewhat more precise diagnosis can be made if continuous FHR monitoring has been used. The cause of the distress may be evident, as with prolapse of the cord or abruptio placentae, or it may be obscure. The hazards of the forceps operation must be balanced against the hazards of the fetal distress before proceeding with the operation.

Maternal indications include coincidental medical disease that contraindicates maternal pushing in the second stage (severe heart disease or pulmonary tuberculosis) or conditions that are better treated by abbreviating labor (hemorrhage from abruptio placentae, eclampsia, intrapartum infection).

Fetopelvic dystocia, or uterine dysfunction, or both are common indications for a mid-forceps operation. It is self-evident that fetopelvic disproportion of a major degree is best treated by cesarean section. When the fetal head rests below the level of the ischial spines due to a minor malpresentation such as (1) a deflexed head or a posterior position of the vertex and (2) a minor degree of pelvic abnormality, mid-forceps delivery should be attempted. In most instances, the operation will be successful; in a few cases a failed "trial" of forceps will suggest that delivery is better effected by cesarean section.

The choice of the appropriate instrument will depend on the position of the fetus and the shape of the pelvis. While the Kielland and Barton forceps are most effective with the transverse position, most obstetricians prefer the Simpson or Tucker-McLean blades for a necessary pelvic rotation and the Simpson instrument for extraction. The Scanzoni operation has been described previously under Persistent Occipitoposterior Position.

Uterine dysfunction (see pp. 205–207) may be due simply to a poor fetopelvic relationship, although in certain instances the dysfunction seems inherent in the uterus. If oxytocin fails to effect descent of the fetal head after mid-pelvic arrest, the mid-forceps operation may be used to compensate for the dysfunction.

The use of regional block *anesthesia* may interfere with the voluntary expulsive efforts of the mother and require the use of mid-forceps to terminate the second stage of labor.

A *2-hour second stage* is the usual length of time compatible with maternal and fetal safety because of the increased risk of rupture of the lower uterine segment if the labor is permitted to continue beyond this point. The mid-forceps operation may be the appropriate method of terminating the second stage. If no evidence of maternal or fetal danger is apparent, the second stage may occasionally be extended beyond 2 hours.

Mid-forceps delivery may also be used as an *elective* procedure. However, in this case, the operation is not justified unless the obstetrician is certain that the procedure will be an easy one.

Prerequisites

Mid-forceps should be used only if certain conditions are fulfilled. The same prerequisites apply as well to the outlet forceps operation.

1. The cervix must be fully dilated. This prerequisite is of great importance, since severe hemorrhage and even maternal death may result from laceration of the cervix and lower uterine segment. On rare occasions, in the most expert hands, and under the most pressing circumstances, forceps delivery may be effected with the cervix dilated only to 8 to 9 cm. when combined with incision of the cervix (Dürhssen's incisions). The full dilatation rule must be violated only under the most unusual circumstances.
2. The forceps should be applied only to a vertex presentation or to a face presentation with the chin in the mother's anterior pelvis. Forceps are not applicable to a brow or a posterior face presentation. They may be used with care with compound presentation.
3. The vertex must be well engaged, a condition usually judged by the pelvic level reached by the presenting part. Engagement usually has occurred when the presenting part has reached the level of the maternal ischial spines (station 0). The presence of severe molding, a large caput, or severe asynclitism may nullify this relationship. There is *no* justification for forceps application if the vertex is not engaged.
4. The obstetrician must have knowledge of the pelvic architecture of the patient and of the precise position of the fetus. If the suture lines and

fontanelles are obscured by molding, he must confirm the fetal position by palpating a fetal ear. The forceps application must be cephalic rather than pelvic; i.e., the forceps must overlie the fetal malar eminences precisely.

5. The fetal membranes must be ruptured to prevent slipping of the forceps on the fetal head.
6. An expert anesthesiologist must be available.

Forceps Application

The details of application of low forceps (prophylactic) and forceps for rotation of the fetal head (Scanzoni maneuver) have been described elsewhere. The technique of insertion and use of mid-forceps is beyond the scope of this book, but the following generalizations can be made.

The forceps must always be applied so that the fetal head is grasped with the long axis of the blades in the sagittal plane. If the forceps is applied otherwise, the compression of the forceps will be exerted on the face or occiput, possibly harming the fetus. Traction is also much less secure and effective than with a good application.

Traction and compression forces of forceps have been measured by a number of investigators [6]. It would appear that no harm is likely to result from moderate traction on the fetal head. (The bravado performances of previous years, when enormous traction was applied to effect delivery are another case.) Indeed, the total compressive force (force of compression multiplied by the time the force is exerted) of an outlet forceps operation may be less than the force exerted by spontaneous delivery on the head by pelvic resistance in the primigravid patient.

The experienced obstetrician will be familiar with one or two instruments and use them for most cases. We prefer the Simpson forceps and occasionally use the Tucker-McLean instrument for rotation operations. For transverse pelvic arrest, an instrument without a pelvic curve is needed, either the Kielland or the Barton forceps. The use of these forceps requires skill, and they should not be used by the occasional operator.

THE DIFFICULT FORCEPS OPERATION VERSUS CESAREAN SECTION

The role of the forceps delivery has undergone periodic change over the centuries, and the present decade is no exception to this rule. At the time forceps were first used, a cesarean section was all but unknown and carried a 100 percent maternal mortality. The use of forceps entailed a much lower maternal and fetal risk than did abdominal delivery. The only reasonable alternative to a forceps delivery of an impacted infant was internal podalic version and extraction or fetal destruction and delivery. Both were hazardous at best for infant and mother. Clearly, forceps were usually superior.

With the problems of hemorrhage and infection largely solved, cesarean section can be performed today with virtually no maternal mortality or perinatal mortality from the procedure. While the forceps delivery enjoys the virtue of avoiding an incision in the uterus, the absence of a more immediate danger to the infant from the forceps operation must be shown to justify the practice. While low forceps, including elective outlet forceps, are indeed safe, the mid-forceps operation is known to be associated with a significant perinatal mortality.

How then can a physician balance the hazards of a difficult forceps operation against the hazards of a cesarean section? He may decide never to use mid-forceps, or he may decide that the risk of rupture of a section scar during subsequent pregnancies precludes the use of this procedure when forceps are a possibility. Neither extreme is wise. One approach is the use of "trial" forceps. Apply the blades and try the extraction. If difficulty is encountered, resort to immediate cesarean section. Rigid rules of procedure are simply not appropriate. Clinical judgment, as inexact as the term is, must be exercised if perinatal mortality is to be lowered without a concomitant increase in the risk of uterine rupture.

Vacuum Extractor

Malmström [7] described the use of the vacuum extractor method of delivery, whereby a flat metal cup of one of various diameters (3 to 6 cm.) is applied and attached to the fetal head by pumping air out of the device, thus creating a vacuum. The vacuum extractor is said to be superior to forceps, since less pelvic space is occupied and lower perinatal mortality and morbidity result. Reports of scalp lacerations, cephalhematoma, and even intracranial hemorrhage dampened the initial and short-lived enthusiasm that greeted the device in the United States. A few American clinics and a number of European clinics continue to find the device better than forceps. These conflicting results have not been adequately explained. Our personal reaction is that the vacuum extractor is not as effective in extraction as forceps and that the hazards associated with its use are as great as with forceps. The last word has not been written about this instrument.

Other Abnormalities of Labor

MULTIPLE PREGNANCY

A multiple pregnancy is one in which more than one fetus develops. The exact incidence of this event is unknown for several reasons. Information collected on birth certificates or in hospital obstetrical units excludes abortion data, and twins are known to abort more frequently than do singletons. Further, the "twin" may be born in an unrecognized form, such as a fetus papyraceus, and the delivery will not be recorded as a twin birth.

From delivery information, it is evident that twinning varies by race and age of the gravida as well as by hereditary factors. Dizygotic twinning is more common in the black race (1 to 73.3) than among whites (1 to 93.3) and even less common in the yellow race. The incidence of twinning increases with maternal age in all races. It is known that twinning is more common in certain families, and a hereditary factor is evident. Whether this factor is passed only through maternal genes or whether the paternal genes also exert an influence is uncertain. All these influences on the incidence of twinning are exerted on the frequency of dizygotic, not monozygotic, twinning, however. Indeed, the frequency of monozygotic twinning is amazingly similar in all races. The recent use of agents

that are effective ovulatory stimulants (gonadotropins, clomiphene) has greatly increased the likelihood of multiple pregnancy, frequently triplets or quadruplets. This effect may be dose-related, or it may depend on an idiosyncratic patient response.

Monozygotic twins result from the division of one fertilized ovum in a very early stage of gestation. Dizygotic twins develop when two separate ova are fertilized by two separate sperm cells. Superfecundation, that is, fertilization of two ova by two separate coital actions during the same menstrual cycle, may explain dizygosity, although one act of coitus is the most frequent explanation. Superfetation, that is, fertilization of two ova released at two different ovulatory cycles, has not been shown to occur in the human. The biology of the two types of twinning is of some importance to the obstetrician because he is the authority most likely to be questioned about the zygosity of a set of twins. He is in the best position to express an opinion on the matter if he carefully examines the placenta at delivery.

Dizygotic twins may be of the same or opposite sex. Two amnions and two chorions are always present, although the placentas may have fused, giving the appearance of one placenta. Monozygotic twins are always of the same sex, but since the splitting of the conceptus may occur at various times, the number of amnions and chorions will vary. If the splitting occurs before the third day after ovulation, two chorions and two amnions will form (Fig. 11-11). If the split occurs after day 3 but before day 8, the twins will have one chorion and two amnions. Rarely, the twinning occurs after day 8, and in this instance the amnion does not split, and the twins are monoamniotic, monochorionic. Most monozygotic twins (about two-thirds) are diamniotic, monochorionic, while most of the remainder are diamniotic, dichorionic. Monoamniotic twins are rare and are particularly susceptible to umbilical cord accidents; two fetuses occupy the same amniotic space, allowing the cords to entwine.

Determination of zygosity is based on the preceding observations when possible and on the other factors as necessary. In the unusual instance of one

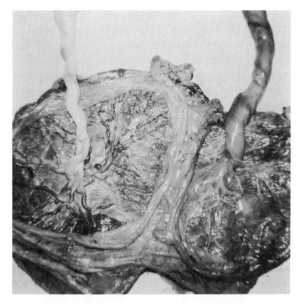

Fig. 11-11. Placenta from dichorionic twin pregnancy. Fetus from placenta on the right died in utero.

amniotic sac, monozygosity is certain. If the membranes separating the two fetal sacs consist of two layers only (two amnions), monozygosity is equally certain. If the membranes can be separated into three or four layers (two amnions plus two chorions, with the chorions often fused), the zygosity cannot be stated with certainty on the basis of this observation alone. If the twins are of unlike sex, dizygosity is certain. With twins of the same sex, other tests must be employed to determine the zygosity. Blood grouping of major and minor factors will enable recognition of zygosity in most cases. While dizygosity can be diagnosed with certainty, identical blood groupings will not permit a definite diagnosis of monozygosity. Subsequent observation of these infants by a pediatrician is necessary to make an accurate diagnosis. Determination of zygosity is of increasing clinical importance as organ transplant surgery becomes more commonplace.

Using these techniques, 668 pairs of twins in a British study were analyzed as follows [8]:

Monochorial and hence monozygotic: 20 percent.

Of unlike sex and dichorial, hence dizygotic: 35 percent.

Of like sex and dichorial, hence zygosity uncertain: 45 percent.

Genotyping allowed 37 percent to be recognized as dizygotic. The remainder (8 percent) were presumed to be monozygotic.

Diagnosis

There is usually evidence of twins on physical examination, and when the diagnosis is missed, it is primarily because the physician has not kept multiple pregnancy in mind. The first clue is a family history of twinning. This information is usually offered by the patient. A finding of major importance is a uterine size larger than the gestational interval suggests. While an unusually large uterus may be due to a gestation of longer length than suggested by the menstrual history or a hydaditiform mole, a multiple pregnancy must always be considered. Careful abdominal palpation will usually reveal the presence of more than two fetal poles, although it is not always possible to identify two fetal heads. Some observers have been aided by the presence of fetal heart rates of differing frequency observed in areas far removed from one another. This sign is of infrequent help in our experience. The definitive diagnosis must be made with the help of an x-ray film or with ultrasonography. While ultrasonography may identify two fetuses as early as the first trimester of pregnancy, x-ray diagnosis is undependable before the sixth month because fetal movements may obscure the ill-defined skeleton. Thereafter, accuracy near 100 percent is possible.

Management

When the diagnosis of multiple pregnancy is established, the gravida should receive extraordinary prenatal attention for many reasons. Acute toxemia of pregnancy is more frequent with twins than with a singleton, and so is hydramnios. The greatly enlarged uterus increases the severity of backache and pelvic pressure, and varicosities and edema of the lower extremities are likely to be unusually severe.

Fetal hazards are even more evident. In addition to the risk imposed if toxemia occurs, premature labor is an ever-present hazard. Indeed, early labor is the major factor in the greatly elevated perinatal mortality associated with multiple gestation. It is the shortened gestation that is lethal, since a twin has a lower perinatal mortality than does the singleton of equal birth weight.

Although not amenable to treatment, the hazard of the "transfusion syndrome" should be recognized; this syndrome occurs only with monochorial twins. When vessel anastomoses develop between the two fetuses, one fetus is likely to become hypervolemic, with cardiac hypertrophy and exaggerated growth; the other becomes anemic and suffers malnutrition and delayed growth. If the syndrome is severe, the second twin may die in utero. If death occurs early, the fetus may be compressed, with the resultant development of a fetus papyraceus. In another example, one infant may require immediate postnatal transfusion, while the other requires phlebotomy to avoid cardiac decompensation. The presence of the rare acardiac monster has also been explained on the basis of the transfusion syndrome. The first twin enjoys a major circulatory advantage, while the second twin is acardiac because of lack of blood flow to develop the heart. The acardiac monster may be so small as to elude recognition at delivery or so large as to cause dystocia. Finally, in rare instances, monozygotic twins remain fused and deliver as conjoined (Siamese) twins. In this instance, survival is the exception.

If the prenatal course is carefully monitored, many of these risks can be avoided. Certainly, acute toxemia of pregnancy can usually be identified in a very early stage, which will allow treatment to be initiated. Persistent acute toxemia poses a therapeutic dilemma, however, since interruption of the pregnancy frequently results in the birth of immature fetuses. Prolongation of pregnancy with persistent toxemia, on the other hand, usually fails to encourage the desired intrauterine growth of the fetuses, and the risk of intrauterine fetal death is always present. Interruption usually is the preferred approach.

Premature labor poses a most common fetal hazard and can be effectively prevented in many cases. The time-honored therapy of prolonged bed rest is of little use for most obstetrical problems, but the tendency of twins to be born prematurely can be effectively reduced by bed rest. A number of clinical trials have established the usefulness of this therapy, but the mechanism of action is unknown. Presumably, the uterus is rendered less irritable in this situation. Of at least theoretical usefulness to prevent premature labor is the avoidance of an orgasmic response; one investigator has shown a "triggering" of labor with orgasm [9]. The precise clinical usefulness of this information is uncertain at the present time.

Management of Delivery

The presentations of twin fetuses are both vertex in one-third to one-half of cases, both breech in about 10 percent, and cephalic-breech in most of the remaining. Shoulder presentations in one or both fetuses is seen in about 10 percent of cases.

Delivery of twins is likely to be complicated by the smallness of the babies, frequent malpresentations, uterine dysfunction from overdistention of the uterus, and occasionally by interlocking twins. A complication of the postpartum period is the uterine atony resulting from overdistention of the uterus. All these factors must be kept in mind as labor begins.

The first stage of labor is frequently uncomplicated, although uterine dysfunction, usually secondary to arrest of dilatation or lack of fetal descent, may occur. Since the fetuses are small, fetopelvic dystocia is uncommon unless the presentation is a transverse lie. While oxytocin may correct the uterine dysfunction, the overdistended uterus with its risk of subsequent rupture should be kept in mind.

The frequent malpresentations usually do not interfere with the progress of labor. Prolapse of the umbilical cord is an ever-present danger when the presenting part does not fit well into the pelvic inlet. If the first twin presents as a transverse lie—an uncommon occurrence—cesarean section may be necessary. With all other presentations, section is reserved for obstetrical indications, with lack of progress of labor being the most common. Many obstetricians feel that an easy forceps delivery is less traumatic to the head of a premature infant than is spontaneous delivery. We agree with this concept and encourage the routine use of outlet forceps in such deliveries.

The method of delivery of the second twin poses a controversy. Certain factors increase the risk for the second twin, e.g., malpresentation, and contraction of the partially emptied uterus, with the risk of placental separation. While undue haste in the delivery of the second twin may result in maternal damage, delivery should be effected within 15 minutes. Occasionally, a second infant will descend rapidly through the pelvis and deliver without difficulty. More often, however, the second twin does not enter the pelvic inlet quickly because of the lack of uterine contractions or because of a malposition. We think it best to encourage the early delivery of the second twin, first by amniotomy; then, if descent does not occur within a few minutes, by breech extraction if the breech presents or by version and extraction if the presentation is vertex or transverse lie. General anesthesia should be used for any intrauterine manipulation.

Analgesia should be kept to a minimum or avoided altogether when premature labor is anticipated. Anesthesia for the first twin should not depress the baby (e.g., general anesthesia) or interfere with the possibility of intrauterine manipulation by providing poor relaxation of the uterus (e.g., conduction anesthesia). Pudendal block anesthesia for the first twin and general anesthesia to allow uterine relaxation for the delivery of the second twin would seem ideal. Circumstances surrounding the birth, however, may suggest a different choice.

Interlocking twins are rare but are usually seen when the first twin presents by breech and the second by vertex. As the first twin delivers, his chin interlocks with the chin of the second fetus who is trying to enter the pelvis. Delivery of the first twin can rarely be completed successfully, and a destructive operation on the first baby may be necessary to allow successful management of the second twin. No effective method is currently available for

detecting the likelihood of this tragic occurrence. Fortunately, the accident is a rare one.

Atony of the uterus in the postpartum period must always be anticipated when the uterus has been overdistended with twins. It may be possible to decrease the risk of this complication by a modest delay in delivery of the second twin. Certainly, the atony can be minimized by the administration of a dilute solution of intravenous oxytocin to be started immediately after the delivery of the second twin. To expedite the oxytocic administration, it may be wise to have an intravenous solution of 5 percent glucose in water running before delivery, adding oxytocin to the solution after delivery. The fundus must be palpated and massaged at frequent intervals following delivery if hemorrhage is to be avoided.

Multiple pregnancy of more than two fetuses presents the same problems as do twins but frequently in an exaggerated form. Triplets occur about once in every 9000 deliveries and quadruplets and quintuplets with great infrequency, except following ovulation-producing drugs.

PREMATURE LABOR

Premature birth is the major cause of perinatal death in the United States. The importance of prematurity as a cause of perinatal death is demonstrated by Chase's [10] estimation that "at the present level of mortality in the United States, an arithmetic increase of 1 percent in infants weighing less than 2,501 gm. at birth causes a relative increase of 10 percent in the first week mortality."

Traditionally, premature labor has been defined as labor that results in the birth of an infant weighing 2500 gm. or less at birth. With the increasing realization that some infants experience intrauterine growth retardation (IUGR) and may be mature but of low birth weight, a new concept developed. *Premature labor* is better defined as labor occurring at less than 37 weeks' gestation. A *low-birth-weight infant* is an infant of whatever gestation who weighs 2500 gm. or less when born. In the majority of instances, premature labor results in the delivery of a low-birth-weight infant, and in the following discussion these two terms are used interchangeably except where noted.

Incidence

The delivery of an infant of low birth weight occurred in 7.8 percent of deliveries in the United States in 1960, but the incidence was only 6.8 percent in whites and 12.7 percent in blacks. A disturbing increase to 8.2 percent for both races was reported in 1964. Since that time, the incidence has decreased with an incidence of 7.1 percent in both races in 1977, 5.9 percent among whites and 12.8 percent among blacks. Why the incidence is so much higher in blacks than in whites has been under constant study. A potent socioeconomic factor is undoubtedly operating, but the possibility that genetic factors are also at work is a reasonable theory. The length of gestation is slightly shorter in blacks than in whites, and this may be genetically determined. The incidence of low-birth-weight infants in Great Britain and other European countries has been consistently lower than in the United States. For one possible explanation of this observation, see the section on Nutrition During Pregnancy in Chapter 3.

Cause

The cause of premature labor in the individual patient is unknown in the majority of instances. However, a large number of factors are known to increase the risk of premature labor, and one or more of these factors may be present in an individual patient. ① *Premature rupture of the membranes* (PROM) occurs in at least 20 percent of patients with premature labor. The cause of PROM is unknown, but a strong socioeconomic effect is indicated by a much higher incidence among lower socioeconomic groups (see Premature Rupture of Membranes). ② *Multiple pregnancy* frequently terminates before 37 weeks' gestation, and low birth weight is commonly noted. ③ *Hypertensive cardiovascular disease* and *acute hypertensive disease of pregnancy* result in premature birth, both because IUGR is sometimes an accompaniment of the disease and because clinical necessity frequently demands premature induction of labor.

Premature induction of labor or early cesarean section may also be necessary with ④ *diabetes mellitus*, but in this case, a larger baby for the shortened length of gestation may result because of the well-recognized macrosomia in infants of diabetic mothers. ⑤ Third-trimester bleeding from *placenta previa* or *abruptio placentae* results in premature spontaneous labor or premature intentional delivery. ⑥ *Cigarette smoking* has been shown to be associated with infants of lower mean birth weight and perhaps also of shortened gestation. ⑦ *Asymptomatic bacteriuria* has been reported to predispose to premature labor [11]. Many investigators have been unable to confirm this relationship, but acute urinary tract infection (and probably also other acute febrile infections) does predispose to premature labor [12]. ⑧ *Uterine abnormalities* such as a septate uterus cause premature labor in many patients. And a large number of cases of premature labor remain unexplained.

Prevention

With the myriad of possible etiologic factors and the infrequency with which a single factor is recognized in the individual patient, the prevention of premature labor has proved an elusive goal. Certain treatments, however, have either been shown to be effective in specific cases or are thought to be effective often enough to warrant their use.

Bed rest is known to delay the onset of labor in patients with a multiple pregnancy and should be prescribed in these gravidas. By inference, bed rest may be useful in any patient threatening to go into labor prematurely. Vigorous antibiotic treatment of pyelonephritis and other acute infections should be prescribed. *Surgical correction* of a uterine abnormality before pregnancy may be beneficial. *Expectant management* of patients with placenta previa has reduced the perinatal mortality with this disease.

The recent introduction of determinations of the lecithin-sphingomyelin (L/S) ratio in amniotic fluid to predict lung maturity has added materially, although indirectly, to the prevention of premature labor. It is now possible to predict with some accuracy when the fetal lung is sufficiently mature to

Table 11-1. Tocolysis Score

Factor	0	1	2	3	4
Contractions	—	Irregular	Regular 10 min.	—	—
PROM	—	—	High or ?	—	Low
Bleeding	—	Spotting; moderate bleeding	Severe bleeding (100 ml.)	—	—
Cervical dilatation (cm.)	—	1	2	3	≥4

PROM = premature rupture of membranes.
Source: After W. Gruber and K. Baumgarten. *Perinatal Medicine*. 4th European Congress of Perinatal Medicine, Thieme, Stuttgart, 1975. P. 356.

allow extrauterine survival. Postponement of a necessary induction or cesarean section, or pharmacologic prevention of premature labor for a period of time, may permit the fetal lungs to mature (see Premature Rupture of Membranes).

Pharmacologic agents that are thought to prevent or delay premature labor are now available for general use or are undergoing clinical trial.

Diagnosis

The diagnosis of premature labor is made on the basis of a history of regular uterine contractions *and* evidence of progressive change in the cervix (effacement, or dilatation, or both). A history of contractions is in itself unreliable, since many patients experience Braxton Hicks contractions during the third trimester without going into labor. If cervical effacement or dilatation accompanies the cramps, premature labor is evident. Some objectivity in the diagnosis can be reached by using a Tocolysis Score (Table 11-1). The probability of stopping labor with betamimetics described below can be estimated from the Tocolysis Score (Table 11-2). It is evident that low scores frequently indicate false labor.

Termination of Premature Labor

Various pharmacologic agents have been used or recommended to arrest premature labor. While the precise physiologic mechanism for the initiation of labor is unknown, certain mechanisms that seem to be related to the onset of labor can be affected by these agents. Alcohol is thought to block the re-

Table 11-2. Probability of Stopping Labor for 1 Week with Betamimetics

Score	1	2	3	4	5	6	≥7
Labor stopped (%)	100	90	84	38	11	7	Never

Source: After W. Gruber and K. Baumgarten. *Perinatal Medicine*. 4th European Congress of Perinatal Medicine, Thieme, Stuttgart, 1975. P. 356.

⊕ Calcium gluconate can be used to reverse the Mg sulfate effect (= Convannya!)

lease of oxytocin from the posterior pituitary gland. Similarly, loading the maternal circulation with a rapid intravenous infusion of fluids is thought to block both the release of antidiuretic hormone and oxytocin from the pituitary gland. Magnesium sulfate ⊕ is thought to reduce uterine contractility and some clinicians have used this drug to attempt labor inhibition. Betamimetic drugs, especially those with beta-2 effects (Terbutaline, isoxsuprine), have also been used to stop premature labor. Progesterone alone has been shown to be ineffective, however. Prostaglandins act as myometrial membrane receptors for various hormones and are thought to be important in the initiation of labor. Various antiprostaglandin drugs (aspirin, naproxen, and indomethacin) act as antiprostaglandins and theoretically might stop premature labor. The antiprostaglandin drugs have the potential for delaying closure of the ductus arteriosus in the newborn and their use is not recommended. These drugs, therefore, will not be discussed further.

Currently, the betamimetics are the most widely

used method for terminating premature labor. Terbutaline, a beta-2 mimetic drug with direct effects on the uterine and lung smooth muscles, with only mild cardiovascular effect, is in the widest use in the United States at the present time. After intravenous hydration with Ringer's lactate solution, and after elimination of patients over 35 years of age and those with a history of cardiac disease or congestive heart failure, the drug is administered subcutaneously and subsequently orally. Maternal side effects include tachycardia, light-headedness, flushing, and, rarely, hypotension. Pulmonary edema has been reported in a small number of these patients but responds well to standard therapy for congestive heart failure. Mild maternal hyperglycemia, plasma volume expansion, and hypokalemia are also seen in patients on Terbutaline. No ill effects on the fetus have been noted to date.

Isoxsuprine (Vasodilan), another betamimetic drug, has also been in common usage for inhibiting labor. This drug has more alpha stimulation with a resultant higher risk of maternal cardiovascular side effects such as hypotension and tachycardia. Frequent monitoring of blood pressure and pulse is necessary. Many other betamimetic drugs have also been used, but none has had frequent usage in the United States.

Alcohol has been shown to decrease uterine contractility through suppression of oxytocin release from the posterior pituitary gland. The drug has been used extensively with uncertain effectiveness and with major side effects, especially severe intoxication with nausea and vomiting in the mother. Long-term use may incur a risk of inducing the fetal alcohol syndrome.

If labor cannot be stopped, certain steps should be taken to protect the fetus. Minimal or no analgesics should be used since depression of the premature fetus may be lethal. Local or conduction anesthesia for delivery is preferred for the same reason. An atraumatic delivery is essential, but neither the use of prophylactic outlet forceps nor low vertical cesarean section has been fully evaluated in this regard. A wide episiotomy is useful to minimize fetal head trauma. The presence of a

pediatrician or other expert in neonatal resuscitation in the delivery room is essential. (Immediate care of the premature infant is discussed in Chapter 13.)

PREMATURE RUPTURE OF MEMBRANES
When the fetal membranes rupture before labor begins, premature rupture of the membranes is said to have occurred. This sequence of events is present in about 15 percent of patients, 30 percent when the infant weighs less than 2500 gms., 13 percent in those above this weight limit [13]. If labor ensues promptly, as it does in 9 out of 10 cases, and if the gestation is at term, little harm results. If, however, labor fails to begin within 24 hours, there is a sharp increase in the risk of infection. This factor results in a sharp increase in the perinatal death risk in the term pregnancy with ruptured membranes beyond 24 hours and, to a lesser extent, in the preterm patient. While the maternal risk is much smaller, amnionitis may lead to serious maternal infection, even septic shock and death.

Pregnancy at Term
Labor ensues within 24 hours in most cases of premature rupture of the membranes when the patient is near term. In many instances, labor will begin spontaneously within 6 hours of the rupture and this event may be awaited. Without evident labor after 6 hours, however, induction with a dilute intravenous solution of oxytocin is indicated. Labor usually begins promptly and delivery occurs within a reasonable number of hours. If labor fails to begin with the induction, the choice between cesarean section and further waiting is not an easy one. Cesarean section is chosen by more and more obstetricians because the hazards of intrauterine infection seem greater than the hazards of unexpected immaturity. This is especially true in centers with excellent facilities for the care of the neonate.

Preterm Pregnancy
The management of premature rupture of the membranes in the premature infant will vary according to a number of factors: the number of weeks of gestation, the risk of infection at the par-

ticular hospital involved with the patient's care, and the degree of sophistication of the neonatal unit that will care for the infant. If a gestation is greater than 34 weeks, and if the L/S ratio is greater than 2, suggesting maturity of the fetal lungs, the patient may be treated aggressively as we have described for the patient at term. Labor should be induced. If the gestation is below the limit of viability (26 weeks?), the physician may choose to recommend evacuation of the uterus by induction of labor to protect the mother from the risks of infection at the cost of fetal loss. The gravida herself may choose to wait for greater fetal maturity even with an increased maternal risk, although such expectant management almost never succeeds if premature rupture of the membranes occurs before 26 weeks' gestation. Before electing to ignore the possibility of fetal survival in such cases, it is best to confirm the gestational interval by B-scan determination of the biparietal diameter.

Between 28 and 34 weeks, some obstetricians now recommend a planned delay of 48 to 72 hours or more before delivery during which time maternal corticosteroid therapy is prescribed to accelerate fetal pulmonary maturation. If necessary, labor may be inhibited with beta-sympathomimetic drugs until the steroids have had a full 48 hours to become effective. This therapeutic regimen should still be considered an experimental one since the proof of better perinatal survival remains elusive and since the effect of steroids or the labor-inhibiting agents on the long-term development of the newborn remains uncertain.

Maternal antibiotics are prescribed for premature rupture of the membranes by many authorities. Others argue that the risk of fetal infection is little reduced by maternal antibiotics and at a cost of confusion over what antibiotics to prescribe for the development of infection in the newborn. If maternal antibiotics are to be used, ampicillin is probably the best choice because of its wide spectrum of activity and because it crosses the placenta easily, unlike many other antibiotics. It has been shown that the risk of amnionitis is less if antibiotics are prescribed for the mother.

The diagnosis of membrane rupture is not always an easy one to make but is often of such great clinical import that efforts should be made to determine whether or not there is amniotic fluid in the vault of the vagina. Methods for detecting the presence of amniotic fluid are described in Chapter 9.

PROLAPSE OF THE UMBILICAL CORD AND OTHER CORD ACCIDENTS

Prolapse of the umbilical cord is said to be present when the cord presents ahead of the presenting part (overt prolapse) or alongside the presenting part (occult prolapse). While the effect of the two varieties is similar, the degree of fetal risk is higher with overt prolapse, since impingement of the cord between the pelvis and the presenting part is apt to be more severe and more certain. Overt prolapse includes those cases in which the cord can be palpated in the vagina, as well as those in which the cord actually extrudes from the introitus. The hazard is primarily to the fetus, but undue haste or unwise interference may also endanger the mother. The accident occurs about once in 200 deliveries.

Etiology

Prolapse of the cord is most frequently seen when the presenting part does not accurately adapt to the pelvic inlet. Breech presentation, especially the footling variety, face position, and transverse lie are the common predisposing factors. Prolapse of the cord occasionally occurs when the vertex fails to engage for whatever reason (e.g., poor flexion of the head, fetopelvic disproportion) and following amniotomy, before the presenting part is well into the pelvis. A recent study related prolapse of the cord to amniotomy in one-fourth of cases [14], although other factors were also sometimes at work. Prematurity is a strongly related factor; birth weight is less than 2500 gm. in nearly one-half the fetuses. Immature gestation combined with possible intrauterine asphyxia from interference with umbilical cord circulation is a deadly combination.

Diagnosis

Diagnosis of cord prolapse is usually easy. A change in the FHR may suggest the diagnosis, which can be confirmed by pelvic examination.

The cord is easily felt if the membranes are ruptured and if pulsations remain. It may be impossible to feel through intact membranes, and experience is necessary to recognize a pulseless cord. If the cord prolapse is through the introitus, anyone can make the diagnosis.

What is most important is that the diagnosis be made early and, indeed, anticipated if possible. Whenever conditions favoring prolapse of the cord are present, special vigilance in monitoring the FHR is required. A pelvic examination must be performed immediately following spontaneous rupture of the membranes in any patient who exhibits a change in FHR pattern following spontaneous rupture. Of great importance in the prevention of prolapse of the cord is the avoidance of amniotomy, except as an emergency measure, before engagement of the presenting part has occurred or with malpresentation of the presenting part at any pelvic level. The risks of amniotomy must at all times be balanced against the gains expected.

Treatment

Treatment of prolapse of the cord is early delivery if the cord continues to pulsate. Delay will pose undue risks for the fetus, but traumatic delivery is dangerous for the mother. Therefore, the best method of delivery is usually cesarean section. Version and extraction may be an acceptable alternative if no fetopelvic disproportion exists, if full dilatation of the cervix has occurred, and if the physician has had experience with this maneuver. The operation is probably best reserved for the multigravida.

If cesarean section is chosen, it must be performed immediately. While the patient is being transferred to the operating room, she should be placed in the Trendelenberg position to minimize fetal pressure on the umbilical cord. A gloved hand should be kept in the vagina to keep the fetal presenting part out of the pelvis and away from the prolapsed cord. No attempt should be made to replace the cord, since more harm than good will usually result. If the cord is pulseless, or if the FHR is markedly slow without periods of recovery, section is not justified, since fetal survival is unlikely.

Prognosis for the infant depends on the rapidity with which the diagnosis is made and treatment begun, as well as on the maturity of the fetus. If the fetus survives the neonatal period, the likelihood of normal brain development is directly related to the degree of maturity, not usually to the degree of asphyxia. This fact should be comforting to the parents of such a child.

RUPTURE OF THE PREGNANT UTERUS

Rupture of the pregnant uterus still accounts for maternal deaths in spite of advances in obstetrical care. While the specific causes of uterine rupture have changed over the past two or three decades, the overall incidence has remained about the same. As cesarean section has replaced the difficult operative vaginal delivery in obstetrical care, the number of uterine ruptures caused by traumatic procedures has decreased, but the number of ruptures through cesarean section scars has increased. Fortunately, the latter occurrence is frequently less life-threatening than the former.

While uterine rupture may occur with an interstitial pregnancy or with abortion induced by hypertonic saline or prostaglandin, the term *uterine rupture* is usually reserved for ruptures occurring after 20 weeks of gestation. The rupture may occur (1) spontaneously in an intact uterus, (2) as a result of trauma, or (3) through a previous cesarean section scar.

Spontaneous Rupture in an Intact Uterus

Rupture of the intact uterus before labor is exceedingly rare and is usually related to previous uterine sepsis, previous curettage, or pregnancy in a poorly developed uterine horn. The author has recently seen a paper-thin uterine horn in a pregnancy interrupted by hysterotomy at four months' gestation. If pregnancy had been allowed to continue in this patient, uterine rupture would surely have occurred.

Rupture of the intact uterus during labor can be due to neglect of a patient with fetopelvic disproportion or to rupture through an area of the cervix where excessive scar tissue has resulted from a previous delivery. The rupture is almost always through the lower uterine segment. A major factor in rupture of the intact uterus is the use of oxytocin for poor labor progress, especially in the older patient of high parity. Even minor degrees of fetopelvic disproportion may cause rupture in a parous uterus if oxytocin produces unusually strong contractions. Indeed, poor contractions in this situation may serve as a "safety valve," and indicate that all is not well in this grand multipara. Recent tabulations of patients with uterine rupture have pointed out the frequency with which oxytocin has appeared in the history of these patients [15, 16]. While oxytocin carefully administered is a safe drug, its use for lack of labor progress in the woman who has had four or more pregnancies is associated with a substantial risk of uterine rupture.

Traumatic Rupture of the Uterus

Abdominal trauma is a rare cause of spontaneous rupture of the intact uterus and should be ruled out in anyone involved in an automobile accident.

A more common cause of traumatic rupture of the uterus is a vaginal operative procedure intended to facilitate delivery of the fetus. As with spontaneous rupture of the intact uterus, traumatic rupture nearly always occurs in the lower uterine segment. While version and extraction or breech decomposition and extraction are the most likely operations to result in uterine rupture, simple breech extraction of a footling presentation, or even the mid-forceps operation, may be at fault. Certain factors predispose to uterine rupture with an operative procedure. If the membranes are intact before the version and extraction or breech decomposition is performed, ample room for intrauterine manipulation exists. If the membranes have been ruptured for some hours, the uterus will have clamped down more tightly on the fetus, allowing much less room for the procedure. Simple breech extraction or a mid-forceps operation is occasionally performed just before full cervical dilatation has occurred, e.g., for prolapse of the umbilical cord, and rupture of the uterus is more likely to occur in this set of circumstances.

The increasingly frequent use of cesarean section in preference to a potentially traumatic vaginal delivery has markedly decreased the number of uterine ruptures from trauma. The obstetrician who chooses a vaginal operative procedure should have a good reason for doing so. He should remember also that vigorous fundal pressure used to complete a difficult vaginal delivery will in itself cause uterine rupture on occasion.

Rupture of the Uterus Through a Cesarean Section Scar

Rupture of the uterus through a previous cesarean section or myomectomy scar accounts for an increasing number of reported cases as the indications for the use of cesarean section are liberalized. Rupture is more likely to occur through a classic cesarean section scar than through a scar in the lower uterine segment. Recognition of this fact has led to an increased use of the lower segment type.

The classical cesarean section incision is made in the contractile portion of the uterus. Formerly, it was made across the top of the fundus (high classical section), but in recent years it has been made almost exclusively through the anterior uterine wall (low classical section). About 1 percent of these low classical incisions will rupture during labor, and a slightly smaller percentage will rupture before labor. The rupture is likely to be a massive rent, with severe maternal symptoms and extrusion of the fetus in most cases. Usually, it is necessary to remove the uterus at the time of laparotomy.

With incision in the lower uterine segment (low flap section), subsequent rupture of the uterus is less frequent and less likely to be overt and massive than with classical incisions; it is more likely to be "silent," or occult. Moreover, rupture almost never occurs before the onset of labor. With an occult rupture, few if any symptoms are experienced, and the defect in the lower segment may be found incidentally at the time of repeat section. Undoubtedly, an uneventful labor and vaginal delivery can occur with an occult rupture, at least in some cases. The rupture typically involves the uterine musculature only, with the fetal membranes and the overlying peritoneum intact. The rent may be safely repaired without hysterectomy following repeat section. If the uterine rupture is massive, however, the rent may do damage to the surrounding tissue, even causing lacerations of the bladder.

The type of delivery performed subsequent to a cesarean section remains a controversial issue, although most obstetricians follow the dictum, "once a section, always a section." Certainly, the maternal and fetal risk of subsequent rupture following a classical incision scar is great. Maternal mortality may approach 5 percent in these cases, while at least half the fetuses die. Moreover, only two-thirds of the accidents can be prevented by repeat section before the onset of labor. One-third of the ruptures occur in the third trimester, before labor begins. The lower-segment rupture, however, is much less frequent than rupture of the upper segment and should be preventable by scheduling repeat section before the onset of labor. Since an unexpectedly small infant will occasionally result from this practice, it is not an altogether desirable one. Increasingly, we use amniotic fluid sampling to determine fetal maturity before scheduling a repeat section. Methods used to analyze the fluid are described in Chapter 12. It seems certain that the combined use of amniotic fluid sampling and repeat section before the onset of labor will lower perinatal mortality and the risk of uterine rupture.

Clinical Picture of Uterine Rupture

Excluding occult rupture, which is usually silent or nearly so, rupture of the uterus produces a catastrophic clinical picture. The patient experiences severe abdominal pain followed by a tearing sensation and a marked decrease in the pain. If the rupture has extended into the broad ligament, subsequent bleeding may be minimized by the restricted space into which it can escape. On the other hand, communication with the peritoneal cavity results in massive hemorrhage and extrusion of the fetus into the cavity. The fetus may then be palpated in greater detail, since only the abdominal wall covers the fetus. A large, hard, globular mass, the contracted empty uterus, may be felt suprapubically. If the rupture has occurred during labor, the presenting part will no longer be palpable in the pelvis; the uterine rent may or may not be palpable.

Shock usually quickly supervenes and becomes profound if bleeding is not controlled. External bleeding may be scant, or it may become more profuse as the clinical course proceeds. If the patient is untreated, death will result in many cases. With adequate treatment, maternal mortality remains about 5 percent if the rupture has occurred through a classical cesarean section scar. Mortality is much higher if the rupture has occurred in an intact uterus.

Treatment

The measures that must be instituted immediately after the diagnosis is made are (1) the treatment of shock with adequate transfusion and ancillary measures and (2) laparotomy to stop the hemorrhage. In most cases, hysterectomy will be necessary, usually of the supracervical type, unless a total hysterectomy is required to stop the bleeding. Ligation of the hypogastric arteries may be preferable to removal of the cervix if the ureters are thought to be vulnerable to damage. In rare cases, the rent in the uterus may be repaired, although this practice is not recommended by most American obstetricians. This technique is most likely to be applicable to a rent through a lower-segment scar. The fetal loss with uterine rupture approaches 75 percent, and immediate laparotomy offers the only possibility of improving this figure.

PLACENTA ACCRETA

Placenta accreta is recognized clinically when the placenta adheres abnormally to the uterus following delivery. An association between placenta previa and placenta accreta has been mentioned by some authors. Pathological examination shows that the decidual layer is defective and the placenta is attached directly to the myometrium. Placenta accreta may be *total*, that is, none of the placenta can be separated from the uterus; or it may be *partial*, that is, only a few areas are adherent, and the remaining placenta is easily separated. If the placental attachment actually invades the uterine musculature, *placenta increta* is diagnosed. If the placenta reaches the serosal surface of the uterus (or, rarely, into the peritoneal cavity), *placenta percreta* is the term used.

Placenta accreta of the complete variety is very rare; placenta increta and percreta are even less common. Placenta accreta of the partial type is more common, although a precise incidence figure cannot be given because of variability in making the diagnosis. If a small area of the placenta is adherent during manual removal of the organ, some obstetricians might employ the term placenta accreta, while others would describe the placenta as merely adherent. In this mild form, the condition is not rare and seldom causes serious harm.

Treatment of total placenta accreta is laparotomy and abdominal hysterectomy. No attempt should be made to create a tissue plane between the placenta and the uterus, since either uterine perforation or severe hemorrhage will ensue. The treatment of lesser degrees of the disease must fit the circumstances. If a small area of adherent placenta can be peeled off the uterus with relative ease, this is the best course to follow. If a larger area is involved, or if removal proves to be difficult, hysterectomy is a wiser choice.

AMNIOTIC FLUID EMBOLUS

Amniotic fluid embolism, though rare, may be a cause of maternal death during labor or immediately following delivery. At autopsy, the diagnosis is confirmed when the pulmonary vasculature is found to contain the particulate matter of the amniotic fluid, i.e., lanugo hairs, desquamated epithelial cells, and, perhaps especially, meconium. The pathophysiologic mechanism causing death remains clouded, but the disease is probably initiated by the leakage of a large amount of amniotic fluid into the maternal circulation. The particulate matter blocks the pulmonary vasculature, and a clinical picture resembling the one noted with pulmonary embolism is initiated, i.e., dyspnea, cyanosis, pulmonary edema, and even death. If the patient survives the initial insult, a disturbance in blood clotting becomes evident. The patient may die of hypofibrinogenemia, which probably results from disseminated intravascular coagulation initiated by thromboplastic material released from the amniotic fluid. Apparently, a few patients have recovered from the disease, but without the pathologic confirmation obtainable only by microscopic examination of the lungs, the diagnosis in these patients remains in doubt.

Amniotic fluid embolism most commonly occurs in the multigravid patient whose labor is tumultuous. The membranes are usually ruptured, and in many cases the amniotic fluid contains meconium. The fetus may be large, or the fetal head may simply fit snugly in the lower uterine segment, thus effectively blocking the escape of amniotic fluid through the vagina. In some fashion, amniotic fluid enters the maternal circulation, either by dissection around the end of the placenta and into the dilated decidual veins or possibly through an open cervical vein. A very strong uterine contraction without the possibility of vaginal egress of the fluid completes the picture. Oxytocin has been implicated in a disproportionate number of cases.

Treatment is usually unsuccessful, since death occurs rapidly. Initially, the disease may be treated, as is pulmonary embolism, with oxygen and other supportive measures. If uncontrollable bleeding supervenes, blood replacement, supplemented by the administration of fibrinogen, may be the most logical course to follow. The therapeutic dilemma of treating shock due to blood loss with a large volume of transfused blood, which in turn will aggravate the acute cor pulmonale that results from the pulmonary blockage, is at present insoluble. If hemorrhage does not occur, cortisone, heparin, and endotracheal intubation may speed resolution of the pulmonary process.

EARLY POSTPARTUM HEMORRHAGE

Newton [17] measured an average blood loss in vaginal delivery of slightly greater than 500 ml. during the first 24 hours. A diagnosis of postpartum hemorrhage therefore requires a blood loss at least in excess of 500 ml. Postpartum hemorrhage may occur in the immediate postpartum period (early postpartum hemorrhage), or it may occur after the first 24 postpartum hours (late postpartum hemorrhage); the latter is discussed in Chapter 14. Although precise criteria for the diagnosis of hemorrhage may be elusive, it is most important to remember that steady modest bleeding can be just as hazardous as a sudden large hemorrhage; indeed, the former is more commonly encountered in clinical practice. Excessive bleeding of any amount must be investigated and treated vigorously *immediately* if unnecessary maternal deaths are to be avoided.

Etiology and Diagnosis

Early postpartum bleeding (that occurring during the first 24 postpartum hours) may be due to uterine atony, lacerations of the birth canal, or other unusual causes, such as retention of placental fragments and blood clotting defects.

Uterine atony can be anticipated in many instances. Overdistention of the uterus (large baby, twins, hydramnios), a prolonged labor, high parity, deep anesthesia for delivery, and the presence of placenta previa or abruptio placentae all predispose to excessive postpartum bleeding due to atony. When uterine atony seems a likely possibility, certain steps should be taken to prevent its development or to minimize its effects. For patients with predisposing factors, 1 to 2 units of blood should be cross-matched, so that immediate transfusion may be started if atony and hemorrhage develop. An intravenous infusion of dextrose in water should be started during labor, with the addition of 10 units of oxytocin to 500 ml. of fluid for rapid administration immediately after delivery of the baby. Routine manual exploration of the uterus to remove any placental fragments remaining after placental delivery can also be recommended. Expert care must be exercised in the management of the postpartum fundus, with judicious massage to maintain uterine tone for at least 2 hours after delivery.

Lacerations of the vagina, cervix, and even the lower uterine segment should be suspected with postpartum bleeding. Indeed, even the episiotomy normally is a major source of blood loss; an average loss of 253 ml. is reported by Odell and Seski [18]. Careful inspection of the vagina, cervix, and the lower uterine segment should routinely follow every delivery, especially an operative delivery. The vaginal canal can be visualized with the help of

an assistant and appropriate vaginal retractors, but careful palpation of the entire vagina is also necessary. The cervix can be visualized by having an assistant exert gentle abdominal pressure downward on the fundus, which will bring the cervix into view. Sponge forceps should be applied to the cervix for retraction, and the cervix should be inspected for lacerations throughout its circumference. All lacerations should be sutured with chromic catgut whether or not they are bleeding. A cervical laceration may occasionally be seen to extend upward into the lower uterine segment; when this is observed, a tamponade should be carefully applied in preparation for abdominal hysterectomy. Palpation of the lower uterine segment will identify the occasional laceration that cannot be visualized.

Retention of placental fragments is a rare cause for early postpartum hemorrhage and can be ruled out by careful manual exploration of the uterus, a procedure that should be routine with vaginal delivery. Focal placenta accreta will also be recognized in this manner and treated appropriately. A blood clotting defect may be suspected when bleeding persists in the absence of any other evident cause, and appropriate tests should be ordered for its identification.

Treatment

The following steps should be taken quickly if a blood loss greater than 500 ml. occurs after delivery. Preferably, the investigation should be completed before the patient leaves the delivery room, to avoid the possibility of a second anesthetic and the trauma of a reexamination.

1. Palpation of the uterine fundus to determine its contractile state.
2. Inspection and palpation of the cervicovaginal canal for lacerations.
3. Manual exploration of the uterus for retained placental fragments and for palpation of the lower uterine segment.
4. Initiation of an intravenous infusion if one is not already running and the addition of 10 units of oxytocin in 500 ml. of normal saline infusion.

5. Cross matching of at least 2 units of bank blood.
6. Collection of 5 ml. of maternal venous blood in a dry test tube for blood clotting determination (see Abruptio Placentae in Chap. 7).
7. Vigorous massage of the fundus if atony is suspected and if lacerations have been sutured.
8. If massage has failed to stop bleeding, bimanual compression of the uterus should be employed by applying pressure vaginally with the right fist against the anterior wall of the uterus and abdominally by compression of the posterior uterine fundus with the palm of the left hand.
9. If bimanual compression has failed to stop the bleeding, preparation for abdominal hysterectomy or hypogastric artery ligation should be begun.
10. The usual measures to treat hypovolemic shock (central venous pressure monitoring, transfusion, morphine, oxygen) must be used early and vigorously. The amount of blood loss is usually underestimated.

Hysterectomy or bilateral hypogastric artery ligation should be used only as a last resort yet early enough to avoid irreversible shock. Multiple transfusions will usually prepare the patient adequately for the necessary surgery. Placenta accreta may also necessitate hysterectomy.

CERVICAL LACERATIONS

A discussion of perineal and vaginal lacerations was included in the section on normal labor, since these are so commonly seen. Cervical lacerations, however, are less common and should be included in a discussion of abnormal labor.

Small cervical lacerations are probably a part of normal labor because of the enormous dilatation the cervix must undergo in such a short time. These lacerations are rarely symptomatic and are therefore usually not diagnosed. Larger tears may occur with spontaneous labor, but they are more frequently noted following forceps usage. The laceration may involve only the periphery of the cervix, or it may extend upward to involve the vagina or even the lower uterine segment. When the laceration involves the lower uterine segment, the diagnosis of a ruptured uterus is warranted. Treatment for this eventuality is instituted as described earlier in this chapter. Hysterectomy is almost always indicated. In some cases, the cervical laceration may occur in an annular fashion, with evulsion of the entire circumference of the cervix. Such lacerations may be caused either by tumultuous labor or, more frequently, by forceps delivery before full cervical dilatation. On occasion, the anterior lip of the cervix may be trapped between the symphysis pubis and the slowly descending fetal head, causing necrosis of this area of the cervix, with subsequent sloughing. Since many of these lacerations are asymptomatic, it is wise to examine the cervix routinely following delivery if subsequent hemorrhage is to be avoided.

Examination of the cervix is carried out with the help of ring or sponge forceps attached to the cervix and gently pulled downward. An assistant should push the fundus down to allow an easier pull on the cervix while a second assistant retracts the perineum and vagina. When a laceration is recognized, interrupted catgut sutures should be used to approximate the edges to prevent subsequent bleeding. Only a minimal number of sutures should be used, since the engorged area may bleed from each suture hole.

INVERSION OF THE UTERUS

On rare occasions following delivery, the uterus may turn inside out, so that the inside of the fundus protrudes into the vagina or through the introitus. This complication is termed *inversion of the uterus*. While an incomplete inversion may occur, in most cases the inversion is complete. The accident usually occurs immediately following delivery (acute). The diagnosis may be missed until a few hours later (subacute), or the condition may be missed for a longer period of time (chronic). Since acute inversion is the most common variety, shock is an early sign in most instances.

Although mismanagement of the third stage of labor (traction on the umbilical cord, vigorous Credé's maneuver) has been etiologically related to acute inversion, the literature, as well as our own experience, suggests the infrequency of these predisposing causes. Multiparity, also said to be a predisposing cause, seems to be an equally unlikely etiological factor, since over half the cases occur in primigravidas. In a recent series of 18 cases with matched controls, Watson et al. [19] noted no etiologic relationship between age, parity, duration of labor, type of delivery, or management of the third stage with inversion of the uterus. What is important is that the diagnosis be made without delay.

Following delivery of the placenta (occasionally, the placenta will remain attached to the inverted uterus), the inverted uterus may be seen protruding from the introitus, or it may be palpated as a large mass in the vagina. Bleeding is sometimes profuse, although some authors have said that the shock usually noted with the condition is out of proportion to the amount of blood loss and may be due to a severe vagal response. Abdominal examination reveals the fundus to be much lower than usual, with a dimpling effect; or it may not be felt at all. Since an occasional case of inversion will apparently produce no symptoms whatsoever, the possibility of inversion is another reason for performing a routine pelvic examination following delivery.

Treatment must be provided quickly. Blood is drawn for type and cross matching, and the patient is transfused as required. Even before the shock is reversed, the uterus is reinverted under light general anesthesia. One hand provides counterpressure abdominally on the fundus. The other hand is inserted into the vagina, and, with well-spread fingers gently pushing on the inner cervical margin, the uterus is pushed upward. The anatomic area inverted last—the cervix and the lower uterine segment—is the first area replaced. The procedure usually is an easy one and should be followed by fundal massage and intravenous administration of oxytocin to keep the uterus firm.

If the diagnosis has been missed and later replacement is not possible because of cervical edema, an operative procedure may be required. The operator may choose an abdominal approach in which an upward pull on clamps attached to the round ligaments and the anterior and posterior walls of the uterus may allow replacement. Failing this, the cervix may be incised longitudinally in its posterior aspect to allow replacement. A similar cervical incision may be made by the vaginal approach but, in this case, on the anterior cervical lip.

ABNORMALITIES OF FETAL HEART RATE

In Chapter 9, the normal FHR pattern was identified as one with a baseline rate between 120 and 160 and with a beat-to-beat variability of 6 to 10 or more beats per minute. Tachycardia (baseline greater than 160 beats per minute) may be present with prematurity, maternal fever, hyperthyroidism, after certain drugs (e.g., atropine), and as a very early sign of fetal hypoxia. It is usually not pathologic and usually demands no treatment unless other abnormal patterns coexist. Persistent bradycardia (baseline less than 120 beats per minute, 100 beats per minute according to some authorities) may be evidence of a congenital heart block in the fetus or may be seen as a very late pattern in a dying fetus.

Periodic Deceleration Patterns

Periodic FHR decelerations have been classified by Hon [20] and Caldeyro-Barcia et al. [21] as: (1) early deceleration, usually thought to be due to head compression, (2) late deceleration, usually thought to be due to uteroplacental insufficiency, or (3) variable deceleration, usually thought to be due to compression of the umbilical cord (Fig. 11-12).

Early deceleration begins with the onset of the uterine contraction and ends with the disappearance of the contraction, usually forming a mirror image of the contraction pattern. Late deceleration has its onset later in the contraction, usually after its peak has been reached, with return to the baseline after the contraction has disappeared. A variable deceleration pattern is recognized by periodic, nonuniform FHR dips having no apparent relationship to uterine contractions. Return to the baseline may occur rapidly or may be greatly delayed with more severe dips.

Another abnormality of great importance, especially when associated with an ominous deceleration pattern, is a decrease in the beat-to-beat variability (BBV). A decrease in BBV in the absence

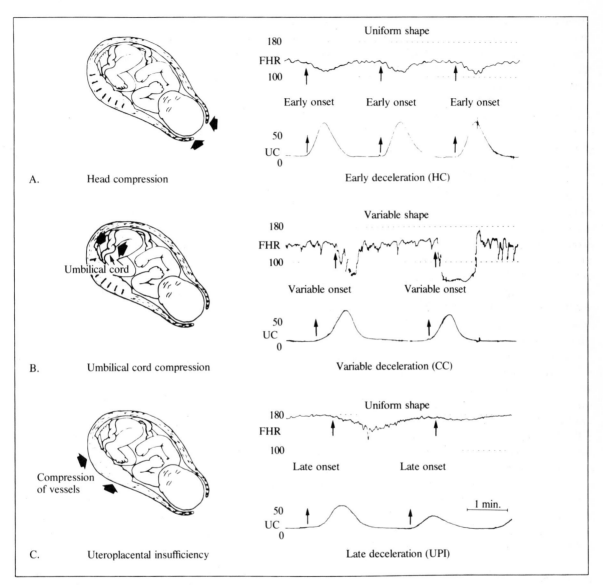

Fig. 11-12. Mechanisms of fetal heart rate deceleration patterns. A. Early deceleration. B. Variable deceleration. C. Late deceleration. (UC = uterine contraction; HC = head compression; UPI = uteroplacental insufficiency; CC = cord compression.) (From E. Hon. An Atlas of Fetal Heart Rate Patterns. *New Haven, Conn.: Harty, 1968. With permission from Corometrics Medical Systems Incorporated, Wallingford, Conn.)*

of other fetal heart rate abnormalities is probably benign [22]. A decrease in BBV is also seen after certain maternal drugs (atropine, barbiturates, meperidine, magnesium sulfate), when the fetus is "asleep," and with fetal asphyxia.

Treatment of Deceleration Patterns
Treatment for the early deceleration pattern is usually unnecessary since the abnormality is not associated with fetal distress.

Treatment for persistent late decelerations includes: (1) discontinuation of oxytocin if the drug is being used; (2) turning the patient on her side to obviate both vena caval and aortal obstruction of blood flow; (3) correction of maternal hypotension, whatever the cause (intravenous fluids, blood transfusion, ephedrine sulfate); (4) administration of oxygen to the mother; and (5) confirmation of the diagnosis of presumed fetal asphyxia by fetal scalp blood sampling (FSBS) if the above measures fail, and especially if the BBV is also decreased.

Treatment for the variable deceleration pattern will depend on the severity of the abnormality. The pattern is usually not ominous if the deceleration lasts less than 60 seconds, is less than 60 beats per minute, if return of the baseline FHR is abrupt, and if the BBV is not decreased. The variable deceleration pattern is more ominous when a return to the baseline is delayed or if late decelerations appear. Treatment may include a change in maternal position, search for a frank or an occult prolapse of the umbilical cord, and, if the pattern is severe, confirmation of the diagnosis of fetal asphyxia by FSBS.

Fetal Scalp Blood Sampling
Sampling of the fetal scalp blood has been described in Chapter 9. The procedure is used to confirm a diagnosis of fetal asphyxia made by recognition of an abnormal FHR pattern (late deceleration, severe variable deceleration). If the pH of the fetal scalp capillary blood falls below 7.25, a repeat sample should be taken within 10 to 30 minutes. If the reading is 7.20 or less, fetal acidosis due to asphyxia should be presumed. Factors that may alter interpretation of the pH reading include severe caput succedaneum, maternal acidosis due to dehydration or other cause, and rare miscellaneous causes. A pH below 7.20 without evident explanation demands immediate delivery of the fetus.

In summary, if the FHR pattern is recognized as abnormal and ominous, FSBS should be used to confirm fetal acidosis or asphyxia. Simple therapeutic measures may reverse the asphyxia, but early delivery is necessary to save the fetus if fetal distress persists.

Cesarean Section
With the increased safety of abdominal delivery and the recognition that difficult vaginal obstetric operations are hazardous to both mother and baby, the incidence of cesarean section in most large clinics has increased significantly in the past decade or two. Improved rates of neonatal survival for the tiny premature infant and the relative safety of abdominal delivery for the pregnant patient have both contributed to this increased cesarean section rate. The rate reported from the Collaborative Perinatal Project on women who delivered during the 1960–1965 period was five percent. Similar university hospitals today report rates of 12 to 20 percent. Although indications for cesarean section have been liberalized, it should be remembered that the maternal mortality rate for cesarean section is 3 to 4 times greater than with vaginal delivery (8–10 deaths per 10,000 versus 2.7 deaths per 10,000). The solution to all obstetrical problems is certainly not cesarean section, and the midforceps operation, at least in the hands of an expert, should not yet be relegated to history as long as certain safeguards are taken with its use.

INDICATIONS FOR CESAREAN SECTION
Table 11-3 illustrates the changes that have taken place in indications for cesarean section over the past 20 years. The major changes illustrated on the table are (1) an enormous increase in the number of cesarean sections done for malpresentation, primarily breech; (2) a manyfold increase in the number done for toxemia; and (3) a substantial increase in those done for failure to progress, fetal distress, and diabetes mellitus. Fewer sections are

Table 11-3. Percentage of Deliveries Accomplished by Cesarean Section for Various Indications

Indication	Collaborative Project[a] 1960–1965 (%)	UCDMC[b] 1977–1978 (%)	Approximate Increase
Repeat	2.3	3.3	1.5-fold
Malpresentation	0.1	2.9	29.0-fold
Failure to progress	1.0	2.2	2.0-fold
Fetal distress	0.3	0.8	2.5-fold
Toxemia	0.05	0.5	10.0-fold
Diabetes mellitus	0.1	0.2	2.0-fold
Placenta previa	0.3	0.2	0.5-fold (decrease)
Abruptio placentae	0.2	0.2	No change
Cord prolapse	0.1	0.2	2.0-fold

[a]From K. Niswander and M. Gordon. *The Collaborative Perinatal Study: The Women and Their Pregnancies*. Philadelphia: Saunders, 1972. P. 379.
[b] University of California at Davis Medical Center.

done today for placenta previa and there has been little change in the number done for abruptio placentae.

1. *Failure to progress* is the most common indication for primary cesarean section, accounting for 25 to 50 percent of all primary cesarean sections. We prefer to use the term "failure to progress" rather than the less exact terms of cephalopelvic disproportion and/or uterine inertia.
2. *Malpresentation* is the second most common indication for primary cesarean section. While most of these babies present by breech, a small number present by transverse lie, brow, or face. Many clinics now perform cesarean section for virtually all breech presentations. A discussion of the use of vaginal delivery versus cesarean section for breech presentation is presented on page 218.
3. *Fetal distress* is an indication for cesarean section in slightly less than 1 percent of our deliveries. The diagnosis of fetal distress is discussed under fetal heart rate monitoring on page 240.

4. *Pregnancy-induced hypertension* is an indication for cesarean section in some patients if the cervix is unripe.
5. Most patients with *placenta previa, prolapse of the cord,* and many patients with *diabetes mellitus* are best delivered by cesarean section.
6. *Herpes vulvitis* is an indication for cesarean section when the disease is active or has recently been active. The section should be performed before membranes rupture or within 4 to 6 hours thereafter because of the risk of ascending infection. While some clinics demand a negative herpes culture from the amniotic fluid before proceeding to cesarean section, the rarity of a positive culture has encouraged us to eliminate this test.
7. *Miscellaneous indications* include failed induction of labor, severe Rh disease, failed forceps, among others.
8. *Repeat* cesarean section accounts for about one-third of all operations. It has been shown that many patients with nonrecurring indications for cesarean section (e.g., placenta previa, cord prolapse, malpresentation) can deliver vaginally, especially if the patient has delivered previous

children vaginally. While a majority of clinics tend to follow the rule "once a section, always a section" because of the risk of rupture of the uterus in a pregnancy subsequent to the use of cesarean section, this dictum is being increasingly challenged. The risk of subsequent rupture of the uterus is particularly low with a low transverse incision.

TECHNIQUES FOR CESAREAN SECTION

1. *Low segment section.* After entry into the peritoneal cavity, an incision is made in the peritoneum overlying the lower uterine segment thus allowing dissection of the bladder off the lower uterine segment. A transverse uterine incision is made in the noncontractile portion of the uterus.

2. *Low vertical section.* In certain special situations (extreme prematurity before the lower uterine segment has formed adequately, transverse lie, and some cases of placenta previa), a low vertical section is performed. The uterine incision is made longitudinally in the anterior wall of the uterus after the development of a bladder flap.

Subsequent rupture of the uterus is much less frequent with a low segment operation than with the low vertical type. Furthermore, rupture with the low segment operation is more likely to be associated with less bleeding and a lower fetal mortality rate. Virtually none of the ruptures with the low segment operation occur before labor, while one-third of the ruptures following a low vertical section occur before labor. Rupture of the uterus is discussed on page 234.

References

1. Friedman, E. *Labor: Clinical Evaluation and Management.* (2nd ed.). New York: Appleton-Century-Crofts, 1978.
2. Hendricks, C., Brenner, W., and Kraus, G. Normal cervical dilation pattern in late pregnancy and labor. *Am J Obstet Gynecol* 106:1065, 1970.
3. Niswander, K. Induction of Labor. In J. Sciarra (Ed.), *Davis' Gynecology and Obstetrics.* Hagerstown, Md.: Harper & Row, 1976.
4. Wetrich, D. Effect of amniotomy upon labor: A controlled study. *Obstet Gynecol* 35:800, 1970.
5. Towbin, A. Hypoxic damage in fetus and newborn: Cerebral hypoxic damage in fetus and newborn. *Arch Neurol* 20:35, 1969.
6. Pearse, W. Forceps versus spontaneous delivery. *Clin Obstet Gynecol* 8:813, 1965.
7. Malmström, T. The vacuum extractor, an obstetrical instrument. *Acta Obstet Gynecol Scand (Suppl)* 4:33, 1954.
8. Cameron, A. The Birmingham Twin Survey. *Proc R Soc Med* 61:229, 1968.
9. Goodlin, R., Schmidt, W., and Creevy, D. Uterine tension and fetal heart rate during maternal orgasm. *Obstet Gynecol* 39:125, 1972.
10. Chase, H. *International Comparison of Prenatal and Infant Mortality: United States and Six Western European Countries.* U.S. Public Health Service Publication No. 1000, Series 3, No. 6. Washington, D.C.: U.S. Government Printing Office, 1967. P. 63.
11. Kass, E. The Role of Asymptomatic Bacteriuria in the Pathogenesis of Pyelonephritis. In E. Quinn and E. Kass (Eds.), *Biology of Pyelonephritis.* Boston: Little, Brown, 1960. P. 399.
12. Niswander, K., and Gordon, M. *The Collaborative Perinatal Study: The Women and Their Pregnancies.* Philadelphia: Saunders, 1973. P. 250.
13. Hertz, R., and Rosen, M. Clinical Management of Premature Rupture of the Membranes. In A. Gerbie and J. Sciarra (Eds.), *Gynecology and Obstetrics*, Vol. 2. Hagerstown: Harper & Row, 1979.
14. Niswander, K., Friedman, E. A., Hoover, D. B., Pietrowski, H., and Westphal, M. Fetal morbidity following potentially anoxigenic conditions: III. Prolapse of the umbilical cord. *Am J Obstet Gynecol* 95:853, 1966.
15. Klein, T., and O'Leary J. Rupture of the gravid uterus. *J Reprod Med* 6:218, 1971.
16. Garnet, J. Uterine rupture during pregnancy: An analysis of 133 patients. *Obstet Gynecol* 23:898, 1964.
17. Newton, M. Postpartum hemorrhage. *Am J Obstet Gynecol* 94:711, 1966.
18. Odell, L., and Seski, A. Episiotomy blood loss. *Am J Obstet Gynecol* 54:51, 1947.
19. Watson, T., Besch, N., and Bowes, W. Management of acute and subacute puerperal inversion of the uterus. *Obstet Gynecol* 55:12, 1980.
20. Hon, E. *An Introduction to Fetal Heart Rate Monitoring.* New Haven: Yale Cooperative Corporation, 1971.
21. Caldeyro-Barcia, R., Ibarra-Polo, A., Gulin, L., Poseiro, J., and Mendez-Bauer, C. Diagnostic and Prognostic Significance of Intrapartum Fetal Tachycardia and Type II Dips. In H. Mack (Ed.), *Prenatal*

Life: Biological and Clinical Perspectives. Detroit: Wayne State University Press, 1970.

22. Goodlin, R. *Care of the Fetus.* New York: Masson, 1978.

Additional Readings

Brenner, W., Bruce, R., and Hendricks, C. The characteristics and perils of breech presentation. *Am J Obstet Gynecol* 118:700, 1974.

Lederman, R., Lederman, E., Work, B., and McCann, D. The relationship of maternal anxiety, plasma catecholamines, and plasma cortisol to progress in labor. *Am J Obstet Gynecol* 132:495, 1978.

Milewich, L., Gant, N., Schwarz, B., et al. Initiation of human parturition. VIII. Metabolism of progesterone by fetal membranes of early and late human gestation. *Obstet Gynecol* 50:45, 1977.

Schrinsky, D., and Benson, R. Rupture of the pregnant uterus: A review. *Obstet Gynecol Surv* 33:217, 1978.

Schwarcz, R., Belizan, J., Cifuentes, J., Cuadro, J., Marques, M., and Caldeyro-Barcia, R. Fetal and maternal monitoring in spontaneous labors and in elective inductions. *Am J Obstet Gynecol* 120:356, 1974.

Weissberg, S., and O'Leary, J. Compound presentation of the fetus. *Obstet Gynecol* 41:60, 1973.

Wheeler, T., and Greene, K. Fetal heart rate monitoring during breech labour. *Br J Obstet Gynaecol* 82:208, 1975.

Zuckerman, H., Reiss, U., and Rubinstein, I. Inhibition of human premature labor by indomethacin. *Obstet Gynecol* 44:787, 1964.

12

INTRAUTERINE GROWTH RETARDATION

Intrauterine growth retardation (IUGR) is a relatively new obstetrical diagnosis that is more or less synonymous with the terms *placental dysfunction, fetal malnutrition,* and *inadequate placenta.* The diagnosis has been made primarily by the pediatrician rather than by the obstetrician, and a well-recognized newborn syndrome has evolved as more neonatologists have become interested in these babies. Recognition by the obstetrician of a fetus with inadequate placental support in utero has been hampered by lack of diagnostic tools. This deficiency is rapidly being corrected and good tools are now at hand to allow increasing accuracy in prenatal diagnosis of intrauterine growth retardation or placental dysfunction. While the problem of making an intrauterine diagnosis is now nearing solution, therapy remains pragmatic with limited choices available. However, even this problem can be attacked more logically now than was possible a few years ago.

What the obstetrician calls IUGR of the fetus, the pediatrician describes as a "small-for-dates" baby. In addition to the obvious discrepancy between newborn weight and length of gestation, certain physical findings are characteristic of such an infant and serve to support the diagnosis. A typical pattern of extrauterine growth further strengthens and confirms the diagnosis.

The small-for-dates baby appears thin and malnourished but more alert than a similar-sized infant of shorter gestation. There may be maceration of the skin, and the skin may also be pale. The fingernails are frequently long, and the scalp hair may be long. There is little vernix caseosa, and the infant may be stained the brownish hue (from meconium) of the scant amniotic fluid. Clifford [1] found that the prognosis for these infants is worsened if they are meconium-stained, and the outlook is frequently desperate when bright yellow staining of the skin, nails, and umbilical cord is present. Neurologic examination aids the pediatrician in determining the gestational age of the child. A more detailed pediatric description can be found in Chapter 13.

The classic obstetrical sign of delayed intrauterine growth is recognition of a uterus size smaller than the gestational interval would suggest. This is assessed by abdominal measurement. The inexactness of this observation is all too evident. In our experience, overestimation of fetal weight by 1000 gm. or more occurred in 15.7 percent of babies of birth weight equal to or less than 2500 gm. [2]. Even when the obstetrician notes a fundus small for gestational age, he is likely to guess that the menstrual dates have been incorrectly remembered and that the gestational interval is in truth shorter than originally calculated. The additional signs of scant amniotic fluid and staining of the fluid are difficult to recognize without a very special diagnostic effort. Amnioscopy for this purpose has failed to gain support in the United States. In the hands of an experienced operator, it is said that when a small obturator is inserted through the cervix with a bright light source for reflection, differentiation of clear amniotic fluid from stained fluid or fluid containing particles of meconium can be made [3]. However, the newer diagnostic tools to be discussed below seem more promising than amnioscopy.

Etiology

There are multiple causes for delayed intrauterine growth, but in practice the etiology remains obscure in at least 50 percent of cases. Lack of adequate placental support for fetal growth might occur at one of a number of points. The mother might simply be insufficiently nourished to supply nutritive support to the fetus. The fetus is usually, but not always, an effective parasite. The blood flow through the uterus might be insufficient to deliver otherwise adequate nutrition to the fetus, as with hypertensive diseases of pregnancy. Instances of this occurring are recognized clinically. The placenta might be too small to support growth of the fetus. While a small placenta is, indeed, often seen in a small-for-dates baby, whether the small placenta causes the delayed fetal growth or simply accompanies it remains unclear. The fetus might not be able to utilize all the nutrients supplied by an adequate uteroplacental circulation. No clear-cut examples of this possibility have been described without an abnormality of the fetus. While congenital malformation (trisomy 18 and 21, Turner's syndrome) or intrauterine infection of the fetus (rubella, cytomegalovirus, syphilis, malaria) are well-recognized causes for small-for-dates infants, these etiologies are outside the limits of the present discussion.

Obstetrical Diagnosis

PREDISPOSING FACTORS

Note must be taken of the patient with a disease or condition that is known to predispose to placental dysfunction. The hypertensive diseases of pregnancy probably head the list and include both chronic hypertension and preeclamptic syndrome. While most babies born of such patients will be of appropriate weight for gestation and at no special risk, placental dysfunction must be assumed to be present until proved otherwise. Patients with closely related diseases such as chronic renal disease are also suspect. A second predisposing cause of placental dysfunction is a poor obstetrical history. Poor reproductive performance may be manifest as a fetal or neonatal death or simply as a premature delivery, and a history of any reproductive failure should suggest the possibility of placental dysfunction in the present pregnancy. The extremely thin patient who gains little or no weight

during pregnancy should have special diagnostic attention. While the majority of diabetic patients have large babies, placental dysfunction may occur in a patient with vascular disease.

Some clinics screen all patients from midpregnancy on for possible placental dysfunction. This approach is discussed under Evaluative Tools for Fetal Assessment. While expensive, it is just such practices that will ultimately allow early recognition of all placental dysfunction and perhaps permit improved treatment for the disease. An analogy to the Papanicolaou (Pap) smear and cancer of the cervix can be drawn. The cost of routine Pap smears is high in terms of the relatively low yield of patients with cancer. Yet society is happy to pay the cost. A similar attitude may develop toward placental dysfunction and other causes of poor pregnancy outcome.

PHYSICAL FINDINGS

The primary physical finding in placental dysfunction is an estimated fetal weight less than the calculated length of gestation would suggest. Unfortunately, many variables make fetal size estimation from abdominal palpation unreliable. These include obesity, poor abdominal relaxation, poor abdominal tone with protrusion of the fundus, and unusual uterine shapes. Nevertheless, a certain degree of accuracy can be attained in correlating fetal size with gestation. At five lunar months the fundus is usually at the level of the umbilicus; at seven months the fundus can be palpated halfway between the umbilicus and the xiphoid process of the sternum. At nine months the fundus is at the level of the xiphoid (see Fig. 3-5). A better method of measuring fundal height (and therefore fetal size) perhaps is quantification of the distance from the symphysis pubis to the top of the fundus. The measurement may be made best with a tape measure. The height of the fundus from the symphysis pubis measured in this fashion approximates in centimeters the gestational age after 20 weeks. An increase of 1 cm. per week in this measurement from 20 to 36 weeks is to be expected. Of particular importance is a comparison of the current measurement with the measurement made at the last office visit.

*the following are the uterus that appears large for gestational age = (1) multiple fetuses.
(2) distended bladder.   (5) hydatid form mole
(3) inaccurate menstrual history   (6) uterine myomas/
(4) hydramnion.   adenomyosis.
                                          (7) a closely attached ?

Cont: (7) ... adnexal mass.
(8) Macrosomia late in pregnancy!

249

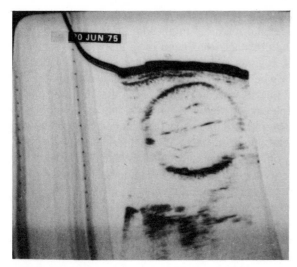

Fig. 12-1. Biparietal diameter measurement. Gray scale. Centimeter scale illustrated. The fetal midline echoes are attributable mainly to the falx and the intercerebral fissure.

With this approach, poor fundal growth can frequently be identified.

LABORATORY TOOLS

Ultrasound Scanning for Diagnosis

Serial ultrasonographic measurement of the fetus is currently the most accurate method for detecting IUGR. The first measurement should be taken between 20 and 24 weeks of gestation if the diagnosis is suspected by that time. Repetition of the examination at monthly intervals will, in most cases, identify the fetus who is failing to grow appropriately. The most widely used measurement at the present time is the biparietal diameter (Figs. 12-1 and 12-2). A more accurate diagnosis of IUGR may be possible with additional measurements. Of current interest is the head-to-abdomen ratio, the head-to-crown-to-rump length ratio, and the total intrauterine volume.

Two types of growth retardation have been identified. With *symmetrical* IUGR, the head-to-abdomen ratio is normal throughout pregnancy but both measurements are smaller than the gestational interval would suggest. With *asymmetrical* IUGR,

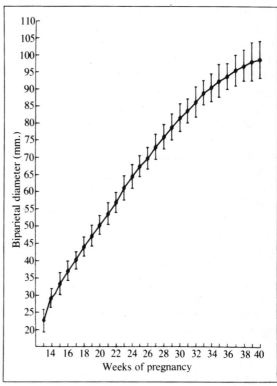

Fig. 12-2. Mean fetal biparietal diameter ± 2 standard deviations for each week of pregnancy. (From S. Campbell and G. Newman. Growth of the fetal biparietal diameter during normal pregnancy. J Obstet Gynaecol Br Commonw *78:513, 1971.)*

the head grows normally for gestational age but the abdomen is smaller than expected. The infants with this type of IUGR have a more favorable prognosis than do those with the symmetrical type.

Tests for Determining Fetal Maturity

When IUGR is suspected late in pregnancy, the finding of a smaller than expected fetus on ultrasound may indicate either IUGR or an error in the presumed gestational interval. The gravida may simply be of shorter gestation interval than her dates would indicate. It is therefore important in some cases to determine if the fetus is sufficiently mature to survive an extrauterine existence. Certain tests can be used for this purpose.

LECITHIN-SPHINGOMYELIN RATIO. This newest test for measuring fetal maturity has proved the most useful. It is based on the relative levels of certain surface-active phospholipids in the amniotic fluid as term is approached. Gluck et al. [4] in 1971, noted an abrupt increase in the amount of lecithin in the amniotic fluid at about 35 weeks' gestation with little or no change in the sphingomyelin. On the basis of 302 amniocenteses, these investigators reported that a sudden increase in the L/S ratio after 35 weeks "heralds maturity of the pulmonary alveolar lining. . . ." Innumerable studies since the original report have confirmed this conclusion. An L/S ratio greater than 2.0 predicts with great accuracy the absence of respiratory distress syndrome (RDS) in the newborn. Recently, Gluck [5] has shown that the presence of phosphatidyl glycerol (PG) in the amniotic fluid of the fetus with a mature L/S ratio improves the accuracy of the L/S ratio in predicting the absence of RDS in the newborn infant.

OTHER TESTS. A number of other tests on amniotic fluid predict with lesser accuracy the maturity of the fetus. These have now been largely abandoned because of the reliability of the L/S ratio, but occasionally they continue to be useful.

Bilirubin is present in the amniotic fluid of all fetuses in a rising level to about 20 to 24 weeks and a falling level thereafter. In the absence of fetal hemolytic disease, the bilirubin will be absent from 36 weeks onward. Absence of bilirubin therefore *suggests* maturity of 36 or more weeks, but exceptions occur. *Creatinine* is seen in ever-increasing levels in the amniotic fluid as a result of increased excretion of creatinine primarily through the fetal kidney. When a level of 2 mg. per 100 ml. or higher is recorded, term gestation can be expected. Yet another test of fetal maturity is the presence of desquamated *fetal cells*. Certain cells, presumably of fetal sebaceous gland origin, appear late in pregnancy and can be identified as orange staining with a 0.1% Nile blue sulfate. When the cells approximate 20 percent or more of all amniotic cells counted, term gestation can be diagnosed.

Assessment of Fetal Condition

Prenatal maternal monitoring of fetal activity during pregnancy has been recommended as a means of evaluating fetal health when IUGR is suspected or when other fetal jeopardy is a likely possibility. While this prenatal history should be asked of all antepartum patients, it is especially important when IUGR is suspected. Indeed, a decrease of fetal activity may be the first evidence of the syndrome. If decreased fetal movement is noted, the fetus should be evaluated immediately by the tools described below. Goodlin and Haesslein [6] have suggested that electronic fetal monitoring during labor may be a less effective tool in reducing perinatal mortality and morbidity than is surveillance of antenatal patients for decreased fetal movements.

ANTEPARTUM ELECTRONIC FETAL MONITORING

Antepartum electronic fetal monitoring (EFM) currently provides the most reliable means of assessing fetal condition when IUGR is suspected. The tests currently used are based on the changes in fetal heart rate described in Chapter 9.

Oxytocin Challenge Test

The oxytocin challenge test (OCT) (also called contraction stress test) is probably the single most reliable test of fetal health with IUGR. The first OCT should be performed as soon as IUGR is suspected, or whenever a compromised fetus is suspected for other reasons (e.g., postmaturity). A negative OCT is reassuring, but repetition of the test at weekly intervals is necessary. A positive OCT demands immediate hospitalization of the mother for further evaluation of the fetus and possible early delivery. The technique of the test is simple: With appropriate recording devices on the abdomen, uterine activity and fetal heart rate are continuously monitored. If no uterine contractions are noted for a 30-minute period, IV oxytocin is started at 0.5 to 1 mU per minute. This dosage is increased as necessary to produce three uterine contractions within a 10-minute period. A normal baseline heart rate and the absence of repetitive late decelerations is read as a negative test. Persistent late decelerations imply placental insufficiency and further evaluation with hospitalization of the mother is indicated.

Nonstress Test

The nonstress test (NST) is a newer technique that may prove to be as accurate as the OCT. This depends on the reactivity of the fetal heart rate to fetal movement. The technique is even simpler than the OCT: With the patient in the lateral decubitus position, the FHR is recorded with an abdominal lead. The mother's perception of fetal movement is recorded on the recording paper and an increase in the FHR of at least 15 beats per minute for 15 seconds or more immediately following the movement is an indication of a reactive, and therefore healthy, fetus. A nonreactive fetus should be checked immediately with an OCT.

Human Placental Lactogen

Human placental lactogen (HPL) is a hormone produced by the placenta and the level of this hormone in maternal urine has been suggested by some investigators as a possible test for fetal health. While some authorities have shown that low levels are indeed associated with placental insufficiency [7], others have found little clinical use for this measurement [8]. In a double-blind study to determine the usefulness of maternal serum levels of HPL in predicting placental dysfunction, Spellacy et al. [7] found good correlation between low levels and fetal risk. Clinical management based on the measured level of HPL significantly lowered the fetal death rate. In a recent report, Spellacy et al. [9] suggested that HPL levels may be used as a screening tool for all pregnancies. A level of less than 4 μcg. per ml. at 28 weeks gestation should alert the physician to proceed to use more definitive measures of fetoplacental function, according to Spellacy.

Serial Estriol Levels

Another currently available test for appraisal of fetoplacental function is a measurement of estriol levels in the urine or serum. The biochemistry of

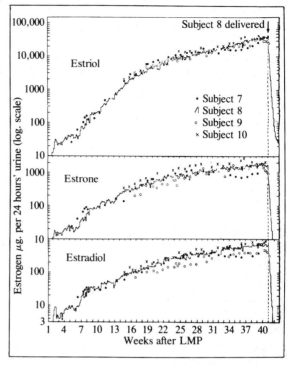

Fig. 12-3. Urinary estrogen excretion during pregnancy, as determined chemically. (From J. Brown. Urinary excretion of oestrogens during pregnancy, lactation, and the reestablishment of menstruation. Lancet 1:704, 1956.)

this compound has been described in Chapter 1. Some clinical laboratories measure and report total urinary estrogens rather than urinary estriol levels since the methodology for the former is much simpler and cheaper. The practical difference is not a great one to the clinician since estriol comprises by far the largest fraction of total urinary estrogen compounds, as seen in Figure 12-3.

Measurement of estriol in a 24-hour collection of urine may be inaccurate due to incomplete collection of the sample. Additionally, a number of factors may interfere with the production or urinary excretion of estriol, and these must be kept in mind when estriol excretion is used as a guide to fetal health. Maternal exogenous corticosteroid administration suppresses fetal adrenal activity, probably by suppression of fetal pituitary ACTH, and lowered levels of urinary estriol result. Ampicillin decreases estriol excretion by interfering with the enterohepatic circulation. Severe maternal kidney disease may decrease urinary estriol levels even with a healthy fetus and placenta. Anencephaly is associated with extremely low levels of urinary estriol. Multiple pregnancy usually results in unusually high levels of estriol because of additional fetal adrenal production of estrogen precursors. Finally, maternal activity affects urinary estriol levels. Bed rest increases estriol excretion, probably because of improved kidney function.

The use of serum estriol levels has obviated some of the shortcomings of the 24-hour urinary levels. The broad spread of normal values, however, limits the usefulness of this test. Since the kidney excretion of creatinine is thought to remain fairly constant throughout the 24-hour period, a determination of an estriol-creatinine ratio in a morning sample of urine has been recommended. While these variations on the 24-hour urine measurement of estriol have their advocates, no one method is used universally.

While a moderately skeptical attitude toward the use of urinary or serum estriol levels to assess fetal well-being and to plan obstetrical management is in order, the test appears to be useful to confirm the validity of the OCT or the NST or to function as a screening test. The following precautions should be taken in the use of the test:

1. Since values in an individual patient may vary as much as 20 percent on successive days, repeated determinations are essential before an adequate interpretation of the results can be made.
2. Since a low value may precede fetal demise by only a short interval (24 hours? 48 hours?), frequent determinations are essential, preferably every day or every other day.
3. A low urinary value in the presence of poor maternal kidney function demands further investigation and a maternal serum level determination.
4. Factors presently known to affect estriol levels

should be excluded. In addition, other as yet unknown extraneous factors may be identified in the future and should be constantly kept in mind.

Estriol levels may be useful for patients with diabetes mellitus, hypertensive disease, suspected postmaturity or suspected placental dysfunction, and a poor reproductive history, as well as for any other patient whose pregnancies are not progressing as expected. Erythroblastosis fetalis apparently cannot be monitored with estriol levels, since very high or very low levels occur in this condition for unknown reasons. The advice given by many authorities that obstetrical management should be based on clinical judgment to confirm abnormal estriol levels is obviously wise.

Amnioscopy

Amnioscopy is used by some clinics, especially in suspected postmaturity, to detect meconium staining in amniotic fluid and, by inference, a compromised fetal condition. With an amnioscope inserted just within the cervix, dilated at least to 1 to 2 cm., amniotic fluid can be visualized as either clear or stained. The risk of accidentally rupturing membranes is apparently small. Little interest in this tool has been generated in the United States.

Amniocentesis

Amniocentesis may be used for the sole purpose of identifying meconium staining. More often, amniotic fluid obtained for other reasons (fetal maturity evaluation) will be discovered to be meconium stained. Whether or not such a finding should precipitate immediate action remains unclear. A recent study concluded that the mere presence of meconium in the amniotic fluid without signs of fetal asphyxia (late decelerations with EFM or other evidence of acidosis) is an unreliable sign of fetal distress and not an indication for intervention [10]. The presence of meconium demands the immediate use of the NST or the OCT. Conversely, the absence of meconium provides a reassuring prognostic sign.

Management of IUGR

The management of IUGR has changed over the past few years because of the increasing ability of the clinician to evaluate fetal condition. Before the newer tests became available, management was primarily based on statistical probabilities. Is the fetus likely to die in utero if not delivered? Is the fetus likely to succumb as a neonate if delivered? Are the risks for the fetus greater from continuing placental insufficiency or from the ravages of immaturity as a newborn? The answer frequently depended on "clinical experience."

If IUGR is diagnosed and if the fetoplacental function tests are reassuring, treatment with bed rest, mild sedation, avoidance of excessive exercise and coitus, and a high protein diet can be recommended and encouraged. These measures increase uterine blood flow.

While clinical judgment is still the final arbiter of a problem in placental dysfunction, this judgment is buttressed by information on fetal well-being (OCT, NST, HPL, estriol levels) and on fetal maturity (L/S ratio and other tests). If the fetus is judged to be in jeopardy but mature, immediate delivery is recommended. If the fetus is in danger but immature, delay in delivery, with frequent monitoring both of fetal health and maturity, may allow successful delivery as soon as maturity is achieved. In some cases, fetal maturity fails to occur before fetal demise.

Delivery is indicated either when intrauterine existence seems jeopardized or when extrauterine existence seems assured. An L/S ratio of 2.0 or greater provides such reassurance. If delivery is chosen, the method of delivery must be selected with care. Abdominal delivery may be the choice if the cervix is unripe, especially if the OCT has been positive. The fetus simply may not tolerate the relative hypoxia produced by uterine contractility. Induction of labor, with careful monitoring of acute fetal condition (EFM), as described in Chapter 9, may be advisable. If heart rate patterns suggesting fetal compromise fail to occur, vaginal delivery may be possible. If a uteroplacental insufficiency (UPI) or severe cord compression FHR

pattern develops, there is still time for cesarean section. In general, the fetus with IUGR tolerates vaginal delivery poorly.

Page [11] has suggested the possibility of feeding a malnourished fetus in utero by injecting nutritive substances into the amniotic fluid. While the concept is an interesting one, this has not been proven to be clinically useful.

Post-Term Pregnancy and Post-Term Dysmaturity

Post-term pregnancy can be defined as that pregnancy that extends beyond 42 weeks (294 days). Four to ten percent of gravida have a pregnancy which extends beyond 42 weeks. Four to seven percent experience a pregnancy of greater than 44 weeks [12]. Since delayed ovulation and subsequent delayed fertilization accounts for about 70 percent of post-term pregnancies, it is apparent that many of these patients will not experience any fetal problems whatsoever [13]. The post-term dysmaturity syndrome, characterized by evidences of placental insufficiency, is said to occur in less than 20 percent of patients with post-term pregnancy. Since post-term dysmaturity is associated with an increased risk of perinatal mortality and morbidity, it becomes important to select out of the group of patients who go beyond 42 weeks those whose fetus is in jeopardy from placental dysfunction.

The characteristics of the post-term dysmature baby are described in Chapter 13. Fetal and placental growth usually cease at about 41 to 42 weeks gestation and there are an increasing number of infarcts found in the placenta. A decrease in amniotic fluid volume occurs with an increased incidence of meconium staining. The result is an increased risk of fetal distress, of meconium aspiration, and of perinatal death or morbidity.

The etiology of post-term pregnancy is unknown. The post-term dysmaturity syndrome is presumed to result from aging of the placenta, which in turn supports the fetus inadequately. It is known that post-term dysmaturity results in a 50 percent risk of recurrence of the syndrome in a subsequent pregnancy. It is also known that the absence of fetal adrenal activity, as with an anencephalic fetus, has frequent association with post-term pregnancy.

The diagnosis of post-term pregnancy begins early during the prenatal course. The physician should use as many tools as he has available to accurately date the early pregnancy. This information may be of great importance in patients who go or seem to go beyond 42 weeks gestation. The following are useful in dating a pregnancy:

1. Menstrual history. Prolonged intermenstrual intervals suggest a longer gestation than dating of the last menstrual period would suggest. Similarly, confusion may result from recent cessation of oral contraception with the known complication of post-pill amenorrhea. In a similar way, a nursing mother with amenorrhea may not know when she became pregnant.
2. Precise identification of date of conception because of a single unprotected act of intercourse.
3. Bimanual examination early in pregnancy will allow fairly precise dating of length of gestation by uterine size.
4. The initiation of fetal movement will be felt by the mother at about 19 weeks in primigravidas and 18 weeks in multigravidas [14].
5. The fetal heart can be heard by a Doppler instrument by 12 weeks gestation or by a stethoscope at 20 to 22 weeks gestation.

When a diagnosis of post-term pregnancy is made with certainty or reasonable certainty, appropriate tests should be done to determine if the fetus is in good condition or if the fetoplacental function is deteriorating. As with IUGR, a history of decreased fetal movements will suggest that the fetus is in trouble. Urinary or serum estriol levels may be determined 3 or 4 times a week. The NST and OCT should be used as described for the fetus with IUGR.

Treatment will depend on the condition of the fetus. With reassuring fetoplacental function tests, labor need not be induced at 42 weeks. Frequent repeat evaluations of fetoplacental function should be made. If the tests suggest a deteriorating condi-

tion for the fetus, delivery should be accomplished with all due speed. Careful EFM should be started simultaneously with induction of labor. The patient should be encouraged to labor off her back and she should probably receive oxygen throughout labor. As soon as it is technically feasible to do so, internal EFM should be initiated since the beat-to-beat variability of the fetal heart rate tracing is more reliable with a direct scalp electrode. Disturbing EFM tracings demand immediate assessment of the fetal acid-base balance with fetal scalp blood sampling. Immediate delivery is indicated for a deteriorating fetal condition. The oropharynx of the infant should be carefully suctioned even before delivery of the body. Neonatal care should begin in the delivery room and this care is described in Chapter 13.

HEMOLYTIC DISEASE OF THE FETUS

Hemolytic disease of the fetus and newborn is an immunologic disorder in which the immune mechanism of the mother is stimulated to produce antibodies that destroy fetal red blood cells. The resulting fetal hemolysis triggers a series of pathologic events that in many instances terminate in the death of the fetus. While many fetal antigens may gain access to the maternal circulation and initiate the process, 98 percent of clinical cases are caused by the Rh or ABO systems. (ABO sensitization is discussed separately under Hemolytic Disease of the Newborn.) The most severe disease and nearly all fetal deaths are associated with the Rh system.

Hemolytic disease of the fetus is genetically induced by the inheritance from father to fetus of a red blood cell antigen (Rh factor) not present in the maternal organism. When the antigen enters the maternal circulation, an immune reaction in the mother produces antibodies that in turn are passed transplacentally to the fetus. In the fetus, the antibody attacks the fetal red blood cells and initiates the pathologic process. Although a number of Rh antigens may cause the disease, the most common is the D antigen, and the following discussion centers around that antigen.

Pathophysiology

The D antigen is present in about 85 percent of Caucasians, 95 percent of blacks, and 99 percent of Orientals [15]. The possibility of an Rh sensitization exists when an Rh-negative woman (d-d, i.e., no D antigen) becomes pregnant by an Rh-positive man (D-d or D-D). This is most likely to occur in the white population. The D antigen is dominant and the inheritance of one D antigen from the father assures that the D antigen will be on the red blood cells of the fetus. If the man is homozygous for the D antigen (D-D), all the children he fathers will be Rh-positive. If he is heterozygous for the trait (d-D), 50 percent of his children will be Rh-positive.

Initial sensitization of the mother by the fetal D antigen inherited from the father is thought to occur usually in the immediate postpartum period after the birth of the first child with fetal-maternal incompatibility. Although small amounts of fetal blood frequently enter the maternal circulation during pregnancy, sensitization usually fails to develop at this time probably because the maternal reticuloendothelial system is able to destroy the foreign cells before the immune mechanism is activated. It is at the time of placental separation that fetal-maternal transfusion first occurs to any significant degree, and it is at this time that sensitization occurs. In a very small number of patients, maternal sensitization does indeed occur during the first pregnancy, due perhaps to passage of a large amount of fetal blood to the mother. In either case, maternal antibodies (IgG) thus formed pass easily across the placenta during a subsequent pregnancy and cause hemolysis of the fetal red blood cells containing the inducing D antigen. The frequency with which immunization occurs in the Rh-negative woman, married to an Rh-positive husband, with an Rh-positive pregnancy, and with no previous transfusions or other potentially sensitizing experiences, has been reported by Freda [16]. During the first pregnancy, 0.3 percent were immunized, 18 percent during the second, 16 percent during the third, and 15 percent during the fourth or higher pregnancy.

Various fetal events occur in response to the maternal antibodies. The fetal red blood cells are rapidly hemolyzed, which encourages a rapid production of new red blood cells, some of which are still immature (erythroblasts) when they are discharged into the fetal circulation. In some instances, destruction of red blood cells is very rapid, but in other cases the hemolysis is less severe and proceeds at a slower rate. In the first instance, severe hemolytic disease may result; in the second, the fetal disease may be mild.

The severity of the hemolytic process may depend on many factors; for example, the number of antibodies present, the type of antibody involved (albumin-active, enzyme-active, and so on). A maternal-fetal incompatibility for a blood group factor other than an Rh factor, notably an ABO incompatibility, may also protect against D-antigen sensitization. If the mother's blood grouping is O Rh-negative (and thus contains anti-A and anti-B antibody), and if the fetal blood grouping is A Rh-positive or B Rh-positive, the fetal cells that enter the maternal circulation may be inactivated by the A or B incompatibility before the D antigen can express itself.

The increase in hematopoiesis that results from the increased hemolysis occurs primarily in the liver, causing an enlargement of that organ. Splenomegaly is also seen as a result of hyperactivity as the spleen attempts to remove the products of hemolysis from the fetal circulation. Hemolysis causes increased production of lipid-soluble indirect bilirubin from heme, and removal of this substance from the fetal circulation is accomplished by transplacental passage to the mother and conjugation and excretion by the maternal liver. The fetal liver is too immature to conjugate this increased load of indirect bilirubin, which is an advantage to the fetus, since only indirect bilirubin is readily transported across the placenta. After birth, however, the inability of the newborn liver to conjugate all the indirect bilirubin formed by continuing hemolysis is a distinct hazard to the infant, since indirect bilirubin in sufficient amount may cause kernicterus, a crippling neurologic disease the details of which are described under Hemolytic Disease of the Newborn. Indeed, the major purpose of exchange transfusion of the Rh-sensitized newborn is removal of indirect bilirubin from the circulation.

While bilirubin production is not damaging to the fetus (as opposed to the neonate), the anemia that results from rapid red blood cell destruction may be the cause of fetal death. In such instances, the mechanism of fetal death is probably cardiac failure due to the anemia; the stillborn infant with hemolytic disease displays massive pitting edema, enlargement of the liver and spleen, and other evidences of cardiac failure (fetal hydrops). In some instances, the fetal anemia is mild enough to permit the continuation of fetal life. When the anemia is judged to be life-threatening, intrauterine transfusion, discussed subsequently, may correct the fetal anemia sufficiently to prevent fetal death.

If the Rh-affected infant survives until birth, various clinical situations may be apparent in the delivery room and in the nursery. In a few instances, massive fetal hydrops will be evident in the live-born, with neonatal death a near certainty. In other cases, the fetus may appear entirely normal at birth, but hepatosplenomegaly, bilirubinemia, and anemia may develop later. Rapid progression of the disease in the newborn demands prompt and aggressive treatment. Of crucial importance is the maintenance of the newborn bilirubin at low levels. Kernicterus may develop in 50 percent of cases if the level exceeds 30 mg. per 100 ml. (see p. 262).

Obstetrical Management of Hemolytic Disease of the Fetus

DIAGNOSIS

The diagnosis of the disease, as well as appraisal of its severity, is based on obstetrical history, maternal Rh antibody titers, and an interpretation of the amount of certain substances in the amniotic fluid.

Obstetrical History

The immunologic basis of the most common form of the disease is a fetal-maternal incompatibility for the D antigen. Since the fetal Rh type cannot be determined directly, the possibility of a fetal-maternal incompatibility must be suspected whenever the mother is D-negative and the father is D-positive. The zygosity of the father is important in certain situations. If he is known to be homozygous for the D antigen (D-D) every fetus he fathers will be Rh-positive and potentially erythroblastotic. If he is heterozygous (D-d), half of his children will be Rh-negative and unaffected. This fact may completely alter the answer the physician will give to an Rh-sensitized patient when she asks: "What are the chances of my successfully completing another pregnancy?" The father is known to be heterozygous if either a previous child fathered by him or one of his parents is Rh-negative. In the absence of this information, the zygosity is less certain, since anti-d serum is not available. The zygosity can be inferred with good statistical accuracy by using other antisera, such as anti-c. The reader interested in more detailed information is referred to an immunologic text. With modern Rh management, however, information regarding the zygosity of the father has only limited value.

The natural history of hemolytic disease of the fetus must also be considered when making the diagnosis. In the absence of prior sensitization caused by the administration of mismatched blood or serum, sensitization rarely occurs during the first pregnancy. It may occur in the immediate postpartum period, and the red blood cells of a subsequent Rh-negative fetus may then be hemolyzed by the D antibodies formed at this time in the maternal circulation. In addition, once the mother has been sensitized by a prior pregnancy, the small number of Rh-positive fetal red blood cells that gain access to the circulation during pregnancy may stimulate an increase in the level of D antibodies, an anamnestic response.

While the severity of the fetal disease varies under these circumstances, two prototypes are recognized. In some pregnancies, the disease is severe and tends to be severe in all future pregnancies with Rh-positive fetuses. In others, the disease is mild and tends to be mild in subsequent pregnancies. It is unusual, for example, for an Rh-negative woman to deliver an infant who is minimally affected once she has experienced a fetal death from erythroblastosis. On the other hand, some Rh-negative women deliver two or three Rh-positive infants, each of whom is only minimally affected or is not affected at all by Rh disease.

Maternal Antibody Titers

Maternal antibody titers are useful in recognizing when sensitization has occurred and, in certain instances, when a fetus has hemolytic disease. They are useless in assessing the severity of fetal disease. Severe disease is rarely seen when the antibody titer is 1:16 or less, but this observation is valid only if the particular laboratory performing the test has confirmed this experience. The presence of any titer is evidence that the mother may have been sensitized to the D antigen. A rise in titer of two dilutions or more during a pregnancy suggests that the fetus has hemolytic disease.

The maternal antibody titer of the Rh-negative women should be determined as early in pregnancy as possible and again at 24 and 36 weeks with the first pregnancy or when sensitization has not been previously identified. If she is known to be sensitized from a previous pregnancy and has a titer higher than 1:16, it is unnecessary to repeat the titer; management will depend on amniocentesis, reproductive history, and other factors.

Amniocentesis

Amniocentesis must be performed on any Rh-negative patient with an antibody titer greater than 1:16 or with a history of delivering an erythroblastotic still-born or a sensitized live-born infant. The test is based on the observations of Bevis [17] and Liley [18] that bilirubinoid substances can be detected in amounts higher than normal in the amniotic fluid of fetuses with hemolytic disease. The amniotic fluid level of the substances is a good predictor of the severity of the fetal disease.

The first amniotic fluid tap should be performed as early as the twenty-fourth to twenty-fifth week if there has been evidence of erythroblastosis in previous children or if the antibody titer is higher than 1:16. If a low antibody titer increases during pregnancy, the need for the tap may be recognized later. Depending on the results of the reading, a second amniocentesis may be performed one to two weeks later. If the difference in optical density at 450 millimicrons (ΔOD_{450}) (see Procedure) has decreased substantially at the second reading, a third test, if necessary, may be performed two to four weeks later. A high, a rising, or a steady ΔOD_{450} should be repeated in one week if an intrauterine transfusion is not indicated immediately.

Liley [19] and others have correctly predicted fetal outcome by the level of the ΔOD_{450} for a specific length of gestation. In normal pregnancy or in mildly affected Rh fetuses, the ΔOD_{450} decreases rapidly as pregnancy progresses, with a negative reading at about 36 weeks in most cases. Moderately severe and severe disease is predicted if the reading can be plotted within certain limits (Fig. 12-4), or if the ΔOD_{450} does not decrease regardless of how low the initial reading is. The limits for predicting severity of disease is illustrated in Figure 12-4 [20]. Liley has constructed a similar graph but on semilog paper. The indications for intrauterine transfusion, premature induction of labor, or expectant management based on amniotic fluid findings are described in the section on obstetrical management.

PROCEDURE. Amniocentesis is performed in any manner consistent with minimal risk to the fetus, with avoidance of needle puncture of the placenta if this is possible. This is best accomplished with the aid of an ultrasonographer who can usually detect placental location as well as identify a pocket of fluid for needle insertion. If ultrasound is unavailable, displacement of the presenting part with the needle inserted just above the symphysis pubis and bladder is currently the favored technique. In later pregnancy, dislodgment of the presenting part can be done with abdominal pressure; during early

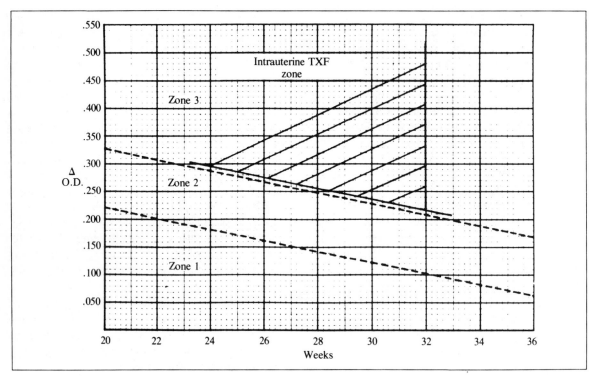

Fig. 12-4. Representation of zones (after Liley) of predicted severity of fetal hemolytic disease by ΔOD_{450} arithmetic scale. (From E. H. Bishop and T. E. Brown, Jr. ACOG Technical Bulletin, No. 17, July, 1972.)

pregnancy, displacement with vaginal pressure may be needed.

A No. 22 spinal needle can be used to remove the fluid. The fluid is shielded from light and transferred immediately to the laboratory. Spectrophotometric scanning over the range of wave lengths from 350 to 700 mμ will include the area surrounding 450 mμ needed for Rh screening. An absence of bilirubinoid material will be identified by a smooth curve throughout the range studied, with a gradual fall in optical density (OD) from the lower end of the spectrum to the upper. The substances in question for Rh disease are termed *bilirubinoid* because the pigments that cause the observed displacement of optical density include not only bilirubin but also related compounds. If these substances are present, there will be a hump in the spectrophotometric reading that will have its peak at or near 450 mμ. The difference between the reading at this peak and the reading if the smooth curve had been maintained is read as differential optical density at 450 mμ (ΔOD_{450}). This

reading is plotted on a graph with weeks of gestation on the ordinate, the ΔOD_{450} on the abscissa, and the zones of severity of hemolytic disease preprinted (Fig. 12-4). Interpretation requires some experience, but it is not complicated.

OBSTETRICAL INTERFERENCE

In hemolytic disease, obstetrical interference consists primarily of intrauterine transfusion and premature induction of labor. Only certain Rh-sensitized patients will be candidates for one or both of these treatment modalities. Phenobarbital administered to the mother for 72 hours before labor may increase fetal liver enzyme activity, thus increasing the excretion rate of conjugated bilirubin in the newborn.

Intrauterine Transfusion

INDICATIONS. The decision to perform intrauterine fetal transfusion is based on the near certainty that fetal death before viability will occur without treatment. Such a prediction can be made if: (1) the initial ΔOD_{450} on the amniotic fluid (with a repeat confirmatory reading a few days later) is in the "severe" zone; or (2) low readings continue to climb, even to the midzone. With these criteria, it is unlikely that a fetus will be transfused unnecessarily. The case for transfusion is strengthened further if the obstetrical history of the patient includes a previously Rh-affected fetus, which is the usual circumstance.

TIMING. The decision to transfuse should come after the twenty-fifth week (before 25 weeks, the transfusion is technically difficult and usually results in fetal death) and before the thirtieth week (the fetus is viable at this point, and the hazard of intrauterine transfusion outweighs the risk of induction and prematurity). The second transfusion is usually performed 7 to 10 days after the first, with two- to three-week intervals between transfusions thereafter. Small amounts of O Rh-negative packed cells are given when gestation is early (about 75 ml. at 26 weeks), with increasing amounts as gestation and the size of the fetus increase (about 150 ml. at 34 weeks).

Among fetuses not hydropic at the time of the first transfusion, a live-born rate of about 50 percent can be anticipated. Death may occur from premature labor, occasionally from intrauterine infection, and most frequently from an unknown cause that is probably related to the transfusion procedure itself. Most deaths from the latter cause occur with the first transfusion and are probably due to the stress of the transfusion on a sick fetus. Subsequent transfusions are rarely associated with fetal death. Delivery after 35 weeks or when maturity is sufficient to assure extrauterine survival is accomplished as described under Delivery before Term.

TECHNIQUE. Fetal transfusion is accomplished by placing a large bore needle in the peritoneal cavity

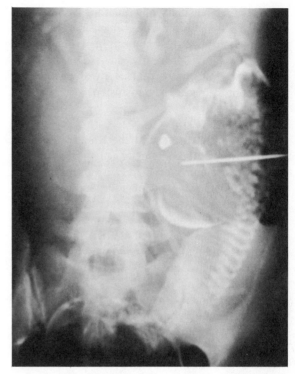

Fig. 12-5. Intrauterine transfusion for fetal hemolytic disease. The needle is in the fetal abdominal cavity, which is outlined by a small amount of dye injected through the needle.

of the fetus. The needle can be inserted with the help of radiography or, more recently, under ultrasonic control. The location of the needle is checked by the injection of 1 to 2 ml. of Hypaque (sodium diatrizoate). If the peritoneal cavity has been entered, a typical x-ray picture of spreading dye will be seen (Fig. 12-5). The dye will appear in a concentrated glob if the fetus has been punctured elsewhere.

When the abdomen is properly entered, the appropriate amount of fresh O-Rh-negative packed red cells previously cross-matched against the mother's serum is injected either through the needle directly or through a plastic tube inserted through the needle and into the fetal peritoneal cavity. About 85 percent of the transfused red blood cells enter the fetal circulation intact. In most cases, the fetus is unusually quiet for 24 hours following the transfusion, after which increasing activity is noted by the mother. In a minority of cases, the fetus apparently dies soon after the transfusion. Fetal movement nearly always occurs throughout the period of transfusion.

Delivery Before Term

In earlier years, delivery of the Rh-affected fetus before term was the only management that offered any improvement over merely awaiting the outcome. Although this is no longer true, there still is a place for premature delivery either by induction of labor or by cesarean section. Almost without exception, the fetus transfused in utero should be delivered prematurely about seven days after the last transfusion and at about 34 weeks' gestation. A fetal maturity estimation must be made to avoid the delivery of a grossly immature infant. The use of amniotic fluid for estimating fetal maturity by L/S ratio measurement is useful in this regard. Ultrasonic measurement of the fetal biparietal diameter may be helpful.

Indications for premature delivery among fetuses not transfused in utero include the following:

1. The fetus is judged to be ill by spectrophotometry but is not a candidate for transfusion.
2. The fetus is discovered to have serious hemolytic disease after the thirty-second week because of late registration for prenatal care or other reasons.
3. The fetus is *not* shown conclusively by spectrophotometry to be unaffected or only mildly affected by the disease.

Induction is initiated with intravenous oxytocin and careful amniotomy if the cervix is ripe, and there are no contraindications to the procedure. Failure to progress with induction, an unripe cervix, an unusual presentation (breech, face, shoulder), or other indication for section demand abdominal delivery. When the decision to deliver prematurely has been made, procrastination should be avoided.

Prophylaxis

Prevention of Rh sensitization has been possible since the mid-1960s. This important discovery has sharply decreased the number of Rh-sensitized fetuses seen. Prevention is based on an important observation made in 1909 that an antigen will not provoke an immune response in the presence of the corresponding antibody that has been passively administered. Freda et al. [21] in 1967 theorized that Rh antibodies might inactivate the Rh-positive cells rapidly enough to prevent a maternal immune reaction under the following conditions: (1) if initial sensitization to the Rh factor occurs in the immediate postpartum period as a result of the entry of large amounts of fetal blood into the maternal circulation, and (2) if passive immunization of the mother is achieved by giving Rh antibodies during this critical period. Extensive clinical experience has demonstrated the correctness of this theory, and passive immunization with fraction II gamma globulin with high Rh-antibody activity is now routine in obstetrical clinics among Rh-negative women who are unsensitized and who have delivered an Rh-positive infant.

Certain criteria have been set up to identify the patients who should receive this prophylaxis:

1. The gravida should be Rh-negative.
2. The postpartum serum of the gravida should not contain Rh antibodies (negative indirect Coombs' test).
3. The infant just delivered should be Rh-positive.
4. The direct Coombs' test in the newborn should be negative.

If these criteria are met, the mother is given 1 ml. of Rh immune globulin within 72 hours of delivery.

This treatment prevents Rh sensitization in almost all patients. Failure to prevent sensitization may be due to an unusually large escape of fetal blood to the maternal circulation. If this circumstance is suspected, the dosage of Rh immune globulin can be doubled or tripled. A Kleihauer stain of the maternal blood to demonstrate fetal cells and to estimate the amount of fetal blood present should precede the administration of the larger dose. If the placental blood is carefully drained before placental delivery, and if care is exercised in effecting placental delivery as atraumatically as possible, less fetal blood will enter the maternal circulation.

The Rh immune globulin should also be given to Rh-negative patients who abort spontaneously or who undergo therapeutic abortion. With an abortion of twelve weeks or less, a micro-dose (50 μg.) can be used; with a longer gestational interval, the full dose (300 μg.) is required. The micro-dose should also be given when amniocentesis is performed on an Rh-negative patient whose mate is Rh-positive.

Recently there has been interest in providing prophylaxis *during* pregnancy to avoid the occasional (1.8 percent of Rh-negative gravida) immunization that occurs during pregnancy, not during the postpartum period [22]. Bowman has recommended a single 300 μg. dose at 28 weeks gestation in the nonimmunized Rh-negative woman.

HEMOLYTIC DISEASE OF THE NEWBORN
Dilip M. Purohit and Abner H. Levkoff

Rh immune prophylaxis has decreased the incidence of hemolytic disease of the newborn due to the Rh(D) antigen. The incidence of other uncommon Rhesus factor incompatibilities due to C, c, e, E antigens, as well as the incidence of ABO incompatibility and incompatibility due to other red cell antigens such as Kell and S, remains unchanged. The perinatal mortality due to Rh disease has dropped from 45 percent in 1940 to 8 percent today because of amniotic fluid analysis, intrauterine transfusion, exchange transfusion, and improved neonatal care [23].

Clinical Manifestations
The clinical manifestations of Rh hemolytic disease in the neonate are secondary to hemolytic anemia and hyperbilirubinemia. Anemia may be severe enough to produce congestive heart failure; such an infant, who may also be hypoproteinemic and edematous is called hydropic. Extramedullary erythropoiesis can result in hepatosplenomegaly. The infant is usually not jaundiced at birth because of the transplacental transfer of unconjugated bilirubin from fetus to mother. The speed at which the level of serum bilirubin rises after birth depends on the severity of the hemolysis.

Unlike Rh disease, in which the first baby is rarely affected, the first baby is not uncommonly affected in ABO disease. With ABO disease, however, the hemolytic process is milder and the babies are not born with hydrops. The commonest disturbance is OA incompatibility. Why immune anti-A and anti-B (IgG) antibodies in addition to natural anti-A and anti-B (IgM) antibodies develop in O mothers is not well understood. Since the IgG antibodies can cross the placenta, the fetus may be affected even in the absence of prior immunization by a previous pregnancy.

Laboratory Studies
In Rh hemolytic disease, the infant exhibits a positive Coombs' test, reticulocytosis, increased nucleated red blood cells, and varying degrees of anemia. There may be thrombocytopenia and leukocytosis. Cord bilirubin, though elevated, is generally under 4 mg. per 100 ml.

The breakdown of heme in 1 gm. of hemoglobin yields 35 mg. of unconjugated lipid-soluble bilirubin, which is then bound by albumin, transported to the liver, and picked up by the hepatocytes for conjugation and excretion into the intestinal tract. The high level of β-glucuronidase in the neonate's intestinal tract deconjugates a portion of the bilirubin, with subsequent reabsorption by the intestinal tract (enterohepatic circulation of bilirubin) (Fig. 12-6). Unconjugated bilirubin not bound to albumin, "free bilirubin," can enter the cells of the body, since this compound is lipid-soluble.

Entry into brain cells produces an encephalopathy associated with yellow staining of basal ganglia (kernicterus). Bilirubin conjugated by glucuronic acid is no longer lipid-soluble and is nontoxic to the central nervous system.

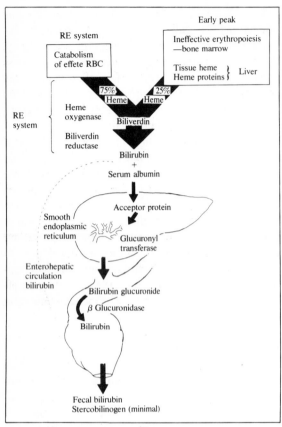

Fig. 12-6. Neonatal bile pigment metabolism. (From M. Maisels. Neonatal Jaundice. In G. Avery [Ed.], Neonatology: Pathophysiology and Management of the Newborn. Philadelphia: Lippincott, 1975.)

The determinants of the level of unbound, potentially toxic bilirubin are the concentration of albumin, and the factors that interfere with the binding of bilirubin by albumin, i.e., drugs, such as salicylates, sodium benzoate, and furosemide, as well as the nonesterified fatty acids associated with inadequate caloric intake. Acidosis reduces the binding capacity of albumin for bilirubin [24].

Ultimately then, the potential hazard of unconjugated bilirubin cannot be determined by serum levels alone. Special tests such as Sephadex gel filtration and peroxidase method determine the unbound fraction, "free bilirubin," whereas hydroxybenzeneazobenzoic acid (HBABA) binding and salicylate saturation index estimate the available albumin binding sites for a given level of serum bilirubin.

Early studies revealed that the incidence of kernicterus increases as the bilirubin levels exceeded 20 mg. per 100 ml. Lethargy, poor sucking, and hypotonia, the initial manifestations of kernicterus, are later replaced by hypertonia and opisthotonic posture. The infant may die of bilirubin encephalopathy and pulmonary hemorrhage. Surviving infants appear to improve for a short while, only to manifest choreoathetosis, deafness, and psychomotor retardation toward the end of the first year. One or more of the factors interfering with bilirubin-albumin binding, such as hypoalbuminemia, acidosis, and starvation, may be present in the sick premature infant. Consequently, these infants are at risk even with levels of bilirubin under 20 mg. per 100 ml.

Management

The treatment of hemolytic disease is designed primarily to prevent the accumulation of bilirubin in amounts that exceed the capacity of albumin to bind it. Bilirubin levels rising at a rate of 0.5 to 1 mg. per 100 ml. per hour will generally necessitate an exchange transfusion. In Rh hemolytic disease, exchange transfusion with 180 ml. per kilogram of fresh Rh-negative blood compatible with baby and mother will remove sensitized erythrocytes and bilirubin at the same time it corrects the anemia. In ABO hemolytic disease where the mother is O and the baby is A or B, an exchange transfusion is performed using group O blood compatible with the baby and the mother. However, because of unavailability of fresh whole blood, often fresh washed group O cells are mixed with plasma that is Group AB or the same as the baby's blood group. Albumin, in a dose of 1 gm. per kilogram given 1 to 2 hours prior to exchange transfusions, enhances by 40 percent the removal of bilirubin from the tissues. Such use of albumin is contraindicated in infants with severe anemia or edema or congestive heart failure because of the dangerous hypervolemia it may produce. If the infant's circulatory status is compromised at birth by severe anemia or hydrops, a smaller transfusion of packed cells may be used to stabilize the infant.

Photo-oxidation of bilirubin occurs when it is exposed to light at wavelength of 450 mμ. At this wavelength, the tetrapyrrole bilirubin is broken down into nontoxic dipyrroles. Clinically, this effect can be accomplished by exposing the infant to fluorescent light (phototherapy). In Rh disease, such phototherapy may preclude the need for repeat exchange transfusions; ABO disease is usually amenable to phototherapy alone. Since the sensitized cells are not removed when phototherapy is used, these infants have to be followed closely for the development of late anemia.

CONGENITAL MALFORMATIONS
Ronald J. Jorgenson

The description of teratology as being the study of monsters, since the word is derived from the Greek *teras,* or "monster," and *logos,* or "treatise," has been modified both by compassion and by an understanding of the biologic bases for aberrant development. Teratology is defined by the modern clinician as the area of medicine that deals with the embryogenesis and classification of congenital defects. This definition rightly implies that the body of knowledge on which the concepts and classifications of congenital defects are based was developed in the field of embryology.

The processes of development that are studied in embryology may be thought to begin with fertilization of the ovum and to continue until birth. The purist may contend that only those processes occurring during the embryonic period of gestation (the fourth through the seventh week) are the subject of embryology, and he would certainly hesitate to extend his concept of embryology to postnatal development. However, the clinician cannot be so rigid in his approach to the study of the developing human and must view embryology in its broadest sense. The obstetrician, in particular, must monitor the mother and child through several critical states of development and must evaluate the regularity of that development at delivery. In the unfortunate instance that the newborn child has a congenital defect, the obstetrician must be competent and supportive in his approach to the family of the child. The confidence required to help the family adjust to their newfound situation is gained in part by familiarity with congenital defects and with their biologic bases.

Etiology of Congenital Defects
The term *congenital defect* refers to morphologic and biochemical abnormalities that are present at birth. The majority of defects discussed here will be morphologic, since biochemical assays are not done routinely on newborns and since it is usually a morphologic defect that prompts laboratory studies. Many of the morphologic defects that are discussed may be thought of as the extremes of continuously variable traits. A structure that it too small or too large may be considered abnormal, but there are intermediate sizes whose normality is difficult to evaluate. Also, defects of several structures may occur simultaneously with predictable consistency. These constellations of defects constitute syndromes and for our purposes here are treated as single congenital defects.

Congenital defects are caused by genetic factors, environmental factors, or both. There is ample evidence that genetic factors may be of major etiologic significance in 30 percent of all congenital defects. Environmental factors may be the primary cause in 10 percent. However, the majority of congenital defects are not due primarily to one or the other set of factors but to an interaction of genes and environment.

Figure 12-7 illustrates the respective roles of heredity and environment in producing congenital defects. Some defects are due to genetic factors for the most part; Down's syndrome (mongolism) is due to an extra chromosome in the 21st pair, and polydactyly (extra digits) may be due to mutant genes. Other defects are primarily due to an environmental agent; the embryopathies of rubella and thalidomide are due to a virus and drug respectively. Neither the genetically determined nor the environmentally determined defects are shown

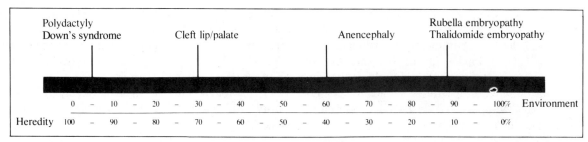

Fig. 12-7. Interaction of genetic and environmental factors in the causation of congenital defects.

at the extremes of the scale. This is to emphasize that neither set of factors operates in a vacuum. The genetic factors are modified by the environment and vice versa. For example, there may be an inherited susceptibility or resistance to thalidomide that results in a more or less severe embryopathy. Conversely, certain manifestations of Down's syndrome may be modified by the environment and environment may even cause the nondisjunction.

The majority of congenital defects are intermediate on this scale, as shown for cleft lip and cleft palate and for anencephaly in Figure 12-7. Orofacial clefting is thought to be due to the interaction of several genes and an unknown number of environmental agents. It is therefore shown as lying closer to the genetic extreme of the scale than to the environmental extreme. Anencephaly may be an isolated trait or may be part of a heritable syndrome. However, a sizable number of cases may be due to environmental factors and anencephaly is shown as having a greater environmental than genetic etiology. Placement of these intermediate defects along the scale is somewhat arbitrary. As our knowledge of the number and relative contribution of etiologic agents increases for the specific defect, its position along the scale will change.

The concentration here on the genetically determined congenital defects does not imply that those that are environmentally determined are less important. It merely reflects two facts: (1) the majority of congenital defects of proved etiology are genetic in nature; and (2) despite the large number of environmental agents being implicated as teratogens, relatively few have been causally associated with specific defects. The emphasis here will be

on an approach to recognizing the etiology of congenital defects and for arriving at specific diagnoses for congenital defects. The etiology is often central to the diagnosis of a congenital defect and the management of the afflicted patient. This will become clear as the reader progresses through these pages.

Genetic Factors in Congenital Defects

A simplistic scheme for categorizing genetically determined defects is shown in Table 12-1. Single-gene defects are the result of a mutant gene at a single locus; that is, the malformation or syndrome is due to information encoded by one gene only. The single-gene defects can be subdivided according to whether the locus is on an autosome or an X chromosome and whether the mutant gene is effective when carried by one chromosome of a pair (dominant) or only when carried by both chromosomes (recessive). Y-linked inheritance and cytoplasmic inheritance have been suggested in man, and there is strong evidence for cytoplasmic genes on a molecular level. However, the impact of these modes of inheritance on the clinical level remains to be demonstrated. The earlier statement that genes do not exist in a vacuum should be recalled. It is probable that each single gene defect is modified by the remainder of the genome and the environment. However, biochemical studies and concordance with Mendel's basic laws confirm that one gene is the major determinant in the single-gene defects. McKusick's extensive *Mendelian Inheritance in Man* lists 1364 documented single-

Table 12-1. Categories of
Genetically Determined Disorders

Single-Gene Disorders (Monogenic)
  Autosomal dominant
  Autosomal recessive
  X-linked dominant
  X-linked recessive
  Y-linked
  Cytoplasmic
Multiple-Gene Disorders
  Polygenic
  Multifactorial
Chromosomal Disorders
  Structural modifications
  Deletions or additions
  Aneuploidies (abnormalities of number)

Table 12-2. Criteria for Characterizing
a Congenital Defect as Genetic

Individual Criteria
  No exogenous agent identified as the cause.
  The defect has a characteristic age of onset.
  The defect is remarkably similar in unrelated persons.
Family Criteria
  The defect occurs in relatives.
  Concordance varies with zygosity of twins.
  Consanguinity is present in the family.
Population Criteria
  Frequency of the defect differs for the sexes.
  Frequency of the defect differs for racial and ethnic groups.
General Criteria
  The defect is known to be genetic in animal models.
  There is biochemical or laboratory confirmation of genetic etiology.

gene defects (malformations and syndromes) and suggests that an additional 1447 may be due to a single gene.

Polygenic defects are those that are caused by two or more genes. In most cases, the number of genes involved is not known with certitude, although estimates can be made. The multiple genes are probably at widely separated loci, and each influences the manifestation of the defect in a unique way. The situation of polygenic inheritance is complicated when environmental factors also modify expression of the defect, i.e., when the defect is multifactorial. A wide range of syndromes and most of the common traits in man (height, intelligence, skin color, and so forth) are polygenic or multifactorial in nature.

Defects that are due to rearrangements of parts of chromosomes, deletions or additions of short segments of chromosomes, and abnormal numbers of chromosomes are in a sense polygenic. There are many loci on each chromosome, and an alteration of morphology or number necessarily involves multiple genes. However, the genes that are involved do not necessarily code information for a single trait and many more genes are involved than the several associated with polygenic defects. As a result, the chromosomal defects produce significant aberrations in multiple systems.

It is not always easy to decide whether a con-

genital defect is genetic or environmental in origin. Table 12-2 lists some of the criteria that may be useful in determining that a defect is genetic. Many of the criteria listed are not conclusive. The fact that no exogenous agent can be causally associated with a given syndrome may indicate only that our knowledge is limited. Also, environmentally caused defects may have a characteristic age of onset, may appear clinically similar in unrelated individuals, may appear in relatives, and by nature or differing life experiences may occur at different frequencies in the two sexes and among racial and ethnic groups. Simultaneous compliance with several of the criteria suggests that the cause of the defect is genetic. Compliance with only one of the very specific criteria, such as positive family history or a pathognomonic laboratory test result, is often sufficient to demonstrate the genetic nature of a defect.

DIAGNOSIS

In practice, it is often familiarity with the defect that leads the practitioner to a correct appraisal of the etiologic alternatives and to a correct diagnosis. However, the number of congenital defects is extensive, and it is unlikely that the practitioner will be personally familiar with more than several of them. It is imperative, then, that the practitioner develop a systematic method for evaluating the patient under his observation who has a rare congenital defect. A method based on the approach used at several birth defects centers follows.

General Information
In addition to the routine medical history and systems review, particular care must be taken to elicit a family history. Details of the technique of obtaining and interpreting a family history may be found in any one of a number of excellent texts on human genetics. National, racial, and religious backgrounds are often not stressed in family histories but are essential here because of the ethnicity of certain genetic disorders. Sickle cell anemia in blacks, Tay-Sachs disease in Ashkenazi Jews, and glucose 6-phosphate dehydrogenase deficiency in Mediterranean Europeans are three of the many disorders with a predilection for specific groups of people.

Correlations Based on Developmental Biology
The earliest possible variation from normal morphogenesis that could account for the observed defect should be identified. Based on this identity, the time of onset of the defect can be calculated and later environmental insults ruled out as causes of the defect. It should be determined whether the defect can be explained on the basis of altered morphogenesis of a single system or of multiple systems. In some cases of multiple-system defects, the possibility must be considered that a primary defect in one system has adversely affected morphogenesis in the others.

SINGLE-SYSTEM DEFECT. A single-system defect is one that results from aberrant development of one progenitor structure or tissue. If one postnatal structure is defective, such as a cleft palate, it is easy to identify the defect as monosystemic. However, it is possible that a defect in one progenitor may cause secondary defects in several surrounding structures. This is still a single-system defect, although it is more difficult to recognize as such.

The various ectodermal dysplasias are excellent examples of single-system defects that involve several postnatal structures. In X-linked recessive hypohidrotic ectodermal dysplasia, the skin, eccrine glands, hair, and teeth are defective (Fig. 12-8). Each listed structure is derived in part from the primitive ectoderm, and the constellation of defects seen at birth or at some time after birth may be attributed to abnormal development of the ectoderm alone.

Two frequently diagnosed single-system defects that illustrate the diversity of these disorders are the Robin anomaly (formerly the Pierre Robin syndrome) and amniotic constriction bands. The Robin anomaly consists of a cleft palate, micrognathia, and glossoptosis (Fig. 12-9). Clefting of the lip is not a feature of the condition, nor are other anomalies that have been mentioned in some case reports. Some researchers contend that the small mandible in the Robin anomaly results in a posterior position of the tongue and that the tongue subsequently interferes with closure of the palate. Others contend that the cleft allows an abnormal tongue posture that results in the lack of normal stimulation for mandibular growth. The arguments about which defect causes the others are circular, and it is equally as likely that a single primary defect elsewhere, such as anomalous stapedial artery circulation or abnormal fetal posture, is responsible for all three clinical manifestations.

Amniotic bands may cause constriction, underdevelopment, or amputation of developing structures, usually the limbs (Fig. 12-10). The primary defect probably is not in the affected limbs but rather is in the amnion, which ruptures prematurely, forming strands of tissue that encircle appendages of the developing embryo and cause the constrictions.

The etiology of single-system defects is usually not clear. Several have been shown to be due to single mutant genes. An environmental etiology has been documented for a few (masculinization of the female fetus due to androgens, deafness due to quinine, and discolored teeth due to tetracyclines). The majority are multifactorial in nature and do not commonly recur in families.

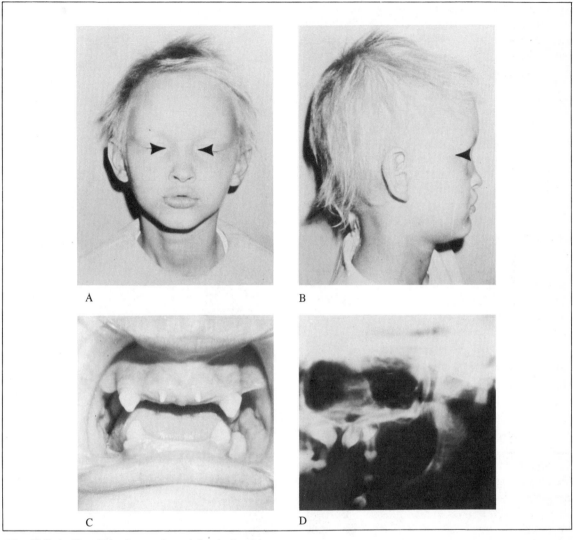

Fig. 12-8. A. Hypohidrotic ectodermal dysplasia with sparse facial and scalp hair. B. Concave profile with everted lips. C. Conical teeth. D. Congenitally absent teeth.

MULTIPLE-SYSTEM DEFECTS. A multiple-system defect is one that is due to abnormal development of more than one primordial tissue or organ. These defects constitute the syndromes (from the Greek words *syn*, "with," and *dromos*, "running together") that are the bane of the diagnostician. The difficulties encountered in diagnosing multiple-system defects (syndromes) rests in part in the lack of specificity of the individual defects; an isolated defect may be a common feature of several syndromes but may not be found consistently in any of them. Diagnosis often depends more on the overall pattern of defects rather than on the presence of one or more pathognomonic defects. In addition, the pattern of defects in a given syndrome may vary markedly from one affected individual to the next.

Another feature that complicates diagnosis is

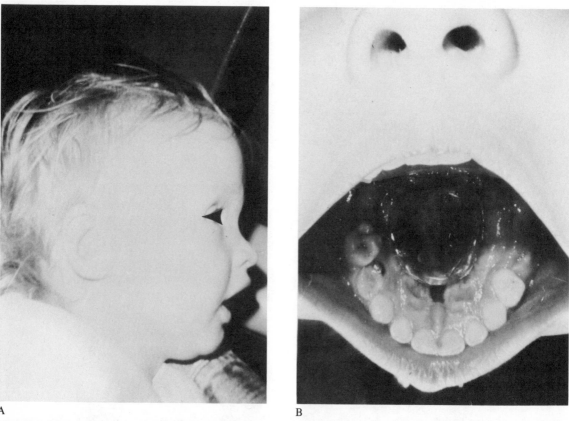

A   B

Fig. 12-9. Micrognathia (A) and cleft palate (B) in the Robin anomaly (formerly the Pierre-Robin syndrome).

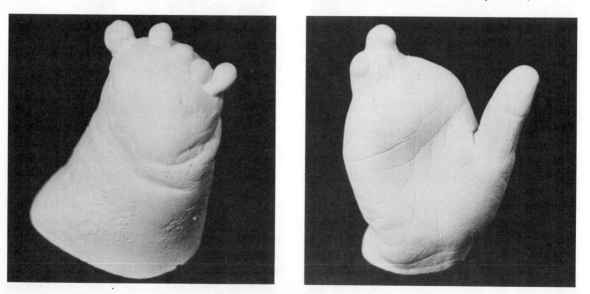

Fig. 12-10. Congenital anomalies of the hand presumed to be due to amniotic constriction bands.

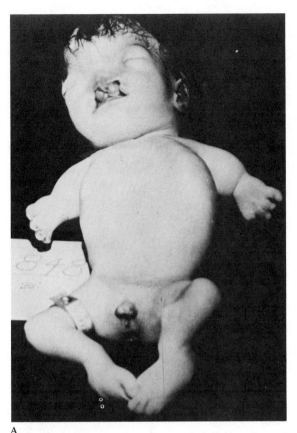

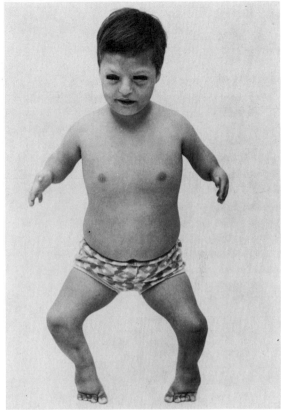

A

B

Fig. 12-11. The Robert syndrome (A) and the pseudothalidomide syndrome (B) have several common features but are distinct entities. Note the genital enlargement and severe lower limb malformations in the Robert syndrome; the absence of these features in the pseudothalidomide syndrome, and the facial hemangioma in the latter. (From D. Bergsma. Limb Malformations. *Original Article Series Vol. X, No. 5, Symposia Specialists, P.O. Box 610397, Miami, Florida 33161.)*

clinical similarity among syndromes. There are more potential teratogens than there are ways for the body to react to an insult; therefore, more than one agent may be responsible for the same defect. For example, cleft lip and palate may be an isolated condition caused by a mutant gene; or it may be polygenic in nature or one defect in a multiple-system syndrome; or it may be caused by a drug (the second most common feature of thalidomide embryopathy is orofacial clefting). In the case of some syndromes, the phenotypes are not identical but are so similar as to complicate the diagnosis. Certain features of the pseudothalidomide syndrome and the Robert syndrome are so striking that the two may be confused by an untrained observer (Fig. 12-11). The absence of severe lower-limb malformations and genital enlargement and the presence of capillary hemangiomas in the pseudothalidomide syndrome serve to distinguish it from the latter.

Minor Defects

The less severe malformations, such as the hemangiomas in the pseudothalidomide syndrome, are often essential components in a differential diagnosis. These minor defects do not constitute serious medical or cosmetic handicaps, but they are frequently associated in predictable patterns with

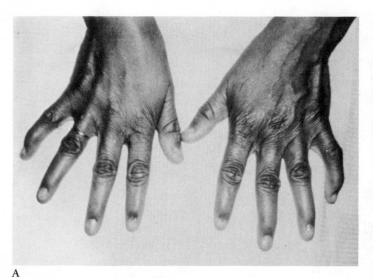

A

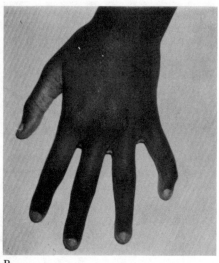

B

Fig. 12-12. Camptodactyly (bent fingers) in mother (A) and daughter (B) may be familial trait rather than an indicator of more severe morphogenetic disturbance.

major defects. They also are superficial and easily evaluated. The finding of one minor defect in a patient is of no serious consequence. However, as the number of minor defects in an individual increases, the likelihood of finding a major defect increases disproportionately. Marden and co-workers [25] have reported that 14 percent of neonates have one minor defect, 0.8 percent have two, and 0.5 percent have three or more. The incidence of major malformations in the 14 percent with one minor defect is no higher than in newborns with no minor defects. The incidence of major malformations in the 0.8 percent with two minor defects is five times that of the population in general, and 90 percent of those with three or more minor defects have a major malformation.

There are two considerations that are important when examining a patient for the presence of minor defects. First, members of the patient's family should be examined to determine whether or not an observed defect is a familial trait. If the defect is found in relatives, it should be assigned less significance than otherwise as an indicator of abnormal morphogenesis (Fig. 12-12). Second, evaluation of the defect should be as objective as possible. Little difficulty with objectivity is encountered when evaluating findings that can be classified as present or absent, e.g., polydactyly (Fig. 12-13).

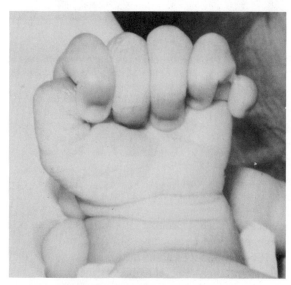

Fig. 12-13. Polydactyly in newborn. This trait is 10 times more common in blacks than whites, may be familial, and is one of many traits that can be scored as absent or present in syndrome identification.

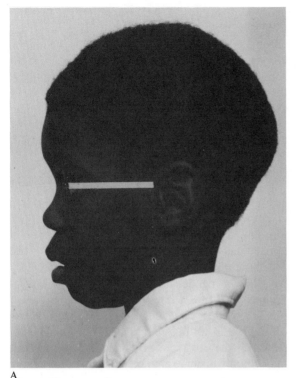

A

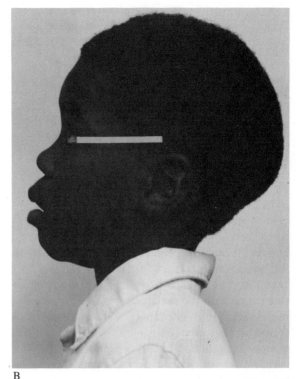

B

Fig. 12-14. Continuously variable traits may be misclassified by the clinician. In this case, ear placement appears normal in A, but may be judged abnormally low in B due to rotation of the head.

Minor defects that represent the extreme ranges of normal variability, on the other hand, are more difficult to assess and should be labeled defects only in a limited sense. Low-set ears, for example, are commonly described in congenital malformation syndromes when, in fact, few data are available on the position of ears in the general population, and actual measurements of ear position are seldom used to confirm a clinical impression (Fig. 12-14). The deceptiveness of clinical impressions was accurately demonstrated by Shapiro and coworkers [26] in an objective study of the height of the palatal vault in Down's syndrome. Nearly every table of clinical findings in Down's syndrome lists a highly arched palate as a consistent feature. Shapiro et al. were able to show that the palates of patients with Down's syndrome were the same height as the palates in age-matched and sex-matched controls. However, the palates in Down's syndrome patients were slightly narrower than those in the controls, and all but a few were significantly shorter than the palates in the controls. A short, narrow palate, then, is interpreted by the majority of clinicians as being highly arched.

Laboratory Tests

Although clinical diagnosis may be subjective, it should not be denigrated. Confirmatory laboratory tests are ordered legitimately only after several potential diagnoses are suggested during physical examination. Unfortunately, there are pathognomonic tests for only a relative few of the multitude of congenital defects in man. The majority of these tests measure a specific enzyme system or survey for a chromosome imbalance. Enzyme systems that function during embryogenesis but do not function postnatally cannot be assayed. Also, it is impossible to assay retrospectively for the majority of environmental agents implicated as potential teratogens. The viruses of toxoplasmosis and rubella, the cytomegalovirus, and the spirochete of syphilis cause prenatal infections and may persist in the blood of the mother or child after birth. However, they are just as likely not to persist.

ENZYME DEFICIENCIES. Specific enzyme deficiencies have been identified for just over 150 heritable defects. Some of these are congenital defects, and most are recessive in nature. Of course, there are confirmatory tests, more or less precise, for a number of heritable conditions that result in the excretion by the body of specific molecules but for which the primary enzyme deficiency is not known. The excreted molecules are presumably involved in some way with the metabolic pathway of the defective enzyme. The mucopolysaccharides excreted in the urine of patients with the various mucopolysaccharidoses are diagnostic aids but certainly are not the deficient enzyme. It may be more convenient to assay for a by-product in the urine or blood than to assay for the enzyme, even when the primary defect is known. The deficient enzymes in homocystinuria and phenylketonuria are cystathionine synthetase and phenylalanine hydroxylase respectively. However, the common assays for these conditions measure homocystine in the urine of suspected cases of homocystinuria and phenylalanine in the blood or phenylpyruvate in the urine of suspected cases of phenylketonuria.

CHROMOSOME ANALYSIS. Laboratory analysis of chromosomes in man has evolved from an academic exercise to a critical diagnostic aid over the past 20 years. A number of congenital defects have been causally related to chromosome imbalance since 1959, when trisomy of chromosome 21 was described in patients with Down's syndrome. Chromosome abnormalities have been found in nearly one-fourth of spontaneous abortions. The frequency of chromosome abnormalities is higher in early abortions than in late abortions; as many as one-third of fetuses aborted in the first trimester have been reported to have abnormal chromosome constitutions. The most common chromosome abnormalities in abortuses are trisomy of the larger autosomes (those in groups A through C), monosomy of autosomes and of the X chromosome, and polyploidy. The most common chromosome abnormalities in neonates are trisomy of small autosomes (those in groups D, E, and G), sex chromosome aneuploidies (excluding the YO constitution), and variations of size and shape.

Chromosome analysis is a time-consuming, costly process, and the clinician should have a sound reason for ordering such an analysis. Chromosome analyses are indicated in some cases and not indicated in others. The clinician should not order a chromosome analysis on a patient with a well-known mendelian syndrome. Mendelian syndromes are those due to a single-gene defect (dominant) or a matched pair of gene defects (recessive). It is not possible to visualize the gene defect with the most powerful microscope, since it may be only a single amino acid substitution in the deoxyribonucleic acid (DNA) chain making up the gene. Even if the gene defect involves the deletion, insertion, or transposition of a segment of DNA, it is impossible to see microscopically. Chromosome studies should not be done in patients with less well-known syndromes but with a family history strongly suggesting mendelian inheritance. It is likely that the syndrome is one of a plethora of poorly documented heritable syndromes, rather than being due to a familial chromosome abnormality. This statement is based on (1) the estimate that the extensive catalogues compiled by McKusick describe only 0.1 to 1.0 percent of the defects in man that could potentially be gene-determined and (2) the observation that only a small percentage of chromosome abnormalities are such that they could simulate mendelian inheritance. Balanced chromosome translocations or mixoploid chromosome constitutions (mosaicism) are two examples of chromosome abnormalities capable of mimicking mendelian inheritance, but each is relatively rare.

One of the hallmarks of chromosomally determined syndromes is that multiple organ systems are involved, especially the head, face, heart, and genitourinary system. It is hard to imagine a chromosome abnormality that affects only a single enzyme or structural protein or that acts only during a limited time of embryogenesis, since a large number of genes are involved with each recognizable morphologic or numeric chromosome abnormality.

Table 12-3 lists the indications for a chromosome analysis. Each of the clinical features listed has a low frequency in the general population but a relatively high frequency in patients with chromosome syndromes. The findings listed are particularly suggestive of chromosome abnormalities when a patient has more than one of the features, especially mental retardation or genital anomalies in association with others. However, patients with one or two features only are not necessarily suspect, since the features may be familial traits or coincidental findings in otherwise normal persons.

Two of the indications for chromosome analysis in Table 12-3 must be singled out for consideration: classic phenotypes and homozygosity for rare recessive traits.

Some clinicians feel it is not necessary to study the chromosomes of patients with classic chromosome syndromes. Others maintain that for academic interest and positive diagnosis, a chromosome survey is mandatory. The latter position seems reasonable, since phenocopies (an abnormal phenotype that closely resembles that of a well-known syndrome) are prevalent in clinical medicine and since translocation syndromes and aneuploid syndromes may be clinically identical. Differences in the recurrence risks of translocation syndromes and aneuploid syndromes may be dramatic. A special situation indicating the need for chromosome studies is the very young mother who has a child with a chromosome syndrome. Such women are often mosaic in their chromosome constitution or carry a balanced translocation, necessitating chromosome studies before genetic counseling. Their risk for transmitting a chromosome imbalance to their next children is much higher

than that of a mother with a normal chromosome constitution.

The Noonan syndrome is a well-known phenocopy of an aneuploid chromosomal syndrome, the Turner syndrome. Some time after

Table 12-3. Indication for Chromosome Studies

General
  Classic phenotypes
  Apparent homozygosity for rare recessive traits
  High fetal wastage
  Parents of child (children) with chromosome disorder
  Family aggregation of chromosome disorders.
  Advanced maternal age
Congenital Anomalies
  Cranium
    Scalp defects (ulcer at vertex, abnormal whorls)
    Craniostenosis
  Ears
    Abnormal size, shape
    Abnormal position (low-set, posteriorly rotated)
  Eyes
    Mongoloid or antimongoloid slant to palpebral fissures
    Microphthalmia, anophthalmia
    Hypotelorism, cyclopia
    Iris coloboma
  High-pitched, weak cry (cat-cry)
  Webbed neck
  Atresia or stenosis of gastrointestinal tract
  Ambiguous genitalia
  Lymphedema
  Skeleton
    Hypodactyly, polydactyly, syndactyly
    Abnormal posture of fingers or toes
    Abnormal dermatoglyphics (high number of arches or ulnar loops, single palmar flexion crease)
    "Rocker-bottom" feet
    Radioulnar synostosis, wide carrying angle
Acquired (Late-Onset) Anomalies
  Severe mandibular prognathism
  Gynecomastia
  Keloids in whites
  Sexual immaturity
  Cancer (leukemia, retinoblastoma, Wilms' tumor, bilateral neoplasms)
  Somatic asymmetry
  Mental retardation
  Antisocial behavior

Turner had described the clinical findings in 45 XO females (the Turner syndrome), a number of cases were reported in males and in females with a normal number of sex chromosomes. Noonan and Emke [27] later supplied the evidence that these pseudo-Turner syndrome patients had an autosomal dominant condition that closely resembled the Turner syndrome but was not identical to it in features or etiology. It is important that the estimates of the recurrence risk for the Turner syndrome in a family differ from those for the Noonan syndrome.

Rare recessive traits are usually due to homozygosity for a mutant gene at a specific locus. However, a chromosome anomaly may be suspected if a rare X-linked recessive disorder occurs in a female or a rare autosomal recessive disorder occurs in a male or female without a family history suggesting recessive inheritance (no parental consanguinity, no affected siblings, parents of widely separated national stock). The suspected chromosome anomaly may be deletion of a segment of chromosome material carryng the specific locus, so that the person is in effect hemizygous for the mutant gene and would manifest the phenotype. A short-arm deletion of a G group chromosome has been suggested as being responsible for hemizygosity for the pyknodysostosis locus in a girl with the classic phenotype of this autosomal recessive syndrome.

Prenatal Diagnosis

Considerable interest has developed recently in the detection of fetal defects before birth. The techniques used more or less widely for prenatal diagnosis include amniocentesis, fetal visualization, maternal serology and urinalysis, and fetal biopsy. The goal of prenatal diagnosis is to confirm that the result of the pregnancy will be a healthy child or to offer the prospective parents the opportunity to terminate a pregnancy that is certain to result in the birth of a child with serious physiologic or cosmetic defects.

Forecasters predict a time when all pregnancies will be monitored by one or more of the prenatal diagnostic techniques, but there are several difficulties to be overcome before this vision becomes reality. Our diagnostic acumen is at the present time crude, as discussed earlier. Not only would diagnostic tests have to be developed for the majority of conditions, but the tests would also have to be proved infallible before the conscientious physician would recommend that a mother and fetus be subjected to them. Further, the technique would have to be risk-free. While a calculated risk may be seen as appropriate in some cases, no risks should be taken when no prenatal defect is suspected and the monitoring is for routine purposes only. Finally, public and individual attitudes toward termination of pregnancy would have to be considered. A psychologically damaging situation would be created by diagnosis of an untreatable defect in a family unalterably opposed to abortion. The difficult problem of judging normality would further complicate the issue. Who would judge which fetus is not normal enough to survive, and by what standards?

The technique for prenatal diagnosis that holds the most promise for the immediate future is amniocentesis. Amniocentesis is defined as the process of aspiration of amniotic fluid and at present refers to the transabdominal aspiration of amniotic fluid (Fig. 12-15). The specimen obtained during the transabdominal puncture consists of amniotic fluid and cells. The fluid is derived in part from fetal urine and consequently may contain enzymes and metabolic products that permit assessment of fetal health. Prenatal diagnoses of conditions such as Tay-Sachs disease and Pompe's disease may be based on amniotic fluid assays but are preferably based on cultivated cells from the specimen.

The cellular component of the aspirated material, composed of desquamated cells from the fetal skin and amnion, is generally more useful than the fluid in diagnosing fetal disease. Being of fetal origin, the cells are useful for determining the sex of the fetus by the presence of sex-chromatin material (Barr body) or Y-chromosome fluorescence. Sex determination does not establish the diagnosis of fetal disease but is useful when dealing with women who are carriers of X-linked recessive disorders such as

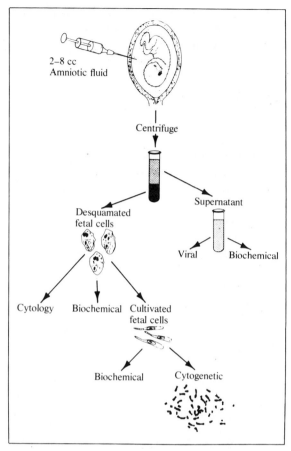

Fig. 12-15. Fluid and cells withdrawn from the amniotic cavity may be used for a variety of specialized assays, as shown here. (From H. Nadler. Prenatal detection of genetic defects. J Pediatr *74:132, 1969.)*

conditions, since the risks for their male children and for their female children are identical.

Cultures of cells derived from the amniotic fluid can be used for chromosome studies. Every recognized abnormality of chromosome number or structure has been identified in amniotic fluid cells. Chromosome analyses are particularly useful and indicated during the pregnancies of women who are beyond 35 years of age, have a history of repeated spontaneous abortion, are known to carry a balanced translocation chromosome, or have had a previous child with a chromosomally determined birth defect. Many health centers routinely offer amniocentesis and chromosome analysis to women over the age of 35 to 40 years because of the relatively high risk for a chromosome abnormality in their offspring (2 to 4 percent) and in light of the proved low morbidity of the procedure.

Amniocentesis can be performed during a limited period of pregnancy only. Two restrictions are placed on its timing. First, transabdominal puncture must be performed at a time when there is sufficient fluid to assure that the fetus will not be injured and that the volume of fluid aspirated will not significantly alter intrauterine pressure. It is generally accepted that the presence of 100 ml. of fluid is sufficient for risk-free amniocentesis. This volume is reached by 14 weeks of gestation; it increases to 250 ml. by 16 weeks and to 350 ml. by 20 weeks. Second, the aspirated specimen must be submitted to the proper laboratory sufficiently early that chromosome studies or biochemical assays can be completed prior to the latest acceptable date for therapeutic abortion, 26 to 28 weeks in most areas. Chromosome studies usually can be completed in two to three weeks, while the length of time required for biochemical assays varies for the particular assay and between laboratories. As much as six to eight weeks may be required for some assays. The opportune time for amniocentesis, then, is from 14 to 20 weeks' gestation.

Genetic Counseling
Congenital defects can be treated by a variety of methods that include surgery, immunization, enzyme or substrate replacement, and diet. Genetic

hemophilia or muscular dystrophy of the Duchenne type. In such cases, the risk of a male fetus being affected is 50 percent, while the risk of a female being affected is negligible, although 50 percent would be expected to be carriers. Abortion of the high-risk male fetus is defensible. Sex determination and abortion of fetuses of one sex or the other for purposes of having a balanced family, on the other hand, are not as readily defensible. It would be a futile exercise to determine fetal sex in women with X-linked dominant conditions or in women who are known carriers of autosomal recessive counseling is usually included in discussions of the treatment of congenital defects, although its usual application results in prevention of defects through family planning rather than treatment of an existing condition.

PREREQUISITES

In 1975, an ad hoc committee of the American Society of Human Genetics defined genetic counseling as:

. . . a communication process which deals with the known problems associated with the occurrence, or the risk of occurrence, of a genetic disorder in a family. The process involves an attempt by one or more appropriately trained persons to help the individual or family to (1) comprehend the medical facts, including the diagnosis, probable causes of the disorder, and the available management; (2) appreciate the way heredity contributes to the disorder, and the risk of recurrence in specified relatives; (3) understand the alternatives for dealing with the risk of recurrence; (4) choose the course of action which seems to them appropriate in view of their risk, their family goals, and their ethical and religious standards, and to act in accordance with that decision; and (5) to make the best possible adjustment to the disorder in an affected family member and/or to the risk of recurrence of that disorder [28].

Thus, there are three prerequisites in the counseling process: an adequate diagnosis, an adequate family history, and a trained counselor.

Adequate diagnosis has been the major emphasis in our discussion of congenital malformations. As has been stated, genetic factors and environmental factors must first be delineated in the etiology of the observed defect. This delineation is often accomplished by verbal history from a family member and may be misleading. It is common for a parent to search through the inconsequential events of pregnancy to find a potential cause of a birth defect and to emphasize that event in the history. Such fallacious thinking is reinforced by the clinician who fails to place the events of the pregnancy in proper perspective. Second, diagnosis must be certain. For this reason, many special investigations, such as enzyme assays and chromosome

studies, are often necessary. The clinician also must train himself to recognize syndromes for which no laboratory tests are diagnostic but for which clinical findings may be relatively pathognomonic.

An adequate family history is essential to the counseling process, especially for traits that may have more than one etiologic background, e.g., cleft lip and palate. A hereditary pattern may be identified on the basis of an adequate pedigree even if an exact diagnosis is not possible. For instance, a history of dwarfism in four consecutive generations of a family with half the children of dwarfed family members being affected regardless of sex and with instances of male-to-male transmission suggests an autosomal dominant syndrome. Regardless of the diagnosis, the recurrence risk can be predicted. However, as mentioned earlier, defects caused by environmental agents and other factors may produce an apparent mendelian pedigree pattern. Thus, counseling on the basis of history alone must be approached cautiously.

A major controversy in clinical genetics today centers on the question of who should be responsible for genetic counseling. The answer should be that each health professional should do the counseling for which he or she is adequately trained. It is virtually impossible for any one person to be trained adequately in each area of genetics, since genetics is a mosaic of so many basic and clinical specialties. Counseling alone incorporates so many specialties that the majority of those concerned feel it must be a team effort.

Genetic counseling can be arbitrarily divided into levels of complexity; it can be done on the basis of pedigree interpretation, on the basis of empirical observations, and by application of statistical techniques. Depending on his level of training in genetics, the obstetrician may be able to deal competently with each of the three levels of counseling. At a minimum he should be trained to deal with simple pedigree interpretations, which for purposes of this discussion includes counseling for well-known mendelian defects with no positive family history.

SITUATIONS PRECIPITATING COUNSELING REQUESTS

Genetic counseling is usually sought after the birth of an affected child, but because of the recent intensive publicity about genetic defects and as a result of screening programs, people are seeking counseling for other reasons. The most common problems for which advice is requested and can be given based on pedigree analysis (level one of genetic counseling) are discussed in the sections that follow.

Carriers of Autosomal Recessive Defects

A person who has a child with a known recessive defect or who has a demonstrably low level of an enzyme known to be associated with a recessive defect is certain to be a carrier of the mutant gene. In the first instance, if future pregnancies are with the same spouse, the risk of recurrence is 25 percent. The risk remains the same regardless of the number and outcome of earlier or subsequent pregnancies. In this instance, 50 percent of the pregnancies will result in unaffected children who will be carriers and can have affected children only if they marry another carrier, a likelihood that is increased by marrying a relative. The remaining 25 percent of the pregnancies will result in normal children who will carry only normal genes. The cannot pass on the defect, nor can any of their children. A person who is identified as a carrier through laboratory screening can have affected children only if the spouse is also a carrier; in this case, the recurrence risk is the same as that described for the parents of an affected child. If the spouse is not a carrier, half the children will be carriers, but none will be affected.

A commonly encountered situation is that of an individual asking for counseling based on the observation of an autosomal recessive defect in a relative. The estimate of the recurrence risk is no more difficult for this person than for the certain carrier, but it usually decreases rapidly as the closeness of relationship decreases. The estimate can be made precisely, but the procedure will not be discussed here.

Relatives of a Person with an Autosomal Dominant Trait

The starting point for counseling when dealing with an autosomal dominant trait is to establish whether the counselee is or is not affected. The affected person will pass the trait on to half of his children on the average. The children may be more or less severely affected than the parent; the variability of dominant conditions is well documented. There is no indication that the manifestations of the trait become more severe in subsequent generations and no indication that those with less severe manifestations pass the gene on less frequently than those with more severe manifestations.

The unaffected person who seeks counseling will usually be the parent or a sibling of an affected person, and the recurrence risk will be negligible. The sporadic nature of the dominant defect must be explained in detail to normal parents of an affected child, and the situation must be examined closely to rule out phenocopies, and reduced penetrance. Again, the recurrence risk in future children of the parents or in the unaffected children of the parents is negligible, whereas the affected person can expect half of his or her children to be affected.

Relatives of a Person with an X-Linked Trait

X-linked dominant traits are rarer than X-linked recessives, and with the exception of modifications on the basis of the sex of future children, persons seeking advice about these conditions can be counseled on the same bases as those concerned about autosomal dominant traits. The modifications are that males affected with an X-linked dominant trait will not have affected sons, but all the daughters of affected males will be affected. The risk for offspring of affected males, then, is negligible for sons and 100 percent for daughters. The recurrence risk for children of an unaffected relative of a male with an X-linked recessive trait also varies with the person's sex. The mother of such a male is certain to be a carrier, and each of her subsequent pregnancies carries a 50 percent risk for male children and a negligible risk for female children. Half the female children, however, will be carriers and capable of passing on the gene. Unaffected brothers of an affected male cannot transmit the gene. However, each unaffected sister has a 50 percent chance to be a carrier. Further, if she is a carrier, she has a 50 percent chance to transmit the gene. Therefore, the likelihood that she will pass the gene to the next generation is 25 percent (the product of 50 percent times 50 percent).

The risks of recurrence of autosomal dominant and X-linked traits are straightforward and can be reviewed in more detail in most texts on human genetics.

Relatives of a Person with a Multifactorial Defect

Many congenital malformations are multifactorial in nature, and counseling in these cases must be based on something other than pedigree analysis. It is common to use empirical data to estimate recurrence risks for multifactorial defects; this is the second of the arbitrary levels of genetic counseling. Personal observation and the experience of others as documented in the literature or through collaborative arrangements must be compiled to develop an expected recurrence risk. Usually, the quoted risk is low (2 to 10 percent), but in some cases the risk may approach that for mendelian defects (25 to 50 percent). Since this type of counseling requires extensive knowledge of specialized literature, it may be best left to the genetics specialist.

Distant Relatives of Persons with Autosomal or X-Linked Recessive Trait

If the carrier status of the person seeking counsel is not known, the third of the levels of complexity of genetic counseling must be used. It also is best left to the genetic specialist, since it requires an extensive knowledge and application of statistics, probabilities, and the laws of chance. The results of the application of these techniques to a clinical situation may be unfamiliar to the nonspecialist (e.g., risk figures of 1 in 128 or 1 in 512) and require elaborate explanations to patients.

References

PLACENTAL DYSFUNCTION
1. Clifford, S. Pediatric aspects of the placental dysfunction syndrome in postmaturity. *JAMA* 165:1663, 1957.
2. Niswander, K., Capraro, V., and Van Coevering, R. Estimation of birth weight by quantified external uterine measurement. *Obstet Gynecol* 36:294, 1970.
3. Saling, E. *Foetal and Neonatal Hypoxia in Relation to Clinical Obstetric Practice.* Baltimore: Williams & Wilkins, 1968.
4. Gluck, L., Kulovich, M., Borer, R., Brenner, P., Anderson, G., and Spellacy, W. Diagnosis of the respiratory distress syndrome by amniocentesis. *Am J Obstet Gynecol* 109:440, 1971.
5. Gluck, L. Evaluation of fetal lung maturation by analysis of phospholipid indicators in amniotic fluid. In *Lung Maturation and the Prevention of Hyaline Membrane Disease, Proceedings of the Seventieth Ross Conference on Pediatric Research,* Ross Laboratories, Columbus, Ohio, 1976. Pp. 47–49.
6. Goodlin, R., and Haesslein, H. When is it fetal distress? *Am J Obstet Gynecol* 128:440, 1977.
7. Spellacy, W., Buhi, W., and Birk, S. The effectiveness of human placental lactogen measurements as an adjunct in decreasing perinatal deaths. *Am J Obstet Gynecol* 121:835, 1975.
8. Josimovich, J., Kosor, B., Boccella, L., et al. Placental lactogen in maternal serum as an index of fetal health. *Obstet Gynecol* 36:244, 1970.
9. Spellacy, W., Cruz, A., and Kalra, P. Oxytocin challenge tests results compared with simultaneously studied serum human placental lactogen and free estriol levels in high risk pregnant women. *Am J Obstet Gynecol* 134:917, 1979.
10. Miller, F., Sacks, D., Yeh, S., et al. Significance of meconium during labor. *Am J Obstet Gynecol* 122:573, 1975.
11. Page, E. Problems of nutrition in the perinatal period. Ross Laboratory's Conference, Nassau, Bahamas, May 11–13, 1969.
12. Hobart, J., and Depp, R. Prolonged pregnancy. In R. Depp and J. Sciarra (Eds.), *Gynecology and Obstetrics,* Vol. 3. Hagerstown: Harper & Row, 1979.
13. Boise, A., Mayaux, M., and Schwartz, D. Classical and "true" gestational postmaturity. *Am J Obstet Gynecol* 125:911, 1976.
14. Rawlings, E., and Moore, B. The accuracy of methods of calculating the expected date of delivery for use in the diagnosis of postmaturity. *Am J Obstet Gynecol* 106:676, 1970.

Additional Readings

Anderson, G. Postmaturity: A review. *Obstet Gynecol Surv* 27:65, 1972.

Crane, J., and Kopta, M. Prediction of intrauterine growth retardation via ultrasonically measured head/abdominal circumference ratios. *Obstet Gynecol* 54:597, 1979.

Hobbins, J., Berkowitz, R., and Grannum, P. Diagnosis and antepartum management of intrauterine growth retardation. *J Reprod Med* 21:319, 1978.

Perkins, R. Antenatal assessment of fetal maturity. *Obstet Gynecol Surv* 29:739, 1974.

Sabbagha, R. Intrauterine growth retardation. Antenatal diagnosis by ultrasound. *Obstet Gynecol* 52:252, 1978.

HEMOLYTIC DISEASE OF THE FETUS AND NEWBORN

15. Landsteiner, K., and Weiner, A. An agglutinable factor in human blood recognized by immune sera for rhesus blood. *Proc Soc Exp Biol Med* 43:223, 1940.

16. Freda, V. Hemolytic Diseases of the Newborn. In D. Danforth (Ed.), *Obstetrics and Gynecology* (3rd ed.). Hagerstown: Harper & Row, 1977.

17. Bevis, D. Composition of liquor amnii in hemolytic disease of newborn. *Lancet* 2:443, 1950.

18. Liley, A. Liquor amnii analysis in the management of the pregnancy complicated by rhesus sensitization. *Am J Obstet Gynecol* 82:1359, 1961.

19. Liley, A. The use of amniocentesis and fetal transfusion in erythroblastosis fetalis. *Pediatrics* 35:836, 1965.

20. Bishop, E., and Brown, T. ACOG Technical Bulletin No. 17, July, 1972.

21. Freda, V., Gorman, J., Pollack, W., Robertson, J., Jennings, E., and Sullivan, J. Prevention of Rh isoimmunization. *JAMA* 199:390, 1967.

22. Bowman, J. Suppression of Rh isoimmunization: A review. *Obstet Gynecol* 52:385, 1978.

23. Queenan, J., and Schneider, J. Practical clinical aspects of Rh-prophylaxis. *J Perinat Med* 1:223, 1973.

24. Maisels, M. Bilirubin. *Pediatr Clin North Am* 19:447, 1972.

CONGENITAL MALFORMATIONS

25. Marden, P., Smith, W., and McDonald, M. Congenital anomalies in the newborn infant, including minor variations. *J Pediatr* 64:357, 1964.

26. Shapiro, B., Gorlin, R., Redman, R., and Brubel, H. The palate and Down's syndrome. *N Engl J Med* 276:1460, 1967. .

27. Noonan, J., and Emke, D. Associated non-cardiac malformations in children with congenital heart disease. *Am J Dis Child* 116:373, 1968.

28. Editorial. *Am J Human Genet* 27:240, 1975.

General Readings

McKusick, V. *Mendelian Inheritance in Man* (5th ed.). Baltimore: Johns Hopkins University Press, 1978.

Gorlin, R., Pindborg, J., and Cohen, M. *Syndromes of the Head and Neck*. New York: McGraw-Hill, 1976.

Smith, D. *Recognizable Patterns of Human Malformations* (2nd ed.). Philadelphia: Saunders, 1976.

Bergsma, D. (Ed.). *Birth Defects Compendium* (2nd ed.). Baltimore: Williams & Wilkins, 1979.

Stanbury, J., Wyngaarden, J., and Frederickson, D. *The Metabolic Basis of Inherited Disease* (3rd ed.). New York: McGraw-Hill, 1972.

Stern, C. *Principles of Human Genetics* (3rd ed.). San Francisco: Freeman, 1973.

Warkany, J. *Congenital Malformations*. Chicago: Year Book, 1971.

13   The Newborn

FETAL ADAPTATION TO EXTRAUTERINE LIFE

Dilip M. Purohit and Abner H. Levkoff

Once the infant is delivered, novel responses are required of him to maintain his independent existence. He must breathe air, change his circulatory pattern, ingest, digest, and assimilate food for activity and growth, maintain his body temperature, limit the invasion of ubiquitous microorganisms, provide new routes for excretion of metabolic end products, restrict the hemorrhage of trauma, resist gravity, and behave in a fashion that ensures maternal caretaking. If the normal course of gestation and labor has not been modified too drastically by medical efforts, the neonate readily faces these challenges.

Breathing

The basic, functional respiratory unit consists of the respiratory bronchiole, alveolar duct, and alveolar sacs [1] (Fig. 13-1). Each component of this unit permits gaseous exchange. During the last trimester of gestation, the lungs undergo an alveolar phase of growth, providing the term fetus with approximately 24 million alveoli, each having a diameter of 50 μ and lined by vacuolated epithelial cells (type II cells), which produce surfactant, and nonvacuolated, flattened cells, which participate in the exchange of gases.

Vascularization of the lung has so developed by 26 to 28 weeks of gestation that there is close approximation of the capillaries to the alveoli at this time. Gaseous exchange can then occur, and extrauterine existence is possible. Nevertheless, infants born at this gestational age are usually capable of only limited periods of breathing because of the difficulty in maintaining expanded alveoli at end-expiration; this difficulty is due to excessive surface tension forces at the air-alveolar interface. With gestational maturation, however, the type II alveolar cells produce a surface tension–reducing substance (surfactant), lecithin, preventing alveolar collapse.

Two biochemical pathways in the production of lecithin have been described [2]. One, utilizing the enzyme methyltransferase, initiates the production of palmitoyl-myristoyl lecithin beginning at 22 to 24 weeks of gestation (Fig. 13-2). This surface-active material is effective in permitting alveolar stability at end-expiration and accounts for the survival of some small human premature infants. Mammals below primates do not have this early surfactant system and cannot survive if prematurely born. Even in the human, the pathway is extremely brittle and is adversely affected by acidosis, hypothermia, and hypoxia.

The second and major pathway utilizes the enzyme phosphocholine transferase to produce dipalmitoyl lecithin. It matures at about 35 weeks' gestation and does not demonstrate the brittleness that characterizes the methyltransferase system. When this pathway matures, the lung is said to be biochemically mature. Anatomically, however, the number and size of alveoli continue to increase until at least 12 years of age, reaching a population of approximately 240 million and a diameter of 200 μ each.

During the intrauterine period, the alveoli are distended with fluid that has a lower pH, a higher osmolarity, a higher sodium concentration, and a lower urea concentration than amniotic fluid. This fluid intermittently flows out of the lungs into the amniotic fluid. At term, this lung fluid amounts to approximately 30 ml. per kilogram of body weight, which is equal to the functional residual volume of air that replaces it when breathing begins.

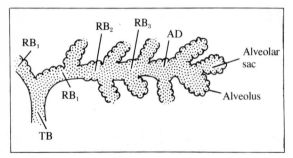

Fig. 13-1. Terminal respiratory unit. (RB = respiratory bronchiole; TB = terminal bronchiole; AD = alveolar duct.) (From G. Cumming and L. Hunt [Eds.]. Form and Function in the Human Lung. Edinburgh & London: Churchill/Livingstone, 1968.)

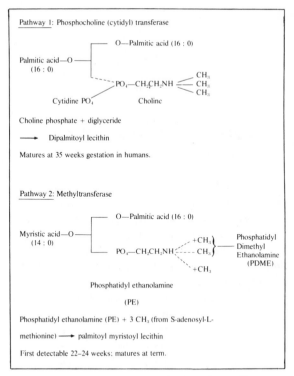

Fig. 13-2. Pathways for synthesis of lecithin in the human fetus. (From L. Gluck and M. Kulovich. Fetal lung development. Pediatr Clin North Am 20:367, 1973.)

INTRAUTERINE RESPIRATORY MOVEMENTS

Respiratory movements have been shown to occur in fetal lambs [3]. Each breathing movement is accompanied by a small to-and-fro movement of tracheal fluid with simultaneous changes in intrathoracic pressures. The net flux of fluid, however, is from lung to amniotic fluid, with the lung secreting up to 100 ml. per kilogram of body weight per day. Since the lung fluid carries surfactant into the amniotic fluid, determination of the lecithin content of amniotic fluid obtained by amniocentesis is used to assess lung maturation. By using the ultrasound A-scan, human fetal breathing movements have been detected as early as 16 weeks of gestation [3]. At term, fetal breathing at a rate of 70 respirations per minute occurs 75 to 80 percent of the time. These respiratory movements have been shown to be depressed by mild hypoxemia, hypoglycemia, hypercapnea, and drugs. Severe hypoxemia produces gasping, with the ingress of large quantities of amniotic fluid.

THE FIRST BREATH

To accomplish initial aeration of the lungs, the expanding thoracic cage must overcome two major resistances, i.e., the surface tension at the air-fluid interface and the elastic resistance of the lung tissue itself [4]. A squeezing action of the birth canal on the thoracic cage in the vaginally born neonate is ssociated with partial expulsion of lung fluid. The recoil of the chest and first breath produce a negative intrathoracic pressure of up to 70 cm. H_2O. As this air reaches the distal lung, the antiatelectatic property of the lecithin present in the alveoli prevents collapse at end-expiration. A portion of the air of each breath remains in the alveoli and begins to establish the functional residual volume. Exhalation against a partially closed glottis during the first seconds of breathing produces a positive intrathoracic pressure of up to 50 cm. H_2O, which helps to prevent the collapse of respiratory units and facilitates the absorption of lung fluid by capillaries and lymphatics (Fig. 13-3). Since the interval between birth and the first breath is so short, neurally transmitted impulses independent of blood chemistry changes may be important in initiating the first breath [5].

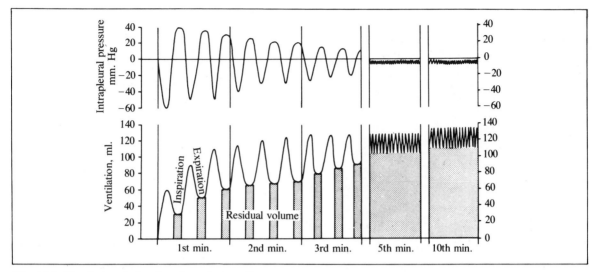

Fig. 13-3. Ventilation during first few minutes after birth. Residual volume increases progressively. Respiratory excursions eventually become quieter from smaller amounts of negative pressure exerted. (From J. Bonica. Principles and Practice of Obstetric Analgesia and Anesthesia. Philadelphia: Davis, 1972.)

Circulatory Changes

FETAL CIRCULATION

During intrauterine life, the placenta functions as an organ of gas exchange. The oxygenated blood from the placenta flows through the umbilical vein to the ductus venosus, which shunts approximately one-half of the umbilical venous blood directly into the inferior vena cava. The oxygenated blood from the inferior vena cava flows across the foramen ovale to the left atrium, whereas relatively less oxygenated blood from the superior vena cava flows into the right ventricle (Fig. 13-4). The pulmonary vascular resistance is high in utero because the pulmonary arterioles are both coiled and constricted. Most of the right ventricular output flows through the ductus arteriosus to the descending aorta. Only 10 to 15 percent of combined ventricular output circulates through the lung.

CHANGES IN PULMONARY CIRCULATION

At birth, the gaseous distention of the lung by the first breath uncoils the pulmonary vasculature and decreases pulmonary vascular resistance. The increased oxygen content of the inspired air and the increased arterial oxygen tension of the blood produces pulmonary vasodilatation. Acetylcholine and histamine are also known to be vasodilatory [6]. In the neonate, the pulmonary vasculature is very labile. Pulmonary vasoconstriction and increased pulmonary vascular resistance can occur in the presence of hypoxia, acidosis, and increased levels of circulating norepinephrine secondary to hypothermia [7] (Fig. 13-5). Elevation of the hematocrit in the newborn, in the presence of neonatal red cells that are less deformable than usual, results in increased blood viscosity, leading to increased resistance to the flow of blood. The viscosity rises exponentially as the central hematocrit goes over 65 vol%. It doubles at a hematocrit of 70 vol% [6]. Studies in newborn lambs have shown a marked increase in pulmonary vascular resistance when the hematocrit reaches this magnitude. High hematocrits are commonly seen in small-for-dates infants who have suffered chronic intrauterine hypoxia.

Infants whose cords are clamped 3 minutes after delivery (late-clamped) have higher hematocrits than those whose cords are clamped 20 seconds after birth (early-clamped). The hematocrit of the early-clamped baby averages 44 vol% at 24 hours versus 72 vol% in late-clamped infants.

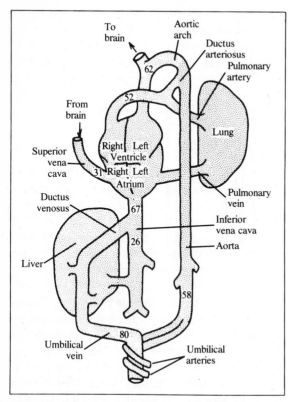

Fig. 13-4. Fetal circulation with levels of percent oxygen saturation. (From S. Korones. High-Risk Newborn Infants. St. Louis: Mosby, 1972. Adapted from J. Lind, L. Stern, and C. Wegelius. The Foetal Circulation. In J. Anderson [Ed.], Human Foetal and Neonatal Circulation, 1964. Courtesy of Charles C Thomas, Publisher, Springfield, Illinois.)

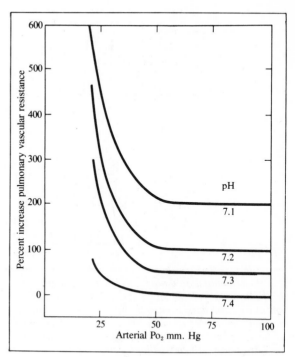

Fig. 13-5. Pulmonary vascular resistance in the newborn calf at varying oxygen tensions and pH. (From A. Rudolph. Response of the pulmonary vasculature to hypoxia and H+ ion concentration changes. J Clin Invest 45:399, 1966.)

CLOSURE OF FETAL CHANNELS

After the cord is clamped, there is decreased blood return to the right atrium. At the same time, since the blood flow to the lungs is established, there is increased blood return to the left atrium. Left atrial pressure is thereby increased, with subsequent closure of the foramen ovale. The foramen can reopen in the first few days of life if an increase in pulmonary vascular resistance produces an increase in right atrial pressure.

The ductus arteriosus is as large as the aortic arch. Increased oxygen tension of the blood and local release of acetylcholine are probably responsible for the contraction of ductal muscle. This im-

mediate functional closure is followed by an anatomic closure during the next few weeks. Thus, fetal circulation, in which both ventricles contributed almost equally to the systemic circulation and worked in parallel, is changed to adult circulation, in which the ventricles pump in series; that is, all the blood pumped by the left ventricle to the systemic circulation must first be pumped by the right ventricle through the lungs to the left side of the heart. The work of the heart is thereby tripled (Fig. 13-6). The median heart rate shortly after birth is 180 per minute and slows to 110 to 140 per minute after the sympathetic activity resulting from the stimuli of labor decreases.

BLOOD GASES

Prior to the onset of labor, umbilical venous blood carrying oxygenated blood has a Po_2 of 30 mm. Hg,

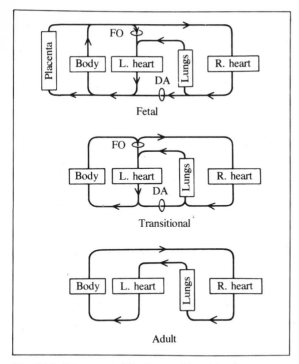

Fig. 13-6. Diagrams of fetal, transitional (early neonatal), and adult (late neonatal) types of circulation. (FO = fossa ovalis; DA = ductus arteriosus.) (From Foetal and Neonatal Physiology *by G. S. Dawes. Copyright © 1968, Year Book Medical Publishers, Inc., Chicago. Used by permission. [After Born, G. V. R., Dawes, G. S., Mott, J. C., and Widdicombe, J. G.:* Changes in the heart and lungs at birth. Cold Spring Harbor Symp Quant Biol *19:102, 1954.])*

a P_{CO_2} of 42 mm. Hg, and a pH of 7.33. At the time of delivery, the umbilical artery values are: P_{O_2}, 10 mm. Hg; P_{CO_2}, 58 mm. Hg; and pH, 7.25. By 60 to 120 minutes, the pH and P_{CO_2} return toward normal values, but the P_{O_2} is only 80 mm. Hg. It may not reach adult levels of 95 to 100 mm. Hg until 72 hours of age because of the small venoarterial mixing through as yet persistent fetal channels.

Thermal Regulation

The fetus has a temperature approximately 0.5°C. higher than that of the mother. The heat output of approximately 25 calories per kilogram per minute is dissipated primarily by way of the placenta, which at term has an umbilical blood flow of 100 ml. per kilogram per minute [8]. The main source of fetal metabolic fuel is glucose, which crosses the placenta by facilitated diffusion. Oxygen consumption of the fetus at term is approximately 4 ml. of oxygen per kilogram per minute, with 1 ml. of oxygen providing 5 calories of heat, depending on the substrate metabolized.

HEAT LOSS AT BIRTH

On delivery into a cool environment, the newborn, who is a homoiotherm, is especially vulnerable to heat loss because of two factors: (1) his body mass is 5 percent that of the adult, whereas his surface area is 15 percent of the adult; and (2) the thickness of the newborn's subcutaneous fat is less than that of the adult, providing less insulation. These factors allow a heat loss per unit of mass that is four times that of the adult. The newborn infant can restrict heat loss by peripheral vasoconstriction and, if neurologically unimpaired, by reducing the radiating surface area by flexing the body.

In spite of the capacity to restrict heat loss, the deep body temperature of the wet newborn falls 2° to 3°C. under the usual conditions of delivery. Under these conditions, a heat loss of approximately 200 calories per kilogram per minute occurs; this is more than twice the capacity of the neonate of 75 calories per kilogram per minute on exposure to cold stress. This initial fall in body temperature (with subsequent return to normal body temperature over the next 6 hours) can be minimized by prompt drying and placement in a warm incubator [9] (Fig. 13-7).

MECHANISM OF THERMOGENESIS

Unlike the adult, who increases heat production by shivering, the neonate responds to cold primarily by nonshivering thermogenesis.

Animals, especially rabbits, have been shown to have metabolically active fat in the interscapular and perispinal areas. It is rich in mitochondria that give the cells a brown color when depleted of lipid. On exposure to cold, the temperature receptors in the skin send impulses to the central nervous system, which in turn stimulates the production

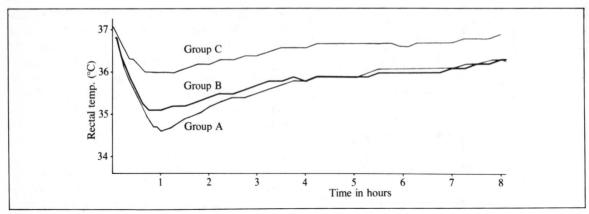

of norepinephrine by the peripheral sympathetic fibers and epinephrine by the adrenal medulla. These catecholamines act on the brown fat and cause hydrolysis of triglycerides, with the recycling of fatty acids into neutral fat. This recycling reaction is exothermic and warms the blood circulating through the brown fat (Fig. 13-8). Under cold stress, as much as 25 percent of the cardiac output may flow through the brown fat. This reaction is oxygen-dependent and also needs a supply of glucose. Hypoxia, hypoglycemia, and damage to the central nervous system can interfere with this protective thermogenic process.

Human neonates have a smaller quantity of brown fat than do experimental animals. However, under cold stress, the nape of the newborn's neck is warmer than other areas. Both norepinephrine and thyroid hormones cause increased heat production in a human neonate; 30 minutes after birth there is a tenfold rise, compared with umbilical vein levels, in the level of thyroid-stimulating hormone. Serum thyroxine and the triiodothyronines also rise after birth, and the human neonate is relatively hyperthyroid during the first few days of life [10]. Iodothyronines act synergistically with catecholamines to increase nonshivering thermogenesis. Thyroid hormones can mobilize fatty acids from body fat stores in response to catecholamines. Thus, thyroid hormones may play a dual role in heat production, namely, substrate mobilization

Fig. 13-7. Mean changes in core temperature after birth. Group A had routine delivery room care plus bath on admission to nursery. Group B had the same care as Group A, but no bath. Group C infants were promptly dried and placed in an incubator at 32 to 35°C. (From T. Oliver, Jr. Temperature regulation and heat production in the newborn. Pediatr Clin North Am 12:765, 1965.)

and potentiation of the catecholamine thermogenesis.

The usual short-term cold stress after delivery has its advantages. Increased secretion of catecholamines on exposure to cold results in increased arterial blood pressure. This reverses the right-to-left shunt at the ductus arteriosus and foramen ovale. Also, the stimulation of peripheral thermal receptors appears to play a role in the initiation of respiration by stimulating central respiratory neurons.

ACUTE COLD STRESS
A newborn infant may be exposed to cold stress in the delivery room, especially when resuscitative procedures are initiated in the absence of a radiant warmer. Moderate cold accompanied by a degree of hypoxia is associated with metabolic acidosis, due to the production of organic anions. A normal infant will hyperventilate and compensate for this type of acidosis unless there is severe hypoxemia and respiratory depression.

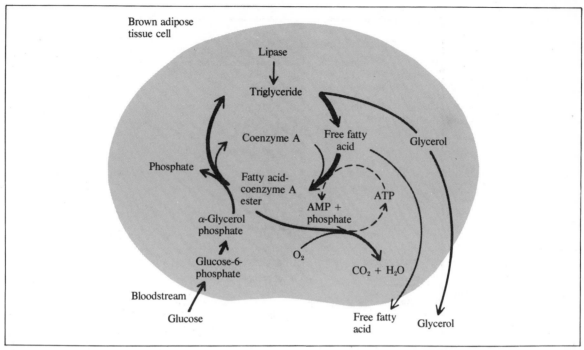

Fig. 13-8. Metabolic pathway for chemical thermogenesis in brown adipose tissue. (From G. S. Dawes. Foetal and Neonatal Physiology. Copyright © 1968, Year Book Medical Publishers, Inc., Chicago. Used by permission. [Redrawn from Dawkins, M. F. R., and Hull, D.: The production of heat by fat. Sci Am 213:62, 1965.])

Susceptibility to heat loss increases in infants with intrauterine growth retardation. The decreased subcutaneous fat in such an infant reduces insulation, and the depleted fat stores limit the substrate available for thermogenesis. Also, the depleted liver glycogen noted in these babies makes them more vulnerable to hypoglycemia; since glucose is needed for recycling fatty acids, the resulting hypoglycemia makes these infants more susceptible to hypothermia.

"Cold injury syndrome" is seen in neonates exposed to severe cold stress who are unable to respond appropriately. These infants appear bright red and lethargic, with a deep body temperature below 32°C. Hypoglycemia, acidosis, and norepinephrine depletion develop, and the infants may die of pulmonary hemorrhage. Management includes slow rewarming, oxygen administration, intravenous fluids, and bicarbonate. Rapid warming with radiant heat may produce apnea.

CHRONIC COLD STRESS

A neutral thermal environment is an environment in which the metabolic rate of the resting individual is minimal as measured by oxygen consumption. In infants weighing less than 1750 gm., maintenance of a neutral thermal environment speeds up growth and significantly reduces mortality [11]. The presence of a normal deep body temperature does not indicate the absence of cold stress, since the core temperature may be maintained by increasing oxygen consumption and peripheral vasoconstriction. To minimize oxygen consumption, incubators have been designed that can automatically regulate the incubator temperature to keep abdominal skin temperature at 36°C. Such an incubator is called servocontrolled.

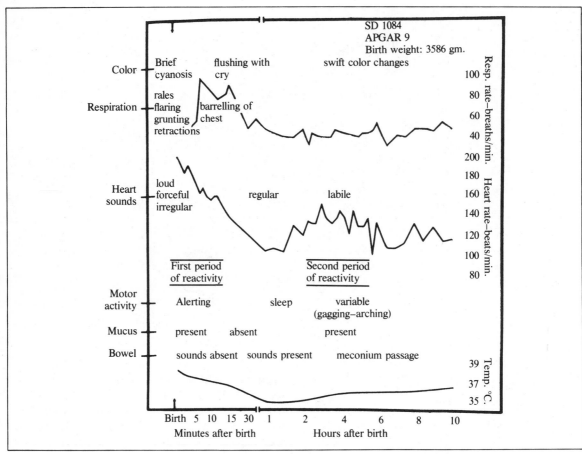

Fig. 13-9. A summary of the physical findings noted
during the first 10 hours of extrauterine life in a repre-
sentative high-Apgar-score infant delivered under spinal
anesthesia without prior premedication. (From M.
Desmond, A. Rudolph, and P. Phitaksphraiwan. The
transitional care nursery: A mechanism for preventive
medicine in the newborn. Pediatr Clin North Am 13:651,
1966.)

Nutrition

As soon as the umbilical cord is cut, the neonate
must depend on his metabolic stores of glycogen
and fat for energy. During intrauterine life, a term
neonate has accumulated total body fat, protein,
and carbohydrate (primarily liver glycogen) equal
to 16, 11, and 1 percent of body weight, respectively. The caloric reserve at birth is enough to
last for 32 days at a metabolic rate of 40 calories per
kilogram per 24 hours, assuming that the neonate
can utilize all his fat and carbohydrate and half his
protein stores, as starvation studies in adults indicate [12].

Following a normal labor and delivery, a newborn infant, if kept in a stable environment, will go
through a characteristic sequence of activity [13]

(Fig. 13-9). Immediately after birth there is a period
of reactivity lasting up to 60 minutes. This is apparently induced by the massive sensory input of labor
and delivery. The next 4 to 6 hours is a sleep
period, after which there is a second period of
reactivity associated with wakefulness, fist sucking, and passage of meconium. The baby is now

ready for feeding. Early feeding at 4 to 6 hours rather than late feeding at 24 hours of age has lowered the incidence of hypoglycemia and hyperbilirubinemia during the first 72 hours of life. The pattern and sequence of the periods of reactivity can be altered by birth injury or maternal medications. A term infant who is not feeding vigorously by the end of 24 hours should be viewed with alarm.

Sucking and rooting reflexes are developed by 32 weeks of gestation, but the coordination between sucking and swallowing develops at 34 weeks. To overcome incoordinated sucking and swallowing, small premature infants are fed via a nasogastric tube. In spite of nasogastric feedings given to the limit of gastrointestinal tolerance, premature infants lose weight initially, and it may take 9 to 12 days before the birth weight is regained. Had the infant remained in utero, he would have gained approximately 350 gm. during this period.

To accelerate the immediate postnatal weight gain, increased protein feedings and supplemental or total parenteral hyperalimentation in the sick prematures have been used. Whether or not such rapid weight gain is advantageous is unknown because the effect of these feeding techniques on brain development has as yet not been determined. The premature infant has been shown to have transient deficiencies of certain enzymes, i.e., cystathionase, tyrosine aminotransferase, and parahydroxyphenylpyruvate oxidase [14]. The enzyme deficiencies can lead to elevated blood levels of tyrosine, phenylalanine, and methionine. Therefore, the high-protein feeding may adversely affect the developing brain in the neonate. Also, because of these enzyme deficiencies cystine, taurine, and histidine are considered essential aminoacids for the neonate in addition to the conventional ones.

A review of the sequence of brain development provides a better understanding of the possible adverse effect of malnutrition. There are two periods when the brain undergoes its most rapid growth. The first is between 12 and 18 weeks of gestation, when growth consists primarily of neuronal multiplication [15]. Placental and maternal restrictive

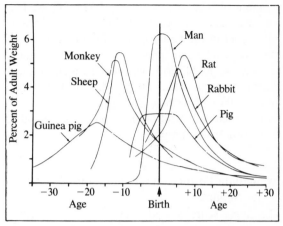

Fig. 13-10. The brain growth spurts of 7 mammalian species expressed as first-order velocity curves of the increase in weight with age. The units of time for each species are as follows: guinea pig: days; rhesus monkey: 4 days; sheep: 5 days; pig: weeks; man: months; rabbit: 2 days; rat: days. Rates are expressed as weight gain as a percentage of adult weight for each unit of time. (From J. Dobbing and J. Sands. Comparative aspects of the brain growth spurt. Early Hum. Dev. 3:79, 1979.)

influences, such as toxemia and malnutrition, do not affect this early phase, but other influences such as irradiation and congenital infections can. The second phase of growth begins in mid-pregnancy and is associated with glial multiplication, dendritic proliferation, and myelinization. Total cell number is reached by 2 years of age, but myelinization continues until the fourth birthday (Fig. 13-10). It is hard to imagine that glial and dendritic proliferation as well as myelinization are not related to intellect. This phase of growth can be restricted by such third-trimester diseases as severe toxemia. Since brain growth continues after birth, it would appear that such infants may be spared permanent neurologic deficits if they are immediately provided with an optimal milieu that allows the brain to catch up.

RESUSCITATION

Neonatal resuscitation is actually "perinatal resuscitation," which begins with prevention and management of fetal distress during labor followed by neonatal resuscitation. It has been estimated that in 50 percent of the neonates requiring resuscitation, the need can be anticipated, and that one infant out of every 40 to 50 births will require resuscitation. Furthermore, at least 50 percent of the babies under 1500 gm. birthweight will require resuscitation. Anticipation and preparation are essential to successful resuscitation.

Immediate Postdelivery Evaluation of the Neonate

The Apgar score is used to evaluate cardiorespiratory and neurologic status of the neonate after birth. Every infant should have a 1- and a 5-minute Apgar score.

during asphyxiation, they can be grouped as follows:

Apgar Score	Signs	Observation
7–10	Reflex activity, heart rate and tone	Good
	Respiration and color	Fair to good
4–6	Reflex activity and heart rate	Good
	Tone and respiration	Fair
	Color	Poor
0–3	Reflex activity and heart rate	Fair to poor
	Tone and respiration	Poor
	Color	Poor

	Score		
Sign	0	1	2
Heart rate	Absent	Below 100	Over 100
Muscle tone	Limp	Some flexion of extremities	Active motion
Respiratory effort	Absent	Slow–irregular	Good cry
Reflex activity (response to stimulation	No response	Grimace	Cough, sneeze or crying
Color	Blue or pale	Body pink and extremities blue	Completely pink

The acronym for Apgar score is:

A–appearance (color)
P–pulse
G–grimace
A–activity (muscle tone)
R–respiration

The score should be given by a person other than the one delivering the baby, usually a nurse trained in Apgar scoring. A score of less than 4 indicates severe asphyxia with depression of cardiopulmonary and CNS function whereas a score of 7 and above is indicative of good condition.

Since the signs disappear in a predictable fashion

The principles of resuscitation fall into the following categories:

A. Airway maintenance
B. Breathing or assisted ventilation
C. Circulation–maintenance of cardiac function and circulation
D. Drugs

The resuscitation is best done under a radiant warmer and at no point should the infant be exposed to cold stress.

Most infants will respond to gentle stimulation, namely, rubbing of the back or gentle slapping of soles of feet or gentle suctioning of nares and oropharynx. If an infant has not responded with crying, good respiratory effort and heart rate over 100 per minute within 15 seconds then more definitive resuscitation procedures should be started. The pharynx should be suctioned before the nose to avoid aspiration.

Moderately Depressed Infant

Most infants who require resuscitation have Apgars of 4 to 6, that is heart rate over 100, irregular or absent respiration, cyanosis or pallor, decreased muscle tone and reflex activity. They respond to bag and mask ventilation with oxygen. Prior to instituting ventilation, upper airways should be suctioned to prevent aspiration. An orogastric feeding tube placed in the stomach will keep the stomach decompressed during bag and mask ventilation. The mask should be a small circular mask that will permit airtight seal and not compress the nares (Fig. 13-11). The bag should be able to deliver up to 100 percent oxygen. Ventilation at a rate of 40 per minute with maximum peak pressures of 40 cm. of water will ventilate respiratory bronchioles and alveolar ducts and improve gaseous exchange. The peak pressure of 60 to 80 cm. of water required to open the atelectatic alveoli poses a risk of pneumothorax. Adequate bag and mask ventilation will result in improvement of heart rate, color, and resumption of respiration usually with initial gasping. Ventilation should be continued until regular respirations are established and color can be maintained, if necessary, with supplemental oxygen.

Bag and mask ventilation is contraindicated when there is meconium stained amniotic fluid and in infants with diaphragmatic hernia. When the amniotic fluid is meconium stained, suctioning of the nasopharynx, prior to delivery of thorax followed by tracheal suctioning if there is meconium in the hypopharynx, will reduce the incidence and prevent the severity of meconium aspiration disease. In infants with diaphragmatic hernia, ventilation is best performed via endotracheal tube to prevent distention of herniated bowel with bag and mask ventilation.

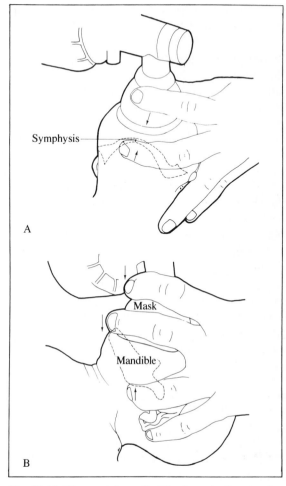

Fig. 13-11. *The mask is applied firmly to the face, and counterpressure is exerted (A) with the middle finger against the symphysis menti, or (B) with the ring finger behind the angle of the mandible. (From K. Niswander.* Obstetric and Gynecologic Disorders: A Practitioner's Guide. *Flushing: N.Y.: Medical Examination Publishing Co., 1975.)*

Severely Depressed Infant

These infants belong to the 0 to 3 Apgar score category with heart rate under 100 per minute (usually under 80 per minute), and are apneic, flaccid, pale, and with minimal or no response to stimulation. Bag and mask ventilation is usually inadequate. They require immediate intubation, and may require external cardiac massage if heart rate is less than 80 per minute.

Technique of Intubation

The infant should receive bag and mask ventilation with 100 percent oxygen until intubation is started. Laryngoscope with No. 0 or No. 1 blade, endotracheal tube, size 2.5 mm. to 4 mm. with soft stylette and size 6 to 8 French suction catheters should be readily available. The infant is held with the head in neutral position, supine with chin pointing upward in the so-called sniffing position. Hyperextension of the neck with retroflexion of the head displaces the larynx anteriorly, making it difficult to intubate.

With the left hand, the laryngoscope blade is inserted along the right angle of the mouth, advanced, and gently brought to midline, thereby pushing the tongue to the left. At first the epiglottis is visualized. The vocal cords are then visualized by lifting the tip of the blade. The glottis and trachea are suctioned if necessary and the endotracheal tube is then passed along the right side of the mouth and inserted to approximately 1.5 cm. beyond the vocal cords. The laryngoscope is then removed. The endotracheal tube stylette is removed and the adapter is placed on the tube. Ventilation is begun with the bag. The chest is auscultated for air exchange to ascertain proper tube placement. After applying tincture benzoin to skin over the upper lip, the tube is secured with adhesive tape taped around the tube and to the skin over the upper lip. The heart rate should be monitored continuously during the procedure by auscultation with stethoscope or by feeling the umbilical cord pulsation. If intubation is unsuccessful on the first try, the infant should be ventilated with bag and mask and oxygen before starting the procedure again.

Cardiac Massage

If heart rate falls below 80 per minute, cardiac massage is required. The hands are wrapped around the infant's chest with thumbs touching over the sternum. Cardiac massage is started by pressing down firmly with thumbs to depress the sternum by ½ inch at a rate of 100 to 120 per minute. The cardiac massage is interrupted every 3 beats for one breath via positive-pressure ventilation. The cardiac massage is continued until the heart rate is over 80 beats per minute with a good femoral pulse.

Drugs

Usually drugs are administered via umbilical vein because of easy accessibility.

1. Epinephrine. If heart rate falls below 50 per minute in spite of ventilation, then 2 ml. of 1-10,000 of epinephrine can be given via umbilical vein or via intracardiac route.
2. Sodium bicarbonate. The acidosis that occurs in the severely depressed infant can be initially treated with 2 mEq per kg. of sodium bicarbonate diluted with at least an equal volume of water for injection and given slowly at a rate of 2 ml. per minute. Bicarbonate is administered only after establishing adequate ventilation.
3. Volume expanders. Hypotension is treated by slow infusion of 10 ml. per kg. of 5% albumin. In case of hypotension due to blood loss, 10 ml. per kg. of blood is transfused using emergency O negative blood or fetal blood obtained by aspirating the vein on the fetal side of the placenta into a 50 cc. syringe whose dead space is filled with heparin.
4. Calcium gluconate. It is administered as a cardiotonic drug in addition to epinephrine. Ten percent calcium gluconate is diluted with equal volume of sterile water for injection and then a dose of 200 mg. per kg. is given at the rate of 2 ml. per minute.
5. Dextrose. In the severely asphyxiated infant who is likely to develop hypoglycemia, 2 ml. per kg. of 25% dextrose can be given via umbilical vein. Glucose provides an energy substrate for heart and brain. It should probably be administered only after adequate resuscitation has been implemented.
6. Naloxon Hydrochloride. Infants who are depressed because of maternal narcotics such as

Demerol or morphine given during labor should be given 0.01 mg. per kg. of naloxon hydrochloride (Neonatal Narcan, 0.02 mg. per ml.) by push infusion via intravenous route.

All neonates receive the following two drugs in the delivery room: Vitamin K_1 oxide 1 mg IM is given to prevent hemorrhagic disease of the newborn. Silver nitrate 1% ophthalmic drops from wax beads are instilled in both eyes to prevent gonococcal ophthalmia. Subsequent saline rinse is avoided.

PHYSICAL EXAMINATION

Initial Physical Examination

The newborn infant should be examined initially in the delivery room and later in the nursery. The Apgar score (see p. 290) constitutes a part of the physical examination after birth. The Apgar ratings of vital signs indicate whether the neonate is successfully adapting to extrauterine life. A low 1-minute score indicates the need for resuscitation. A low 5-minute score reportedly correlated well with neurologic deficits in the 1-year-old infant. However, a poor correlation between a low 5-minute score and neurologic function (including a Stanford-Binet IQ Test) at 4 years of age has recently been noted [16]. A brief physical examination is also performed at birth to detect life-threatening disorders.

Inspection and auscultation of the chest in a normal infant reveals a respiratory rate under 60 per minute, with no retractions, grunting, or rales. The heart rate is 120 to 180 per minute. The infant who is not obtunded has good muscle tone, a position of flexion, and symmetrical movements. Passing a catheter into the stomach through the nares rules out such life-threatening disorders as choanal atresia and tracheoesophageal fistula. A stomach aspirate of more than 20 ml. of clear fluid, especially if it is bile-stained, points to the possibility of upper gastrointestinal tract obstruction. Patency of the anal canal can also be ascertained by passing the catheter into the anus. A scaphoid abdomen should suggest the possibility of diaphragmatic hernia. Genitourinary malformations at times are associated with either a single umbilical artery or low-set ears.

At the end of the examination, if the infant appears stable, he is transferred for transitional care to the low-risk nursery. If the infant has cardiorespiratory distress, he is sent to the intensive care nursery.

Physical Examination in the Nursery

It is preferable to place the dried neonate under a radiant warmer to ensure better observation and prevent heat loss. The infant may be examined within the first 12 hours of life. On admission, weight, heart and respiratory rates, and temperature are obtained by the nursing personnel. Bathing the baby is deferred until the temperature is stabilized at 98°F. Average head circumference is about 33 to 35 cm. at birth. Chest circumference is about 2 to 3 cm. less than that of the head. Head circumference decreases in the first 24 to 48 hours as the molding and scalp edema subside.

POSTURE

The infant's intrauterine posture is commonly maintained after birth. He lies with his neck flexed, arms by the side of trunk, elbows, thighs, knees, and ankles flexed, and fists clenched. Asphyxiated infants are often hypotonic. Tone is also poorly developed in prematures.

SKIN

Skin pallor can be due to anemia or decreased tissue perfusion. Anoxia may produce cyanosis, but, if severe enough, it will produce pallor due to circulatory failure. In the presence of decreased oxygenation of hemoglobin, the normal pink color changes to a deep ruddy hue before cyanosis supervenes.

Evaluation of skin temperature may lead to an important clue. The feet of the infant with sepsis are colder than his abdomen. Increased environmental temperature produces warm hands and feet in an infant. The vernix caseosa is scanty in prematures and postmatures.

Most of the skin lesions seen in the neonate are transient. Venous stasis in the presenting part caused by pressure of the birth canal during labor and delivery can produce transient cyanosis, ecchymosis, or petechiae. Mongolian spots are bluish pigmented areas seen on the buttocks, thighs, and back of black infants. They subside any time from within a few months to up to 4 years. Small capillary nevi are often seen on the nape of the neck (stork bites) and upper eyelids. They disappear in a few years. Milia, which are whitish papular lesions seen on the nose, cheeks, and chin, histologically are epidermal keratogenous cysts. Miliaria crystallina, on the other hand, are vesicular lesions seen on the face and indicate distended sweat glands.

Erythema toxicum, a benign rash of unknown etiology, appears as erythematous macular or papular lesions resembling fleabites. Differentiation from staphylococcal infection is made by Gram stain. Wright's stain of the scrapings from the lesion shows eosinophils.

Transient neonatal pustular melanosis is manifest by vesicopustular lesions without surrounding erythema. Characteristically they appear on chin, neck, nape, lower back, and shins. The pustules disappear in 24 to 48 hours, followed by pigmented macules that disappear in 3 weeks to 3 months. The lesions are more common in black than white neonates [17].

HEAD

The head may undergo extreme molding in vertex delivery. Caput succedaneum, a soft-tissue swelling of the scalp, subsides within a day or two. Anterior and posterior fontanelles are open and may bulge if intracranial pressure is increased. Extreme head molding and overlapping of the sutures may be associated with intracranial bleeding. Cephalhematoma is discussed under Birth Injuries.

EAR AND EYES

Establishing the patency of the ear canal is all that is generally necessary in the ear examination. Visualization of the eardrum is usually not attempted in routine physical examinations. By looking through the magnifying lens of the otoscope, one might note the ocular red reflex. Its absence indicates intraocular disease such as cataracts and tumors. Placing the infant in a sitting position will commonly cause him to open the eyes for examination. Even in the presence of closed lids, a blink reflex to a light beam will indicate sensitivity to light.

Subconjunctival hemorrhage due to venous stasis occurs during delivery. Chemical conjunctivitis due to silver nitrate prophylaxis, when present, subsides in the first two to three days. A purulent eye discharge, especially if seen thereafter, should alert the examiner to possible infection with gonococci, staphylococci, or gram-negative organisms.

MOUTH

Macroglossia may be due to lymphangioma or hemangioma of the tongue, hypothyroidism, or Beckwith's syndrome (visceromegaly and hypoglycemia). Glossoptosis, cleft palate, micrognathia, and respiratory difficulty occur in the Pierre Robin syndrome. Whitish epithelial inclusion cysts, known as Epstein's pearls, are transient lesions on the palate. Natal teeth are occasionally present and, when loose, should be removed because of the danger of aspiration.

EXTREMITIES

Grapelike supernumerary digits hanging by a stem from the lateral border of the hand are commonly seen. The commonest fracture is of the clavicle, which produces asymmetry of movements as well as crepitation. Congenital dislocation of the hip, seen almost entirely in white babies, is diagnosed during abduction of the thighs when the femoral head slips back into the acetabulum, producing a "click."

ABDOMEN

The liver edge can normally be palpated midway between the lower costal margin and the umbilicus. Since kidneys can best be palpated in the unguarded abdomen of the newborn, the presence and size of these organs should be ascertained in this examination. As the bladder is an abdominal organ in the neonate, its distention can be easily palpated.

EXTERNAL GENITALS

The labia minora are well covered by labia majora in a term neonate but not in a premature infant. A whitish, mucoid vaginal discharge, which may become bloody due to withdrawal of maternal hormones, is commonly seen. A redundant segment of the hymen may be seen as a mucosal tag protruding out of the external genitalia. It disappears in a few weeks.

In a term infant, the testes are in the scrotum. At times, there is a small hydrocele that may communicate with the peritoneal cavity. The penis is completely covered with prepuce, which is not retractile. Absence of preputial skin on the ventral surface of the penis indicates the presence of hypospadias. Such infants should not be circumcised at birth, since the preputial skin is required during plastic repair of the hypospadias. Indeed, there is no medical indication for routine circumcision, nor is it necessary to retract the foreskin for cleaning in the neonatal period. During the first year of life, the adhesions between the prepuce and the glans will resolve, allowing retractile foreskin by the end of the first year. An enlarged penis or clitoris or ambiguous external genitals may be due to the adrenogenital syndrome.

CARDIOVASCULAR SYSTEM

Both femoral and radial pulses are felt at birth. Although the absence of femoral pulses may indicate coarctation of the aorta, they are difficult to discern on the first examination. At a systolic pressure below 40 mm. Hg, femoral pulses disappear. The heart rate varies between 120 and 150 per minute but may go as high as 200 per minute during crying and transiently as low as 100 per minute. The systolic blood pressure, which is normally elevated after birth, declines to 50 to 60 mm. Hg by the second day of age. Splitting of the pulmonic second sound occurs after postnatal decrease in pulmonary vascular resistance. Systolic murmurs are often transient and are usually not associated with underlying disease.

NEUROLOGIC EXAMINATION

The neurologic examination entails the assessment of muscle tone and reflex activity. These parameters are affected by gestational age (see the next section). Observation is made for alertness, symmetry of movements, posture, muscle tone, sucking, swallowing, and the Moro reflex. Sucking should be tested by a sterile nipple rather than an unclean finger. The coordination of sucking and swallowing takes place at 34 weeks of gestation. With the infant supported in the supine posture, the Moro reflex is elicited by sudden lowering of infant's head to the mattress.

In addition to the traditional neurologic evaluation, which also has prognostic implications, a second method of neurobehavioral assessment has been developed [18]. In general, it evaluates the infant's adaptive response to various stimuli such as cuddling and sounds. This system gives additional dimension to the evaluation of neurological function.

Chronic use of narcotics by the mother may result in the development of withdrawal symptoms in the infant, manifested by irritability, hyperactivity, sweating, diarrhea, and vomiting during the first days of life.

GESTATIONAL AGE

The evaluation of physical characteristics, reflex activity, and muscle tone are used in the assessment of gestational age of the newborn. Muscle tone develops in a cephalad direction, whereas reflexes develop in a caudad direction. The method for assessing gestational age from these factors is shown in Table 13-1 and Figure 13-12. The birth weight and gestational age can then be plotted on the Lubchenco grid and the infant classified as normal for gestational age, small for gestational age, or large for gestational age.

Posture: Observed with infant quiet and in supine position. Score 0: arms and legs extended; 1: beginning of flexion of hips and knees, arms extended; 2: stronger flexion of legs, arms extended; 3: arms slightly flexed, legs flexed and abducted; 4: full flexion of arms and legs.

Square window: The hand is flexed on the forearm between the thumb and index finger of the examiner.

Table 13-1. Scoring System for External Criteria

External Sign	Score[a]				
	0	1	2	3	4
Edema	Obvious edema of hands and feet; pitting over tibia	No obvious edema of hands and feet; pitting over tibia	No edema		
Skin texture	Very thin, gelatinous	Thin and smooth	Smooth; medium thickness; rash or superficial peeling	Slight thickening; superficial cracking and peeling, especially of hands and feet	Thick and parchmentlike; superficial or deep cracking
Skin color	Dark red	Uniformly pink	Pale pink; variable over body	Pale; pink only over ears, lips, palms, or soles	
Skin opacity (trunk)	Numerous veins and venules clearly seen, especially over abdomen	Veins and tributaries seen	A few large vessels clearly seen over abdomen	A few large vessels seen indistinctly over abdomen	No blood vessels seen
Lanugo (over back)	No lanugo	Abundant; long and thick over whole back	Hair thinning, especially over lower back	Small amount of lanugo and bald areas	At least ½ of back devoid of lanugo
Plantar creases	No skin creases	Faint red marks over anterior half of sole	Definite red marks over > anterior ½; indentations over < anterior ⅓	Indentations over > anterior ⅓	Definite deep indentations over > anterior ⅓
Nipple formation	Nipple barely visible; no areola	Nipple well defined; areola smooth and flat, diameter < 0.75 cm.	Areola stippled, edge not raised, diameter < 0.75 cm.	Areola stippled, edge raised, diameter > 0.75 cm.	
Breast size	No breast tissue palpable	Breast tissue on one or both sides, < 0.5 cm. diameter	Breast tissue both sides; one or both 0.5–1.0 cm.	Breast tissues both sides; one or both > 1 cm.	
Ear form	Pinna flat and shapeless, little or no incurving of edge	Incurving of part of edge of pinna	Partial incurving of whole of upper pinna	Well-defined incurving of whole of upper pinna	
Ear firmness	Pinna soft, easily folded, no recoil	Pinna soft, easily folded, slow recoil	Cartilage to edge of pinna but soft in places; ready recoil	Pinna firm, cartilage to edge; instant recoil	
Genitals Male	Neither testis in scrotum	At least one testis high in scrotum	At least one testis right down		
Female (with hips ½ abducted)	Labia majora widely separated, labia minora protruding	Labia majora almost cover labia minora	Labia majora completely cover labia minora		

[a]If score differs on two sides, take the mean.
Source: From L. Dubowitz, V. Dubowitz, and C. Goldberg. Clinical assessment of gestational age in the newborn infant. *J Pediatr* 77:1, 1970. Adapted from Farr and Associates, *Develop Med Child Neurol* 8:507, 1966.

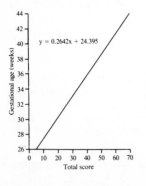

$y = 0.2642x + 24.395$

Graph for reading gestational age. Total score derived by adding score from external and neurologic criteria.

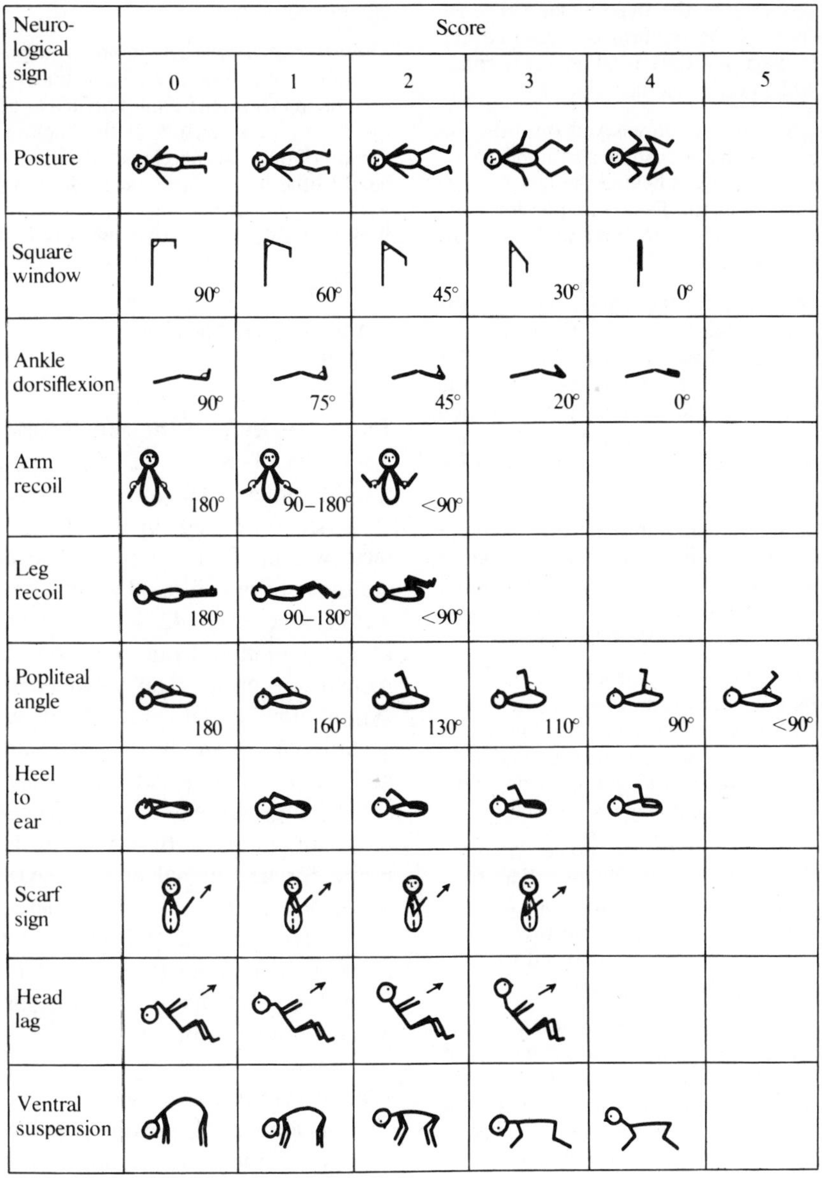

Neurological sign	Score 0	1	2	3	4	5
Posture						
Square window	90°	60°	45°	30°	0°	
Ankle dorsiflexion	90°	75°	45°	20°	0°	
Arm recoil	180°	90–180°	<90°			
Leg recoil	180°	90–180°	<90°			
Popliteal angle	180	160°	130°	110°	90°	<90°
Heel to ear						
Scarf sign						
Head lag						
Ventral suspension						

Fig. 13-12. Scoring system for neurologic criteria. For legend see following page. (From L. Dubowitz, V. Dubowitz, and C. Goldberg. Clinical assessment of gestational age in the newborn infant. J Pediatr *77:1, 1970.)*

Enough pressure is applied to get as full a flexion as possible, and the angle between the hypothenar eminence and the ventral aspect of the forearm is measured and graded according to diagram. (Care is taken not to rotate the infant's wrist while doing this maneuver.)

Ankle dorsiflexion: The foot is dorsiflexed onto the anterior aspect of the leg, with the examiner's thumb on the sole of the foot and other fingers behind the leg. Enough pressure is applied to get as full flexion as possible, and the angle between the dorsum of the foot and the anterior aspect of the leg is measured.

Arm recoil: With the infant in the supine position, the forearms are first flexed for 5 seconds, then fully extended by pulling on the hands, and then released. The sign is fully positive if the arms return briskly to full flexion (Score 2). If the arms return to incomplete flexion or the response is sluggish, it is graded as Score 1. If they remain extended or are only followed by random movements, the score is 0.

Leg recoil: With the infant supine, the hips and knees are fully flexed for 5 seconds, then extended by traction on the feet, and released. A maximal response is one of full flexion of the hips and knees (Score 2). A partial flexion scores 1, and minimal or no movement scores 0.

Popliteal angle: With the infant supine and his pelvis flat on the examining couch, the thigh is held in the knee-chest position by the examiner's left index finger and thumb supporting the knee. The leg is then extended by gentle pressure from the examiner's right index finger behind the ankle, and the popliteal angle is measured.

Heel to ear maneuver: With the baby supine, draw the baby's foot as near to the head as it will go without forcing it. Observe the distance between the foot and the head as well as the degree of extension at the knee. Grade according to diagram. Note that the knee is left free and may draw down alongside the abdomen.

Scarf sign: With the baby supine, take the infant's hand and try to put it around the neck and as far posteriorly as possible around the opposite shoulder. Assist this maneuver by lifting the elbow across the body. See how far the elbow will go across and grade according to illustrations. Score 0: elbow reaches opposite axillary line; 1: elbow between midline and opposite axillary line; 2: elbow reaches midline; 3: elbow will not reach midline.

Head lag: With the baby lying supine, grasp the hands (or the arms if a very small infant) and pull him slowly toward the sitting position. Observe the position of the head in relation to the trunk and grade accordingly. In a small infant the head may initially be supported by one hand. Score 0: complete lag; 1: partial head control; 2:

able to maintain head in line with body; 3: brings head anterior to body.

Ventral suspension: The infant is suspended in the prone position, with examiner's hand under the infant's chest (one hand in a small infant, two in a large infant). Observe the degree of extension of the back and the amount of flexion of the arms and legs. Also note the relation of the head to the trunk. Grade according to diagrams.

If score differs on the two sides, take the mean.

COMMON NEONATAL PROBLEMS

Postmaturity and the Small-for-Dates Infant
The older classification of prematurity by a birth weight under 2500 gm. has been replaced by a classification based on gestational age as well as birth weight. Preterm, term, and postterm infants are those born before 38 weeks, between 38 and 42 weeks, and after 42 weeks of gestation respectively, counting from the first day of the last menstrual period. The word *postmature* is used synonymously with the word *postterm*. When gestational age and birth weight are considered together, the infants can be classified as follows: small for gestational age (SGA), i.e., those under the tenth percentile by weight for gestation; appropriate for gestational age (AGA), i.e., those between the tenth and ninetieth percentile; and large for gestational age (LGA), i.e., those over the ninetieth percentile (Fig. 13-13) [19]. Of all low-birth-weight infants (<2500 gm.), approximately 60 percent are preterm.

POSTMATURE INFANTS
The incidence of postmature births is approximately 3 percent. These infants are large and may cause dystocia, especially in the primigravida. Although the majority of these infants are normal, a significant proportion (15 percent) suffer from placental insufficiency and intrauterine weight loss as manifested by decreased or absent vernix, no lanugo hair, long nails, abundant scalp hair, desquamation, and parchment-paper skin (collodion

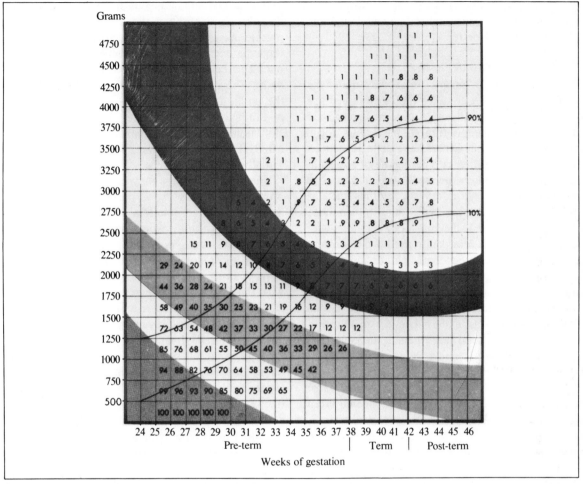

Fig. 13-13. Newborn classification and neonatal mortality risk by birth weight and gestational age. Curvilinear zones of mortality rates are obtained by connecting blocks having similar mortality rates. (From L. Lubchenco, D. Searls, and J. Brazie. Neonatal mortality rate: Relationship to birth weight and gestational age. J Pediatr 81:814, 1972.)

skin). The term *dysmaturity*, which has been used to describe these babies, should be discarded because growth retardation may accompany any gestational age.

Clifford [20] originally described the placental dysfunction syndrome in postmature infants in whom placental function failed to satisfy fetal oxygen needs and needs for other nutrients. It is now obvious that the syndrome may be seen in term, preterm, and post-term infants. Depending on the amount of hypoxia and growth retardation, postmature babies may have loose skin and meconium staining of amniotic fluid, placental membranes, umbilical cord, skin, and nails. Aspiration pneumonia or hypoglycemia may develop in these infants, and they may manifest signs of hypoxia of the central nervous system. The overall mortality is approximately 35 percent, but with the widespread use of biochemical and biophysical monitoring for assessing fetal well-being, and with improved neonatal intensive care, the fetal and neonatal outcome will change for the better.

SMALL-FOR-DATES INFANTS

By definition, small-for-dates infants are under the tenth percentile by weight for their gestational age on the Lubchenco grid, or 25 percent lighter than the mean birth weight (fiftieth percentile) for a given gestational age. Others have defined them as those infants under the third percentile or two standard deviations below the mean weight. Since infants born at high altitude, e.g., in cities such as Denver, are known to be smaller at birth than those born at sea level, and since most of the infants with intrauterine growth retardation are born at or near term, the widely used tenth percentile on the Denver grid is in fact approximately equivalent to the third percentile at sea level [21].

The etiologic factors in small-for-dates infants may be classified as maternal (e.g., malnutrition and toxemia) and fetal (e.g., genetic defects such as Down's syndrome and achondroplasia). Even though placental insufficiency is thought to be etiologic, placental factors are poorly defined. Size and gross pathologic changes in the placenta often have not correlated well with placental insufficiency. The mother who has once given birth to an infant with intrauterine growth retardation is more likely to do so again in future pregnancies. Socioeconomic and cultural factors appear to play an important role in determining the size of the infant at birth.

The development of various organs in growth-retarded infants depends on the gestational age at which the "insult" took place. The head circumference and length of small babies afflicted by third-trimester influences are less affected than weight, so-called asymmetric growth retardation. On the other hand, with first-trimester insults, such as congenital rubella, all growth parameters are severely affected.

Clinically, infants who suffered third-trimester insults present with a characteristic appearance. Most of them are born at or near term. They are active and alert, unless depressed by perinatal hypoxia. The subcutaneous fat is decreased, and the ribs show through the thin, loose skin. The muscle mass over the cheeks, arms, buttocks, and thighs is decreased. The abdomen may be scaphoid. The head looks larger than the rest of the body. There may be a widening of the sutures of the skull, the result of relatively unimpaired growth of brain associated with retarded growth of the skull bones. Unless the neonatal course is complicated, they nurse well and may not have the usual initial weight loss.

The neonatal course may be complicated by the problems resulting from perinatal hypoxia, superimposed on chronic fetal malnutrition. As a result, the meconium aspiration syndrome, central nervous system hypoxia, hypoglycemia, polycythemia, and pulmonary hemorrhage may develop. Polycythemia (central hematocrit > 65 vol%), along with the less deformable neonatal red blood cell, can cause an inordinate rise in blood viscosity and vascular resistance, resulting in sludging of red cells in different organs; this may be followed by lethargy, tremors, seizures, cyanosis, cardiorespiratory distress, increased pulmonary vascular resistance, and right-to-left shunting through the ductus arteriosus. The treatment consists of partial exchange transfusion with plasma to lower the hematocrit, keeping the blood volume constant.

Hypoglycemia and Hypocalcemia

Homeostasis of glucose and calcium metabolism is essential for normal neuromuscular function. In the neonate, aberrations in glucose and calcium metabolism are often secondary to acute or chronic perinatal distress.

Neonatal hypoglycemia has been defined as two consecutive blood glucose values under 30 mg. per 100 ml. in term infants and under 20 mg. per 100 ml. in low-birth-weight infants. Glucose transferred from mother to fetus that is not metabolized is stored as glycogen in the liver, heart, and skeletal muscle and is the primary source of energy during the first hours of life. The glycogen stores are depleted in infants with intrauterine growth retardation. After birth, the combination of a relatively large, metabolically active, glucose-dependent brain, depleted hepatic glycogen stores, and functionally immature neoglucogenesis predisposes these neonates to hypoglycemia within the first 24 hours of life [22]. Furthermore, in the presence of anoxia, on a molar basis, the energy derived from anaerobic glycolysis is 1/18th that of the aerobic metabolism of glucose. Consequently, there is a rapid depletion of hepatic glycogen, leading to hypoglycemia.

Hypoglycemia may also be seen in infants of diabetic mothers. Here, it is mainly due to the neonatal hyperinsulinemia (maternal hyperglycemia → fetal hyperglycemia → hyperplasia of pancreatic beta cells → hyperinsulinemia). Hypoglycemia in infants may be manifested by apnea, limpness, sweating, twitching, and convulsions. Untreated, hypoglycemia may lead to permanent central nervous system damage and thereby constitutes one of the medical emergencies of the neonatal period.

Neuronal integrity can be maintained in the presence of anoxia as long as the circulatory system can supply glucose to the brain and carry hydrogen ions away from it. The circulation persists until the myocardial glycogen is depleted, at which time the heart ceases to contract. In experimental animals exposed to anoxia, the survival time has been shown to correlate directly with myocardial glycogen content.

Umbilical-vein serum calcium levels in term and premature infants are higher than those of their mothers. In a nondistressed neonate, the serum calcium falls 1.0 to 1.5 mg. per 100 ml. within 48 hours. In term infants born after perinatal distress, hypocalcemic tetany with calcium levels under 8 mg. per 100 ml. and increased serum phosphorus may develop. The mechanisms involved are (1) a transient hypoparathyroidism secondary to hypoxia and (2) endogenous release of phosphorus as a catabolic response to anoxia.

Hypocalcemia due to similar mechanisms may also develop in premature infants born after perinatal distress. Hypocalcemia occurs frequently in infants whose birth weight is under 1800 gm. and whose 1-minute Apgar score is low [23]. Recurrent apnea is a common manifestation in such infants. Thus, perinatal hypoxia may be a common denominator of recurrent apnea and hypocalcemia (Fig. 13-14).

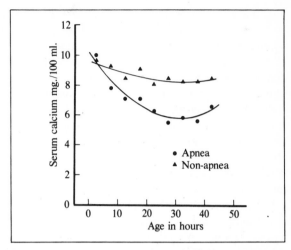

Fig. 13-14. Mean calcium values of all observations on 27 neonates, 14 with recurrent apnea and 13 without apnea. (From J. Gershanik, A. Levkoff, and R. Duncan. The association of hypocalcemia and recurrent apnea in premature infants. Am J Obstet Gynecol 113:646, 1972.)

Respiratory Distress

Perinatal hypoxia, acidosis, pulmonary vasoconstriction, and delayed resorption of lung fluid either alone or in combination play a role in each of the following forms of respiratory distress in the neonate.

HYALINE MEMBRANE DISEASE

Hyaline membrane disease is seen in neonates born prematurely. It is also seen in infants of diabetic mothers, who also are often born prematurely. The incidence is approximately 15 percent in infants under 2500 gm.

The prematurely born infant is handicapped by a nonrigid thoracic cage and the brittle methylation pathway for surfactant production. The compliant thoracic cage prevents the development of appropriate negative intrathoracic pressures necessary to overcome the resistances mentioned previously, impairing initial attempts at aeration. If the infant has suffered perinatal hypoxia and acidosis, the surfactant synthesis is depressed, leading to diffuse expulsive collapse of alveoli. The subsequent series of events includes capillary leakage into alveolar ducts, formation of fibrin membrane, increasing hypoxemia and acidosis due to intrapulmonary shunting of blood (perfusion of collapsed alveoli), and increasing pulmonary vasoconstriction. Although the membrane that lines the partially open alveolar ducts is the hallmark of the disease, the alveolar collapse is the basic physiologic derangement.

It has been shown that maturation of surfactant synthesis is delayed in infants born to Class A, B, and C diabetic mothers. This is possibly related to the inhibitory effect of insulin on surfactant synthesis. Thus, the earlier delivery required for their survival makes them vulnerable to hyaline membrane disease. Gestational age assessed by measurement of fetal biparietal diameters does not necessarily correlate with the degree of lung maturation. Therefore, amniocentesis to measure lecithin content may be essential.

Accelerated maturation of surfactant synthesis is associated with maternal vascular disease, e.g., toxemia, and with prolonged rupture of membranes associated with amnionitis. In the latter instance, increased corticosteroid production by larger-than-usual adrenals may account for the observed acceleration of surfactant synthesis [24]. Controlled studies have shown a reduced incidence of hyaline membrane disease in premature infants born before 32 weeks of gestation whose mothers received parenteral betamethasone 24 hours prior to delivery [25].

TRANSIENT TACHYPNEA OF THE NEWBORN

Transient tachypnea, a relatively benign form of respiratory distress, is seen in infants with a mean weight greater than 2.4 kg. There is a significant number of smaller premature infants in this group as well and a relatively high incidence of low Apgar scores. The clinical picture at birth includes grunting, retractions, tachypnea, and cyanosis in room air. Grunting and retractions subside during the first 24 hours, and cyanosis improves with the ad-

ministration of oxygen. The clinical condition is usually markedly improved by the end of the week. Chest x-rays show hyperinflation of the lungs, with increased bronchovascular markings extending into the periphery and the presence of pleural and interlobar effusion. Resorption of interstitial pulmonary fluid is thought to be delayed, as evidenced by the ease with which the blood can be oxygenated with increased ambient oxygen. The exact mechanism of pulmonary edema is not known.

FETAL ASPIRATION SYNDROME

Unlike hyaline membrane disease, the fetal aspiration syndrome is more common in postmature infants. The fetus who is subjected to acute hypoxemia will gasp and inhale amniotic fluid, which, unlike lung fluid, contains hair, squamous cells, and vernix. If hypoxemia is severe enough, reflex dilatation of the anal sphincter and passage of meconium will increase the amount of debris in the amniotic fluid. After birth, this debris-filled fluid reaches the lung with initiation of respiration and produces foreign-body alveolitis. This series of events is more apt to occur in a postmature infant whose aging placenta predisposes him to additional hypoxemia during labor. In utero passage of meconium and meconium aspiration disease rarely occur before 34 weeks of gestational age [27].

In the presence of massive aspiration, the course is downhill over a period of several days in spite of the relatively good initial blood oxygenation. Recovery from this disease requires removal of the offending material by macrophages and may take several weeks. In a prospective study of meconium-stained infants it was concluded that deep suctioning of the nasopharynx, prior to delivery of the thorax, coupled with tracheal suction under direct vision if meconium was still present in the hypopharynx, significantly reduced the incidence of meconium aspiration syndrome and prevented the severe disease [26].

The association of necrosis of the papillary muscles of the heart, cardiomegaly, congestive heart failure and murmur of atrioventricular insufficiency has recently been described in severely asphyxiated neonates with meconium aspiration disease [28, 29].

PERSISTENT FETAL CIRCULATION

Persistent fetal circulation (persistent pulmonary hypertension) is a form of respiratory distress seen mostly in term infants. Clinically, the infant has respiratory distress and cyanosis that are not relieved appreciably by oxygen therapy. In some infants there is no apparent lung disease, clinically or radiologically, and it is difficult to distinguish them from those with congenital cyanotic heart disease. However, the majority of infants either have perinatal asphyxia, meconium aspiration disease, pneumonia (especially due to Group B streptococci), nonspecific pulmonary parenchymal changes, or diaphragmatic hernia with hypoplastic lungs. Cardiac catheterization or echocardiogram, or both, reveal a persistent increase of pulmonary vascular resistance as evidenced by high pulmonary pressure and right-to-left shunting through a patent ductus arteriosus. The resultant hypoxia and acidosis may require respiratory therapy in addition to oxygen. Recently, drugs such as tolazoline and hyperventilation alkalosis have been used to decrease the high pulmonary vascular resistance in these infants [30, 31].

Although the majority of such infants recover within a week, mortality may be as high as 20 percent. Increased thickness of the media and narrowing of the lumen of pulmonary vessels has been found in some neonates dying of this disorder. In an attempt to explain the pathogenesis, pregnant rats were exposed to either 13 percent or 20 percent ambient oxygen during the last 10 days of gestation. The progeny of the hypoxic mothers had marked thickening of the muscularis of the smaller pulmonary arteries, which is evidence that chronic hypoxia plays a role in this disease [32]. The occurrence of persistent fetal circulation in the neonates born to mothers who received indomethacin, a prostaglandin synthetase inhibitor, during pregnancy, has indicated that such drugs may also play a role [33, 34].

Birth Injuries

Birth injuries sustained during labor and delivery are secondary to mechanical trauma or hypoxia. Only mechanical injuries are discussed here. Eighth in rank among the causes of neonatal mortality, they are responsible for 2 percent of overall neonatal mortality [35]. The common predisposing factors are birth weight over 9 pounds, prematurity, cephalopelvic disproportion, prolonged labor, and abnormal presentation. The injuries can be broadly classified as soft-tissue, skeletal, visceral, and neurologic.

SOFT-TISSUE INJURIES

Localized ecchymosis, facial petechiae and subcutaneous fat necrosis are commonly seen. Traumatic fat necrosis is manifested by the development of erythematous hard plaques of varying size on the cheeks, buttocks, thighs, and back between 6 and 10 days of age. They gradually subside.

SKELETAL INJURIES

Fracture of the clavicle and cephalhematoma with or without skull fracture are seen commonly. In cephalhematoma, there is subperiosteal bleeding over a cranial bone, often the right parietal bone. The swelling does not cross the suture line. Hyperbilirubinemia and anemia are commonly seen in the presence of a large hematoma. These loculations of blood resolve gradually and should not be aspirated.

Clavicular fracture can occur after difficult delivery in vertex presentation or delivery of a breech with an extended arm. The infant fails to move the ipsilateral upper arm, but movements at the elbow and wrist are normal. Differentiation from brachial palsy and a fractured humerus is accomplished by x-ray study. Pinning the shirt sleeve of the affected arm to the mattress with the arm abducted and the elbow flexed 90 degrees will provide adequate immobilization to alleviate pain and permit callus formation, which occurs in 7 to 10 days.

VISCERAL INJURIES

Although they are relatively uncommon, rupture of the liver, spleen, adrenal gland, kidney, or gastrointestinal tract may cause sudden deterioration in the condition of the newborn and subsequent death. The associated peritoneal hemorrhage can at times produce bluish discoloration of the overlying abdominal skin.

NEUROLOGIC INJURIES

Facial nerve palsy, brachial plexus palsy, spinal cord injury, and intracranial hemorrhage constitute the major neurologic injuries. The facial nerve can be traumatized by forceps application or by prolonged pressure of the maternal sacral promontory during spontaneous delivery. As compared with the unaffected side, the face on the affected side appears smoother, and the nasolabial fold is less pronounced. The mouth is drawn to the normal side during crying, and there may be inability to close the eye on the affected side.

The brachial plexus may be injured during the delivery of a large infant who is hypotonic because of asphyxia. Brachial plexus injury may also be associated with a breech delivery with extended arm or shoulder dystocia. Depending on the spinal roots involved, the brachial palsy may be designated as Erb-Duchenne paralysis, with paralysis of the upper arm caused by fifth and sixth cervical nerve injury, or Klumpke's paralysis, with paralysis of the lower arm due to eighth cervical and first thoracic nerve involvement. Klumpke's paralysis is sometimes associated with ipsilateral Horner's syndrome due to damage to the fibers of the cervical sympathetic chain.

Longitudinal stretching, torsion, and excessive flexion of the head during difficult delivery predisposes to spinal cord injury. Hypotonia, secondary to perinatal hypoxia, increases the risk by facilitating separation of bony segments of spine and overstretching of the soft tissue and cord. It has been estimated that 75 percent of cord injuries occur with breech deliveries. The roentgenogram taken before breech delivery may show hyperextension in utero with the fetal face looking upward ("stargazing" fetus). If the hyperextension persists during labor, as seen in a roentgenogram obtained at the onset of labor, the incidence of cord injury in the vaginally delivered neonate is 25 percent [36]. No cord injury is seen in such infants delivered by cesarean section. The infant with a damaged cord appears as a floppy baby and may die due to damage of the vital centers. At postmortem examination, the presence of cervical epidural hemorrhage should suggest an underlying cord injury.

Intracranial hemorrhage in the term infant is commonly associated with extensive molding and rupture of the major venous sinuses (Fig. 13-15). In the past, the subdural hemorrhage occurring in the posterior fossa had a grave prognosis. Early neurosurgical intervention with evacuation of clots by suboccipital craniectomy may change the outlook of the condition [37].

In the preterm infant, intracranial bleeding, primarily intraventricular, is commonly due to hypoxia [38]. Besides causing loss of autoregulation of cerebral blood flow and thereby making the infant vulnerable to sudden increases in blood pressure or blood volume, hypoxia can cause venous thrombosis in the terminal vein. Indeed, sudden death on the third or fourth day of life of the asphyxiated premature baby is usually due to sudden rupture of a hemorrhagic terminal-vein infarct into the ventricles.

Neonatal Infections

Infection probably accounts for at least 20 percent of neonatal deaths. Of the humoral antibodies present in the mother, only IgG crosses the placenta. In utero, the fetus produces small quantities of IgM in the last trimester. Perinatal infection intensifies IgM production. Increased levels of cord blood IgM (>20 mg. per 100 ml.) have been shown to be associated with intrauterine infections [39]. Further identification of infection can be made by demonstrating the presence of antigen-specific IgM by a fluorescent technique.

The defense system of the term infant is not fully mature as evidenced by opsonic activity and complement content that are insufficient for optimal phagocytosis. The infrequency of breast feeding today further compromises the infant's resistance to infection. Macrophages and secretory IgA antibodies are two main factors in breast milk that offer protection against enteric pathogens [40].

Infection may be acquired transplacentally in utero, during the process of labor and delivery, or during the stay in the nursery. The common transplacentally acquired infections are viral, protozoal, and spirochetal. Of the viral and protozoal infections, rubella, cytomegalovirus, and toxoplasmosis

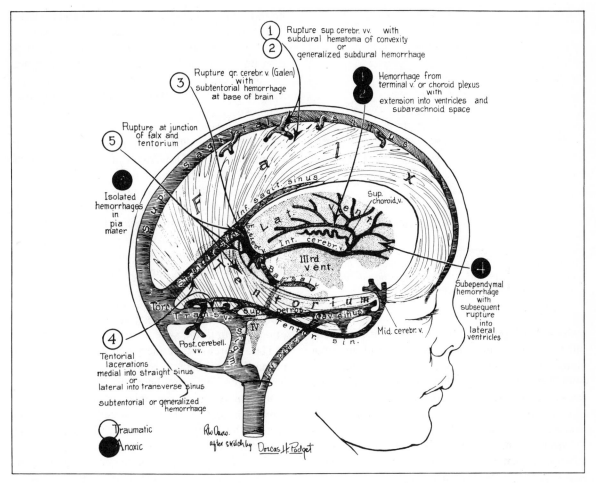

Fig. 13-15. Intracranial dural and venous relationships, showing frequent sites of injury and common sources of hemorrhage in newborn infants. Traumatic lesions are indicated by black numbers on white and asphyxial (anoxic) lesions are shown by white numbers on black. (From E. Haller, R. Nesbitt, Jr., and D. Anderson. Clinical and pathologic concepts of gross intracranial hemorrhage in perinatal mortality. Obstet Gynecol Surv 11:179, 1956. Copyright © 1956, The Williams & Wilkins Co., Baltimore.)

are the most frequent. Herpes simplex, another viral infection, is transmitted before birth by ascent from an infected cervix or by contamination of the baby at the time of delivery. The eponym TORCH (*t*oxoplasmosis, *r*ubella, *c*ytomegalovirus, *h*erpes simplex, and *o*ther viruses) has been used to designate these congenital infections, since their clinical manifestations are similar [41]. The manifestations include hepatosplenomegaly, jaundice, thrombocytopenia with or without purpura, chorioretinitis, intrauterine growth retardation, and intracranial calcification. The pathogenesis of transplacental fetal infection is depicted in Figure 13-16.

It has now become apparent that a newborn infant who seems normal at birth may be infected with cytomegalovirus and manifest psychomotor retardation at a later date. The same is probably true of other congenital infections, making the clinically apparent infection only the tip of the

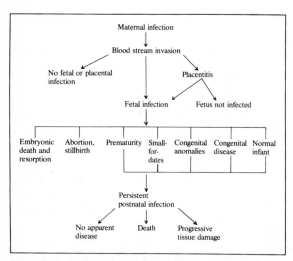

Maternal infection

Blood stream invasion

No fetal or placental   Placentitis
infection

Fetal infection   Fetus not infected

Embryonic   Abortion,   Prematurity Small-   Congenital Congenital Normal
death and   stillbirth   for-   anomalies   disease   infant
resorption   dates

Persistent
postnatal infection

No apparent   Death   Progressive
disease   tissue damage

Fig. 13-16. Pathogenesis of transplacental fetal infection. (From J. Klein and S. March. Infection in the newborn. Clin Obstet Gynecol *13:322, 1970.)*

iceberg. The approach to eradication of congenital infection lies in prevention; for example, immunization of prepubertal females against rubella; cesarean section delivery when herpetic lesions are found on the cervix; and avoidance of consumption of undercooked meat during pregnancy for prevention of toxoplasmosis.

The fetus may be infected by an organism ascending through the birth canal at the time of delivery, especially after prolonged rupture of the membranes and amnionitis. The infection may also be acquired during the passage through the birth canal. Beta-hemolytic streptococci, the predominant pathogen before 1940, was superseded in the late 1940s by coliform bacilli. Later, in 1950, the incidence of staphylococcal infection increased, but the coliform bacilli again assumed first place in 1960. The common bacterial pathogens at present are the gram-negative bacilli (*Escherichia coli, Pseudomonas, Klebsiella*) and the group B beta-hemolytic streptococci. *Listeria monocytogenes,* gonococci, and staphylococci constitute most of the remaining bacteria responsible for infection.

The infection may be manifested by septicemia, meningitis, pneumonia, or pyelonephritis. In addition to prolonged rupture of the membranes (> 24

hours), difficult labor, and low birth weight, obstetrical manipulations and perinatal asphyxia are other predisposing factors. A high index of suspicion on the physician's part, coupled with apnea, lethargy, poor feeding, vomiting, diarrhea, fever, or hypothermia in the neonate, leads to early clinical diagnosis.

Approximately half the bacterial infections of the neonate are caused by gram-negative bacteria, apparently due to the low levels of IgM present in the newborn. Since the course of the disease with these organisms can be fulminating, leading to meningitis or endotoxic shock, treatment should be initiated early after appropriate diagnostic procedures are accomplished. Such procedures include blood culture, lumbar puncture, suprapubic bladder aspiration for urine culture, and a chest roentgenogram. The antibiotics of choice for initial use are penicillin and kanamycin or penicillin and gentamicin; these will cover both gram-positive and gram-negative organisms until the specific organism is identified.

The source of nursery-acquired infection is primarily the hospital personnel. However, other infants, fomites, humidification equipment, or the mother may be responsible. Bacteria like *Pseudomonas* and *Serratia* ("water bugs") proliferate in humidifying equipment. Good handwashing technique by nursery personnel is the primary method of preventing the spread of bacterial infection in the nursery. It must be remembered that infants with congenital infections such as rubella can transmit their infection to susceptible hospital personnel.

Maternal Attachment
Maternal attachment is the foundation for optimal maternal caretaking. The planning for and confirmation and acceptance of pregnancy, plus the awareness of fetal movements, plays a role in the development of this bond. The mother's behavior in the first few minutes on being presented with her baby shortly after birth is predictable. She begins with fingertip touching of the infant's extremities and proceeds in the next few minutes to massage and encompass the trunk with her palm. The mother has a special interest in eye-to-eye contact

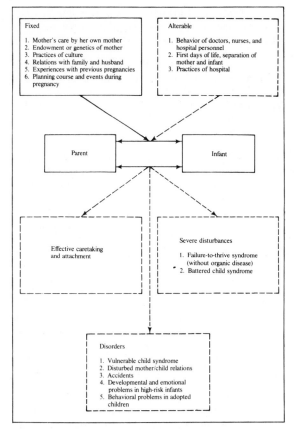

<table>
<tr><th>Fixed</th><th>Alterable</th></tr>
</table>

Fixed
1. Mother's care by her own mother
2. Endowment or genetics of mother
3. Practices of culture
4. Relations with family and husband
5. Experiences with previous pregnancies
6. Planning course and events during pregnancy

Alterable
1. Behavior of doctors, nurses, and hospital personnel
2. First days of life, separation of mother and infant
3. Practices of hospital

Parent

Infant

Effective caretaking and attachment

Severe disturbances
1. Failure-to-thrive syndrome (without organic disease)
2. Battered child syndrome

Disorders
1. Vulnerable child syndrome
2. Disturbed mother/child relations
3. Accidents
4. Developmental and emotional problems in high-risk infants
5. Behavioral problems in adopted children

Fig. 13-17. Hypothesized diagram of the major influences on maternal behavior and the resulting disturbances. Solid lines represent unchangeable determinants; dotted lines represent alterable determinants. (From M. H. Klaus and J. H. Kennel. Maternal-Infant Bonding. *St. Louis: Mosby, 1976.)*

affectional attachment occurred ranged from a few days to as late as nine weeks.

Unlike lower animals, human neonates are not programmed primarily by instinctive behavior. Their intellectual development depends on the process of learning that in turn depends on the sensory input provided by the mother, which in turn depends on maternal attachment.

It would appear that the maternal attachment process is a highly vulnerable one during the early neonatal period. Even the suggestion to the mother by the physician that her baby is abnormal may interfere with the process. Obviously, complete removal of the baby to the intensive care nursery will interfere with many of the normal contacts between mother and infant that would normally occur during the first few hours of life. In animals, this period of contact appears to be extremely critical, and separation during this time causes a total collapse of the mothering response. Studies in humans have shown that early contact between the mother and the infant as well as extended contact later during the hospital stay, instead of brief contacts only during feedings, help in fostering a positive mother-infant relationship. Therefore, the current hospital routines that curtail such early and extended contacts should be revised [43].

It is felt that the single most important factor that predisposes to a breakdown in maternal attachment in human beings is the lack of nurturing the mother had as a growing child [44] (Fig. 13-17). Failure to thrive due to child neglect and the battered child syndrome represent two clinical entities known to be due to maternal detachment.

with the infant. She positions her face in such a manner that her eyes and those of the infant meet fully in the same vertical plane of rotation. This eye-to-eye contact may be one of the major factors responsible for initiating maternal caretaking responses. A study of modal responses of primiparous women whose mean age was 24 years and whose mean educational level was 2.7 years of college showed that the feeling of simple caretaking evolved into positive feelings of affection at the beginning of the third week [42]. The time at which

References

FETAL ADAPTATION TO EXTRAUTERINE LIFE
1. Charnock, E., and Doershuk, C. Developmental aspects of human lung. *Pediatr Clin North Am* 20:275, 1973.
2. Gluck, L., and Kulovich, M. Fetal lung development. *Pediatr Clin North Am* 20:267, 1973.
3. Dawes, G. Prenatal life: Fetal respiratory movements rediscovered. *Pediatrics* 51:965, 1973.
4. Avery, M. *The Lung and Its Disorders in the Newborn Infant.* Philadelphia: Saunders, 1968.
5. Bonica, J. *Principles and Practice of Obstetric*

Analgesia and Anesthesia, Vol. 1. Philadelphia: Davis, 1967.

6. Dawes, G. *Fetal and Neonatal Physiology.* Chicago: Year Book, 1968.

7. Klaus, M., and Meyer, B. Oxygen therapy for the newborn. *Pediatr Clin North Am* 13:731, 1966.

8. Adamson, K., Jr. The role of thermal factors in fetal and neonatal life. *Pediatr Clin North Am* 13:599, 1966.

9. Oliver, T., Jr. Temperature regulation and heat production in the newborn. *Pediatr Clin North Am* 12:765, 1965.

10. Erenberg, A., Phelps, D., Lam, R., and Fisher, D. Total and free thyroid concentrations in neonatal blood. *Pediatrics* 53:211, 1974.

11. Silverman, W. *Dunham's Premature Infants.* New York: Harper & Row, 1964.

12. Heird, W., Driscoll, J., Jr., Schullinger, J., Grebin, B., and Winters, R. Intravenous alimentation in pediatric patients. *J Pediatr* 80:351, 1972.

13. Desmond, M., Franklin, R., Valbora, C., Hill, R., Plumb, R., Arnold, H., and Watts, J. The clinical behavior of the newly born. *J Pediatr* 62:307, 1963.

14. Raiha, N. Biochemistry and nutrition of premature infants. *Pediatrics* 53:147, 1974.

15. Dobbing, J. Later growth of the brain. *Pediatrics* 53:2, 1974.

PHYSICAL EXAMINATION OF THE NEWBORN

16. Drage, J., Berendes, H., and Fisher, P. The Apgar Scores and Four-Year Psychological Examination Performance. Pan American Health Organization Scientific Publication No. 185, 1969. P. 222.

17. Ramamurthy, R. S., Reveri, M., Esterly, N. B., Fretzin, D. F., and Pildes, R. S. Transient neonatal pustular melanosis. *J Pediatr* 88:831, 1976.

18. Brazelton, T. *Neonatal Behavior Assessment Scale.* London: Spastics International Medical Publications, 1973.

COMMON NEONATAL PROBLEMS

19. Battaglia, F., and Lubchenco, L. A practical classification of newborn infants by weight and gestational age. *J Pediatr* 71:159, 1967.

20. Clifford, S. Postmaturity with placental dysfunction: Clinical syndrome and pathologic findings. *J Pediatr* 44:1, 1954.

21. Usher, R. Clinical and therapeutic aspects of fetal malnutrition. *Pediatr Clin North Am* 17:169, 1970.

22. Cornblath, M., and Schwartz, R. *Disorders of Carbohydrate Metabolism in Infancy.* Philadelphia: Saunders, 1976.

23. Gershanik, J., Levkoff, A., and Duncan, R. The association of hypocalcemia and recurrent apnea in premature infants. *Am J Obstet Gynecol* 113:646, 1972.

24. Naeye, R., Harcke, H., Jr., and Blanc, W. Adrenal gland structure and hyaline membrane disease. *Pediatrics* 47:650, 1971.

25. Liggins, F., and Howie, R. The Prevention of RDS by Maternal Steroid Therapy. In L. Gluck (Ed.), *Modern Perinatal Medicine.* Chicago: Year Book, 1974.

26. Carson, B. S., Losey, R. W., Bowes, W. A., and Simmons, M. A. Combined obstetric and pediatric approach to prevent meconium aspiration syndrome. *Am J Obstet Gynecol* 126:712, 1976.

27. Matthews, T. G., and Warshaw, J. B. Relevance of the gestational age distribution of meconium passage in utero. *Pediatrics* 64:30, 1979.

28. Setzer, E., Ermocilla, R., Tonkin, I., John, E., Sansa, M., and Cassady, G. Papillary muscle necrosis in a neonatal autopsy population: Incidence and associated clinical manifestations. *J Pediatr* 96:289, 1980.

29. Donnely, W. H., Bucciarelli, R. L., and Nelson, R. M. Ischemic papillary muscle necrosis in stressed newborn infants. *J Pediatr* 96:295, 1980.

30. Purohit, D. M., Pai, S., and Levkoff, A. H. Effect of tolazoline on persistent hypoxemia in neonatal respiratory distress. *Crit Care Med* 6:14, 1978.

31. Peckham, G. T., and Fox, W. W. Physiologic factors affecting pulmonary artery pressure in infants with persistent pulmonary hypertension. *J Pediatr* 93:1005, 1978.

32. Goldberg, S., Levy, R., Siassi, B., and Belten, J. Maternal hypoxia-neonatal vasculature effect. *Pediatrics* 48:528, 1971.

33. Levine, D. L., Fixler, D. E., Morriss, F. C., and Tyson, J. Morphologic analysis of the pulmonary vascular bed in infants exposed in utero to prostaglandin synthetase inhibitors. *J Pediatr* 92:478, 1978.

34. Csaba, I. F., Sulyok, E., and Ertl, T. Relationship of maternal treatment with indomethacin to persistence of fetal circulation syndrome. *J Pediatr* 92:484, 1978.

35. Valdes-Dapena, M., and Arey, J. The causes of neonatal mortality: An analysis of 501 autopsies on newborn infants. *J Pediatr* 77:366, 1970.

36. Bresnan, M., and Abroms, I. Neonatal spinal cord transection secondary to intrauterine hyperextension of the neck in breech presentation. *J Pediatr* 84:734, 1974.

37. Serfontein, G. L., Rom, S., and Stein, S. Posterior fossa subdural hemorrhage in the newborn. *Pediatrics* 65:40, 1980.

38. Volpe, J. J. Neonatal intracranial hemorrhage. *Clin Perinatol* 4(1):77, 1977.
39. Alford, C. Immunoglobulin determinations in the diagnosis of fetal infection. *Pediatr Clin North Am* 18:99, 1971.
40. Welsh, J. K., and May, J. T. Anti-infective properties of breast milk. *J Pediatr* 94:1, 1979.
41. Nahmias, A. The TORCH complex. *Hosp Pract* 8(May):65, 1974.

MATERNAL ATTACHMENT

42. Robson, K., and Moss, H. Patterns of maternal attachment. *J Pediatr* 77:976, 1970.
43. Lozoff, B., Brittenham, G. M., Trause, M. A., Kennel, J. H., and Klaus, M. H. The mother-newborn relationship: Limits of adaptability. *J Pediatr* 91:1, 1977.
44. Klaus, M., and Kennell, J. Mothers separated from their newborn infants. *Pediatr Clin North Am* 17:1015, 1970.

14

The Puerperium

The puerperium is defined as the six-week period following delivery. This definition implies that the anatomic and physiologic changes that occurred in the maternal organism during pregnancy have returned to the nonpregnant status at six weeks. We will first discuss the normal physiologic changes that occur during the puerperium and then describe some of the pathologic developments of this period.

Expected Physiologic Changes of the Puerperium

UTERUS

As might be expected, the most dramatic physiologic changes of the puerperium occur in the uterus. The uterus rapidly shrinks in size following the delivery of the fetus and the placenta. If uterine contractility is normal, the uterus immediately after delivery can be felt as a hard, globular mass arising from the pelvis and extending about half the distance between the symphysis pubis and umbilicus. The uterine wall, which is about 5 mm. thick in late pregnancy before the onset of labor, is now about 5 cm. in thickness and tightly contracted to control bleeding from the many vessels opened by separation of the placenta from its uterine bed. In due course, the blood vessels will thrombose and in this way minimize blood loss. In the first hour or so after delivery, uterine contractions must provide the hemostatic effect.

The uterus rapidly decreases in size over the next few days and weeks and cannot be felt by abdominal palpation after the seventh to tenth postpartum day. At six weeks, this process of *involution* is usually complete, and the uterus has returned to its prepregnant size. Uterine involution occurs apparently as a result of shrinking of individual muscle cells with a loss of protein, primarily actomyosin, and not as a result of diminution in the number of cells. The exact cellular mechanisms that accompany this remarkably rapid catabolism are unknown.

The placenta separates in the decidua, and the decidua remaining in the uterus functions as two layers. The layer lining the uterine cavity becomes necrotic and in due time is sloughed with the lochia. The residual layer adjacent to the myometrium contains the remaining portions of the endometrial glands, and the cells lining these glands rapidly proliferate to reepithelialize the inner uterine surface. The placental site is characterized by many thrombosed veins and an absence of epithelium. This site is reepithelialized both by an ingrowth of epithelium from the decidua surrounding the site as it grows under the decidua being sloughed and by proliferation of the endometrial glands underlying the placental site itself. While the placental site is not totally reepithelialized for about six weeks, the remainder of the endometrial cavity is covered by epithelium by the end of two to three weeks. Subinvolution of the placental site is a well-recognized clinical entity and is discussed under Postpartum Bleeding.

CERVIX AND VAGINA

The cervix undergoes equally rapid involution from the soft, bruised, flabby structure seen in the patient immediately after delivery to an organ constricted to the point where only one finger can be inserted through it at the end of one week. At six weeks, the cervix has usually not healed completely but rather remains engorged, with areas of pseudoerosion (downgrowth of endocervical epithelium onto the ectocervical surface) frequently seen. A few weeks later, the cervix is involuted to its maximum point, although the organ may remain chronically infected and require treatment. The cervix rarely resumes its pregravid appearance spontaneously; rather, the external os assumes a "fish-mouth" shape due to lacerations.

The vagina shrinks rapidly, although, like the cervix, it does not involute to its pregravid size. The normal rugae, which disappear with delivery, begin to return at about three weeks. The pelvic muscles surrounding the vagina gradually recover much of their former tone, although the parous vagina is rarely as muscular as the nulliparous organ. Hymenal tags remain as remnants of the hymen.

ABDOMINAL WALL

The muscles of the abdominal wall were forced to stretch noticeably to accommodate the enlarged pregnant uterus. Following delivery, the abdominal wall remains distressingly flabby, with no apparent muscle tone at all. Involution of this structure takes many weeks for completion and in many women remains forever incomplete. Exercises designed to strengthen the abdominal musculature are recommended for all patients. The extreme abdominal relaxation normal at this time assumes clinical importance with intra-abdominal disease. If evidences of surgical abdominal disease are present, the abdominal musculature simply cannot contract sufficiently to provide the muscular rigidity and rebound tenderness usually noted with intra-abdominal disease.

URINARY TRACT

Probably as a result of bruising during the passage of the fetus through the birth canal, the postpartum bladder has poor muscle tone and may overdistend in the postpartum patient without producing the usual symptoms suggesting a full bladder. This fact has important implications in the postpartum care of the bladder. A second factor influencing bladder physiology is the diuresis that occurs within a day following delivery and persists for a number of days as the body excretes the water held as interstitial fluid and increased blood volume during pregnancy. The urine may contain large

amounts of lactose, probably originating in the breasts. Acetonuria may also develop following a long hard labor, perhaps as a result of low food intake.

BREASTS

The hormone control of breast development and lactation is complex. It is an over-simplification to say that estrogen stimulates ductal development or that progesterone stimulates alveolar development, since the addition of prolactin or somatomammotropin increases these effects. The presence of these hormones during pregnancy accounts for the breast growth that occurs at this time. The exact role of human placental lactogen remains obscure.

The milk flow, which does not begin until the postpartum period, may be initiated by a drop in the level of serum estrogen that accompanies delivery of the placenta. This drop may permit an increase in the secretion of prolactin from the anterior pituitary gland, which in turn stimulates milk secretion from the epithelial cells of the acini. The secretion distends the distal tubules in the ducts, but actual movement of the secreted milk into the sinuses from which it is suckled is dependent on the release of oxytocin from the posterior pituitary gland, the "milk let-down" phenomenon. This effect is induced by oxytocin-mediated contraction of the myoepithelial cells surrounding the alveoli. It is easy to understand that many factors might interfere at various points in this complex hormonal mechanism directed toward inducing lactation.

Colostrum, a substance much like breast milk except that it contains more globulin and less sugar and fat, is secreted in the immediate postpartum period and even during pregnancy. Antibodies present in the colostrum may be important in passively immunizing a newborn infant against certain infectious diseases.

During the second or third postpartum day, the breasts become greatly engorged and full. This engorgement does not occur simultaneously with milk production, since the milk appears on the fourth or fifth day. Suckling induces further lactation in two ways: it increases actual milk production and increases the secretion of oxytocin from the posterior pituitary gland, which induces milk let-down. Engorgement of the breasts produces discomfort, heaviness, and a general feeling of lassitude, but it does not produce the so-called milk fever of previous generations. Fever means infection somewhere in the mother, and a search should be made for its cause. Many drugs are secreted in breast milk, so that care should be taken with maternal drug therapy [1]. Sedatives and laxatives maternally administered are two examples of drugs that may produce obvious effects on the suckled newborn.

WEIGHT LOSS

The gravida loses about 12 to 13 pounds (5.4 to 5.9 kg.) of weight as the fetus, placenta, and amniotic fluid are expelled. Fluid loss through increased urinary flow and diaphoresis during the first few postpartum days account for at least another 5 pounds (2.27 kg.). Subsequent weight loss of a lesser degree will occur when breast involution is complete.

Postpartum Care

IMMEDIATE CARE

Immediate postpartum care is crucial if the patient is to recover from delivery quickly and completely. During the first postpartum hour, the uterus must be kept well contracted if bleeding is to be minimized. The open sinuses in the placental sites are not yet thrombosed and will bleed copiously if they are not constricted by intertwining, tightly contracted uterine muscle cells. In most instances, the uterus will contract spontaneously after delivery of the placenta. Almost continuous gentle palpation of the postpartum fundus should be performed, however, since relaxation even for a few seconds may allow a blood loss of 500 to 1000 ml. If the uterus has a tendency to relax, digital massage will usually induce a contraction. It is also wise to administer a dilute solution of oxytocin intravenously in this circumstance, or indeed in any patient who has exhibited a predisposing cause of postpartum hemorrhage, such as an overdistended uterus from twins, abruptio placentae, or a history of postpartum bleeding with a prior pregnancy.

Should bleeding occur, the obstetrician must determine its source by careful inspection for lacerations of the birth canal as well as by palpation of the fundus.

SUBSEQUENT CARE

Subsequent postpartum care will involve many organ systems.

General Measures

BED REST. Bed rest is enforced for a brief time only, just long enough to allow the new mother to recover her strength through sleep and to recover from the effects of any analgesic or anesthetic agents that she may have received during labor. As soon as she wants to ambulate, she should be helped to the bathroom. Since she may not recognize her own lack of strength, it is mandatory that she not attempt to get out of bed without the help of an attendant. Early ambulation has been shown to decrease the incidence of subsequent thrombophlebitis and pulmonary embolism, and the practice should be encouraged. Similarly, bladder and bowel dysfunction are minimized if the patient can use the bathroom instead of the bedpan.

DIET. A full diet may be given as soon as the mother wants it and as soon as the danger of nausea seems to have passed. It may be wise to start with fluids and progress to more substantial food, but the normal hunger of a postpartum patient must be recognized. Especially if she is nursing, a good diet should be encouraged. This is not the time to prescribe a weight-reducing diet.

Genitourinary Tract

The genital tract should be treated as if it were an open wound—which, indeed, it is. The normal bacterial flora of the vagina can be expected to enter the uterus almost immediately, but these organisms are usually not pathogenic. Prophylaxis against infection can be maximized with careful perineal care directed toward avoiding fecal or other contamination that may infect an episiotomy or perineal laceration or ascend to infect the uterus.

The patient must be told that after each urination and bowel movement, she should wash the vulva carefully from front to back to avoid contamination. The vagina should not be invaded except for a crucial and essential pelvic examination.

The urinary tract is especially likely to require attention. The bladder may become overdistended because of the lack of bladder sensation experienced by most patients. Edema around the urethra may make urination difficult or impossible. Careful appraisal by abdominal palpation of the degree of bladder distention should be made, and a history of urination should be taken at least every 4 hours for the first postpartum day or two. If the bladder seems distended and the patient is unable to void or to void only in small amounts, she should be catheterized, with due care to minimize the risk of introducing infection. Patients receiving intravenous fluids or who had heavy analgesia or anesthesia that may take some time to wear off should be examined more often than every 4 hours.

Breasts
Care of the breasts will depend on whether or not the mother desires to nurse. If she chooses to nurse, the baby should be put to the breast about 12 hours after delivery and at 4-hour intervals thereafter. The 2:00 A.M. feeding may be omitted if desired. Before nursing, the nipples should be cleansed, and the nursing time should be limited to no more than 3 minutes on each breast. This time can be gradually lengthened to a maximum of 10 minutes on each breast. A vigorous newborn can easily empty the breast in this length of time, and longer intervals lead to sore and cracked nipples. After nursing, it is again wise to cleanse the nipples thoroughly and apply commercial nipple cream to keep them soft. Should a crack develop in a nipple, every effort should be made to encourage rapid healing. Not only will nursing be painful with a cracked nipple, but a break in the skin of the nipple frequently precedes breast infection. A crack will usually heal if the baby is not allowed to nurse on the breast for 8 to 24 hours. Nipple creams will aid the process. The opposite breast must not be nursed for more than the usual time, since prolongation of nursing will expose that nipple also to the possibility of cracking. We have found nipple shields of little use, since the nipple may be painfully sucked into the plastic shield and give the patient little more comfort than unprotected nursing.

A typical nursing mother will become very discouraged the first few days about whether or not she can nurse successfully. The baby may be too sleepy to nurse, the nipples may be sore, or her milk may seem slow to come in. She should be cheerfully encouraged to persist, since nursing is usually successfully well established after a few days. Cracked nipples are frequently the major obstacle.

Should the patient choose not to nurse, she should be reassured that stopping the milk flow is not a major problem. During the stage of engorgement, her heavy breasts should be well supported with a well-fitting brassiere. She may require ice packs or small doses of analgesics to achieve comfort during a 12- to 24-hour period. The mere avoidance of emptying the breasts will quickly stem most of the milk flow. Although a little milk may leak for several days or weeks, this is usually not a disturbing symptom. The use of hormones (estrogens or testosterone) has been advocated to prevent or minimize lactation. The current favorite is Deladumone, a combination of testosterone and estradiol, given intramuscularly during the second stage of labor. We prefer to avoid using hormones. In our experience, most of the preparations fail to provide relief of the engorgement process, and the subsequent painless expulsion of milk is usually not a disturbing symptom even without the hormone. Secondary engorgement and lactation may occur 7 to 14 days following the discontinuance of these medications in many patients, causing symptoms that may be every bit as severe as the initial ones.

Afterpains
Afterpains are noted especially by the multigravid patient. Their cause is unknown. Presumably, the multigravid uterus contracts less effectively postpartum than does the primigravid uterus, and the contraction, followed by relaxation and contraction again, is experienced by the patient as pain. The symptoms are most likely to occur during nursing, when the oxytocin released as a result of suckling causes the uterus to contract. Symptoms can be re-

lieved by analgesic drugs if necessary, and they usually disappear within a day or two.

Bowel Function

Bowel function may be sluggish for the postpartum patient just as it was during pregnancy. Most obstetricians prescribe a stool softener daily beginning the first postpartum day until the patient has a normal bowel movement. If this medication fails, the patient may be given a clear water enema on the third postpartum day. After discharge from the hospital, continued use of the stool softener may be required for a week or two, after which time bowel function usually returns to the prepregnant pattern.

Lochia

Lochia is the vaginal discharge experienced by the postpartum patient. The discharge is composed of blood, shreds of membrane, and necrotic decidua with leukocytic infiltration. For the first two or three days, blood predominates (*lochia rubra*). As the amount of blood decreases, the discharge color changes to a whitish hue (*lochia alba*). Small irregular amounts of vaginal bleeding may persist for a variable length of time, occasionally until the six-week checkup. Anything more than a slight bloody discharge should be considered abnormal and reported to the obstetrician.

Menstruation

Menstruation recurs on the average about six to eight weeks after delivery in women who are not nursing. Wide variation in the time of reappearance of the menses in lactating women has been reported, with an average of three to four months. While lactation amenorrhea confers a degree of contraceptive protection, dependence on this contraceptive measure should be discouraged because of its uncertainty. Ovulation has been reported to occur as early as the forty-second postpartum day in lactating women [2].

Length of Hospitalization

Postpartum hospitalization currently averages only two to three days in most American hospitals, primarily because of cost. While an occasional patient will require a longer hospital stay because of a complication, most women are happy to leave the hospital for the comfort of home. Early discharge, however, increases the need for the exhausted postpartum patient to have help at home. If the patient is allowed to rest for long periods while most of the household chores are left in the hands of another person, she will recover much more quickly from her labor experience than otherwise. In the long run, her family is much better off when she has adequate rest during the recovery period.

Postpartum Office Visit

The postpartum office visit should be made four to six weeks after delivery. The visit has several purposes. A pelvic examination is performed to detect abnormalities that may have been induced by pregnancy and delivery, notably cervical infection. Some patients will require cervical cautery for chronic infection, but this should be postponed for another month or two until pelvic engorgement has totally disappeared and when the Pap smear is known to be negative. The condition of the episiotomy should be noted, and if pelvic relaxation has occurred, the degree should be recorded. Reassurance that no discomfort will be experienced with the first intercourse after delivery is of great importance to some patients. Last, and perhaps most important, contraceptive advice should be offered if it has not been provided during the hospital stay.

Complications of the Puerperium

POSTPARTUM BLEEDING

Immediate postpartum hemorrhage has been discussed in the chapter on abnormalities of the third stage of labor. Late postpartum hemorrhage is bleeding that occurs after the first 24 hours, caused either by a retained placenta or placental fragment or, just as often, by subinvolution of the placental site. The bleeding typically occurs 7 to 14 days after delivery and often with no warning whatsoever. Whether or not the patient bled excessively after the delivery of the placenta is *not* important, since no correlation between the two types of hemorrhage is evident. When the patient reports bleeding, it is frequently massive, requiring removal to the hospital, perhaps even by ambulance. The immediate therapeutic problem is often blood loss and shock, which must be treated with adequate blood replacement. Vaginal bleeding may decrease, or, more typically, continue, until operative treatment.

With the patient in good hemotologic condition and under general anesthesia, a careful pelvic examination is performed. On rare occasions, the bleeding source will be a genital tract laceration. The cervix will usually be patulous and the uterus, enlarged and boggy. Careful curettage may produce a placental fragment, or the scrapings may contain only necrotic decidua from a poorly involuted placental site. In either case, bleeding usually stops promptly, usually without recurrence. Special care should be exercised during the curettage to avoid perforation of the uterus, which is especially soft at this time. Rarely, a submucous myoma or other unusual cause may explain the bleeding.

The patient is placed on a broad-spectrum antibiotic, and recovery is rapid. Discharge from the hospital is usually possible after 24 to 48 hours. Rarely, bleeding will not be controlled by curettage, and hysterectomy or hypogastric artery ligation will be necessary. In most of these cases, placenta accreta will be found in the specimen.

HEMATOMAS

Hematomas of the genital tract are an occasional complication of delivery. The most common location is the vulva or the lower vagina, although rare instances of high vaginal hematomas with retroperitoneal dissection above the brim of the pelvis have been reported. With hematoma formation above the pelvic fascia, the only evidence of disease may be shock secondary to blood loss. Vulvar or vaginal hematoma is first suspected when the patient complains of extreme pain near the episiotomy site that no analgesic medication will relieve. Examination reveals a distinct and sometimes massive swelling of the vulva or lower vagina. The area is exquisitely tender and may contain a large clot. Unless the hematoma is very small, the patient should be moved to the operating room, where incision and evacuation of the hematoma is performed. If a bleeding site is identified, a ligature is placed around the torn vessel, or, typically,

bleeding will be controlled by mattress sutures placed at the base of the hematoma. A small drain may prevent recurrence. A tight vaginal pack for 12 to 24 hours may provide hemostasis.

The hematoma site is more frequently opposite the episiotomy incision than in it, and it apparently results from tearing of a deep vessel by overstretching of the vaginal outlet. Although the complication is unusual, early treatment is necessary, since fatal hemorrhage into a hematoma can occur and because necrosis of the skin overlying an untreated large hematoma can be expected.

POSTPARTUM INFECTION

Puerperal morbidity is recognized when a postpartum patient's temperature is elevated to 100.4°F. (38°C.) on two or more of the first 10 postpartum days, excluding the first day. Infection of the genital tract is the most common of a number of causes of puerperal infection.

Infection of the Genital Tract (Puerperal Fever)

The story of the discovery of the cause of puerperal infection is one of the most interesting episodes in the history of medicine. Against strong resistance from within the profession, Semmelweiss and Holmes independently in the mid-nineteenth century recognized that the cause of puerperal sepsis, whatever its nature, was transmitted from patient to patient or from autopsy room to lying-in ward, usually on the hands of the physician. This observation, together with many important subsequent studies, provided the basis for the virtual eradication of the epidemic form of this highly lethal disease. The recent development of effective antibiotic therapy has made treatment of the disease, once it develops, possible. But the prevention of infection by the methods suggested by these medical pioneers remains the major deterrent against the disease.

Two forms of the disease are recognized: (1) the epidemic form, caused almost exclusively by beta-hemolytic streptococci from an exogenous source, and (2) the sporadic form, frequently caused by bacteria normally present in the vagina or on the surrounding perineal area.

The epidemic form of the disease is, fortunately, rare, but an occasional serious outbreak is still reported. The cause is nearly always to be found in the hospital environment, in the throats or infected skin wounds of the labor attendants. Labor and delivery room personnel should be screened on a daily basis to exclude anyone with a pharyngitis due to a streptococcus or with an infected laceration or other skin lesion, however minor. If careful aseptic technique at delivery is added to this precautionary measure, epidemics of puerperal sepsis should be eliminated.

ETIOLOGY. It is uncertain what factors cause the sporadic type of puerperal infection to develop, since an organism from the normal bacterial flora of the vagina or lower bowel may be the etiologic agent. Poor aseptic technique or poor postpartum perineal care may allow the introduction of bacteria from the perineal area, accounting for many of the infections. Droplet infection from the throat of a labor attendant may be the source of infection. Poor management of the third stage of labor with hemorrhage or with retention of placental fragments may also be a predisposing factor, as may premature rupture of the membranes. Certainly, minimal tissue damage and minimal blood loss during labor and delivery are important desiderata. As indicated, the microorganisms most frequently responsible for sporadic puerperal infection are normal flora of the vagina or of the lower bowel (anaerobic streptococcus, alpha-hemolytic streptococcus, *Escherichia,* or other coliform bacilli, *Clostridium perfringens*), but an exogenous organism may be responsible (staphylococcus). A wide variety of causative organisms makes culture essential for treatment to be appropriate.

CLINICAL COURSE. Endometritis is probably the primary pathologic reaction in most, if not all, cases of puerperal sepsis; in most instances, the disease does not progress beyond this stage. The disease usually occurs on the second or third postpartum day (with severe disease, the onset may be within the first 24 hours) and is manifested by a minimal fever, vague lower abdominal pain or cramps, and perhaps by a foul-smelling vaginal discharge. The examiner will note mild tenderness of the fundus, which may be somewhat less involuted than expected. Recovery is usually rapid even without treatment.

When endometritis progresses to a more serious stage, it may do so very rapidly, or progression may occur over a number of days. Spread of the infection may occur via the veins, with a resulting thrombophlebitis. Less frequently, the spread follows lymphatic channels, sometimes subsequently involving the venous system. The ovarian veins provide a common route of spread. If the left ovarian vein harbors the infection, subsequent involvement is of the left renal vein; the vena cava is affected if the right ovarian vein carries the infection. With spread from the endometrium via the uterine veins, the iliac vessels may be affected, but this is much less common than is ovarian vein spread. Thrombosis probably develops in the veins as a protection against spread of the infection toward the heart. Septic emboli, however, may be released from the clot, enter the circulation, and lodge in the lungs, heart valves, kidneys, or other locations.

With pelvic thrombophlebitis, symptoms of severe infection are noted, including chills and a fluctuating temperature that may reach levels of 104° to 105°F. (40°C.). The diagnosis is difficult to make by physical examination, since only generalized tenderness will usually be present at pelvic examination. A venogram with a radio-opaque dye may provide diagnostic help. A definite diagnosis may not be made until pulmonary embolism occurs.

Lymphatic spread results in parametritis, since the loose connective tissue between the leaves of the broad ligament is involved, and peritonitis follows spread to the peritoneum. If the parametritis (pelvic cellulitis) is mild, the slight temperature elevation and paracervical tenderness on pelvic examination may provide the only clues to diagnosis. With severe disease the temperature is higher, perhaps 102°F. (38.9°C.), and there is abdominal tenderness and varying degrees of broad-ligament induration on pelvic examination. The course of the disease is toward gradual resolution of the cellulitis or toward abscess formation.

With the development of an abscess, the temperature is elevated further, and the patient appears more "toxic." The abscess may point at various locations, e.g., over Poupart's ligament or in the cul-de-sac; rarely, it may rupture into the peritoneal cavity, which is a highly dangerous development. Intra-abdominal rupture requires immediate laparotomy and removal of the pelvic organs.

Peritonitis may be limited to the pelvis, or it may become generalized. With widespread disease, the patient appears very toxic, with a high fever. The abdomen is exquisitely tender, but muscle spasm may be absent because of the relaxation of the abdominal musculature that follows delivery. Paralytic ileus develops, and vomiting and abdominal distention are prominent symptoms. Death may ensue rapidly if antibiotic treatment is not started. A pelvic abscess may form in the cul-de-sac, usually with eventual fluctuation and drainage through the rectum. Blood cultures are usually positive with peritonitis or with any serious spread of infection beyond the endometrium.

TREATMENT. Endometritis is common and may be so mild as to require no therapy. The usual course of the disease is toward rapid resolution, and unless the signs and symptoms suggest progression, no antibiotic need be prescribed. Careful monitoring of such a patient is clearly mandatory, since delay in treating a spread of the disease may prove costly.

If parametritis develops, or if the infection spreads elsewhere, vigorous therapy should coincide with a thorough investigation. Cultures from the uterine cavity, taken transcervically, are essential, since a specific antibiotic for the offending organism must be started as soon as possible. A blood culture should be taken repeatedly at the time the temperature spikes, since this procedure may allow identification of the causative organism. The culture technique should be appropriate for both anaerobic and aerobic organisms. While direct smear of the material from the uterus may give information that allows a specific choice of antimicrobial drugs, a wide-spectrum antibiotic will usually be prescribed in large doses until the results of the cultures become available and a more specific drug can be given. If *C. perfringens* is suspected as being the causative organism because of the development of tissue crepitation or because the direct smear has suggested it, massive doses of penicillin should be started *at once,* since toxic shock may be a clinical manifestation of *C. perfringens* infection. Infection with this organism usually follows procedures in which tissue destruction played a major part, with resultant tissue devitalization.

Anemia is treated with blood transfusions, since infection in the anemic patient is especially serious. The patient is placed in a semi-Fowler's position, so that pus will collect in the pelvis rather than in the upper abdomen.

Periodic pelvic examinations should be performed to detect an enlarging, tender tumorlike abscess that is usually palpated either lateral or posterior to the cervix. The hardness of the tumor will be replaced by a softer feel as the abscess becomes fluctuant, usually over a period of 7 to 10 days. As the abscess extends downward into the pelvis, and as fluctuation develops, drainage is mandatory. Premature attempts at drainage may be damaging, however, and should be avoided. The abscess is drained as follows: Under general anesthesia, the fluctuant area is palpated, usually posterior to the cervix, and a large needle is inserted for positive identification of the abscess cavity. Incision and digital breakdown of any pockets of pus are followed by insertion of a soft rubber drain, which is sutured and left in place for a few days. If drainage is complete, dramatic improvement in the clinical condition of the patient is usually observed.

The patient with a pelvic infection should be isolated from the remaining patients on the postpartum floor, and isolation precautions should be observed. If the patient's condition will permit, it is usually best, because of the danger of spread of the infection, to transfer her to a hospital floor that does not house other postpartum patients. Relaxation of these measures may lead to an epidemic of the disease, even in this day of effective antibiotic therapy. Specific therapy cannot replace good public health measures.

INFECTION IN THE EPISIOTOMY SITE. Postpartum infection developing in the episiotomy site is surprisingly rare considering the impossibility of keeping this area completely free from bacteria. Inspection of the normal episiotomy will reveal induration, slight redness, and some soreness on the third or fourth postpartum day, but this is not clinical infection. Tiny pustules may develop at the sites of suture holes, but these disappear spontaneously without any problems. Of greater significance is the unusual development of infection deep in the perineal tissue, with exquisite soreness, marked swelling and redness, and slight purulent drainage, accompanied by generalized fever. While a hot sitz bath or other local heat will encourage resolution of the infection if it is of minor degree, with more severe disease it is best to cut a suture or two to encourage drainage of the trapped purulent material. Indeed, the episiotomy may break down and drain spontaneously if surgical drainage is not provided. Subsequent hot sitz baths will aid the quick resolution of the infection. An antibiotic is usually not necessary. When all infection is gone, secondary closure of the episiotomy will be required. While less functional impairment will result with early secondary closure (7 to 10 days after surgical drainage), many obstetricians prefer to delay closure for six weeks to assure that reinfection has not occurred.

Infection of the Urinary Tract

Trauma inflicted on the base of the bladder as the fetus descends through the pelvis results in edema and even extravasation of blood in the area of the bladder trigone. This damage, coupled with the poor bladder tone normally present in the postpartum woman, frequently results in inability of the pregnant woman to void. The needed catheterization introduces bacteria that flourish in a damaged bladder that may retain urine, and cystitis is a frequent result. The asymptomatic bacteria noted in many pregnant women may cause cystitis even in the absence of catheterization. Infection may be limited to the bladder or may ascend, causing a pyelonephritis that is usually unilateral. The resul-

tant symptoms will depend on the extent of the disease.

Simple cystitis will produce dysuria, frequency, and urgency, sometimes with a low-grade fever. Since these symptoms may be present even when an infection cannot be identified, it is important to confirm the clinical impression of cystitis by identifying white blood cells in a catheterized urine sample. Culture of the urine is also necessary, although a therapeutic delay of 24 to 48 hours will result if the culture report is awaited before initiating treatment. Upper urinary tract infection usually presents a more dramatic clinical picture, with a high fever (102° to 104°F. [38.9 to 40°C.]) and marked tenderness over one or both costovertebral angles. While the symptoms of lower urinary tract infection are usually also present, this is not universally so. The patient may look surprisingly well between temperature spikes, a fact that suggests urinary tract infection instead of genital tract disease.

Treatment usually provides dramatic and rapid relief of symptoms. Although it is best to use an antibiotic specific against the offending organism, delay for identification of the organism is unwise. Since most postpartum urinary tract infection is caused by *E. coli* or one of the related coliform organisms, a favorable therapeutic response to a sulfonamide can usually be expected. Ampicillin or tetracycline are also appropriate drugs for this purpose. Since tetracycline is secreted in breast milk and may yellow the infant's teeth, the drug should not be used if the mother is breast feeding. An organism resistant to these drugs will usually respond to more specific therapy. An increased oral fluid intake should also be encouraged, and it may be wise to provide continuous bladder drainage by catheter until the patient is voiding regularly and in large amounts.

Infection in the Breast

The incidence of postpartum infection in the breast varies remarkably over time. There may be no cases for months, and then a number of cases may appear simultaneously. Since the infection usually occurs from the tenth to the twentieth postpartum day, the relationship between the infection and hospitalization for delivery may not be appreciated. Nevertheless, it is known that the carrier for the causative organism is usually the baby's throat, and it is likely that outbreaks of mastitis follow outbreaks of staphylococcus infection in the nursery.

The development of mastitis usually requires the presence of a cracked or fissured nipple, together with an infant carrier of the offending organism. The infection is introduced periductally rather than through the lactiferous tubules and is usually periductal in location. The importance of nipple care and the prevention or rapid healing of cracked nipples is evident. Of equal importance is the recognition and treatment of hospital epidemics of staphylococcus infection. Early isolation of an infant with an infected cord or an unexplained fever is essential to the prevention of hospital epidemics.

With mastitis, the breast becomes sore, red, and swollen, and a generalized reaction of chills and fever to about 101° to 102°F. (38.9°C.) is common. The diagnosis is usually very obvious to an experienced clinician, although local findings are occasionally obscure. Rapid resolution of the disease follows the administration of an appropriate antibiotic, and recurrence is rare if the antibiotic is continued for a week or more. The choice of antibiotic will depend on the strain of staphylococcus prevalent. (Rare causes due to other organisms, notably streptococci, are recognized.) Penicillin is highly effective unless the particular strain is penicillin-resistant. Discontinuance of nursing is usually necessary because it is painful. In a mother extremely eager to resume nursing, twice-daily emptying of the breast will maintain the milk supply until nursing can be resumed.

If the disease does not respond to an antibiotic, or if the physician sees the patient some days after the onset of mastitis, a breast abscess may be noted. The area of redness and tenderness is usually larger and better circumscribed than with mastitis. Fluctuance will usually be seen as well as felt. Surgical drainage, combined with appropriate antibiotic treatment, is essential and is carried out as follows: Under general anesthesia, an adequate radial incision is made overlying the abscess. The incision is made in radial fashion to minimize damage to the breast lobules. Lobules are drained with the examining finger, and a soft rubber drain or gauze packing is inserted to maintain drainage.

Thombophlebitis and Pulmonary Embolism

An unusual and serious complication in the postpartum patient is the development of femoral, saphenous, or popliteal vein thrombophlebitis. The term *thrombophlebitis* implies the presence of an inflammation of the venous wall as well as the presence of a clot in the vein. The older term, *phlebothrombosis,* referring to the presence of a clot in the vein without an accompanying infective process. We are unable to recognize such a disease state and thus will only use the term *thrombophlebitis*.

ETIOLOGY. Factors that predispose to femoral vein thrombophlebitis are operative or traumatic delivery and delayed ambulation following delivery. The incidence of the disease has decreased as early ambulation has been practiced and fewer difficult operative deliveries have been performed. Pelvic vein thrombophlebitis is usually the result of extension of pelvic infection, but femoral vein disease may also extend upward into the pelvic veins.

CLINICAL FEATURES. Thrombophlebitis may occur in the superficial saphenous venous system, due apparently to pressure from a stirrup delivery; it occurs most frequently in the patient with varicose veins. The affected area is tender, warm, and well localized. Treatment consisting of leg elevation and local application of heat is usually sufficient, and recovery occurs in a few days. Thromboembolism is rare.

Thrombophlebitis of the deep veins, which may be less obvious clinically, is potentially lethal. The leg may be painful, slightly swollen, and tender. Pain may be elicited along the path of the vein. The calf will be tender to pressure, and dorsiflexion of the foot causes pain in the calf (Homan's sign), due apparently to stretching of the affected veins. In a few acute cases, there may be a reflex arterial spasm, causing a pale, severely swollen extremity. A venogram may be diagnostic. In some cases, local symptoms or signs are absent or overlooked, and the first evidence of the disease is an embolus to the lung.

TREATMENT. As indicated, treatmen of a superficial, well-localized thrombophlebitis of the saphenous vein is local heat and elevation of the leg. If the deep veins are involved, more aggressive management is necessary. The leg should be elevated and bed rest strictly enforced. An elastic bandage should be applied from ankle to groin. Anticoagulant therapy is initiated with heparin in appropriate doses rather than with bishydroxycoumarin (Dicumarol). More rapid anticoagulation is achieved with heparin, which is an important factor is preventing thromboembolism. After initial anticoagulation is effective, or while it is being achieved, Dicumarol may be started for longer-term therapy. Heparin must be given parenterally, but Dicumarol can be given by the oral route. Most clinicians prefer Dicumarol therapy for this reason. Since Dicumarol takes 36 to 72 hours to achieve maximum effect, however, early therapy with heparin with later replacement by Dicumarol is the therapeutic program most often chosen.

If rapid correction of anticoagulation is needed because of clinical bleeding or because urgent surgery is required, protamine sulfate provides rapid reversal of heparin activity. Vitamin K will reverse the anticoagulant effects of Dicumarol, but the effect will not be immediately apparent, requiring 4 to 8 hours. (A second disadvantage of Dicumarol is that in the prepartum period it easily crosses the placenta and may cause a bleeding disorder in the fetus. Heparin does not cross the placenta in significant amounts and therefore does not harm the fetus.)

Ligation of the vena cava may be necessary in some patients; if anticoagulant treatment proves ineffective, and there are repeated episodes of pulmonary embolism, no nonsurgical therapy is available. Similarly, showering of septic emboli may not be terminated by anticoagulation, and inferior vena caval ligation may be lifesaving.

References

1. The Medical Letter, March 15, 1974.
2. Sharman, A. *Ovulation in the Postpartum Period.* Excerpta Medica International Congress Series No. 133. Amsterdam: Excerpta Medica, 1966. P. 158.

Additional Readings

Courtney, L. Amniotic fluid embolism. *Obstet Gynecol Surv* 29:169, 1974.

Gainey, H. Postpartum observation of pelvic tissue damage: Further studies. *Am J Obstet Gynecol* 70: 800, 1955.

Jewett, J., Reid, D., Safon, L., and Easterday, C. Chiidbed fever—a continuing entity. *JAMA* 206:344, 1968.

Newton, M., and Bradford, W. Postpartal blood loss. *Obstet Gynecol* 17:229, 1961.

Pearson, H., and Anderson, G. Bacteroides infections and pregnancy. *Obstet Gynecol* 35:31, 1970.

Williams, J. Regeneration of the uterine mucosa after delivery with especial reference to the placental site. *Am J Obstet Gynecol* 22:664, 1931.

15   Diseases of the Placenta

Diseases of the Trophoblast

Hydatidiform mole, chorioadenoma destruens (invasive mole), and choriocarcinoma can all be considered degenerative diseases of the trophoblast. Their neoplastic activity probably arises from the invasive potential of the trophoblast from which they are derived. Histologically, they possess the feature of trophoblastic proliferation to varying degrees. While hydatidiform mole frequently assumes a benign clinical course, chorioadenoma destruens is locally invasive, and choriocarcinoma metastasizes wildly. Chorioadenoma destruens and choriocarcinoma are frequently preceded by a benign form of trophoblastic disease, although this is not uniformly true. While hydatidiform mole can usually be contained and cured, on occasion, if untreated, it rapidly assumes malignant potential and kills. It is not always possible to assess the malignant potential of an individual lesion by its histologic appearance. Trophoblastic tumors therefore should be considered potentially invasive.

While the three lesions have many factors in common, their pathologic features, clinical course, and treatment vary sufficiently to warrant separate discussion of each entity.

HYDATIDIFORM MOLE

Hydatidiform mole is an uncommon complication of pregnancy in most areas of the world, with a hospital incidence in the United States of about 1 in 1500 to 2000 deliveries. For an as-yet-unexplained reason, the disease is many times more common in certain areas of the world, notably in certain countries in the South Pacific. Poor socioeconomic conditions have been said to explain this unusual incidence, but other factors also seem to be operating.

Histogenesis

The histogenesis of hydatidiform mole, according to Reid and Benirschke [1], is related to lack of proper development of the villous circulation. With inadequate villous circulation, edema of the villous stroma appears. As the process continues, cystic degeneration of the villi occurs, resulting in the typical grapelike gross appearance of hydatidiform mole. Evidence to support this hypothesis is found in pathological material from blighted ova: the villi accompanying such a failed pregnancy frequently are edematous, and hydropic degeneration, even to the point of cyst formation, is seen. It is Reid and Benirschke's view that hydatidiform mole might be considered the end stage of a blighted ovum that has failed to abort. It is not difficult to include the factor of malignant potential in this theory, since the early trophoblast is known to possess strong invasive potential.

Pathologic Features

Microscopically, the lesion is characterized by (1) edema of the villous stroma with hydropic degeneration, (2) proliferation of the chorionic epithelium, and (3) absence, or near absence, of villous blood vessels. Of greatest variability from one mole to another is the degree to which the layers of the chorionic epithelium proliferate. While proliferation in some moles may be minimal, consisting sometimes only of a thin layer of both cytotrophoblast and syncytiotrophoblast, in others there is a marked overgrowth, with piling up of trophoblastic cells. It has been suggested that the degree of trophoblastic proliferation may be directly correlated with malignant potential, but this is not a settled issue [2].

Grossly, hydatidiform mole has a highly typical

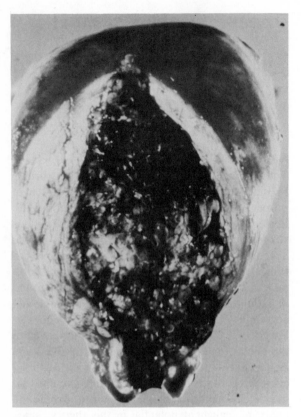

Fig. 15-1. Gross appearance of hydatidiform mole. The uterus has been surgically opened.

appearance, resembling a cluster of grapes (Fig. 15-1). The hydropic vesicles may measure 2 to 3 mm. or more in diameter. The grapelike mass covers the endometrial cavity and may extrude through the cervix more or less in toto or in small pieces. It is usually covered with varying amounts of blood and fibrin and is unmistakable in appearance. If the mass is carefully studied, a small degenerating fetus will sometimes be found among the hydropic villi. On rare occasions, a full-term fetus can coexist with a fully developed hydatidiform mole.

In many cases, lutein cysts form in the ovaries of patients with mole and sometimes attain a diameter of 10 cm. or more (Fig. 15-2). The ovarian enlargement is thought to result from stimulation of the ovarian lutein cells by the high levels of chorionic gonadotropin produced by the mole. The cysts are usually asymptomatic and invariably regress with removal of the mole, although, rarely, they may undergo torsion. Their presence may be useful in differentiating a mole from an early normal pregnancy. No surgical excision is indicated, since regression can be expected.

Clinical and Laboratory Diagnosis

The most consistent early symptom of hydatidiform mole is vaginal bleeding. Unfortunately, this is also the major symptom of threatened abortion, the disease most commonly confused with a mole. Typically, the bleeding is minimal but persistently recurrent over a long period of time. Occasionally, it is profuse. Anemia may result from long-continued bleeding. The uterus frequently is larger than the expected size for the gestational interval. This sign is most likely to be noted very early in a pregnancy but is not diagnostic, since other causes must be excluded. Multiple pregnancy, for example, is characterized by a similar disparity in uterine size and gestation, and an even more common cause for confusion is a disparity between menstrual data and actual length of gestation. Uterine fibroids may also cause uterine enlargement of greater magnitude than is usual for the gestational interval.

Evidence of acute toxemia of pregnancy develops in about 20 percent of the patients with molar pregnancies. While proteinuria and hypertension may be mild, the disease occasionally presents in a severe form, even to the point of convulsions. The presence of acute toxemia is so rare before the twenty-fourth week in normal pregnancy that its appearance may be taken as good evidence of a mole if renal causes of the disease complex can be ruled out.

Hyperemesis gravidarum is seen in about 30 percent of molar pregnancy patients and its presence should alert the clinician to the possibility of a molar pregnancy. In about 10 percent of patients with a mole, evidence of hyperthyroidism is present.

The passage of a typical grapelike cluster from the vagina can make the diagnosis. While this

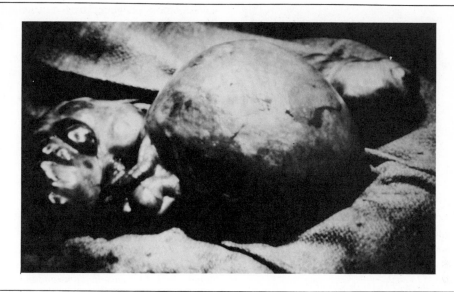

Fig. 15-2. Theca lutein cysts on either side of the uterus and hydatidiform mole in the uterus.

helpful event occurs uncommonly, it is a most useful sign. Intrauterine infection may develop when the mole becomes large, since the necrotic central tissue provides an ideal culture medium. Septicemia is a rare complication of the infection.

Certain laboratory tools may also be useful in arriving at a diagnosis.

URINARY OR SERUM LEVELS OF HUMAN CHORIONIC GONADOTROPIN (HCG). Care in the interpretation of HCG levels is necessary, and a single elevated reading is never diagnostic. High levels of HCG are reached with early pregnancy, especially between the eleventh and twelfth weeks, and with multiple gestation. The usefulness of the test therefore may be limited to a gestation longer than 12 weeks. With a mole, unlike a normal pregnancy, the HCG level remains persistently high or even increases.

RADIOGRAPHIC STUDIES. A simple flat plate of the abdomen may reveal a fetal skeleton, thus in effect ruling out hydatidiform mole (rare instances of the

coexistence of a mole and a normal fetus have been reported). Injection of radiopaque iodine into the uterus may reveal the typical "moth-eaten" appearance of the mole. This test is diagnostic.

ULTRASONOGRAPHIC SCAN. The characteristic appearance of a mole revealed by this method can also be considered diagnostic (Fig. 15-3). This is the safest, most reliable test.

To summarize the diagnostic signs of hydatidiform mole:

1. Look for vaginal bleeding, unusual uterine enlargement, and the development of acute toxemia in early pregnancy. Fetal heart sounds will be absent when a Doppler instrument is used to detect them.
2. Use an ultrasonographic scan or inject a radiopaque contrast medium into the uterus. Either of these tests is diagnostic.
3. Look for persistent or increasingly higher levels of HCG after the twelfth week of pregnancy. This provides presumptive evidence of the presence of a mole.
4. A single roentgenogram showing a fetal skeleton will usually rule out a molar pregnancy when

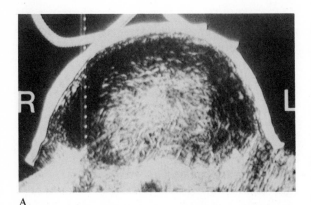

A

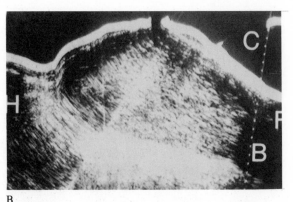

B

Fig. 15-3. Hydatidiform mole. Sonograms were obtained with the conventional (i.e., "black and white") equipment. A. Transverse scan through the uterine fundus. B. Sagittal scan through the midline. (B = bladder; H = [mother's] head; F = [mother's] feet; C = centimeter scale.) On this medium-to-high "gain setting" (i.e., machine sensitivity), the molar "cluster of grapes" shows up as numerous uniform echoes through the uterus. (A normal placenta would produce a similar appearance, but other normal intrauterine structures would be recognized.) The echographic appearance is typical and has been dubbed "snowstorm." Decreases in the gain settings decrease the number and prominence of the echoes.

other diagnostic tests are inadequate. Absence of a skeleton is not diagnostic, however.

Treatment

Treatment of a patient with hydatidiform mole should always be preceded by a chest roentgenogram and an HCG titer. These will provide baseline values against which subsequent tests can be more meaningfully interpreted.

UTERINE EVACUATION. When the diagnosis has been made, the uterus should be emptied in the most expeditious and safest manner, usually by suction curettage. The cervix is often dilated sufficiently to obviate the need for instrumental dilatation, although use of a laminaria tent for presurgical dilatation is recommended. A large (12-mm. or larger) suction curette is best. The curette is introduced into the massive tissue, and the material is quickly removed by the negative pressure. Bleeding, although sometimes significant, is much reduced as compared with bleeding with previously used methods.

Following evacuation of the uterus, the uterine wall should be carefully scraped with a sharp curette to reduce the likelihood of missing some tissue. Since the uterus is soft and easily penetrable, the suction curette, as well as the sharp curette, should be used with care. The administration of a constant intravenous drip of dilute oxytocin during and after the procedure will not only reduce the amount of bleeding encountered but will also minimize the risk of uterine perforation with the curettes.

Although previously used with some frequency, simple dilatation and curettage (D&C) or an abdominal hysterotomy have been largely replaced by suction curettage. If the suction apparatus is not available, a D&C should be performed, with the risk of heavy bleeding sometimes encountered firmly in mind. Occasionally, the bleeding will be so heavy as to require uterine packing, with a subsequent D&C a day or two later. The bleeding may be so brisk as to require an immediate abdominal hysterotomy. Indeed, abdominal hysterotomy should perhaps be utilized as the primary procedure when the uterus is larger than 14 weeks' gestational size and when a suction machine is unavailable. Abdominal hysterectomy has a definite but small place in the treatment of the patient with a large mole who wishes to be sterilized. If infection is present in the uterus, appropriate antibiotic treatment is indicated.

Chemotherapy

The chemotherapy of hydatidiform mole and other trophoblastic disease is based on the somewhat selective response of trophoblastic tissue to folic acid antagonists. Either methotrexate or actinomycin D is the usual drug of choice. Pretreatment evaluation of liver, kidney, and bone marrow function is essential, since the drugs are highly toxic. Periodic repetition of these organ function tests is necessary to control drug dosage. Especially to be feared are bone marrow depression and intestinal hemorrhage. If the therapeutic response is favorable, the HCG titer should begin to decrease within a week, and regression of the lung changes should be demonstrated radiographically soon thereafter. A permanent remission is recognized by a negative HCG titer for 12 months. Most patients will respond favorably to this therapy, but a few will require more complicated treatment including triple-drug therapy with methotrexate, actinomycin-D, and chlorambucil.

PROGNOSIS. Simple complete evacuation of the mole will result in clinical cure in about 85 percent of patients, but choriocarcinoma will develop in about 1.5 to 2.5 percent. The mole will recur in the remainder, but cure in this group can be expected with repeat evacuation or chemotherapy. Whether or not the likelihood of persistent disease can be reduced by the prophylactic administration of chemotherapy is unclear. While some authorities prefer to use routine methotrexate both before and after evacuation of the mole, others prefer a careful follow-up evaluation of each patient before deciding on chemotherapy [3]. The issue is unsettled. Methotrexate chemotherapy is not innocuous and carries a definite mortality.

Follow-up

Careful follow-up examinations and tests are essential to the successful management of these patients. Physical examination is useful and may reveal uterine enlargement that suggests persistent disease or the presence of metastatic lesions. However, repeated measurements of urinary or serum HCG titers, usually performed by radioimmunoassay, provide the major element in the follow-up evaluation. The titration should be performed every two weeks for two months and monthly thereafter for a year. When a mole is present, unlike the situation in normal pregnancy, the HCG levels may not fall to zero rapidly; indeed, the level is zero in only 75 percent of patients at the end of 40 days. The presence of HCG beyond this time should arouse suspicion of persistent disease. Any elevation of HCG titer should be viewed with great alarm.

If the HCG titer suggests persistent disease, a repeat D&C should be performed. A repeat chest roentgenogram and brain and liver scans may reveal metastatic disease. With the diagnosis of persistent or recurrent disease established, chemotherapy is mandatory and curative in most cases. With persistently elevated titers, chemotherapy should be utilized even in the absence of a microscopic diagnosis. The hazards of chemotherapy in this instance are more than outweighed by the hazards of delay. Hysterectomy may be performed for persistent local disease if subsequent pregnancy is not an issue. The surgery does not, however, replace chemotherapy.

It is evident that the possibility of pregnancy during the follow-up period would lead to a confusing differential diagnosis between persistent or recurrent disease and pregnancy. For this reason, pregnancy is absolutely contraindicated until the absence of persistent disease seems a virtual certainty. The patient should be placed on a combination oral contraceptive medication for a year, since this method of contraception provides the greatest degree of pregnancy protection.

CHORIOADENOMA DESTRUENS
(INVASIVE MOLE)

Invasive mole is the diagnosis usually made when hysterectomy has been performed for "benign" trophoblastic disease that persists after treatment. In some cases, a hysterectomy may have been performed because of tumor perforation of the uterus with peritoneal spillage, or hemorrhage. Distant metastases, especially to the lungs, may, rarely, occur. Microscopically, the tumor has an abundance of trophoblastic cells, frequently in sheets, and in numbers far exceeding those seen with benign mole. There are usually villous structures to be seen, which is not the case with choriocarcinoma. The tumor penetrates the myometrium and may be found in the subserosal area, in the parametrium, or even in the peritoneal cavity.

Invasive mole is much more rare than benign mole but more common than choriocarcinoma. The tumor is well treated by hysterectomy, not only to effect a cure but also to prevent complications caused by uterine perforation by tumor and hemorrhage. Chemotherapy with folic acid antagonists is also effective primary treatment.

CHORIOCARCINOMA

Choriocarcinoma is a very rare malignant tumor of trophoblastic origin that occurs only following a pregnancy except for the uncommon case arising in a teratoma in either a male or female. Although the relationship is not always immediately apparent because of a long dormant period, 40 percent of choriocarcinomas follow a molar pregnancy, 40 percent follow abortion, and 20 percent follow a pregnancy that appeared to be normal in all other respects. The diagnosis in the latter group may be particularly difficult to make because the tumor is unexpected.

Pathologic Features

Grossly, the choriocarcinoma forms a tumor mass, with extensive necrosis and hemorrhage. Microscopically, there is no villous formation. The tumor is composed of trophoblastic cells of either cytotrophoblastic or syncytial origin. The cells occur in large masses or sheets that may be obscured by necrosis and hemorrhage in the lesion. The individual cells show marked mitotic activity. The degree of anaplasia is not a reliable criterion on which to base prediction of malignant potential. The stimulus that causes the trophoblast to assume such a malignant character is unknown.

While the primary lesion may be in the uterus, the first clinical evidence of the disease may arise from a metastatic lesion located in any one of several organs, notably the lungs or the vagina but also the brain, kidney, liver, and other organs. The disease is blood-borne, and the microscopic picture usually includes invasion of blood vessels.

Clinical Features and Diagnosis

The clinical picture may begin simply with a history of continued vaginal bleeding following evacuation of a molar pregnancy. Alternatively, there may be no symptoms but simply an elevation of the HCG titer. In some cases, the initial complaints will be caused by perforation of the uterus by the rapidly growing tumor, with intraperitoneal bleeding. Cough and hemoptysis may suggest lung metastasis, while neurologic complaints may emanate from a rapidly growing brain lesion. Such complaints in a postpartum patient should always arouse the suspicion of choriocarcinoma.

The diagnosis may be obscure in many cases. Dilatation and curettage should always be performed when choriocarcinoma seems a possibility. The scrapings are not always diagnostic. The tumor may be present in the myometrium but not in the endometrium and may thus be missed. A normal trophoblast may be misread as choriocarcinoma on occasion. A diagnosis of choriocarcinoma is made in the absence of normal trophoblastic tissue and with a persistently high or rising HCG titer. A local vaginal lesion may be examined by biopsy. Symptoms from distant lesions will require appropriate investigation.

Prognosis and Treatment

Death in an untreated patient can be expected within a few months and is usually caused by hemorrhage from blood-vessel invasion. Before chemotherapy became available, most patients succumbed to this disease. The advent of chemotherapy has almost totally reversed the outlook, with survival of at least 2 out of 3 patients.

Treatment by hysterectomy is occasionally curative if the disease is limited to the uterus. Surgery still has a limited role in therapy for uncon-

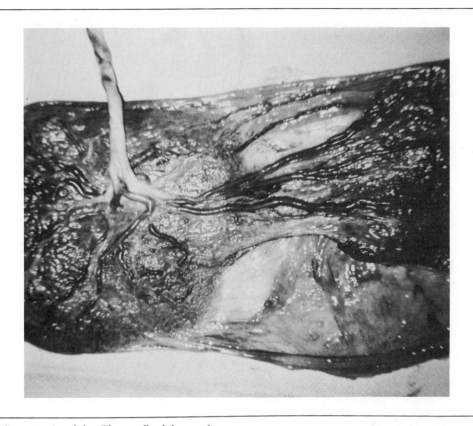

Fig. 15-4. Succenturiate lobe. The smaller lobe can be seen on the left. The blood vessels that connect the accessory lobe with the placenta are also seen.

trolled bleeding, for uterine perforation, and for diagnosis when curettage fails in this respect. The chemotherapeutic agents most often used are methotrexate or actinomycin D. Therapy is complex, and serious side effects are the major concern. It should be instituted by someone thoroughly familiar with the drugs and their potential toxicity.

Other Diseases of the Placenta

The placenta is a flat, discoid organ that averages about one-sixth the weight of the fetus of normal gestation at term. With syphilis, diabetes mellitus, and severe erythroblastosis, the placenta is greatly increased in weight, attaining a ratio to the fetus's weight as high as 1:3, 1:2, or, in rare cases, 1:1.

The normal organ is usually 15 to 20 cm. in diameter and from 2 to 3 cm. thick. Variation from these measurements occurs with certain placental abnormalities.

ABNORMAL PLACENTAL FORMATIONS

Placenta Succenturiata

Although the placenta is usually a single, discoid organ, one or more accessory lobes may occasionally develop (a common finding in other primates), a condition called placenta succenturiata (Fig. 15-4). The clinical importance of this condition is two-fold. Blood vessels connecting the accessory lobe to the placenta pass through the membranes. If they are torn during labor, at the time of rupture of the membranes, they may bleed. Also, the accessory lobe may not be delivered with the placenta, and retention in the uterus may cause serious maternal hemorrhage. If the placenta is

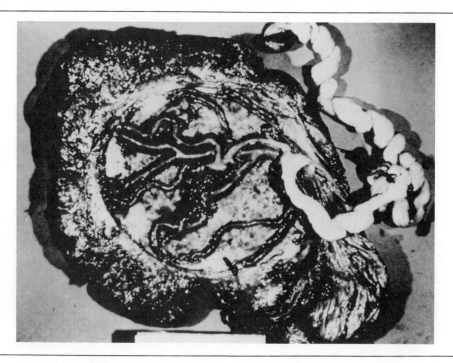

Fig. 15-5. Circumvallate placenta.

routinely examined after delivery, an accessory lobe will be suspected if torn blood vessels are noted on the edge of the placenta. Manual removal of the accessory lobe is mandatory. Physicians who routinely explore the uterine cavity manually following delivery will discover an accessory lobe in this way.

Placenta Membranacea

Placenta membranacea occurs when a thin placenta covers the entire intrauterine surface. The condition results from failure of the chorion laeve to atrophy as it should. Why this occurs remains a mystery. Bleeding in the third trimester may result from the separation of the placenta at the lower uterine pole as prelabor development of the lower uterine segment and cervical effacement occur. Placenta membranacea frequently fails to separate completely following delivery of the fetus, and manual removal is usually required. The adherence of the placenta may make this procedure unusually difficult.

Placenta Circumvallata

Placenta circumvallata occurs with some frequency, although the reported incidence depends on the criteria used to make the diagnosis (Fig. 15-5). Placenta circumvallata is recognized when the fetal surface of the placenta is smaller than the maternal surface, resulting in a whitish ring formation at a variable distance from the placental margin. The fetal blood vessels extend only to the edge of the ring and not to the placental margin. The ring is formed by a double fold of amnion and chorion, with degenerated decidua between the folds. The decidual surface of the placenta lying peripheral to the ring undergoes varying degrees of necrosis. A variety of the condition in which the ring forms at the edge of the placenta is called *placenta marginata*. The ring may extend a full 360 degrees, or it may be incomplete in certain instances.

The cause of placenta circumvallata continues to

be a matter of controversy, with some investigators suggesting that the original chorionic plate was too small, thus forcing the placenta to extend outward to provide adequate maternal-placental exchange. Others think the condition results from frequent marginal placental bleeding during pregnancy. Certainly, bleeding commonly occurs with the condition, but whether it results from the pathologic condition or whether it causes the pathologic condition is unclear.

The clinical significance of the circumvallate placenta lies in its predisposition to cause bleeding during pregnancy—in effect, a marginal placental separation. The risk of premature labor may be slightly increased. While the placental separation may occasionally be sufficient to endanger the fetus, in most cases the importance of the bleeding lies in the confusion it causes in the differential diagnosis of second- or third-trimester bleeding due to placenta previa or to premature separation of the placenta.

TUMORS AND CYSTS

A variety of tumors of the placenta have been described. Although all tumors are uncommon in this location, the most frequently noted placental tumor is chorioangioma. This blood vessel tumor of unknown histogenesis is usually small and does not interfere with pregnancy. The occasional tumor of larger size (5 cm. in diameter or more) may cause hydramnios. Metastatic tumors in the placenta have been described but are rare. Malignant melanoma is the commonest variety reported, but any tumor that is spread by a hematogenous route may lodge in the placenta.

Placental cysts are occasionally seen on the fetal surface of the placenta and are thought to be of chorionic origin (Fig. 15-6). They exert no known clinical effect.

CIRCULATORY DISTURBANCES

Circulatory disturbances of the placenta are commonly referred to as *infarcts,* but the term includes a number of varying disturbances of varying etiologies that are better described with a more specific terminology. Grossly, they may all look the

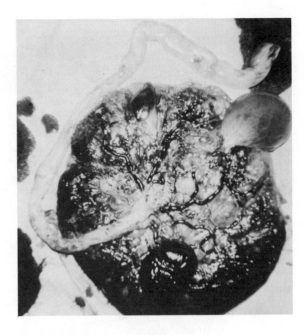

Fig. 15-6. Placental amniotic cyst.

same, with small areas of placental degeneration that in extreme cases may even include the deposition of calcium (Fig. 15-7).

The villi receive their blood supply from the intervillous pool and the maternal spiral arteries of the decidua. If a thrombus develops in the spiral artery, or if it ruptures, thus producing decidual bleeding and necrosis, the blood supply to that area of the villous structure is compromised. An infarct of the villus results. At first, the infarct is red, but it gradually turns whitish; the white infarct is familiar to those who have studied the placenta at delivery. Surrounding villi may not be involved.

A second type of placental damage results from fibrin deposition or thrombus formation in the intervillous space, frequently overlying the syncytium of the villus itself. The etiology of the fibrin deposition is unknown, but it may result from stagnation of blood in the intervillous space. As the fibrin deposit covers the syncytium, the blood supply to the villus is blocked, and syncytial damage results. These fibrin depositions are frequently confused grossly with true infarcts.

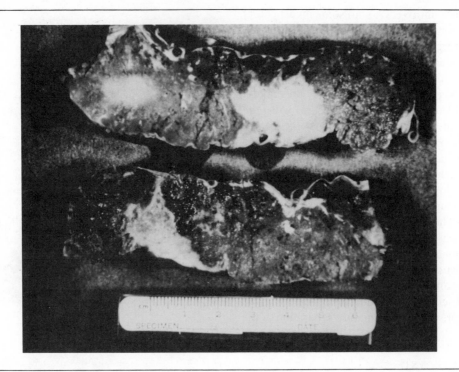

Fig. 15-7. Old "infarct" of the placenta.

There is usually little clinical significance either to true infarct formation or to deposition of fibrin in the placenta. The normal placenta has enormous reserve, and the pathologic process is usually not great enough to use up this reserve. Occasionally, fetal malnutrition or hypoxia results from extensive placental disease. With chronic hypertensive disease or acute toxemia especially, the placental changes may be great enough to compromise the fetus.

ABNORMALITIES OF THE UMBILICAL CORD
The umbilical cord averages about 50 cm. in length, but the length varies, commonly between 30 and 100 cm. Much shorter or much longer cords are occasionally seen. A long cord predisposes to various abnormalities, including knots and entanglements with various fetal parts. An unusually short umbilical cord will occasionally prevent descent of the fetus through the pelvis, a circumstance that should be diagnosable by observing fetal heart rate changes consistent with cord compression or hy-

poxia. Rupture of the cord and even inversion of the uterus have been etiologically related to an excessively short cord.

Knots and Entanglements
The most common fetal entanglement with the cord is a nuchal one, although coiling around an arm or a leg is not uncommon. A nuchal cord occurs in at least 20 percent of deliveries. It is not often responsible for fetal compromise, even when two or three loops are wrapped around the neck. In the unusual instance of monoamniotic twins in which both fetuses occupy the same amniotic sac, cord entanglements may be lethal and are probably the major cause of fetal demise in this instance.

True knots in the cord occur because of fetal movement (Fig. 15-8). They are rarely damaging to the fetus but may become tightened and cause fetal death. False knots are due to kinking of the cord

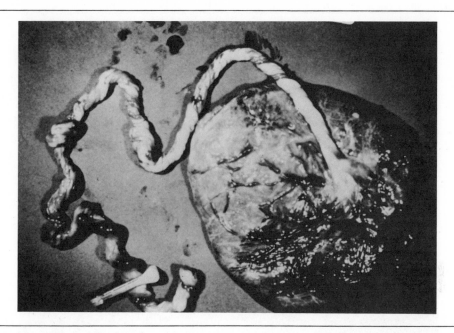

Fig. 15-8. True knot of the umbilical cord.

with adherence of two surfaces and do no harm. Torsion of the cord occasionally occurs and is frequently associated with fetal death. Whether the torsion precedes fetal demise or results from agonal movements of the fetus from other causes is uncertain. Hematoma of the cord probably results from a rupture of a varix and is uncommon. Excessively thick cords or very thin ones can be considered normal variations and are related to the amount of Wharton's jelly that surrounds the vessels of the cord.

Abnormal Insertions

Insertion of the umbilical cord into the placenta is either central or somewhat eccentric in most cases. In a few instances, the cord is inserted at the margin of the placenta. This is called *battledore insertion* but has no recognized clinical significance. In about 1 percent of placentas, the umbilical cord vessels do not insert directly into the chorionic plate but traverse a portion of the membranes before reaching the placenta. This is called *velamen-tous insertion* (Fig. 15-9). Such an insertion will ordinarily do no harm. However, if the fetal membranes containing the fetal vessels happen to overlie the internal os of the cervix, *vasa previa* is present, i.e., the vessels present in front of the fetal head. In this instance, spontaneous or artificial rupture of the membranes may tear a fetal vessel, resulting in exsanguination of the fetus. Usually, the condition is unrecognized and mistaken for a marginal separation of the placenta, and a fetal death results. Microscopic examination of a blood smear taken from the vagina may reveal large numbers of nucleated red blood cells and permit the diagnosis to be made. In rare instances, the fetus may be born alive but require an immediate blood transfusion to correct anemia. Rarely, an astute obstetrician will feel the vessel overlying the fetal head and pulsating simultaneously with the fetal heart. If vasa previa is diagnosed in this manner, an immediate cesarean section is mandatory.

Tumors

Tumors of the umbilical cord are rare, but myxomas and myxosarcomas have been recog-

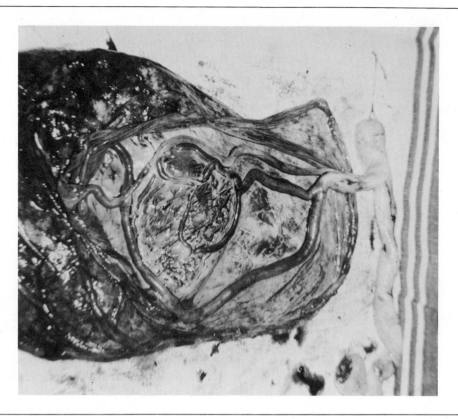

Fig. 15-9. Velamentous insertion of the cord. Note extension of the vessels on the right beyond the placental edge and through the fetal membranes before they join the umbilical cord.

nized. Cysts of the cord are not rare. Some apparently develop from the epithelium of embryonic remnants in the cord, while others may be caused by liquefaction of Wharton's jelly.

Single Umbilical Artery

The umbilical cord normally contains two arteries and one vein, which are surrounded and supported by a gelatinous substance known as Wharton's jelly. In about 1 percent of fetuses, only one umbilical artery can be distinguished. This finding is of great clinical importance, since between 20 and 40 percent of such fetuses will be found to harbor a congenital anomaly, frequently a major one. The genitourinary and cardiovascular systems are most commonly involved [4]. Multiple organs may be affected. From this observation, it is clear that the obstetrician has an obligation at delivery to examine a cross section of the umbilical cord and to determine the number of vessels it contains. If less than three vessels are evident, the pediatrician should be alerted to make an exhaustive search for an anomaly.

DISORDERS OF THE AMNION

Hydramnios → *What catation*

Hydramnios is the term used to describe an excessive amount of amniotic fluid. *Polyhydramnios* is a synonymous term. Since the definition does not include a precise identification of what the normal amount of amniotic fluid is, it is evident that a wide

Poly hydramnios is not asc. w/ Renal agenesis.

+ polyhydramnion is asw :=
1. Maternal Diabetes
2 Neural tube defect of the infants
3 hemolytic dis .
4 Usophageal atresia .

divergence in incidence will be reported from clinic to clinic. An incidence of somewhat less than 1 percent is reasonable.

The amniotic fluid volume increases from an average of about 200 ml. at 16 weeks' gestation to about 1000 ml. near term, although there is a wide variation in the "normal" amount noted at term. Hydramnios is usually clinically evidenced when the amount of fluid volume reaches about 3000 ml.; lesser volumes of about 2000 ml. may justify the diagnosis. Much larger volumes have been recorded in individual patients. The fluid may collect over a relatively long period of time (chronic hydramnios) or it may accumulate within a few days (acute hydramnios). Chronic hydramnios is far more common than the acute form.

ETIOLOGY. The normal circulation of the amniotic fluid is not clearly understood, but it seems certain that there is a relatively large turnover of amniotic fluid. Experiments have indicated that about 500 ml. of fluid is swallowed daily by the fetus; this amount is probably matched by the volume of urine excreted by the fetus. The fluid is probably formed by the amniotic cells, but the fetus "circulates" the fluid.

Hydramnios occurs with some regularity in fetuses who are unable to swallow, i.e., those with esophageal or duodenal atresia. It is presumed that the inability of the fetus to swallow its normal amount of amniotic fluid accounts for the excessive accumulation. Anencephalic fetuses and those with spina bifida also are frequently seen with hydramnios. The usual explanation given for this relationship is that the exposed meninges excrete fluid into the amniotic sac. Fetal kidney defects, on the other hand, may be associated with lower amounts of amniotic fluid than normal (oligohydramnios). In this case, the fetal anuria prevents the excretion of urine in the amniotic fluid. This oversimplified explanation of the etiology of hydramnios does not allow for the many exceptions.

DIAGNOSIS. The diagnosis of hydramnios may be very easy in extreme cases or missed completely with smaller volumes of fluid. Major fetal anomalies are said to be present in 20 to 25 percent of cases of hydramnios and are especially frequent with extreme degrees of the disease. Hydramnios is greatly increased in frequency in maternal diabetes mellitus and may herald incipient fetal demise in such cases. Twin pregnancy increases the incidence of hydramnios. Severe fetal hydrops from erythroblastosis fetalis also is associated with hydramnios. Whenever any of these conditions is suspected based on maternal history, hydramnios should be looked for.

In most instances, the only early evidence for hydramnios is excessive uterine enlargement, which may be noticed by the patient or first observed by the physician. The differential diagnosis between twins or an excessively large baby and hydramnios can usually be made on the basis of physical examination. The fetal parts may be felt less distinctly, and the fetal heart sounds may be difficult to elicit. The fetus is unusually ballotable from side to side. Hydramnios usually occurs a number of weeks before term and a suspicion of the disease should prompt confirmation by real-time sonography or B-scan. A plain x-ray film will reveal a great discrepancy between fetal and uterine size. The fetus may display unusual extension of its extremities due to more than ample space, and an abnormal lie (e.g., a transverse lie, breech) is common. A fetal abnormality may be diagnosable by ultrasonography or by x-ray.

On rare occasions, the disease may be heralded by the onset of respiratory symptoms, dyspnea, and even cyanosis, or with edema of the vulva and lower extremities. Abdominal pain may result from uterine overdistention, and pelvic discomfort may be greatly increased. The patient may be able to tolerate the symptoms, but in some instances therapeutic relief is mandatory.

TREATMENT. The treatment of hydramnios will vary from active intervention to mere watchful waiting. When the symptoms demand relief, the patient should be hospitalized. Bed rest may relieve the symptoms. Diuretics, salt restriction, and similar measures are unsuccessful and should not be prescribed. If immediate relief is necessary, the amniotic fluid may be drained, usually transabdominally but occasionally transcervically. While transcervical amniotomy carries the risk of prolapse of the umbilical cord because of the usual unengaged abnormal lie, if labor is to be induced, this may be the preferred technique. More frequently, the fluid is drained through a No. 18 spinal needle inserted transabdominally. The fluid is withdrawn slowly (500 ml. per hour) in an attempt to prevent abruptio placentae from too rapid reduction in uterine size. A total of 1500 to 2500 ml. may be withdrawn successfully. Labor usually ensues, since the overdistended uterus has caused prelabor changes in the lower uterine segment even with early gestation, the rule with hydramnios. If labor does not ensue, it may be necessary to repeat the amniocentesis every day or two, since the fluid will reaccumulate rapidly.

If the hydramnios does not cause such symptoms, the onset of labor may be awaited without further therapy. Premature labor is to be expected because of the prelabor changes in the cervix and lower uterine segment caused by uterine overdistension. The mother must be warned about the poor fetal prognosis. The expected perinatal death rate is nearly 50 percent, with death caused either by a fetal anomaly or by the effects of immaturity. Uterine dysfunction should be expected because of the uterine overdistention, and postpartum uterine atony and subsequent hemorrhage should be anticipated by the administration of a dilute solution of intravenous oxytocin immediately after delivery.

It should be remembered that amniocentesis is performed only for maternal distress. While labor usually coincidentally ensues, the induction of labor is not the reason for the amniocentesis. With an anencephalic fetus, labor may not ensue after release of amniotic fluid, and this anomaly should be suspected under these circumstances.

Oligohydramnios

Oligohydramnios, a decreased amount of amniotic fluid, is rarely observed. It may be associated with renal agenesis in that the lack of fetal urine may

explain the decreased amount of amniotic fluid. Moderate degrees of oligohydramnios are observed with the postmature syndrome. This is a logical association, since the amount of amniotic fluid normally decreases from about 38 weeks on until delivery. With postmaturity, the scanty amniotic fluid may be meconium-stained, and the infant may be dehydrated. The postmature syndrome is discussed in Chapter 12.

References

1. Reid, D., and Benirschke, K. Gestational Trophoblastic Disease. In D. Reid, K. Ryan, and K. Benirschke (Eds.), *Principles and Management of Human Reproduction.* Philadelphia: Saunders, 1972. P. 286.
2. Hertig, A., and Sheldon, W. Hydatidiform mole, pathologicoclinical correlation of 200 cases. *Am J Obstet Gynecol* 53:1, 1947.
3. Brewer, J., Torok, E., Webster, A., and Dolhart, R. Hydatidiform mole: A follow-up regimen for identification of invasive mole and choriocarcinoma and for selection of patients for treatment. *Am J Obstet Gynecol* 101:557, 1968.
4. Woodling, B., Kroener, J., Puffer, H., Furukawa, B., Anderson, G., Ochoa, R., and Warner, N. Gross examination of the placenta. *Clin Obstet Gynecol* 19(1):21, 1976.

Additional Readings

Benirschke, K. A review of the pathologic anatomy of the human placenta. *Am J Obstet Gynecol* 84:1595, 1962.
Chun, D., Braga, C., Chow, C., and Lok, L. Treatment of hydatidiform mole. *J Obstet Gynaecol Br Commonw* 71:185, 1964.
Delfs, E. Quantitative chorionic gonadotropin: Prognostic value of hydatidiform mole and chorionepithelioma. *Obstet Gynecol* 9:1, 1957.
Malkasian, G., and Welch, J. Placenta previa percreta. *Obstet Gynecol* 24:298, 1964.
Moya, F., Apgar, V., James, L., and Berrein, C. Hydramnios and congenital anomalies: Study of a series of 74 patients. *JAMA* 173:1552, 1960.
Murray, S. Hydramnios: A study of 846 cases. *Am J Obstet Gynecol* 88:65, 1964.
Naftolin, F., Khudr, G., Benirschke, K., and Hutchinson, D. The syndrome of chronic abruptio placentae, hydrorrhea, and circumvallate placenta. *Am J Obstet Gynecol* 116:347, 1973.

Pritchard, J.   Fetal swallowing and amniotic fluid volume. *Obstet Gynecol* 28:606, 1966.

Spellacy, W., Gravem, H., and Fisch, R.   The umbilical cord complications of true knots, nuchal coils and cords around the body. *Am J Obstet Gynecol* 94:1136, 1966.

Wigglesworth, J.   Vascular anatomy of the human placenta and its significance for placental pathology. *J Obstet Gynaecol Br. Commonw* 76:979, 1969.

Wilson, D., and Raalman, R.   Clinical significance of circumvallate placenta. *Obstet Gynecol* 29:774, 1967.

Zaron, D., Imbleau, Y., and Zaron, G.   The radiographic diagnosis of molar pregnancy. *Obstet Gynecol* 35:89, 1970.

Contraceptive techniques have been known to man for centuries. Until recent decades, however, the motivation for their use was always personal—avoidance of a pregnancy that might result from a socially unacceptable liaison or might otherwise be disadvantageous to the couple involved. Society needed people, and contraceptive or abortifacient practices were condemned by the social group and, on occasion, severely punished. The social good was served by fertility, not by limitation of fertility.

The recent sharp decline in death rates resulting from the control of disease changed societal needs. The "population explosion" that followed the lowering of the death rate without a concomitant decrease in birth rate frightened all segments of society. Uncontrolled fertility became clearly recognized as no longer advantageous to the social group. Recognition of these facts has led to the widespread sanction of contraceptive practices. This societal endorsement encouraged the search for safer and more effective techniques, resulting in a wide variety of contraceptive methods with newer and better techniques of continuing probability.

Familiarity with all the useful techniques presently available is of importance to the student for many reasons. There is an enormous demand from patients for contraceptive information. Virtually all Americans who cohabit use contraception either for family limitation or for family spacing, and most seek medical advice about contraception. While not all physicians may supply contraceptive advice, because of the widespread usage of the various contraceptive methods, few will fail to encounter at least an occasional complication caused by contraceptives.

Contraception

For each technique, we will attempt to describe the site and mechanism of contraceptive action, the degree of effectiveness, the advantages and shortcomings, and the hazards and contraindications of the device. Finally, we will outline an approach to the choice of the best contraceptive technique for the individual patient. This choice is ultimately made by the patient and her husband.

The techniques currently in use can be classified either as traditional or new. Traditional methods include coitus interruptus, postcoital douching, and prolonged lactation. The condom, the diaphragm, vaginal spermicides, and the "rhythm" method are also traditional. The new methods include oral contraception and the intrauterine device (IUD).

The relative frequency of the use of these various methods has changed remarkably. Surveys in 1955 showed that about 25 percent of contraceptive users employed a diaphragm, 25 percent used the condom, and 25 percent depended on rhythm [1]. A survey in 1976 by The Center for National Health Statistics [2] revealed that nearly half of the married women in the United States who were contraceptive users chose oral contraception. About 13 percent wore an IUD, and about 25 percent used the diaphragm or the condom. Only about 8 percent depended on the rhythm method. While these United States figures cannot be applied to the world, a similar change in the prevalence of various devices has occurred in most countries.

A major factor in the discussion of contraception is the effectiveness of a particular device, a statistical description of the degree of protection it offers against pregnancy. While such a description would seem easy, this is not the case, and totally reliable

Table 16-1. Approximate Failure Rate of Various Contraceptive Techniques

Technique	Pregnancies per 100 Woman-Years	
	Theoretic Failure Rate	Actual Use Failure Rate
Oral contraceptive (combined)	0.34	4–10
Condom + spermicidal agent	Less than 1	5
IUD	1–3	5
Condom	3	10
Diaphragm with spermicide	3	17
Spermicidal foam	3	22
Coitus interruptus	9	20–25
Rhythm	13	21
Chance (sexually active)	90	90

figures on all devices are simply not available. The reasons for this lack are many. First, the *use effectiveness* of a device, which is the degree of protection offered under the imperfect conditions of human utilization, differs from the *theoretical effectiveness,* the degree of protection that might result if the device were *always* used in a flawless manner. The use effectiveness varies with patient motivation and ease of use, as well as with the inherent protection provided by the device itself (Table 16-1). Second, large populations are essential to the evaluation of a technique, and a certain percentage of patients in large-scale studies inevitably disappear from the follow-up, leaving a sizable number of "unknowns" with regard to pregnancy protection. A third factor that accounts in a major way for the lack of precise information on effectiveness is a statistical one. How does an investigator handle the data on the patient who drops from the study for various reasons and is lost to follow-up? Or the one who becomes pregnant because she failed to use the device properly? Or the patient who must be dropped from the study because of an adverse reaction, or who decides to discontinue for a personal reason?

While it is beyond the scope of this book to describe the mathematical tools used to calculate and describe contraceptive effectiveness, two commonly used methods will be mentioned briefly. The Pearl formula, which has been used widely and re-

quires the most simple calculations, reports the use effectiveness in terms of failure rate per 100 woman-years of exposure according to the following formula:

$$\text{Pearl index} = \frac{\text{number of pregnancies observed} \times 1{,}200}{\text{patients observed} \times \text{months of exposure}}$$

The life-table analysis is a second method intended to overcome certain mathematical shortcomings of the Pearl index, but this tabulation requires a more complex set of calculations. The method allows the determination of the cumulative failure rate for a contraceptive device, together with the rates of patients discontinuing the study for each of many reasons (e.g., accidental pregnancy, planned pregnancy, medical advice, complication of the device). Since the two methods do not give precisely the same results, the effectiveness of any particular device in the sections that follow will be reported according to the life table analysis when this is available.

TRADITIONAL METHODS

Coitus Interruptus

In coitus interruptus, the oldest contraceptive method still in common use, the male is required to withdraw the penis from the vagina before ejaculation, a feat not willingly learned or practiced by many men. While the method has no recognized physical hazards, it may have an adverse emotional impact on one or both partners (e.g., concern over lack of female orgasm or worry over male failure and a resultant pregnancy). This method has particular advantages. It requires no devices or chemicals and is thus available under *all* circumstances and at no cost. When used optimally as the only method, coitus interruptus has a failure rate of 9 pregnancies per 100 woman-years and a rate of 20 to 25 in actual studied use. When used on a one-time basis or in conjunction with other methods, the failure rate will be considerably lower.

Postcoital Douching

Postcoital douching with various substances enjoys very little popularity today but was in widespread use only a few years ago. Since sperm appear in the cervical mucus within 90 seconds of ejaculation in some cases, the method has extremely poor results.

Lactation

Through suppression of ovulation, lactation provides pregnancy protection in the postpartum period. Particularly in developing countries, lactation has had an important demographic impact. In Rwanda, 50 percent of nonlactating women were found to have conceived by four months postpartum, while 50 percent of lactating women had conceived at just over eighteen months postpartum [3]. There is great variability in the time of onset of ovulation during lactation. Among 500 lactating patients who became pregnant, the pregnancy rate was 13.2 per 100 woman-years of exposure during the first postpartum month, with a maximal rate of 62.4 reached during the sixth month [4].

Condom

The condom is an ancient device, having first been described by Fallopius in 1564 for the prevention of syphilis. Subsequently, the contraceptive properties of a male sheath were appreciated, and with the discovery of the vulcanization process for rubber in the nineteenth century, the widespread use of this cheap, effective contraceptive became possible.

The effectiveness of the condom is greatly affected by motivation, since it is so closely time-related to the sex act. Among highly motivated couples, a pregnancy rate of 2.6 per 100 woman-years of exposure has been reported. Exclusive of failure to use the device, pregnancies are due primarily to unacceptable variations of sex technique. Rupture of the condom is unusual. Users should be cautioned to avoid any penile insertion before placement of the device, and withdrawal after ejaculation before the erection is lost is essential. The rubber must be held in place during withdrawal to avoid slipping of the condom.

The advantages of the condom are its low cost, ready availability as a nonprescription item, potential availability even with unexpected coitus, and partial protection against venereal disease, especially gonorrhea. Its major disadvantages are dulling of sensation for some users and the close time relationship to penile insertion. There are no known hazards or contraindications.

The Diaphragm

Although various devices to prevent pregnancy by covering the cervix had been used previously, the modern diaphragm was described in 1882 by Mensigna. Diaphragms in contemporary use vary little from the original design. The modern prescription includes the use of vaginal spermacidal jelly or cream with the diaphragm. The device prevents pregnancy by the dual mechanism of a partial physical barrier between the sperm and the cervix and the spermicidal action of the vaginal jelly. Use of the diaphragm without the jelly is associated with a high failure rate. The device has a theoretical effectiveness that should approach that of the condom; used consistently, failure rates of 2 to 3 pregnancies per 100 woman-years have been reported. In usual practice, however, much higher rates are experienced.

The diaphragm is a dome-shaped device with the dome molded of a thin layer of latex surrounded by a firm rim formed by a circular-shaped, rubber-covered spring. The device is squeezed to allow insertion into the vagina, where it assumes its original shape with release, since it fits the contours of the organ. The diaphragm is available in diameters

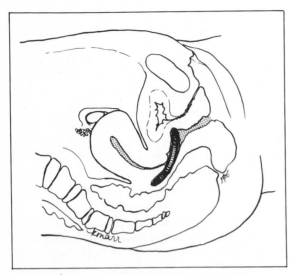

Fig. 16-1. Proper placement of contraceptive diaphragm. (From K. Niswander. Obstetric and Gynecologic Disorders: A Practitioner's Guide. *Flushing, N.Y.: Medical Examination Publishing Co., 1975.)*

from 45 mm. to 105 mm. and must be fitted by the physician to the individual patient so that it covers the cervix.

After a careful pelvic examination, the distance between the posterior fornix of the vagina and the posterior aspect of the symphysis pubis is estimated. A properly fitting diaphragm is the largest one that will fit comfortably between these two landmarks. If it is too large, it will be uncomfortable; if it is too small, it may dislodge. With the patient in the supine position on the examining table, the patient squeezes the diaphragm so that it can be inserted into the vagina. The patient directs the device toward the sacrum so as to enter the posterior fornix, not the anterior fornix (Fig. 16-1). The rim is tucked snugly behind the symphysis pubis, and the index finger palpates the cervix, which should be covered by the soft latex dome. Before insertion, an appropriate amount of jelly is placed on the surface that will lie against the cervix and around the rim for lubrication to ease insertion. The patient is instructed to insert the diaphragm before going to bed and to delay removal for at least 6 to 8 hours following intercourse. During this time the spermicidal jelly inactivates the sperm. If a second co-ital episode occurs before the six-hour interval, an additional insertion of spermicidal jelly without removal of the diaphragm should precede the event.

The diaphragm is safe and has no known hazards. If used correctly and regularly, the failure rate is very low (theoretical rate, 3.0 per 100 woman-years; use effectiveness, 17). It can be employed well before the coital episode, and it does not interfere with sensation as the condom does. While many women cannot tolerate the necessary genital manipulation essential for the use of the device, the insertion becomes routine for others. The one relative contraindication of the employment of the diaphragm is severe pelvic relaxation, especially cystocele, which precludes a good fitting. With mild relaxation, the use of a Matrisalus diaphragm may be possible. This device is shaped like a Smith-Hodge pessary and will dislodge less easily than the conventional round diaphragm.

Vaginal Chemical Contraceptives

Spermicidal chemical products may be used alone as well as with a diaphragm. While such agents have been marketed in many forms, the vaginal contraceptive foam is apparently more effective than the cream product. The foam is inserted into the vagina a short time before intercourse (no longer than 1 hour). It spreads quickly and covers the vagina and cervix. If a second coital episode occurs, it should be preceded by a second application of the chemical. While theoretically as effective as the diaphragm and jelly or condom, in practice, pregnancy rates have been higher with these chemicals, varying from 2 to 38 per 100 woman-years. The lower rates have been experienced in highly motivated populations, just as is the case with other contraceptive methods.

The major advantage of this technique is its simplicity and low cost. There are no known hazards associated with the method, although mild vaginal or penile irritation is occasionally reported. An advantage of unknown effectiveness is a certain degree of protection against venereal disease.

Rhythm Method

The rhythm method depends on the predictability of ovulation, an uncertain premise on which to base a contraceptive practice. The only advantage the method enjoys is approval by the Roman Catholic Church, a major factor in areas with a dominant Church influence. Indeed, it is the only contraceptive method approved by the Church.

The method is based on certain physiologic probabilities: (1) that ovulation occurs 12 to 16 days before the first day of the following menstrual period and (2) that the life span of the ovum is 24 hours and of sperm, 48 hours. It is essential that careful recording of the menstrual dates be maintained for at least a year before the method is used. In this way, the longest and shortest cycles that are likely to occur can be recognized. Abstinence is practiced during the time that ovulation might occur, with intercourse permitted only during the "physiologically sterile" period.

Using the preceding physiologic assumptions, the unsafe period is calculated as follows: Ovulation is likely to occur no earlier than 16 days before the shortest cycle and no later than 12 days before the longest cycle. Subtract 18 days (16 days plus the 2 days of sperm survival) from the expected first menstrual day of the shortest cycle and 11 days (12 days minus the 1 day of ovum survival) from the longest cycle. These dates should encompass all possible pregnancy exposure dates. Intercourse is permitted during the period not included in the unsafe time.

The more irregular the menstrual dates, the more uncertain the protection and the longer the period of abstinence. A cycle that occurs regularly at 28-day intervals would require abstinence only from day 10 through day 17. A cycle length varying from 25 to 32 days would require abstinence from day 7 through day 21. Most couples find a long period of abstinence intolerable, thus accounting for many of the failures. The unpredictability of the physiologic parameters measured accounts for the other failures. Pregnancy rates of from 13 to 21 per 100 woman-years can be expected.

Attempts to improve the predictability of the time of ovulation have included measurements of basal body temperature (BBT), the recognition of changes in the vaginal smear, and other methods. The BBT is known to assume a biphasic curve, with the temperature rise occurring at about ovula-

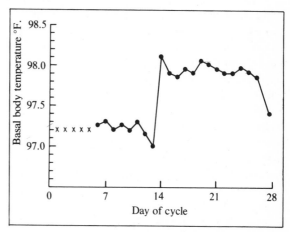

Fig. 16-2. Typical ovulatory biphasic temperature curve. (From K. Niswander. Obstetric and Gynecologic Disorders: A Practitioner's Guide. Flushing, N.Y.: Medical Examination Publishing Co., 1975.)

tion time and the higher temperature persisting until menstruation (Fig. 16-2). If careful recording of the woman's temperature at the same time every morning under basal conditions is maintained, a sustained rise of temperature for three days is good evidence that ovulation has occurred and that the remainder of the month is a safe period. Pregnancy rates of as low as 6 to 7 per 100 woman-years have been reported if intercourse is permitted only between the temperature rise and the subsequent menstrual period. Only a few days of intercourse are allowed, however, and an enormously strong motivation is necessary for success.

MODERN METHODS
Intrauterine Devices
Although the use of IUDs for various gynecologic ills goes back 2000 years, the modern era of contraception, with the placement of an IUD for this purpose, began in 1929 with Gräfenberg [5], a German gynecologist, and in 1934 with Ota [6], a Japanese physician, each of whom reported a large series of patients with failure rates of 1 to 2 percent. Opposition of leading gynecologists to this form of contraception was based on the presumed high risk of pelvic inflammatory disease, and the devices were largely abandoned. Since over 50 percent of

gynecologic disease in that era was of an inflammatory nature even among nonusers of IUDs, however, the relationship of an IUD and pelvic infection was never well established.

A resurgence of interest in the IUD as a contraceptive device occurred in the late 1950s, and a proliferation of devices resulted, with innumerable reports in the medical literature. The search for the perfect instrument resulted in a variety of sizes and shapes, but all the devices were made of inert plastic materials, since minimal tissue reaction was considered desirable. Recent investigators have questioned this concept, however, and the newest devices are based on the idea of incorporation of a material to induce purposeful tissue reactivity to compensate for a smaller and therefore a more acceptable device. More will be said of these newer copper-containing devices later.

MODE OF ACTION. The mode of antifertility action of the IUD is uncertain, but the site of action is almost certainly the endometrial cavity. Experiments in the human have shown that neither ovulation nor steroidogenesis in the ovary is affected by an IUD; tubal peristalsis seems unchanged; there is no pituitary inhibition; and sperm migration into the upper female tract occurs in the presence of an IUD. Changes in the glycogen metabolism of the endometrium have been described, and the IUD consistently causes an increase in the number of inflammatory cells, both in the endometrium itself and in the intrauterine fluid. Infection per se seems an unlikely explanation for the antifertility action, however, since uterine culture with an IUD in place was sterile in all patients in a recent study after 46 days of use, while bacteria were recovered from 100 percent of uteri in the first 24 hours of emplacement [7]. The best theories of action are that the inflammatory cells may engulf the fertilized ovum or that the endometrium is "out of phase" and therefore unreceptive to the ovum.

The most frequently used devices are shown in Figure 16-3. The larger the device, the higher the effectiveness but at the cost of a higher expulsion rate. The smaller, medicated devices (Cu-7, Progestesert-T) seem to provide the answer to this

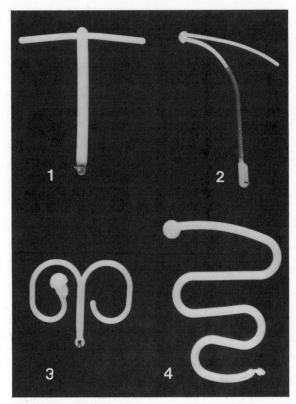

Fig. 16-3. Intrauterine devices in common usage: (1.) Progestasert-T, (2.) Cu-7, (3.) Saf-T-Coil, and (4.) Lippes Loop.

paradox, high effectiveness with a low expulsion rate. The Lippes Loop has enjoyed the widest popularity over the years, but the medicated devices are enjoying increasing usage. The Cu-T device recently introduced into the United States will undoubtedly gain wide acceptance.

EFFECTIVENESS. The reported cumulative pregnancy rate per year for the Lippes Loop D is 2.7 per 100 woman-years [8]. Similar figures for the Cu-7 are 1.6 for nulliparas and 1.9 for multiparas and for Progestesert-T 2.6 and 1.8, respectively. If pregnancy occurs with the IUD in place, the risk of spontaneous abortion is substantially higher than if the pregnancy had occurred after expulsion of the IUD. Removal of the device, if the tail can be visualized, apparently reduces the risk of abortion from about 50 percent to about 25 percent. Also, failure to remove the device has resulted in fatal septicemia in midpregnancy. If the tail of the device is not visible and cannot be easily reached, termination of the pregnancy with removal of the device at the time of surgery should be offered to the patient. No teratogenic effect from an IUD remaining in the uterus throughout pregnancy has been recognized. The IUD apparently does not reduce the risk of occurrence of a tubal pregnancy as it does with an intrauterine gestation. Thus, a pregnancy with an IUD in place occurs in the tube in about 1 of every 20 intrauterine pregnancies, 5 to 10 times the usual incidence.

COMPLICATIONS. Apart from accidental pregnancy, the major hazard of the IUD is infection. Expulsion, bleeding and pain, and perforation of the uterus are usually less serious complications.

Pelvic infection should be suspected in an IUD-wearer who complains of fever, pelvic pain, abdominal tenderness, cramping, or unusual vaginal bleeding. If pelvic examination reveals pelvic tenderness, especially cervical motion tenderness, or other evidences of infection, the IUD should be removed. Cervical culture is indicated and an appropriate antibiotic should be started immediately. In a few instances, a unilateral ovarian abscess has developed after IUD use [9]. Unilateral salpingo-oophorectomy or even hysterectomy may be required to control the infection.

Expulsion of an intrauterine device is more likely to occur when the device is made of soft material, when the shape can be easily changed to a linear form, or when the cervix is soft, as it is during the postpartum period. The Lippes Loop D has an expulsion rate of 12.7 per 100 woman-years. The expulsion rate with the Cu-7 is 8.0 in nulliparas and 5.7 in multiparas and with the Progestesert-T is 7.4 and 3.1, respectively [9]. Most expulsions occur during the first three months of usage, and reinsertion after expulsion increases the expulsion rate to 30 to 35 percent. Palpation of the tail of the device is an important safeguard since 20 percent of expulsions in one large series were unnoticed. With the precaution of palpating the tail before use, the expulsion should be discovered early enough to prevent most pregnancies.

Removal of an IUD at the patient's request is performed in about 5 to 20 percent of patients during the first year and in somewhat fewer in the second year. While some of these removals are for pregnancy or personal reasons, most are for bleeding, pain, or both. Most such removals are made during the first few months of use, but bleeding may be a problem for much longer periods.

Perforation of the uterus is a major, although infrequent, problem associated with the IUD. The incidence is low with many of the devices (1.2 per 1000 patients with the Lippes Loop D, 0.6 per 1000 with the Cu-7) but higher with others (1 per 350 patients with the Dalkon shield, now no longer available). It is thought that the perforation occurs at the time of insertion of the device, although the accident may not become evident for many months. The complication is not always preventable, but the incidence can be lowered if (1) the uterus is sounded before IUD insertion to determine the direction of the cavity, and (2) the tenaculum on the cervix is pulled in such a manner as to straighten the cervical canal and uterus. Perforation is also more common if the IUD is inserted in the immediate postpartum period.

Since perforation is usually asymptomatic, the complication is first suspected when the tail of the device cannot be palpated or when pregnancy occurs. The new IUD user must be carefully instructed on how to palpate the IUD tail. If perforation is suspected and pregnancy is not a likely possibility, the endometrial cavity should be probed and the device removed if it is felt. If the IUD is not located, ultrasonographic and x-ray help should be requested. Removal of the device from the peritoneal cavity can sometimes be accomplished through a laparoscope, or through a cul-de-sac incision if the device is lying behind the uterus. In certain instances, laparotomy may be required. Although an IUD lying free in the peritoneal cavity rarely produces symptoms or serious disease, removal is probably the best management.

ADVANTAGES AND SHORTCOMINGS. The major advantages of the IUD are convenience, the lack of need for repeated action to assure contraception, the high degree of effectiveness, and the apparent safety of the device. An increased risk of nongonococcal pelvic inflammatory disease among IUD users seems well established from recent data. Expulsion or necessary medical removal of the IUD is common, but the patient who retains the device is well satisfied with this method of contraception.

METHOD OF USE. Contraindications to the use of the IUD for contraception include:

1. Suspected pregnancy. It is best to insert the device at the end of the menstrual period.
2. Acute or subacute pelvic infection.
3. History of an infected abortion or postpartum endometritis during the preceding six to eight weeks.
4. Distortion of the endometrial cavity, usually by a myoma.
5. Suspicion of uterine malignancy, especially uterine bleeding.

Relative contraindications include:

1. History of pelvic infection.
2. History of an ectopic pregnancy.
3. Valvular heart disease.

Personal experience, as well as the availability of new devices, will dictate the particular IUD to be used. Nearly all currently available devices are inserted in much the same way, however. It is best to insert the device at the time of the menstrual period or immediately thereafter, since the cervix is more patulous at that time. A careful history and physical examination should rule out the contraindications for use of the device.

Using sterile technique, the vagina is cleansed with an antiseptic solution, and the anterior lip of the cervix is grasped with a tenaculum. The direction of the cervical canal, previously determined by bimanual pelvic examination, is confirmed by the

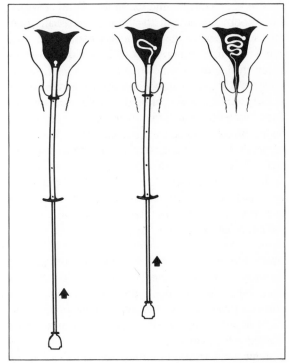

Fig. 16-4. Insertion of Lippes Loop. (From K. Niswander. Obstetric and Gynecologic Disorders: A Practitioner's Guide. Flushing, N.Y.: Medical Examination Publishing Co., 1975.)

uterine sound. The depth of the uterus is likewise determined with the sound. Since nearly all devices are made of polyethylene or other plastic material and have a "memory," the device recovers its shape after being pulled up through a hollow tube by means of a string attached at the lower end of the device. When the device has been pulled entirely within the tubing, the tubing is inserted into the uterus, and the plug in the tubing is pushed in a fashion to extrude the device from the tubing and into the endometrial cavity (Fig. 16-4). The tubing is carefully removed from the cervix, and the device should remain in the uterus. The string or tail attached to the device is cut to about an inch length to allow both easy removal, should this be necessary, and palpation of the string by the patient herself so that she can be certain that the device is in the uterus. Occasionally, dilatation of the cervix to 7 to 8 mm. may be required, and if the usually mild cramps are severe, paracervical anesthesia may be necessary. The insertion of a Lippes Loop is illustrated in Figure 16-4.

The Cu-T device has been used widely outside the United States but has only recently been introduced here. The Cu-T has a slightly wider insertion diameter than the Cu-7, and has therefore been recommended for use in the multipara by some authorities. The cumulative pregnancy rate for the Cu-T has been reported to be between 1.0 and 2.6 per 100 woman-years [10]. The device seems certain to gain wide acceptance.

The mode of action of copper on fertility is thought to be local in the endometrial cavity, with leukocytic infiltration the likely mechanism of the antifertility. While the copper gradually dissolves or is dissipated, there is no evidence that absorption into the maternal organism causes any ill effects. The dissolution of the copper, however, is an important consideration, since the small T device without copper has an unacceptably high pregnancy rate. The Cu-T exerts satisfactory antifertility action for at least two to three years following insertion, and further investigations of the duration of its contraceptive activity are under way.

Oral Contraception

MECHANISM OF ACTION. Oral contraceptives are potent steroid medications. The clinician must know something of the physiology of steroid contraception to minimize its hazards. He must be able to make an informed choice when the patient who is having side effects on a particular medication is switched to another medication, and he must know the physiologic effects of each medication to make an appropriate choice. In short, he must understand how each type of the presently available oral contraceptive agents functions and be able to prescribe each type intelligently.

A brief review of the physiology of contraceptive medication is in order. The usual reason for giving "the pill" is to prevent pregnancy. This may be accomplished either by inhibiting ovulation or by changing other physiologic parameters so that pregnancy will not ensue even if ovulation occurs. It is known that an estrogen alone or a progestin alone will prevent ovulation if a large enough dose is given; the effect is apparently mediated at the level of the hypothalamus or higher nerve centers. Small doses of the progestins, however, prevent pregnancy not primarily by inhibiting ovulation but by altering endometrial metabolism and the type and amount of cervical mucus. Although an estrogen alone or a progestin alone will prevent ovulation, most marketed pills contain both substances for reasons to be discussed.

Although estrogen alone prevents ovulation, it causes an unacceptably high rate of vaginal bleeding, and it is marketed only in combination with a progestin. A progestin alone is an effective antifertility agent but is also associated with a high number of days of vaginal bleeding, as well as with a somewhat lessened antifertility activity, especially if the dosage is low. Such a medication has recently become available on the United States market. Combination therapy, which typically is a combined estrogen and progestin compound taken for 20 or 21 days beginning on day 5 of the menstrual cycle, depends primarily on the antifertility effects of progestin, that is, its antiovulatory effect and the effect of changes on the endometrium and the cervical mucus. The estrogen is added only to decrease the number of days of vaginal bleeding experienced by the patient.

EFFECT OF ORAL CONTRACEPTIVES ON VARIOUS ORGAN SYSTEMS. In addition to their antifertility activity, oral contraceptives exert effects on many other organ systems. It is important for a number of reasons that the physician prescribing oral contraception be familiar with these effects. Unpleasant or even hazardous side effects may result from the action of the pills on certain organs. Diagnosis of disease in various organ systems may be complicated when the patient is on oral contraception, since organ function test results are sometimes substantially altered by such medication. Contraindications to the use of pills are frequently based on the effect of the pills on a particular organ system.

EFFECTS ON REPRODUCTIVE ORGANS. The oral contraceptives have specific effects on the various parts of the reproductive tract.

Ovary. The major effect on the ovary is prevention of ovulation through a marked decrease in follicle-stimulating hormone, although this does not occur with absolute consistency, especially with sequential therapy. This action has the beneficial effect of decreasing the number of functional ovarian cysts. The appearance of an ovarian mass in a patient using oral contraception is likely to indicate a tumor rather than a functional cyst.

Endometrium. Combined therapy usually produces secretory activity, which proceeds to pseudodecidual changes, glandular suppression, and stromal edema. Prolonged therapy or therapy in hypersensitive women may cause marked glandular suppression and amenorrhea. More is said of this symptom later. Abnormal bleeding may result from certain endometrial effects.

Myometrium. Leiomyomas may enlarge greatly or may slow in growth with combined oral contraceptive therapy. This effect is dependent on the relative amounts of progestin and estrogen. Because of the variability of this effect, some consider the presense of leiomyomas a relative contraindication to oral contraceptive administration.

Cervix. An increase in cervical mucus, combined with an increased frequency of polypoid hyperplasia, can be expected with oral contraception. There is no evidence that the medication increases the risk of the development of carcinoma of the cervix.

Vagina. Earlier reports that vaginal candidiasis is exacerbated by oral contraceptive medication have not been confirmed.

Breasts. Breast tenderness is a well-recognized side effect of oral contraception and apparently is an estrogen effect. If oral contraceptives are given to postpartum patients, milk production and quality are occasionally adversely affected (in about 10 percent of patients), a fact that must be discussed with a postpartum patient before prescribing such medication. The problem is less serious in a woman with well-established lactation.

EFFECTS ON OTHER ENDOCRINE ORGANS. Oral contraceptives stimulate the release of certain hormones and inhibit the release of others.

Adrenals. Estrogen increases the amount of circulating transcortin that binds cortisol. A decrease in urinary metabolites of cortisol (17-ketosteroids, 17-hydroxysteroids, aldosterone) may result.

Thyroid. As with pregnancy, estrogen causes an increase in thyroxine-binding globulin, with changes in thyroid function tests similar to those induced by pregnancy. There is, however, no recognized change in thyroid function.

Pancreas. A rise in the plasma insulin level occurs in some patients on oral contraception. This rise is followed in short order by a rise in fasting blood glucose or an abnormal glucose tolerance test result. In most patients, these tests revert to normal following discontinuation of the medication. These effects are particularly likely to be observed in patients who are older, obese, of higher parity, or with a family history of diabetes mellitus or an obstetrical history of excessively large babies or unexplained fetal deaths—in short, in patients in whom diabetes mellitus is more likely to develop. Whether oral contraceptive medication merely identifies the population in which diabetes mellitus is likely to develop in later life or is actively diabetogenic is uncertain. The effects on carbohydrate metabolism are apparently mediated by the progestin content of the pills or by a synergistic action between the estrogen and progestin components.

Hypothalamic-Pituitary Function. Inhibition of ovulation by oral contraceptives apparently occurs at the level of the hypothalamus by an inhibition in the release luteinizing releasing factor. If the progestin component of the medication is too high, or if the physiologic mechanism of ovulation is not functioning well before medication, prolonged amenorrhea during medication or postmedication amenorrhea may result. This side effect is discussed under Postmedication Amenorrhea.

EFFECTS ON BLOOD AND BLOOD COAGULATION. A minimal increase in certain blood clotting factors

(factors VII, IX, and X, fibrinogen) has been reported with oral contraception. Although such changes have been described as constituting a "hypercoagulable" state, most investigators believe these changes to be of no clinical importance. The overall effect of the medication on salt and water metabolism is probably salt and water retention, which may account for the weight gain observed in some patients on oral contraceptives.

EFFECTS ON THE CARDIOVASCULAR SYSTEM. A slight increase in systolic and diastolic blood pressures occurs in women on oral contraceptive medication. This is mediated through the estrogenic component of the pill [11]. The increase in blood pressure is marked in a rare patient and hypertension is recognized as early as one to three months or as long as years after the initiation of contraception. The mechanism is unknown but may be due to changes in the renin-angiotensin-aldosterone system. Cessation of estrogen treatment results in a decline of blood pressure to normal in most patients. Whether the pill identifies a group of women likely to develop subsequent hypertension or whether the effect is simply a drug-related phenomenon is not known.

EFFECTS ON THE LIVER. Certain liver tests, especially those measuring bile excretion such as Bromsulphalein (BSP) excretion, may reach abnormal levels in oral contraception, but this has no known clinical significance. Patients who have experienced idiopathic recurrent jaundice of pregnancy may run an increased risk of jaundice during oral contraception. Severe liver disease is an absolute contraindication to oral contraception.

EFFECTS ON THE SKIN. Chloasma, hyperpigmentation of the skin of the face in a butterfly distribution, is seen in some patients on oral contraception and in some pregnant patients. The lesion is apparently innocuous but distressing. It disappears slowly after discontinuation of medication.

EFFECTS ON THE CENTRAL NERVOUS SYSTEM. A variety of symptoms possibly referrable to the central nervous system have been reported with oral contraception. Nausea and vomiting, depression, loss of libido, and headache are the major ones. While the symptoms are undoubtedly often emotionally induced, headache in particular must be noted, since patients on oral contraception do experience an increased risk of cerebrovascular accidents. Discontinuation of the medication in patients who complain of headache should be considered if another explanation for the headache cannot be elicited. Nausea and vomiting are more frequently noted during early cycles and are probably related to the estrogen content.

EFFECTS ON THE KIDNEY. Ureteral dilatation occurs with oral contraceptive medication but produces no known ill effect.

OTHER SIDE EFFECTS. Because of the potency and widespread physiologic effects of oral contraceptives, it is not surprising that serious complications have been recognized with their use. Side effects of a less serious nature are also important, since they may cause a patient to discontinue medication.

Vascular Complications. An increase in the risk of venous thrombosis and pulmonary embolism in women on oral contraceptives has been well established by a number of retrospective epidemiologic studies [12]. Superficial thrombophlebitis apparently occurs three times as often in oral-contraceptive users as in a similar population of women not taking a contraceptive pill. Deep thrombosis or pulmonary embolism is three to eleven times as frequent in pill users. The increased risk apparently occurs only during ingestion of the medication and for a short time after discontinuation; the risk is unchanged by the length of time the medication has been used. There is good evidence that the estrogen component of the pill is the etiologic factor, and some investigators have suggested that there is a dose relationship. Pills containing no more than 50 μg. of estrogen probably carry a smaller risk than do those with a larger amount.

Thrombotic stroke is also seen among pill takers

about six times as frequently as expected. The risk of myocardial infarction in patients using oral contraception is increased about four-fold, especially in those over the age of 35. Cigarette smoking increases this risk substantially in the woman over 30.

When considering these risks, the physician must remember that pregnancy itself increases the risk of thromboembolism substantially. Much of the data relating the pill to thromboembolism were collected when commercial products contained much larger amounts of estrogen than they do presently. The risks associated with the currently used medications are uncertain but are thought to be substantially less. While these side effects must be seriously considered before prescribing medication, it should be remembered that mortality from thromboembolic disease among pill users is only about 3 per 100,000 women per year. The high risk of death from the pregnancy itself in almost every age group must be balanced against these risks.

Postmedication Amenorrhea. A small number of women will experience amenorrhea following cessation of medication. In most instances, the period of amenorrhea will not exceed six to nine months; on occasion, it may last much longer. The symptom is more likely to occur with medication in which progestin predominates and is apparently due to an effect of the medication on the hypothalamus. Almost half of the patients who experience postmedication amenorrhea have had a history of irregular menses before starting the pill. It is possible that the amenorrhea might have eventually developed even without the use of oral contraception. These facts suggest that if oral contraception is to be used at all in patients with a history of irregular menses, it should not be progestin-dominant but rather an estrogen-dominant medication.

Minor Side Effects. Intermenstrual bleeding occurs fairly frequently with combination pills due to the progestin dominance of many of these pills. The treatment of this complaint will depend on the degree to which it disturbs the patient. If she can tolerate the bleeding and if it is not copious in amount, no treatment is prescribed. The complaint fre-

quently disappears in later months of drug use. If the bleeding is upsetting to the patient, a switch to a more estrogen-dominant pill may cause the symptom to disappear. At no time should the medication be stopped in mid-cycle without prescribing another method of contraception.

Nausea and vomiting are related primarily to the estrogen component of the pill prescribed. While the complaint usually subsides after a month or two of medication, a change to a less estrogen-dominant pill may be tried.

Weight gain is more frequently seen in pill users than is weight loss, although both have been reported. The cause of the weight gain has not been definitely established, but paradoxical effects of progesterone on water and salt metabolism have been reported. Treatment of the symptom has not been satisfactory.

Carcinogenesis. No definite carcinogenic effect of oral contraceptive medication has been established. While a higher incidence of carcinoma of the cervix has been suspected among pill users than among women using other contraceptive devices, the validity of the idea has been questioned. A second study showed that women who choose oral contraceptives are more likely to exhibit cervical dysplasia *at the time of the initial examination* than are women who choose a diaphragm [13].

The role of estrogen in inducing malignancy in the endometrium or in the breasts has been studied for many years with inconclusive findings. Two recent reports, however, have demonstrated an increased risk of the development of endometrial carcinoma in women who have taken exogenous estrogens for prolonged periods [14, 15]. The recent discovery of an increase in the incidence of vaginal carcinoma among young girls whose mothers ingested stilbestrol during their pregnancies suggests a hazard if oral contraception fails to prevent pregnancy. The risk, however, is small and seems to be associated only with synthetic estrogen, which is not used in contraceptive medications.

CONTRAINDICATIONS TO THE USE OF ORAL CONTRACEPTION. Absolute contraindications to oral contraceptive medication include:

1. A history of thrombophlebitis, pulmonary embolus, cerebral apoplexy, or coronary artery disease.
2. Markedly impaired liver function.
3. Known or suspected carcinoma of the breast, uterus, or ovary, and other possibly estrogen dependent malignancies.
4. Undiagnosed genital bleeding.
5. Pregnancy.
6. Hepatic adenoma.

Care in the prescription of oral contraception should be exercised under the following circumstances:

1. Leiomyomas of the uterus.
2. Hypertension.
3. Epilepsy.
4. Menstrual irregularity (see Postmedication Amenorrhea).
5. A history suggesting the possibility of diabetes mellitus (see Pancreas).
6. A history of migraine headaches.
7. Age 35 or over, especially if obese, hypertensive, diabetic, or heavy smoker.
8. Heavy smoking, especially if over 35 years of age.

CHOICE OF MEDICATION. The choice of medication is of increasing importance as more information on the physiologic effects of the various ingredients of contraceptive pills is collected. Certainly, a physician should have a special reason for prescribing a pill with an estrogen content greater than 50 μg., since there is strong evidence that such medication is associated with a higher risk of serious side effects. A history of past illness should identify the patient with a contraindication to any contraceptive medication, and a history of irregular menses should preclude a progestin-dominant type of medication because of the risk of postmedication amenorrhea.

After a careful pelvic examination (including a Papanicolaou smear), breast examination, and blood pressure recording, a low-dose medication should be prescribed (e.g., norethindrone 1 mg.

and mestranol 50 μg.) and the patient should be instructed to return to the physician's office in three months. At that time, a pelvic and breast examination, blood pressure determination, and a functional inquiry relating to pertinent organ systems are indicated. A urine dipstick for glucose and, if necessary, a 2-hour postprandial blood sugar should be recorded. If all is well, the patient can be continued on the medication to return for an examination at least annually unless a complaint arises. An annual history and physical examination is recommended. There is no benefit in intermittent therapy, since periodic exposure to pregnancy carries as great a risk as continued contraceptive treatment.

Medications currently available in the United States are listed in Table 16-2. Table 16-3 gives the etiology of some of the side effects. If the patient's complaint seems to be caused by progestin, a change to a more estrogen-dominant medication is appropriate. A similar change from an estrogen-dominant to a progestin-dominant medication is necessary if the patient has experienced an estrogen side effect, e.g., severe breast tenderness. Some authorities have preferred to start on a sequential medication all women who have irregular menstrual periods or whose fertility is unproved even though their periods are regular to minimize the risk of postmedication amenorrhea. Since such medication is no longer commercially available, an estrogen-dominant pill should be used in women with oligomenorrhea as the initial medication.

HOW TO HELP THE PATIENT CHOOSE A CONTRACEPTIVE METHOD

There is no one contraceptive agent that is satisfactory for all users. The wide variety of drugs or devices available, however, allows an intelligent choice for an individual patient based on her peculiar needs. The pros and cons of all methods must be explained to each patient to help her make a wise choice.

Foremost in the minds of most women is the question of safety. Tietze has estimated the risk of dying from various contraceptive practices and compared these risks to the mortality rate associ-

Table 16-2. Examples of Commercially Available Oral Contraceptives

Progestin (mg)	Estrogen (mcg)	Trade Name	Dominance
Norethindrone (0.35)	—	Nor-QD	P
Norgesterol (0.5)	Ethinyl estradiol (50)	Ovral	P
Norethindrone acetate (1.0)	Ethinyl estradiol (20)	Loestrin 1/20 Zorane 1/20	—
Norethindrone (1.0)	Mestranol (50)	Ortho-Novum 1/50 Norinyl 1/50	—
Norgestrel (.30)	Ethinyl estradiol (30)	Lo-Ovral	—
Norethindrone (0.5)	Ethinyl estradiol (35)	Modicon Brevicon	—
Norethindrone (1.0)	Mestranol (80)	Ortho-Novum 1/80 Norinyl 1/80	E
Norethindrone acetate (1.0)	Ethinyl estradiol (50)	Norlestrin 1 Zorane 1/50	E
Norethynodrel (2.5)	Mestranol (100)	Enovid-E	E

This list is intended to provide examples of oral contraceptive medications currently available in the United States. It is not a complete listing. Medications usually progestin dominant are marked "P"; those usually exerting primarily an estrogen effect are marked "E." The individual patient herself, however, is the ultimate test of hormone effect.

Table 16-3. Side Effects of Oral Contraceptive Medication

Excess Estrogen	Deficient Estrogen	Excess Progesterone	Deficient Progesterone
Nausea and vomiting	Early cycle spotting and breakthrough bleeding	Depression	Late cycle spotting and breakthrough bleeding
Headache		Weight gain	
Cyclic weight gain	Amenorrhea	Oligomenorrhea or amenorrhea	Excessive withdrawal bleeding
Nervousness			
Heavy withdrawal bleeding			

Source: K. Niswander. *Obstetric and Gynecologic Disorders: A Practitioner's Guide.* Flushing, N.Y.: Medical Examination Publishing Company, 1975.

ated with no contraceptive, i.e., due to pregnancy itself (Fig. 16-5). In all age groups (except oral contraceptive users over the age of 40 who smoke), the risk of dying from pregnancy among noncontraceptive users is greater than the risk of death associated with any contraceptive practice. In patients under 30 years of age, all methods of contraception carry about the same mortality risk. A smoker who is over 30 years of age and on oral contraception has a greatly increased mortality risk. *It is important to point out that a traditional barrier method of contraception with abortion back-up for the small number of failures provides the very safest method of contraception available with 100 percent effectiveness.* Not all patients, of course, will accept this alternative.

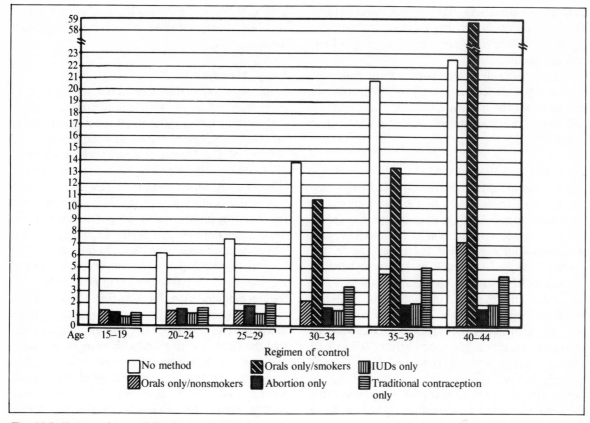

Fig. 16-5. Estimated annual deaths per 100,000 nonsterile women. (Modified from C. Tietze. Fam Plann Perspect *9:74, 1977.)*

To the patient who is interested in effectiveness above all, the contraceptive pill may be the logical choice. She must, however, be informed that potent and effective drugs carry a degree of risk of complications not experienced with other devices.

If a patient desires convenience above all other considerations, she may wish an IUD. She must know that the IUD is less effective than the regularly taken pill and that a small risk of perforation and of infection exists. She must know that a substantial number of patients will experience spontaneous expulsion or will require removal of the device by the physician.

If the patient desires safety above other considerations, she may wish to use the diaphragm or condom. The diaphragm does not interfere with sensation as the condom may, and its use is not so closely related in time to penile penetration. The condom, however, can be used with little or no medical advice, while the diaphragm requires a fitting.

If she chooses to conform to the moral standard of no artificial contraception, she must be carefully instructed on the rhythm method. The poor effectiveness experienced by most patients with this method should be drawn to her attention.

For a patient who wants a high degree of effectiveness without the hazards of contraceptive drugs, a combination of methods may be desirable. For example, a regularly used condom with the application of vaginal foam with every penetration should provide nearly 100 percent effectiveness. The addition of the rhythm method to absolutely regular use of the diaphragm and jelly provides excellent effectiveness.

In the final analysis, the patient must make the contraceptive choice based on what she is told and knows about the options available. Most patients will find a method suitable for their individual needs.

POSTCOITAL MEDICATION

In a number of animal breeds, estrogen in high dosage prevents implantation of the fertilized ovum. Diethylstilbestrol (DES) in large dosage has apparently prevented implantation in the monkey, and this successful experiment led to its use in the human. Data are less reliable in the human because of the lack of laboratory controls, but there is evidence that DES in a dose of 25 to 50 mg. daily for five days, beginning within 24 hours of coitus, will prevent pregnancy [16]. A recent compilation of the literature suggests a pregnancy rate of 0.3 to 0.03 percent among patients so treated [16]. Nausea from the medication is experienced by half the patients. The nausea is so severe in some cases that the regimen cannot be completed. There is some evidence that the risk of ectopic pregnancy is slightly increased with the treatment.

Such treatment is obviously of an emergency nature and should be reserved for cases of rape or similar situations. Dilatation and curettage or menstrual extraction within 24 hours of sexual exposure is a more certain method of preventing implantation. Theoretically, failure of the method might jeopardize the female fetus because of a risk of masculinization. Further, a risk of cervical or vaginal adenosis or even carcinoma of the vagina in the female offspring of a mother treated with DES to prevent abortion has been reported. This method of contraception should not be used in a patient who is unwilling to accept abortion if pregnancy is not prevented.

Recently, the Copper-7 IUD has been shown to be an effective postcoital contraceptive device when inserted within 24 hours of exposure [18]. The device should not be used in cases of rape or with multiple sex partners because of the risk of venereal disease leading to pelvic inflammatory disease.

Legal Abortion

Legal abortion is the intentional termination of pregnancy before viability in a manner consistent with current law or custom. At the present time in the United States, the law, as established by an opinion of the United States Supreme Court in 1973, essentially sanctions abortion on demand [17]. The restrictive state laws passed in the mid-nineteenth century permitting abortion only when the life of the mother was in danger were in effect in most states until the late 1960s. Beginning in 1967, one state after another passed liberalized abortion laws that typically permitted danger to the health of the mother as well as to her life to be considered in the recommendation for abortion. In a few instances, the new state laws sanctioned abortion on demand. Then, in 1973, the Supreme Court ruled that the state laws restricting abortion were unconstitutional on a number of grounds, thus in effect providing abortion on demand. While certain restrictions on this freedom have been imposed in certain states, the availability of abortion for an unwanted or inadvisable pregnancy is a reality in many geographic areas. Certain inconsistencies in the delivery of abortion care to patient populations still exist, but abortions are more common than before the court decision.

Abortion laws in other countries have changed in much the same manner as in the United States, although much earlier in many cases. A particularly instructive example is Japan, where the legalization of abortion after World War II had a major demographic impact. The birth rate decreased from 33.0 per 1000 population in 1949 to a low of 16.9 in 1961. In later years, contraception also played a role in lowering the birth rate, but without the widespread availability of abortion, the Japanese economic and social history of the postwar era would have been very different.

In Czechoslovakia and Hungary, abortion was legalized in 1956 and 1957. In Czechoslovakia, the number of abortions increased from a few thousand to a level of about 90,000, where it stabilized. In Hungary, the number of legal abortions increased even prior to the modifying law and reached a level of about 160,000 in 1960, a figure exceeding the number of live births. Since that time, the number of abortions has decreased, and in 1976 there were 520 abortions per 1000 live births.

The Scandinavian countries passed liberalized abortion laws in the late 1930s, with subsequent amendments during the succeeding years. The administrative procedures were so involved, however, that few early abortions resulted, and the many late abortions performed were associated with a high maternal mortality. These countries now have about 300 abortions per 1000 live births.

The British Abortion Act of 1967 in effect created abortion on demand in that country, and large numbers of abortions have been performed. In countries such as France and Italy, where abortion is not sanctioned or has only recently been sanctioned (i.e., in France), the number of illegal abortions has been estimated to approach a number equal to the number of live births. It is readily apparent that women will seek and obtain abortion no matter what the law permits. The primary question is whether the abortions will be done safely by qualified professionals in hygienic surroundings or unsafely in sordid circumstances by unlicensed practitioners.

The influence of readily available legal abortion on the illegal abortion rate, maternal mortality, and population growth is important to determine, but the secretive aura surrounding abortion even today seriously interferes with the collection of reliable data for such a determination. Gold et al. [19] have reported a decline in the number of deaths from illegal abortion in the United States from 39 in 1972 to 3 in 1976, an effect that seems directly attributable to the increased availability of legal abortion. If abortion simply replaces contraception as a form of birth control, little is accomplished.

INDICATIONS

The older term *therapeutic abortion* is still applicable in the few instances in which the health of the mother is best served by abortion. While these instances are infrequent, the importance of abortion to the individual patient under such circumstances is sufficiently great to warrant a brief discussion of the medical indications for abortion. The emotional, social, and economic indications will also be outlined.

Medical Indications

Few diseases are likely to cause death in pregnancy when the woman receives up-to-date medical treatment. In certain instances, however, the treatment must be heroic. Occasionally, it is unsuccessful in preventing maternal death. Furthermore, most patients and their physicians take into account factors other than mortality in assessing pregnancy risk. Will prolonged hospitalization be required? Will the patient be able to care for her child after birth? What are the economic and social consequences of the therapy in the successfully completed pregnancy, including the effects on siblings? And, especially, are a woman and her husband willing to assume the risks involved in having the child?

Women with Class III and Class IV heart disease or with a history of congestive heart failure during a previous pregnancy should be offered abortion if pregnancy occurs. Certain severe congenital heart diseases, especially when the patient is cyanotic, may require abortion. The pregnancy outcome is particularly ominous if the hematocrit has increased to compensate for the relative lack of oxygen.

The patient with severe hypertension, especially if the disease has seriously affected the myocardium, retina, or kidneys, should be offered abortion. Any severe renal disease, whether it is caused by hypertension, chronic nephritis, or associated with other syndromes such as generalized lupus erythematosus, may require abortion.

Cancer of the breast is said to progress more rapidly during pregnancy, but the evidence is unconvincing. Invasive cancer of the cervix during pregnancy must be treated aggressively, and abortion is the usual consequence. Carcinoma in situ of the cervix requires close surveillance but no pregnancy interruption.

Abortion is required for only the most incapacitating disease of the lungs, rarely for pulmonary tuberculosis. Ulcerative colitis that has its onset during pregnancy or is aggravated by early pregnancy may be best treated by abortion in some patients. Individual circumstances may indicate abortion for a number of other diseases.

Fetal Indications

An abortion may be requested because of the likelihood of severe fetal abnormality related to genetic factors, drug ingestion, or maternal infection during pregnancy. The indications for such abortions are discussed in Chapter 12.

Psychiatric Indications

Before abortion laws were changed, psychiatric illness was a frequent indication for abortion, usually based on the suicidal potential of the woman if the pregnancy continued. It seems likely that most of these patients were aborted for sociopsychological reasons rather than true psychatric disease. Most psychiatrists, however, feel that patients with certain psychiatric diagnoses do indeed require abortion (e.g., severe depression). One investigator reported, however, that patients who required abortion most urgently for psychiatric disease also responded most poorly to this therapy [20]. He felt that these same patients would have responded equally poorly, from an emotional point of view, to the continuation of the pregnancy.

Psychosocial Indications

While there is little disagreement over the medical indications for abortion, there is a marked polarity of views with regard to abortion for social or emotional reasons. Some believe every woman should be able to choose whether or not she wants to bear a child. These advocates point out that the fertilized ovum or fetus is not capable of independent life; that no woman should be forced by her biologic nature to bear a child she does not wish to care for; that the fetus is part of her body and that she should have control over her own body. The population explosion has provided strong demographic support for this view. Others argue that the fetus has a right to be born independent of his mother's wishes. The Supreme Court has supported the former point of view, and this view is currently the law of the land.

Social or emotional disruption by a pregnancy is the indication for most abortions. Typical examples are the widow with teen-aged children who becomes pregnant or the 17-year-old teenager who wants to continue her education rather than raise an out-of-wedlock child. While abortion is a far less satisfactory solution of such problems than is contraception, imperfect answers are sometimes required in an imperfect world.

Techniques

When the decision for abortion has been made, the best technique must be selected from the variety available. The choice will depend primarily on (1) the length of gestation, (2) whether or not an accompanying sterilizing operation is to be performed, (3) the presence or absence of a pathologic condition of the uterus, and (4) a diagnosis that contraindicates a particular technique. The earlier the abortion is performed, the safer the procedure. Mid-trimester abortion is more hazardous than a first-trimester procedure. The techniques currently available to procure an abortion include (1) suction abortion, (2) dilatation and extraction (D&E), (3) intra-amniotic injection of hypertonic saline or prostaglandin, and (4) hysterotomy or hysterectomy. Vaginal prostaglandin suppositories are also available but are not in common usage for intentional abortion.

The length of gestation is a major factor in the choice of technique. Suction abortion is indicated up to the twelfth week (to the fifteenth week with an experienced operator). The use of suction abortion after 12 weeks is associated with an increased blood loss and risk of uterine preforation. D&E can be used between the fifteenth and twentieth weeks. Intra-amniotic injections can be performed as early as the fifteenth week, although delay until the sixteenth or seventeenth week will result in fewer complications. Hysterectomy is useful only when an injection technique has failed or in the unusual patient with placenta previa. Hysterectomy is indicated in a pregnant woman with significant uterine disease (e.g., myomata). Laparoscopic or mini-laparotomy sterilization can be combined with suction abortion, but the recent Federal guidelines on sterilization will not permit this combined therapy on federally funded patients (see Sterilization).

Abortion by a Procedure Through the Cervix
Whether suction abortion or a D&E is planned, it is wise to insert a laminaria tent into the cervix 6 to 18 hours before the procedure. Laminaria tents are fashioned from *Laminaria digitata*, a seaweed obtained from Japanese ocean waters, and are effective cervical dilators because of their intense hygroscopic properties. Without anesthesia, the laminaria tent, which is about 3 mm. in diameter, is inserted into the cervix so that just the tip is visible at the external os. Two or more tents are used for a D&E. In the next few hours, the tent absorbs water and dilates the cervix so that at surgery a dilatation of 10 to 12 mm. or more is observed. The trauma of instrumental dilatation is avoided.

If suction abortion is to be performed, the laminaria tent is removed from the cervix and the cervix sounded for direction. After any necessary additional dilatation, the largest suction curette that can be used is inserted through the cervix and carefully passed to a point near the fundus. By a rotary and to-and-fro motion, the uterus is emptied of its contents with the suction machine. The uterine cavity should be carefully and sharply curetted to assure that all material has been removed. The uterus should be sounded to be certain that it has not been perforated.

D&E has been shown to be safer than intra-amniotic injection techniques for pregnancy interruption between 15 and 20 weeks. Only very experienced operators should attempt it, however, since perforation of the uterus and incomplete emptying is more commonly encountered than with earlier gestations. If a D&E is to be performed, the uterine size is determined by bimanual pelvic examination. The anterior lip of the cervix is grasped with a tenaculum and the cervix sounded to ascertain the direction of the canal. Further dilatation is rarely needed since several laminaria placed the evening before the procedure have usually procured adequate dilatation. With a sponge forceps or a specially designed forceps, the uterus is emptied of its contents. A large curette is used to complete the procedure. Bleeding is sometimes brisk.

It may be necessary to use general anesthesia for either of these operations unless laminaria dilatation of the cervix has been employed. We perform all of our suction abortions under paracervical anesthesia and the patients rarely have any significant pain. D&E is more painful and may require general anesthesia. Both procedures are performed on an outpatient basis and the patient goes home 2 to 4 hours following the procedure. Complications are rare. Prophylactic antibiotics may reduce the incidence of postabortal infection but we do not use them.

An occasional patient will report bleeding and cramps one to three days after the procedure. Since endometritis is the usual cause of these symptoms, a trial of antibiotics is indicated unless severe bleeding is present. If necessary, it is usually easy to pass a curette through the cervix to complete the procedure without cervical dilatation. Unless a patient has a fever, she is not admitted to the hospital. If an infection appears to be serious, or if the patient's condition appears to be deteriorating, she should be admitted for more intensive antibiotic therapy and careful observation.

If perforation of the uterus occurs with the suction curette, it is probably best to perform an immediate laparotomy, since the bowel may have been damaged. If, on the other hand, perforation occurs with a blunt instrument, we have rarely found it necessary to open the abdominal cavity. It has been our practice to watch such a patient in the hospital for 48 hours, and if she does well, no laparotomy is performed.

Intra-Amniotic Injections
PROSTAGLANDIN. The amniotic sac is punctured with a 20-gauge needle inserted transabdominally after using a local anesthetic in the skin of the abdomen. Forty mg. of prostaglandin $F_{2\alpha}$ is injected over a 5-minute period into the amniotic sac. A test

dose of about 4 mg. is injected initially to prove the absence of intravascular injection. Such an injection may evoke contraction of all the smooth musculature and procedure bronchospasm, hypertension, and gastrointestinal symptoms. A history of bronchial asthma should especially alert the operator to the possibility of bronchospasm. Intravenous atropine is an antidote. Within 30 minutes of completion of the injection, uterine activity can be appreciated. Abortion occurs on an average of about 16 hours later. Some investigators have reported a shortened injection-abortion time with the insertion of a laminaria tent into the cervix before the injection [21]. Others have recorded no such effect [22]. There is general agreement that dilute intravenous oxytocin speeds hypertonic saline abortion but this association is less certain with prostaglandin than with saline. A significant number of patients require a D&C because of incomplete passage of the placenta. This complication is more common with prostaglandin than with saline.

With the recommended dosage the severe gastrointestinal symptoms, fever, or both, reported with higher doses of prostaglandin, occur only rarely. The incidence of gastrointestinal symptoms is minimized by pretreatment with prochlorperazine maleate (Compazine). Spontaneous cervical lacerations have also been recorded, but very uncommonly.

HYPERTONIC SALINE ABORTION. Techniques vary substantially for the hypertonic saline procedure. Our technique is to enter the amniotic sac transabdominally with a No. 20 spinal needle after using a local anesthetic in the skin as with the prostaglandin procedure. A few to 100 ml. of fluid is removed, and 120 to 150 ml. of a 20% saline solution is injected slowly into the amniotic sac. Placement of the needle is checked every 5 or 10 ml. to be certain that it is still in the amniotic sac. The stylette is reinserted into the needle before withdrawal from the amniotic sac.

Complications during the procedure are rare. Typically, the patient has no uterine cramps for a number of hours, the latent period. Labor ensues, and delivery usually occurs in about 24 hours. The placenta is retained after the fetus is passed in 15 to 20 percent of patients. After attempting to expel the placenta with periodic pressure on the fundus for an hour or two, the patient can be examined in the treatment room where the placenta usually can be removed with a large sponge forceps. Occasionally, a D&C under anesthesia is required. A few patients may run a postabortal temperature, usually because of endometritis. These patients usually respond quickly to an appropriate antibiotic.

The major complication of hypertonic saline injection is intravascular escape of sodium chloride during injection. Resulting neurologic symptoms of headache, dizziness, and loss of consciousness may ensue. Treatment with a rapid intravenous infusion of 5% glucose in distilled water is usually effective. The complication is a rare one. Many clinics, including our own, treat the injected patient with a dilute intravenous oxytocin drip to shorten the injection-abortion interval. Care must be exercised to avoid water intoxication with oxytocin, since the drug is an antidiuretic. Careful measurement of urinary output will show oliguria before the symptoms of headache, convulsions, and coma ensue. If intravenous fluids are limited to 1500 to 2000 ml. in a 24-hour period and discontinued after no more than two days of therapy, this complication should not occur.

Contraindications to the use of hypertonic saline injection include kidney disease, because of the potential for poor excretion of sodium, and heart disease, because of the risk of precipitating heart failure. A number of recent papers have emphasized the frequent development of changes in the blood clotting and lysing systems with hypertonic saline abortion. For this reason, patients with any blood coagulopathy should be aborted by some other technique.

HYSTERECTOMY AND HYSTEROTOMY. Hysterotomy is rarely employed today. A failed injection procedure or placenta previa may occasionally necessitate its use. Abdominal hysterectomy may be the method of choice for pregnancy interruption if there is uterine disease, usually myomas, which will require subsequent hysterectomy.

CONTRAINDICATIONS

There are few physical contraindications to the abortion, although there are contraindications to many particular techniques.

The major contraindications to saline abortion include cardiac disease, renal disease, and hematologic disease of the blood clotting–lysing systems. A relative contraindication to prostaglandin use is bronchial asthma. Hysterectomy has few contraindications, but the greatly increased maternal mortality associated with this operation compared to that with simpler abortion techniques precludes its use unless uterine disease is an overriding consideration.

COMPLICATIONS AND MORTALITY

The major complications have been listed with the description of each procedure. The risk of maternal death can be documented only by a study of large numbers of abortions, since the risk is of very low magnitude. A vital question is the relative risks of death from legal abortion and from pregnancies that are allowed to continue.

Overall maternal mortality for the United States was 15 per 100,000 live births in 1973; the reported death rate associated with legal abortion was 1.4 per 100,000 abortions in 1977 [24]. Biases inevitably enter comparisons of these figures, however. A number of deaths from illegal abortion are included in the overall maternal mortality figure (4 in 1977); these deaths might not occur with readily available legal abortions. Overall maternal mortality includes deaths from medical complications as well as complications associated with the third trimester (toxemia, third-trimester bleeding), and these complications are unusual among abortion patients or are excluded by definition. What can be concluded from these figures is that legal abortion is probably as safe as, or safer than, carrying a pregnancy to term. Figures from Central European countries confirm this estimate.

Table 16-4. Mortality Risk with Legal Abortion at Various Gestational Intervals

Weeks of Gestation	Death Rate*
≤8	0.6
9–10	1.7
11–12	2.7
13–15	7.5
16–20	14.6
≥21	20.5
Total	2.6

*Death-to-case rate for legal abortions, United States, 1972–1977 among 4,888,617 abortions. From Center for Disease Control. *Abortion Surveillance, 1977.* Atlanta. Issued September, 1979.

The specific effect of liberalizing abortion laws on maternal mortality was studied in New York at the time of the change of the law. Using the figures for the first four months of each year, 1969, 1970, and 1971, a decrease in the number of abortion-related as well as non-abortion-related deaths was experienced with the liberalization [23]. A decrease in the number of patients admitted to hospitals for septic abortion was also noted. There were about 700 fewer births each month, and the number of children born out of wedlock decreased. Whether or not all of these decreases resulted from the abortion law change is impossible to say, but the evidence for such a relationship is compelling.

Easier to determine are the relative risks of maternal death from early abortion as compared with later abortion and from various methods of abortion. Table 16-4 illustrates the effect of weeks of gestation on the mortality rate. With a gestation of eight weeks or less, the death-to-case rate for legal abortions was 0.6 per 100,000 abortions in the United States from 1972 to 1977. If the gestation was 16 to 20 weeks, the risk was 14.6 per 100,000 abortions. As can be seen from Table 16-5, curettage or dilatation and evacuation result in a much lower death rate than do intrauterine instillations or hysterotomy or hysterectomy. Table 16-6 shows that the weeks of gestation are a much stronger determinant of risk of death than is the type of pro-

Table 16-5. Mortality Risk Associated with Various
Legal Abortion Techniques

Type of Procedure	Rate*
Curettage/dilatation and extraction	1.5
Intrauterine instillation	13.5
Hysterotomy/Hysterectomy	43.6

*Death-to-case rate for legal abortions, United States, 1972–1977
among 4,888,617 abortions. From Center for Disease Control.
Abortion Surveillance, 1977. Atlanta. Issued September, 1979.

cedure used to procure the abortion, excluding
hysterotomy and hysterectomy, both of which carry
enormously increased death risks. Dilatation and
evacuation seems to be slightly safer than instillation techniques and prostaglandin overall seems
slightly safer than the hypertonic saline instillation
technique.

EMOTIONAL EFFECTS
The emotional impact of abortion has been inadequately studied, but the impact of refused abortion
has been even more neglected. The most objective
studies have suggested that serious regret or actual
deterioration of the patient's emotional condition
rarely occurs following abortion. Refused abortion,
however, is more likely to be followed by undesirable effects, as judged by one major Scandinavian
study. Of 294 patients refused abortion and studied
a number of years later, nearly one-fourth had

made an inadequate adjustment to the refusal,
while over one-half had experienced insufficiency
reactions during an 18-month follow-up period but
eventually adjusted to the situation [25]. In another
Scandinavian study, 120 children born following a
refused abortion were followed to 21 years of age
and compared with a carefully matched control
group [26]. The children of the study group were
more likely to have required psychiatric services,
were more commonly involved in antisocial acts,
and were more likely to have done poorly in school
than the children in the control group. The poor
social progress for these children was probably due
to the adverse effects of being unwanted children.

ABORTION COUNSELING
The need for counseling when an abortion decision
is to be made seems self-evident, but the nature of
the counseling is crucial if an appropriate decision
is to be reached and a minimum of subsequent regret experienced.

The patient who seeks advice regarding an unwanted pregnancy may have one or more of a
number of motivations. She may have already
made up her mind to have an abortion. She may be
seeking abortion because a parent, husband, or
lover wants her to have the procedure, while she
herself is uncertain or opposed. In some cases, she
is truly undecided and wants help in arriving at the
best choice from a number of alternatives, all of
which may be unattractive to her. In a few cases,

Table 16-6. Mortality Risk of Legal Abortion Associated with Various Techniques at Varying Gestational Intervals

Type of Procedure	Weeks of Gestation						Total
	≤8	9–10	11–12	13–15	16–20	≥21	
Curettage	0.5*	1.6	2.9				1.2
Dilatation & evacuation				6.7	12.9	16.7	8.3
Instillation				9.6	15.4	24.7	14.1
Saline				2.5	19.3	20.6	15.5
Prostaglandin & other agents				32.6	6.1	40.5	10.8
Hysterotomy/Hysterectomy							45.3

*Death-to-case rate for legal abortions, United States, 1972–1977 among 4,888,617 abortions. From Center for Disease Control. *Abortion Surveillance, 1977.* Atlanta. Issued September, 1979.

she may want information about what her child's fate will be if the child is immediately put up for adoption. Most patients find themselves in a psychosocial dilemma and need counseling before the pregnancy decision can be made.

The counselor must make every attempt not to prejudge the situation or impose on the patient the solution he or she might make in a similar set of circumstances. The community resources available to the patient should be described. Interviews with others involved (the consort, a parent) should be arranged if the patient wishes, but the primary agent in the decision is the patient herself, except under the most exceptional circumstances. The help of a psychiatrist or other expert should be sought when the circumstances seem to demand it.

When the decision is made, whether it be for abortion, for marriage and delivery in an unmarried patient, or for delivery and adoption of the child, it is important to support the patient's choice. Indeed, support at this time may make the difference between ultimate satisfaction with the decision or bitter regret. Contraception should be discussed at the abortion interview, since some patients will not return for contraception counseling after the procedure.

Sterilization

Voluntary sterilization by mechanical blockage of the fallopian tubes or the vasa deferentia for the purpose of family size limitation began in the 1940s, although mutilating castrating operations for sterilization or other reasons have been known for hundreds of years. At the present time, enormous numbers of sterilizing operations are being done not only in the United States but also in developing countries. That this method of contraception should have become so widespread in such a short time suggests that it has fulfilled a great need for those desiring to terminate childbearing. The operation is legal in all 50 states.

Operative sterilization should be utilized only when permanent sterilization is desired, since reversibility is difficult and frequently impossible to provide. This is not to suggest, however, that a physician's refusal to perform an operation re-

quested by a young patient or couple is usually justified. Surprisingly few patients seriously regret the operation in later years, and the number upset over additional pregnancies who have been refused the requested operation is undoubtedly great. The physician has a responsibility to point out to his patient the irreversibility of the procedure and the hazards entailed in its performance, but he has no moral right to refuse to perform the operation just because he thinks he knows better than the patient what the future may hold. As with most treatments in medicine, the informed patient should be allowed to make the choice.

FEMALE STERILIZATION

Various techniques of sterilization can be performed on the female. Some are more appropriate for use during the puerperium than others. All currently used techniques attempt to obstruct the fallopian tubes, so that the ovum and the sperm are kept apart.

Older methods that still have applicability in many situations include the Pomeroy, Madlener, and Irving techniques. These usually require a transabdominal approach, although the vaginal route through the cul-de-sac is sometimes used. With the Pomeroy technique, a segment of the tube is double-ligated with plain catgut, and the ligated portion is excised. The end result is a discontinuity of the tube for a distance of about 2 cm. With the Madlener procedure, a tubal segment is ligated with nonabsorbable suture, and the ligated portion is crushed with a hemostat but not excised. Obstruction without excision is the end result. With the Irving technique, the proximal section of the divided tube is buried in the uterine wall, while the distal segment is buried under the peritoneum of the broad ligament. The Irving technique is more time-consuming than the others, but there are virtually no failures. The Pomeroy procedure fails in about 1 of 350 patients, while the Madlener technique fails somewhat more frequently. If the vaginal operative approach is chosen, the Pomeroy technique is usually used, although fimbriectomy may be the choice. Any of these methods may be used during the postpartum period, as well as when pregnancy has been a remote event (interval sterilization).

Laparoscopic sterilization has become a standard operative procedure except during the postpartum period. The technique is a satisfactory adjunct for the postabortal patient who desires an associated sterilizing operation. Either a closed or an open technique can be used. The closed technique is as follows: With the patient under general anesthesia (a few laparoscopists use local anesthesia) and with the patient's bladder empty, pneumoperitoneum is effected by the introduction of carbon dioxide into the peritoneal cavity through a Verres needle puncture site at the inferior aspect of the umbilical rim. A sharp trocar is introduced into the peritoneal cavity to allow insertion of the laparoscope.

The open technique of laparoscopy is as follows [27]: A small transverse skin incision is made at the lower rim of the umbilicus and the incision is extended into the peritoneal cavity, thus allowing insertion of the laparoscope by direct visualization. Pneumoperitoneum is accomplished through the laparoscope rather than through the needle as with the closed technique. In either case, the pelvic organs are visualized and a second puncture is made in the lower abdomen for insertion of the sterilizing instrument. Under direct visualization, tubal continuity is interrupted. We prefer to apply a plastic ring (Falope ring) to a loop of each tube. Alternatively, each tube may be fulgurated at two points, the first 1 cm. from the uterine cornua and the second 1.5 cm. distally, taking care to include a portion of the tubal mesentery in the fulguration. The tube between the two points of the fulguration is transsected with the cutting corner of the cautery. After due delay to observe for possible bleeding, the instruments are removed and the carbon dioxide is expelled. A failure rate similar to that with the Pomeroy procedure has been reported. The prime advantage of the Falope ring technique is the absence of risk of damage to nearby organs by accidental arching of the diathermy current.

Vaginal sterilization can be accomplished in at least two ways. The peritoneum can be entered through an incision in the posterior cul-de-sac and the Pomeroy procedure performed on the tubes after direct visualization. To obviate the occasional difficulty of visualizing the tubes through this colpotomy approach, some operators have suggested visualization of the tubes through a culdoscope, with the insertion of a tubal clamp alongside the culdoscope and withdrawal of the grasped tubes together with the culdoscope into the vagina, where tubal ligation can be completed.

Mini-laparotomy is chosen by more and more surgeons for female sterilization. With the catheter continuously draining the bladder, a tiny transverse incision is made just above the symphysis pubis and the peritoneal cavity is entered. The uterus is manipulated by moving a tenaculum or other device previously placed on the cervix, thus allowing each tube to be visualized. A segment of each tube is grasped with a clamp and doubly ligated with chromic No. 0 catgut suture according to the Pomeroy technique. The failure rate is that associated with the Pomeroy technique. Lubell and Frischer [28] recorded a pregnancy rate of 2 to 4 per 1000 procedures. This method enjoys one advantage over laparoscopic tubal sterilization. Only a small segment of the tube is damaged and reanastomosis is easier, should this be necessary, than following tubal fulguration where the damage is more extensive.

The hazards of general anesthesia and the transperitoneal operative approach are small but significant and include infection and embolization. Special hazards of laparoscopic sterilization include bleeding from the tubal stump, bowel or skin injury from the cauterization current, trocar injury, and respiratory embarrassment from the pneumoperitoneum. Major complications are reported to occur in about 0.6 percent of patients sterilized by laparoscopy [29].

MALE STERILIZATION

Although the precise figures are not available, it would appear that three-quarters of the sterilizing operations performed in the past few years in the United States have been on males. In India, an even higher percentage of sterilizations are on males. The procedure is usually done in the physician's office under local anesthesia and consists of small scrotal incisions and ligation of each vas deferens at two points with transection between the points of ligature. The cut ends are usually cauterized. The mortality is virtually zero, although a few complications such as hematoma formation can occur. The overall failure rate is probably less than 1 percent. Although operative reversibility is sometimes successful, the patient should regard the procedure as permanent.

NEW STERILIZATION TECHNIQUE

A number of promising new approaches to sterilization, all intended to simplify the procedure, are under study. One such method employs the injection of a sclerosing agent through the cervix to cause occlusion of the tubes. While many agents tried cause scar tissue in the endometrium as well as in the tube, one agent, quinacrine chloride, acts selectively on the tubal mucosa and is particularly promising [30]. Zinc inhibits the occlusive action of quinacrine, and the unique absence of zinc in the intramural portion of the tubes allows occlusion only at this point. Accidental spillage in the peritoneal cavity seems innocuous. In clinical trials, a 90 percent success rate has been achieved with two applications of the drug. With improvements in technique to raise the success rate, this method of sterilization appears promising.

References

CONTRACEPTION

1. Ryder, N., and Westoff, C. Reproduction in the United States 1965. Princeton, N.J.: Princeton University Press, 1971.
2. Pratt, W. Patterns of aggregate and individual changes in contraceptive practices: United States, 1965–1975. U.S. Department of Health, Education and Welfare Publication No. (PHS) 79-1401, 1979; revised 1980.
3. Bonte, M., and VanBalen, H. Prolonged lactation and family spacing in Rwanda. *J Biosoc Sci* 1:97, 1969.
4. Martinez-Manautou, J., Gordillo, J., and Rudel, H. W. Contraceptives and lactation. *Rev Invest Clin* 18:195, 1966.
5. Gräfenberg, E. Die intrauterine Methode der Konzeptimsverhutung. Third Congress of the World League for Sexual Reform, 1929, pp. 116–125. In C. Tretze, *Intrauterine Contraceptive Rings: History and Statistical Appraisal.* Excerpta Medica International Congress, Series No. 54. Amsterdam: Excerpta Medica, 1962.
6. Ota, T. A study on the birth control with an intrauterine instrument. *Jap J Obstet Gynec* 17:210, 1934.
7. Mischell, D., Bell, J., Good, R., and Moyer, D. The intrauterine device: Bacteriologic study of the intrauterine cavity. *Am J Obstet Gynecol* 96:119, 1966.
8. Edelman, D., Berger, G., and Keith, L. Intrauterine devices and their complications. Boston: G.K. Hall, 1979. Pg. 20.
9. Taylor, E., McMillan, J., Greer, B., et al. The intrauterine device and tubo-ovarian abscess. *Am J Obstet Gynecol* 123:338, 1975.
10. Tatum, H. Clinical aspects of intrauterine contraception: Circumspection 1976. *Fertil Steril* 28:3, 1977.
11. Spellacy, W. The effect of intrauterine devices, oral contraceptives, estrogens, and progestens on blood pressure. *Am J Obstet Gynecol* 112:912, 1972.
12. Vessey, M., and Doll, R. Investigation of relation between use of oral contraceptives and thromboembolic disease: A further report. *Br Med J* 2:651, 1969.
13. Stern, E., Clark, V., and Coffelt, C. Contraceptives and dysplasia: Higher rate for pill choosers. *Science* 168:497, 1970.
14. Smith, D., Prentice, R., Thompson, D., and Herrman, W. Association of exogenous estrogen and endometrial carcinoma. *N Engl J Med* 293:1164, 1975.
15. Ziel, H., and Finkle, W. Increased risk of endometrial carcinoma among users of conjugated estrogens. *N Engl J Med* 293:1167, 1975.
16. Morris, J., and van Wagenen, G. Interception: The use of post ovulatory estrogens to prevent implantation. *Am J Obstet Gynecol* 115:101, 1973.

LEGAL ABORTION

17. Roe vs. Wade. Supreme Court 93:705, 1973.
18. Population Reports, Series J, No. 9, January, 1976, pg. 141.
19. Gold, J., Smith, J., Cates, W., and Tyler, C. The Epidemiology of Abortion in the United States. In G. Zatuchni, J. Sciarra, and J. Speidel (Eds.), *Pregnancy Termination: Procedures, Safety, and New Developments.* Hagerstown: Harper & Row, 1979.
20. Ekblad, N. Induced abortion on psychiatric grounds. *Acta Psychiatr Scand* (Suppl) 99:1, 1955.
21. Hale, R., and Pion, R. Laminaria: An underutilized clinical adjunct. *Clin Obstet Gynecol* 15:829, 1972.
22. Hanson, F., Haslett, E., and Sacks, D. Laminaria

digitata in saline abortions. *Obstet Gynecol* 43:761, 1974.

23. Pakter, J., and Nelson, F.   Abortion in New York City: The first nine months. *Fam Plann Perspect* 3:5, 1971.

24. Center for Disease Control.   *Abortion Surveillance, 1977.* Atlanta. Issued September, 1979.

25. Höök, K.   Refused abortion: A follow-up study of 249 women whose applications were refused by the National Board of Health in Sweden. *Acta Psychiatr Scand* (Suppl) 168:1, 1963.

26. Forrsman, H., and Thuwe, I.   One hundred and twenty children born after application for therapeutic abortion refused. *Acta Psychiatr Scand* 42:71, 1966.

STERILIZATION

27. Hasson, H.   Open Laparoscopy. In J. Phillips et al. (Eds.), *Laparoscopy*. Baltimore: Williams & Wilkins, 1977.

28. Lubell, I., and Frischer, R.   Does mini-laparotomy for sterilization have a place in your practice? *Contemp Obstet Gynecol* 14:39, 1979.

29. Israel, R.   Current concepts in female sterilization. *Clin Obstet Gynecol* 17:139, 1974.

30. Davidson, O., and Wilkins, C.   Chemically induced tubal occlusion in the human female following a single instillation of quinacrine. *Contraception* 7:333, 1973.

Additional Readings

Quinones, R., Alvarado, A., and Ley, E.   Tubal electrocoagulation under hysteroscopic control (three hundred and fifty cases). *Am J Obstet Gynecol* 121:1111, 1975.

Shepard, M.   Female contraceptive sterilization. *Obstet Gynecol Surv* 29:739, 1974.

Index

Friedman curve, 170